BODYBUILDING PHYSIOLOGY AND TRAINING

MASSIMO SPATTINI, RICCARDO GASPARI
With contributions from Federico Focherini

BODYBUILDING
PHYSIOLOGY AND TRAINING

From training VOLUME and INTENSITY to FREQUENCY

Foreword by Samir Bannout

edra PUBLISHING
esteri

Original title
Massimo Spattini, Riccardo Gaspari
Bodybuilding – Allenamento ed esercizi
Dal volume di allenamento alla frequenza passando per l'intensità

ISBN 978-88-6895-200-6
eISBN 978-88-6895-201-3

Book Publishing Manager: Costanza Smeraldi, Edra S.p.A.

Project Manager: Elisa Bechi, Edra S.p.A

Paper, printing and Binding Manager: Paolo Ficicchia, Edra S.p.A.

Translation: LIFE SHPK, Tirana, Albania

Proofreading of Translation: Margherita Zottola

Layout: T&T studio s.a.s, Milano

Copyediting: ALTER EDOM s.r.l., Noventa Padovana (PD), Italy

Cover: Roberta Venturieri, Edra S.p.A

Cover images: the portrait of Riccardo Gaspari and Giorgio Mesghetz, of Dr. Massimo Spattini and Terenzio Maggio, of Federico Focherini and Angelo Bani; other images from Shutterstock | © Superstar

ISBN: 978-19-5726-038-9
eISBN: 978-19-5726-060-0

edra
PUBLISHING

Edra Publishing US LLC
3309 Northlake Boulevard, Suite 203
Palm Beach Gardens, FL, 33403
EIN: 844113980
info@edrapublishing.com
www.edrapublishing.com

Printed in Italy by Rotomail Italia S.p.A., Vignate - September 2023

Table of contents

Foreword

Over the years I have been researching everything related to bodybuilding and focusing on healthy nutrition in general.

Muscle building is not an exact science but there are ways that have proven to be more effective than others in building the body.

I have trained with lighter weights and higher reps, I have also tried using heavy weights with shorter durations. Finally, I decided to listen to my own body by giving it what it needs.

I have trained with many great champions such as Mike Mentzer and Casey Viator, both heavily into the heavy duty principles introduced to them by Arthur Jones, the founder of Nautilus equipment in the late 70's and early 80's. Mike was a huge advocate of this concept of training and I spent years around Mike discussing everything about building muscles. I also trained with the great Serge Nubret, who believed in high repetitions with longer durations and focused much more on details. He also followed the Keto diet.

I also trained alongside Arnold Schwarzenegger, Franco Columbu and Danny Padilla for years and discussed their concepts of training and dieting repeatedly.

I found out after extensive experience that my body is more responsive to heavier weights with shorter duration, but training the body part twice weekly prior to competitions was more productive and effective to get a more chiseled physique, and I realized that altering my nutritional plan was more necessary in the final weeks to achieve that super sharp muscularity.

Nowadays, after further experiment I now that to put on quicker quality muscle mass, it's definitely more effective to train the body-part once weekly, of course in super intense style.

Personally, I didn't like the idea of counting sets and reps, therefore I listen to my body needs, which means, if I stop at 12 reps or nine reps it doesn't matter and even if I did three sets or four sets that didn't matter either as long as I reach the maximum pump which is the main mission in each of my workouts. I've come to realize it's very important to allow the muscles to relax and give plenty of time and at least 72 hours for complete recovery before working it again.

I personally feel, paying more attention to exercise mechanics and the intensity level during each and every exercise is more necessary than following repetitive exact rules. Also, I trained each workout differently so I don't do the same workout routine exactly as I did the workout before, for example if I did incline bench on Monday then I may do decline on Thursday and so on, instead of doing pec deck, I would choose to do incline or decline dumbbell flies.

In the past years I have trained with Dr. Massimo Spattini for a few contests prep and we both applied this kind of method together… it was very effective and got me on the stage in excellent condition… so the bottom line is LISTEN to your body and also listen to Dr. Spattini's advice because he is heavily experienced in the field and I sincerely want you to follow in his footsteps due to his extensive knowledge in the muscle world.

Dr. Spattini brilliantly merges his knowledge of the hypertrophy mechanism of muscles with his personal experience of bodybuilding. He has proven his expertise in the field both with his own body and with his outstanding work creating hundreds of champions. This book has been co-written with bodybuilding champion and trainer Riccardo Gaspari and with Mr. Universe Federico Focherini.

In this book you will find scientific principles, practical advice and workout plans compiled from the extensive experience of those who have dedicated their lives to the art and science of bodybuilding.

"If you wanna know how to get muscles, you have to learn from the athletes that built themselves and are able to show you how."

Samir Bannout
Mr. Olympia 1983

Introduction

This volume aims to explain the importance of training techniques and methods for those looking for a notable hypertrophic response within body recomposition.

This text is aimed at all athletes and enthusiasts who seek to achieve a realistic goal, with long-lasting results, and who recognize the fundamental importance of their health in terms of both sports and psychophysical well-being.

Too often, the world of bodybuilding and fitness is the victim of myths or false beliefs: we strongly believe in providing correct information, in in-depth study, in personal experimentation and in constant research; on the other hand, we do not believe in passing trends, nor do we do business risking people's health.

In recent years, in the seductive perspective of proposing fast results with little effort, unfortunately, there has been a real demonization of high-volume training in favor of techniques that require very little of it. It is true that the intensity of training is a fundamental variable that normally must be inversely proportional to the volume. However, we believe a compromise is possible to optimize results without penalizing volume. This work reports the results of the most accredited research and the best scientific studies carried out on the volume and intensity of training, all enriched by personal experiences and training plans, to understand the fundamental aspects and the great importance that both the volume and intensity of traning have, while understanding how to use them and, above all, how to derive maximum benefits.

We consider it appropriate to highlight that scientific contributions, although abundant, have been limited to give space to the knowledge acquired in the field. We recognize that, contrary to the deterministic reductive principle, a holistic approach that takes into account individual experiences, observation of the results and all things related is more important than reporting experimental scientific works, which, while partially satisfying our need for knowledge, have the great limitation of constituting only a small part of the great mosaic and often lead to conflicting conclusions. This text, however, goes far beyond this purpose and even becomes a sort of encyclopedia of the various training systems, techniques and exercises for bodybuilding, which are described and analyzed in their specific characteristics.

Weight training and the programs proposed in this book are not only aimed at young, performing male or female athletes, but also at enthusiasts over 40. This volume will help anyone to improve their state of psychophysical well-being: let's remember that weight training helps prevent sarcopenia, osteoporosis, metabolic syndrome and osteoarthritis, and has positive influences in reducing cardiovascular risk, cancer prevention, blood pressure reduction and weight control; in addition, many positive correlations with mood improvement have been highlighted.

Massimo Spattini and Riccardo Gaspari

We dedicate this book to Davide Antoniella,
who, despite his illness, gave his availabily
and contribution until the end
to complete this work

CHAPTER 1

The muscular system

The **muscle** is a contractile organ that performs a motor function in animals. It consists of muscular tissue capable of contracting, determining the intrinsic movement of some organs or the movement of limbs, and, in general, locomotion. This property is due to the structures of the muscle tissue, both morphological and chemical. There are three types of muscle tissue (**smooth, striated, cardiac**) (Fig. 1.1), all of which have, to some extent, elongated, contractile and elastic cells, called *muscle fibers*.

Smooth muscle tissue is present in involuntary muscles, and **striated tissue** in voluntary muscles; **cardiac muscle tissue** is an exception, as it is striated and involuntary.

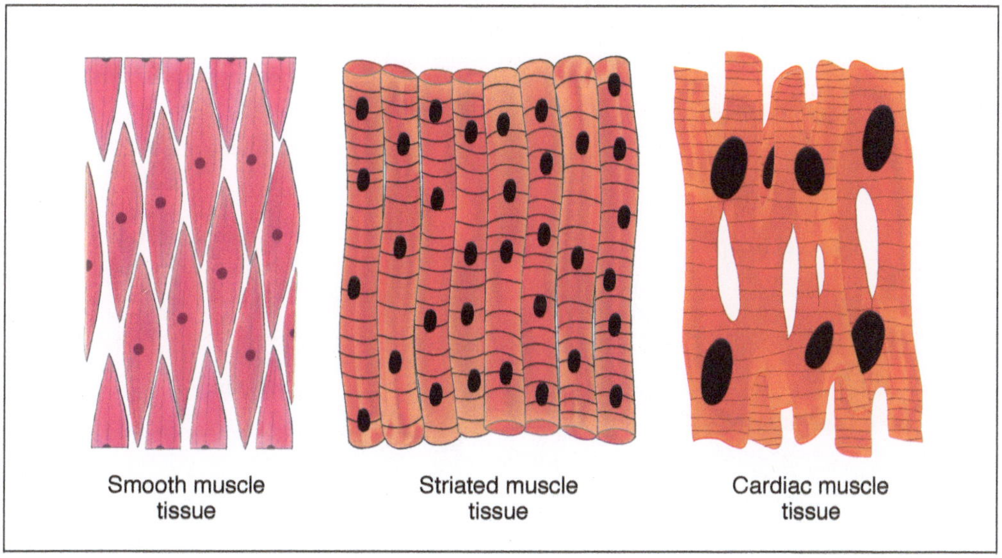

Figure 1.1 Types of muscle tissue.

Striated muscle is made up of a long series of *fibers*. Each of these is made up of other thinner filaments, called myofibrils, which are composed of two proteins, *actin* and *myosin*. At the ends of the muscle bundle, there are tendons, which connect the muscle to the bones.

When we decide to make a movement, we send an electrical impulse to the muscle through the nervous system. This impulse comes from the brain and causes the actin and myosin filaments to slide. In this way, the filaments shorten, causing the contraction of the entire muscle bundle that moves the bones.

The muscle exerts effort, thus requiring energy expenditure. This energy is supplied by a phosphorus compound, called adenosine triphosphate (ATP), produced by a cellular organelle called the mitochondria starting from the sugars that reach the muscle through the blood. The mitochondrion can produce ATP in two different ways: in the first case it uses oxygen, which is aerobic work; in the second case it resorts to lactic acid, thus resulting in an anaerobic workout. There are **more than 600** muscles and they make up about 40% of our body weight (Fig. 1.2); from the large

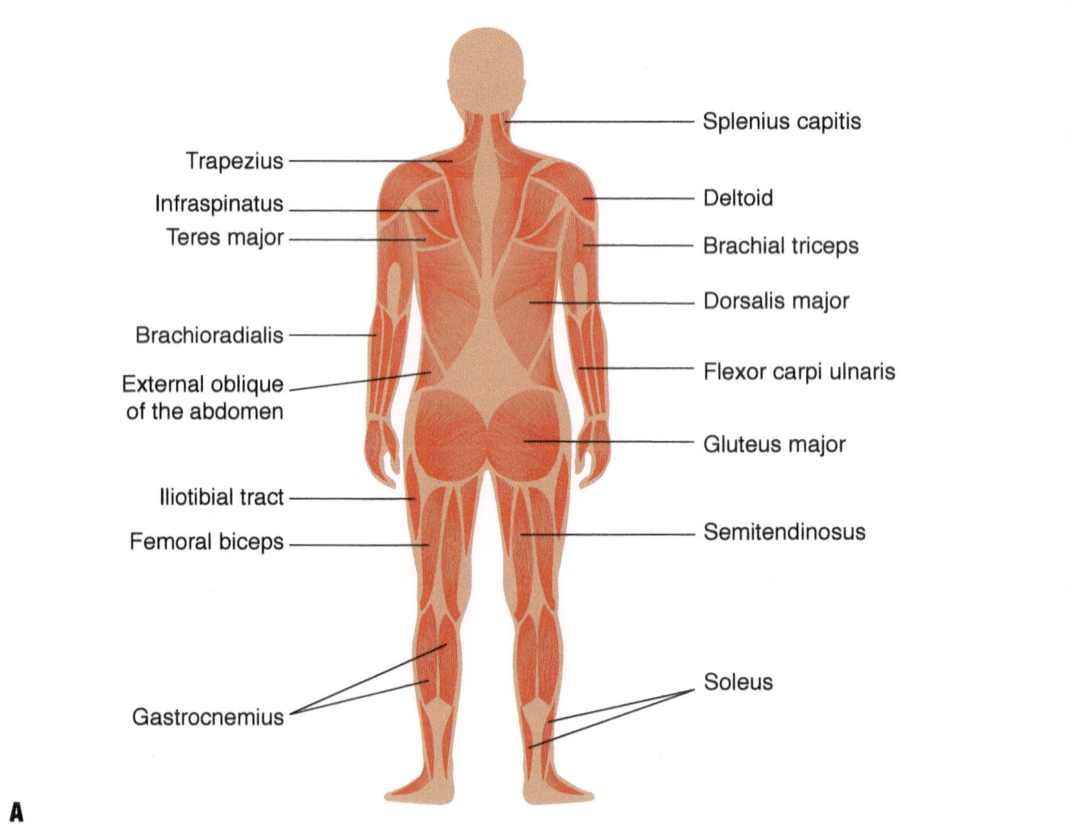

Figure 1.2 The major muscles of the body.

muscles of the shoulders and legs to the small muscles located in the eye sockets that move the eye, *each one contributes to the body's extraordinary range of motion* and have the ability to *contract* and *release* successively.

Muscles are connected to the bones through robust formations of fibrous tissue, called *tendons*, which shorten when the muscle contracts, resulting in the convergence of the two bones on which they are inserted and, consequently, movement.

Muscles can be subdivided into *deep muscles* when they are connected/attached only to bones, and *superficial muscles*, when one of the attachment points is the skin. The latter are the muscles of the face, or mimics, as their contraction changes the construct of the skin of the face, producing facial expressions.

Skeletal muscles are *voluntary muscles*, which means that they contract on our command, although they can also contract following an involuntary reflex stimulus.

On the other hand, **smooth muscles** are *involuntary* and found in visceral structures. *Without our intervention*, they allow automatic motility of the organs, that is,

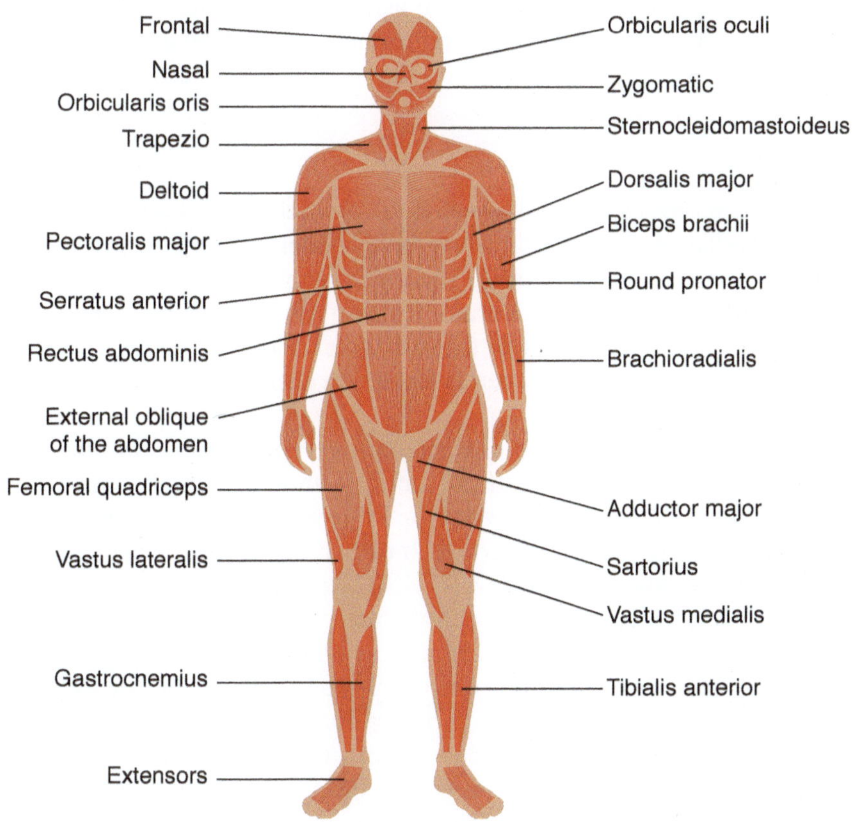

B

the one that regulates the progression of food in the digestive tract or that controls changes in the size of the arterial vessels for the regulation of blood circulation. These are muscles that contract less quickly than skeletal ones, but in which the state of contraction can last longer.

The **third type of muscle tissue** is found exclusively in the heart and constitutes the myocardium. *It combines the characteristics of striated and smooth muscles*, and is therefore capable of rapid and repeated, but involuntary contraction.

Trauma

Excess lactic acid in the muscle can cause a contracture. In this case, one or more muscle fibers remain blocked and hardened to the touch. Although it often causes acute pain, a contracture has limited duration. Rest and massages are required to increase blood flow.

Muscle fibers can also tear. In this case, depending on the extent of the damage, stretching or a tear may occur. Cold compresses, immobilization, and rest are required for thorough healing.

In certain cases, serious injuries, such as tearing of muscle and supporting connective tissue, may occur, thus requiring immediate medical attention and possible surgery.

Muscle fibers

With the due limitations dictated by generalization, there are two basic types of muscle fibers (or cells) of the skeleton: **slow-twitch fibers** (type I, toned, red) and **fast-twitch fibers** (type II, phasic, white). The identification of these two types of muscle fibers was made possible by a laboratory technique called *muscle biopsy*. During a muscle biopsy, a sample of muscle tissue is taken using a needle inserted into the muscle. The fragment of tissue taken is placed on a slide and colored, to then be observed under a microscope.

Each type of fiber has its own characteristics. Type I fibers contract more slowly than type II fibers, they have many mitochondria and have a high aerobic capacity, so they are resistant to fatigue; moreover, type I fibers have a smaller cross-section than type II fibers. Type II fibers are divided into two subgroups: type IIa and type IIx. Type IIa fibers are called "oxidant fast-twitch", because they have a greater quantity of mitochondria; type IIx fibers are called "fast-twitch glycolytic". However, type IIa fibers do not have the same aerobic capacity as slow-twitch fibers.

Regarding the distribution of the two types of fibers, the following two considerations apply. The first is that in each individual the distribution of slow and fast fibers is different in different muscles; for example, the relationship between the two types of fibers is different between the biceps and quadriceps, as well as between the deltoids and triceps. The second consideration is that in the same muscle of different individuals it is very likely that there is a different percentage of the two types of fibers; one person may have a high percentage of type II fiber in the quadriceps, while another may have a low one. As an indication, strength athletes such as weightlifters have 60-90% fast-twitch fibers in the muscles that are used mostly for their sport.

On the other hand, endurance athletes such as long-distance runners probably have 60-90% slow-twitch muscle fibers in their most stressed muscles.

Coaches should know that **training can modify the metabolic structure of the fibers**. With training, type IIa (intermediate) fibers gradually take on the characteristics of IIx (fast) fibers or type I (slow) fibers. It should be noted that in trained people type IIx fibers are larger than type IIa fibers: the transformation of IIa into IIx, with training, contributes to the increase in the volume of the trained muscle, called *muscle hypertrophy* (increase in the size of cells but not in their number).

The characteristics of the types of fibers and their response to training are very complex, and to highlight them it is necessary to consult specific treatises. It is important to underline that, in an individual, the composition of muscle cells is genetically determined; with training, it is possible to partially change the percentage of fiber by changing one type of fiber into another. However, without a doubt, the starting percentage does affect performance and coaches must design individual training programs and understand the reasons why different people respond differently to the same training program. There are no major differences between males and females regarding the distribution of the different types of muscle fibers, but from various studies, it seems that men have a slightly lower percentage of type I fibers than women, while type IIa fibers are higher in men than in women. Apart from this, male muscles are physiologically identical to female ones.

Skeletal muscles

Although type II fibers contract faster than type I, both slow-twitch and fast-twitch types always contract via the same mechanism. Muscles are made up of many single muscle fibers. By observing a muscle fiber under a microscope, it can be seen that it is made up of numerous repetitive elements, called sarcomeres. In addition, chains of proteins called myofibrils are found throughout the muscle fiber. In a myofibril, there are numerous proteins, but the only ones that are important in the contraction process of a muscle are the aforementioned actin and myosin, also known as *contractile proteins.*

Muscle contraction

In order for a muscle to contract, there must be a sufficient amount of ATP in the vicinity of the actin and myosin proteins, and a command must be given by the central nervous system (CNS). When these two factors are present, the thin ends (heads) of the myosin attach themselves to the actin, forming an actin-myosin cross-bridge, a process explained in the "flowing filament theory".

The energy of the ATP causes the ends of the myosin to rotate towards the center of the sarcomere, dragging the actin filament attached to them, so that the actin slides inwards, towards the center of the sarcomere.

This process causes each sarcomere to shorten along the entire muscle; since all sarcomeres shorten at the same moment, there is a reduction in the length of the entire muscle fiber. When many fibers are shortened, there is a muscle contraction, which, therefore, consists of the simultaneous shortening of a large number of fibers of the same muscle. Even though the single fiber shortens when it contracts, muscle contraction does not always involve the shortening of the entire muscle. The *concentric contraction* is the one that involves the shortening of the muscle; the *eccentric contraction* is the one that occurs when the resistance is greater than the developed force, so the muscle actually stretches; the *isometric contraction* is the contraction of individual fibers, without changes in the length of the entire muscle. In summary, muscle contraction is an interaction between the actin and myosin proteins, which causes the contraction of individual muscle fibers, stimulated by a nerve impulse and maintained by the energy of ATP.

Force of contraction

When a muscle fiber contracts, it exerts force. Since the skeletal muscles function according to the "all or nothing" criterion, when a single fiber contracts, it generates the maximum force it is capable of, that is, it is not able to dose the contraction force (as, instead, occurs in the cardiac muscle). The amount of force produced during the contraction of a muscle depends on two factors: (1) the size of the individual fibers (the larger the fiber, the stronger it is); (2) the number of muscle fibers contracting simultaneously.

The force generated by muscle contraction is also linked to the speed of movement around the joint and the initial length of the "belly" of the muscle. The force-speed relationship is such that the faster the movement, the lower the force generated by the contracting muscle. For example, the bicep develops greater force during contraction if the rotation speed around the elbow is 60 degrees per second, compared to how much it develops if the speed is 180 degrees per second. The strength-to-length relationship indicates that a muscle generates maximum force when it begins to contract at a length equal to 1.2 times its resting length. This explains why some athletes, such as baseball or golf players, do some light stretching exercises before starting the swinging movements.

Muscle fiber size

The force generated by a fiber is proportional to its section, but not directly proportional: the same fiber, when it widens, exerts a greater force than when it is narrower; however, bodybuilders, who are certainly stronger than untrained people, are weaker than weightlifters with the same transverse muscle area. This is due to the hypertrophy, partly of a sarcoplasmic type, of the bodybuilder compared to the myofibrillar one of the weightlifter. An interesting study by the University of Copenhagen, in Denmark, showed that the water content and measurements of the quadriceps muscles remain increased for 52 hours after performing 3 series of leg extensions. The cross-sectional area increases by 16% and the water content by 7%, while the water content of the patellar tendon decreases by 14%.

Furthermore, the force exerted by a muscle of a certain section is the same in males and females. Men are generally stronger because they have a greater amount of muscle tissue. In any case, women react just as well as men to a strength training program, so it appears that this type of training is an important component of a physical wellness program in both sexes.

Motor units

In each muscle, the fibers are stimulated individually or in groups. The nerve connected to the spinal cord together with the muscle fibers it stimulates are called the motor unit. Drive units have different sizes. Some motor units, where the nerve stimulates only 5-10 fibers, are associated with small and delicate movements, such as moving the eyes, blinking and painting. However, there are also motor units that consist of a nerve and 500-1000 fibers which are needed for activities such as weightlifting, football, and jumping.

Regardless of their size, the drive units consist of type I fibers and type II fibers. When the fibers of a motor unit contract, all the muscle fibers of this unit contract together, developing maximum strength (all or nothing); the total force developed depends on how many drive units contract simultaneously.

Abilities, strength and endurance

Professional bodybuilders should form their knowledge on two fundamental bases: **exercise technique** and **training technique**. In this regard, we consider it useful to remind the reader of the general meanings attributed to the words ability, power, strength and endurance. In this brief introduction, these words are examined according to common sense for each gymnastic-sport discipline, so that the reader understands that the training methodology, although having common bases, varies according to the needs of each discipline.

Therefore, it is important to remember that all the energy mechanisms of cardiorespiratory and muscular metabolism, namely the aerobic, the anaerobic lactacid and the anaerobic alactacid, have characteristics of trainability both for capacity and for power. **Alactacid power** (sometimes identified with explosive force) is linked to the maximum expenditure of energy in the minimum amount of time; **aerobic capacity**, also called endurance, is linked to the minimum expenditure of energy in the maximum amount of time. These are the two extremes, in relation to time, of the physical-sporting performance of a human being.

As for **strength**, let's introduce the topic with an example: the weightlifter can derive general benefit from the strength and muscular endurance that is performed in aerobic gymnastics with weights or resistance bands. This benefit, however, is not specific to their sporting performance needs. The same goes for a track sprinter, who obviously needs to keep the white fibers hyper-efficient, especially with elastic, fast and reactive strength training, which is very often ballistic.

Let's consider the simple and valid definition of "strength" by the founding fathers of Physical Education: the muscular possibility of opposing or overcoming resistance in the form of an opposing mass. When we examine the amount of resistance and the time and the speed of execution, then we are looking at the various "types" of strength.

So, if you engage in activities in which a muscle group opposes any resistance (even the force of gravity), a force is applied. There are two situations that characterize the muscular "state": tone and trophism. The **tone**, as it is known, is the minimum basal tension, continuously present, which allows the muscle fibers to respond effectively to a stimulus of contraction; it never disappears, except in particular relaxation activities, and tends to increase with physical activity of any kind, but can sometimes be unbalanced by hypokinesia, hypertrophy and/or CNS disorders. Trophism expresses the muscle quality of effectively matching stimuli of high content and energy consumption within the muscle fiber itself.

The various and essential **types of force** are briefly summarized below:

- *maximum* or *maximal force*: maximum force value that can be expressed with the contraction of all muscle fibers;
- *static force*: a force that is expressed with the least muscular excursion, mostly balancing (as in gymnasts); it is of fundamental importance, as it stimulates the gamma circuit and the extrapyramidal system;
- *fast force*: application of force with muscle contractions and decontractions, dependent on the speed of execution; its development is most useful at a young age;
- *elastic force*: an application of a force that exploits the elastic quality of the muscle;
- *reactive force*: the application of a force that exploits the quality of muscular reaction to stimuli that are sometimes unrepeated, and sometimes close to each other in rapid succession.

When we try to make the applications of these forces last over time, obviously without an excessive decrease in effectiveness, we refer to "resistance to force".

This brings us to a classic training theory: **resistance**. The definition describes resistance as the ability to prolong any physical activity over time. This definition is adaptable to speed (endurance to speed), strength (endurance to strength) and aerobic metabolism (endurance), and highlights a fundamental common aspect. Resistance is a concept of capacity, or autonomy. Therefore, it is linked to knowing how to exploit energy for as long as possible without wasting it.

From a lexical point of view, the fundamental difference between capacity and resistance consists in the fact that the former is like a reservoir, and the latter is the ability to use it without waste for as long as possible. The first is an ever-present developable quality, the second is an action that can be improved with a training technique and through psychological factors.

Another useful parallel is the division of motor skills into conditional and coordinative. The former largely depend on the purely energetic and mechanical possibilities of the locomotor system, as well as, obviously, on the psychological conditions of the athlete or student; they are strength, endurance and speed.

The latter, understood as the "ability to organize and control movement", largely depends on the athlete's or student's cognitive-operational and psychomotor conditions, as well as on their psychological conditions. **Coordination skills** were summarized by Dietrich D. Blume in 1981, as follows:

- coupling;
- differentiation;
- preservation of balance;
- orientation;
- rhythm;
- reaction;
- change.

Every athlete should keep in mind that, in all this, psychological conditions, motivation and mood play a fundamental role in the result of the activity itself. What we define and indicate as physical (motor) abilities is also a result of a possibility of an individual disposition aimed at movement, without which the "master" of the movement itself is missing, even though their body, that is the subject, is present.

At this point, it is beneficial to recall the psychomotor factors described by the S. and E. Fabbri brothers in the 1970s, at the height of psychomotor skills:

- breathing education and control;
- static, static-dynamic and dynamic balance;
- definition and coordination of laterality;
- sensorimotor coordination;
- space-time structuring;
- control of psychosomatic tone and relaxation;
- global and intersegmental postural perception;
- general dynamic coordination.

CHAPTER 2

Terminology

Position terminology identifies the location of various parts of the body. The **terms of movement** indicate the displacement of a body part and the direction in which such displacement occurs. Both refer to the subject in an upright position, with the upper limbs adhering to the sides of the trunk and the palms facing outwards.

Position terminology

The position of any part of the human body can be defined by referring to **three planes** (two vertical and one horizontal) perpendicular to each other (Fig. 2.1):

- the **median** (vertical) **sagittal plane** runs anteroposteriorly and divides the body into two almost symmetrical halves, or antimers. The median sagittal plane is flanked by infinite paramedian sagittal planes that have two sides: the one that

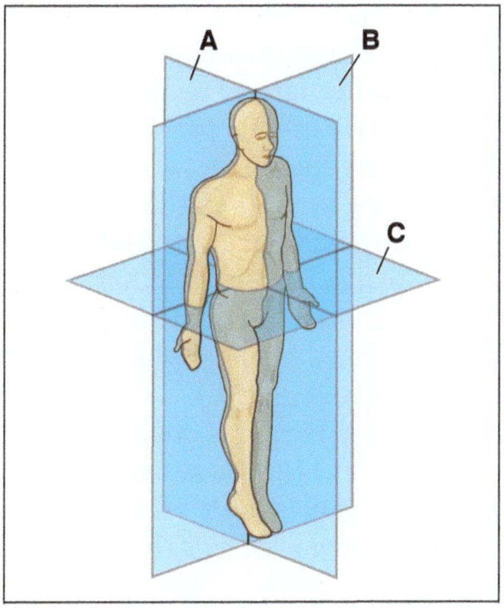

Figure 2.1 (**A**) Median sagittal plane. (**B**) Longitudinal plane. Translated anteriorly and posteriorly, it takes on the respective denomination of *frontal plane* and *dorsal plane*. (**C**) Transverse plane.

turns towards the median sagittal plane is called *medial*, and the opposite one is called *lateral*;
- the **longitudinal** (vertical) **plane** is perpendicular to the sagittal plane and divides the body into two halves. In an upright position, the side that turns forward is called *frontal*; the one that turns posteriorly is called *dorsal*;
- the **transverse** (horizontal) **plane** is parallel to the support surface in the standing position. The infinite transverse planes have two sides: the upper one is called *cephalic*, while lower one is called *caudal*.

In the case of moving parts, such as limbs, additional terms are used to establish the greater or lesser proximity of a point with respect to the median sagittal plane. The *proximal* term indicates a part closer to the median sagittal plane, while the term *distal* indicates a part located at a further distance.

Movement terminology

The direction of movements is indicated by the axis around which they take place. The axes derive from the intersection of two planes and are as follows:

- **sagittal axis**: the intersection between the median sagittal plane and the transverse plane;
- **vertical axis**: the intersection between the median sagittal plane and the frontal plane;
- **transverse axis**: the intersection between the frontal sagittal plane and the transverse plane.

The movements that take place around the transverse axis are called **flexion** (the moving part moves away from the frontal plane) and **extension** (the moving part approaches the frontal plane). The movements that take place around the sagittal axis are called **lateral inclination** when they refer to the spine (head and trunk), **abduction** (the mobile part moves away from the sagittal plane), and **adduction** (the mobile part approaches the sagittal plane), in the case of the limbs. The movements around the vertical axis are called **torsion** in reference to the spine and **rotation** when they take place in the limbs (*external rotation*: movement directed towards the dorsal plane; *internal rotation*: movement directed towards the frontal plane). The rotation movement of the two most distal segments of the upper limb (forearm and hand) is called **pronosupination** (*supination* when directed outward and **pronation** when directed inward).

All the movements previously described take place around an axis and are in relation to a plane (*simple movements*). However, there are movements in which both the axes and the planes are variable in the different stages of execution; they are *complex* or *combined movements* (for example, circumduction is a complex movement of the limbs).

Table 2.1 Motor skills

Coordination skills	Conditional skills	Auxiliary skills
Space-time orientation	Strength	Joint mobility
Adaptation and switching abilities	Speed	Muscle extensibility
Ability to combine movements	Resistance	Muscle elasticity
Differentiation ability		Flexibility
Motor reaction		
Rhythmic skills		
Vestibular ability		
Imagination and motor creativity		
Motor memory		
Motor coordination		
Ability to anticipate		
Ability to represent mental movement		
Motor timing		
Body expression		

Motor skills

Motor skills are divided into **coordinative, conditional** and **auxiliary** (Table 2.1). For the most part, we will talk about the conditional ones, but also involve the auxiliaries and, to a certain extent, the coordinative ones.

Resistance

The ability to extend physical work over time, coping with the onset of fatigue (long, medium, short endurance and speed).

Strength

The ability to overcome resistance or to oppose it with muscular effort (maximum strength, speed strength and strength resistance). It has great room for improvement.

Speed

The ability to perform a gesture (a motor act) in the shortest time possible. It depends on reaction time, speed of the individual movement, frequency and width of the movement. It is the most difficult to train.

CHAPTER 3

The muscles of the body

Chest muscles

They are divided into intrinsic and extrinsic muscles, based on their points of insertion and origin.

Intrinsic muscles

The levatores costarum (or levator costae) are paired muscles which number twelve on each side and are located deep in the back, near the spine. They have a triangular shape, originating from the apex of the transverse processes of C7 to T11 vertebrae and the ribs below. They are inserted at the upper edge of the underlying rib. Each of the four lower muscles, called levatores costarum longi, divides into two fasciculi, one of which is inserted as described above. The other passes down to the second rib below its origin. They are controlled by the cervical nerve and help elevate the ribs during respiration.

Intercostal muscles

They occupy the intercostal spaces, there are 11 on each side, and are divided into medium, internal, and external (Fig. 3.1). The external intercostal muscles extend from the rib tubercles to the costal cartilages, originate from the lower edge of each rib and terminate at the upper edge of the rib below.

The middle intercostal muscles occupy the space from the middle axillary line to the sternum. They originate from the lower edge of the ribs and end at the upper edge of the underlying ribs.

The internal intercostal muscles extend from the costal angle to the sternum. The intercostal vessels and nerves run in the thin space between these muscles. By contracting, the intercostal muscles raise and lower the ribs.

Subcostal muscles

They are found in the inner and posterior parts of the chest wall, near the costovertebral joints. They originate from the inner surface of the ribs and are inserted into the inner surface of the underlying rib. They work by lowering the ribs.

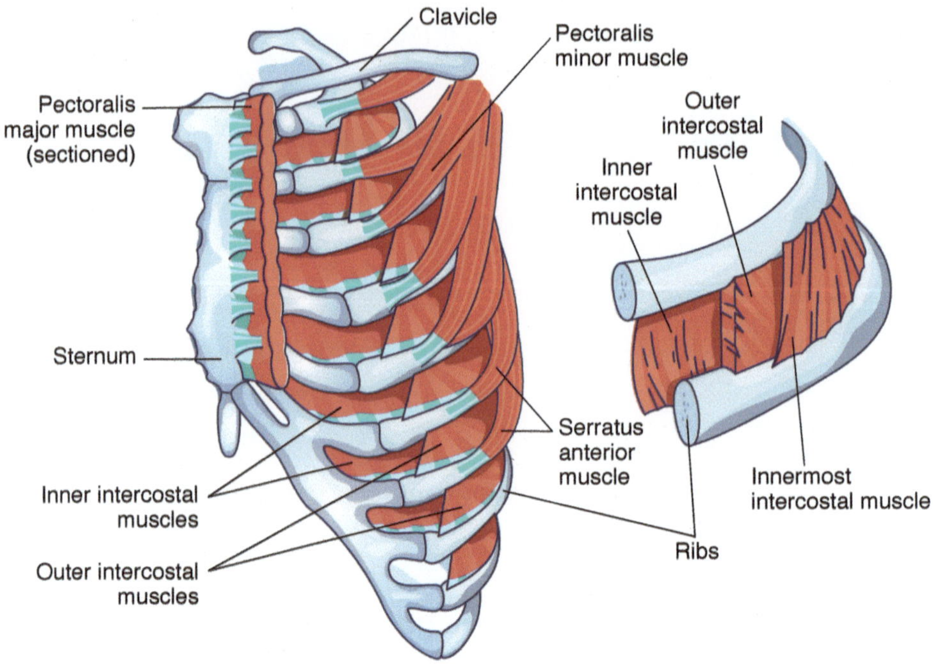

Figure 3.1 Intercostal muscles.

Transversus thoracis muscle

It is located on the inner side of the anterior chest wall. It originates from the posterior side of the body and from the xiphoid process and is carried upwards and laterally, to insert itself on the lower margin of the costal cartilages from the second or third up to the sixth. Its action consists in lowering the rib cartilage.

Thoracoappendicular extrinsic muscles

They originate from the ribs and the sternum and reach the bones of the thoracic girdle and the humerus.

Pectoralis major muscle

It is located anteriorly in the thorax and forms most of the anterior wall of the axilla. A clavicular, a sternocostal, and an abdominal part are distinguished. The bundles of the three parts converge in a flattened tendon, entering the lateral margo of the bicipital sulcus of the humerus. The upper face of the muscle lies deep underneath the mammary gland, while the deep face covers the sternum, the pectoralis minor and the external intercostals. The pectoralis major adduces and rotates the humerus internally or raises the trunk taking a fixed point on the humerus.

Pectoralis minor muscle

It is located deep in the pectoralis major, originates from three tendon digitations from the second, fourth and fifth ribs, and the three bundles converge in a belly which is inserted on the coracoid process of the scapula. Together with the pectoralis major it forms the anterior wall of the axillary cavity and covers the ribs, the serratus anterior and the intercostal muscles. By contracting, it lowers the shoulder and raises the ribs.

Subclavian muscle

It has a cylindrical shape and is located between the clavicle and the first rib, from which (including the cartilage) it originates, and is inserted into the sulcus of the lower face of the clavicle. It relates to the subclavian artery and vein and to the brachial plexus. It works by lowering the collarbone.

Serratus anterior muscle

It is located in the lateral wall of the thorax, originates by means of digitations from the external face of the first ten ribs, and it inserts at the anterior surface of the scapula. It is divided into three parts according to the points of insertion: the superior part originates from the first two ribs, the intermediate part from the second, third and fourth ribs, and the inferior one from the lower ribs.

Spinoappendicular muscles

They originate from the spine and reach the bones of the thoracic girdle and the humerus.

Trapezius muscle

It is located in the nuchal region and in the dorsal part of the chest. Its bundles converge towards the shoulder and its superficial fascia is inserted into the integuments. The deep fascia is connected to the supraspinatus, levator scapulae, splenium capitis and splenium cervicis muscles. Its contraction elevates and adducts the shoulder, and extends the head by rotating it to the opposite side.

Latissimus dorsi muscle

It covers the lower-lateral part of the back and the lateral part of the thorax. It originates from the spinous processes of the last six thoracic vertebrae and from the lumbar vertebrae. Its bundles surround the foramen rotundum, inserting themselves into the bicipital groove of the humerus. With its superficial part, the latissimus dorsi comes into contact with the trapezius and integuments. By contracting, it adducts and rotates the humerus. If it takes a fixed point on the humerus it raises the trunk and the ribs.

Rhomboid muscle

It is located in the lower part of the nuchal region and in the upper part of the back. It originates from the interspinous ligaments of the last cervical vertebrae and inserts itself on the vertebral margin of the scapula. It is covered by the trapezius and, its contraction slides the scapula medially.

Levator scapulae muscle
It occupies the lateral-posterior region of the neck, originates from the transverse processes of the first four cervical vertebrae, and moves to the medial angle of the scapula. It is covered by the trapezius and the sternocleidomastoid. Its action consists in lifting and medially moving the scapula.

Spinocostal muscles
These are large, thin muscles, with a quadrilateral shape. They are found in the middle layer of the back muscles.

Serratus posterior-superior muscle
It originates from the apex of the spinous processes of the seventh cervical vertebra. The muscular belly is divided into four digitations, which are fixed at the upper edge of the ribs from the second to the fifth. It works by elevating the ribs.

Serratus posterior-inferior muscle
It originates at the level of the spinous processes of the last two thoracic vertebrae and the first three lumbar vertebrae, it lies under the latissimus dorsi muscle muscle, and, when it contracts, it lowers the ribs.

Diaphragm muscle
It is an asymmetric, broad and flattened muscle that separates the thoracic cavity from the abdominal cavity. Its surface, similar to a dome, is rather irregular and, on the thoracic side, has a depression on which the heart rests. The inferior vena cava, the azygos vein, the great and small splanchnic nerves, and numerous other vessels pass through the diaphragm. It is crossed by the esophagus and nerve formations. Depending on the insertion points, a lumbar, a rib and a sternal part can be distinguished in the diaphragm. The two diaphragmatic sides are covered by a thin sheet called the diaphragmatic surface, which merges with the pleura in the thoracic cavity and with the peritoneum in the abdominal cavity. The upper surface is related to the base of the pericardium and the pulmonary bases, and the lower face covers the liver, stomach, spleen, pancreas, kidneys and adrenal glands. When it contracts, it lowers and raises the lower ribs, increasing the volume of the thoracic cavity and abdominal pressure.

Muscles of the upper limb

They are divided into extrinsic, which have an insertion on the upper limb but originate in the torso, and intrinsic, which have both the origin and the insertion on the limb.

Deltoid muscle
It is part of the shoulder muscles, which originate from the thoracic girdle and have an insertion on the humerus. Here, the deltoid covers the lateral part of the shoul-

der, its shape resembles the Greek capital letter delta, with the base at the top and the apex facing down, and is flattened. It originates from the anterior margin of the clavicle, from the acromion, and from the spine of the scapula; its bundles are inserted through a robust tendon into the deltoid tuberosity of the humerus. The deltoid has a superficial face in relation to the superficial sheet of the deltoid fascia and a deep face covered by the deep sheet of the deltoid fascia. It is innervated by the axillary nerve (C4-C6) and it can abduct the arm up to 90°.

Supraspinatus muscle

It is located in the supraspinatus fossa of the scapula, from which it originates, and has a triangular prismatic shape. Its bundles run laterally until they enter the upper facet of the greater tubercle of the humerus. The upper fascia of the muscle is close to the trapezius and deltoid muscles, with the interposition of the supraspinatus fascia. The lower face enters into the capsule of the shoulder joint, where its tendon is inserted. It is innervated by the suprascapular nerve (C5) and it abducts and rotates the arm outwards. In addition, it performs a stabilizing action on the shoulder joint.

Infraspinatus muscle

It occupies the infraspinatus fossa, from which it originates, and it is flat. Its bundles end in a tendon, which, adhering to the fibrous capsule of the shoulder, inserts itself on the middle facet of the greater tubercle of the humerus. The superficial part faces the trapezius and the deltoid, and the deep part faces the infraspinatus fossa. It is innervated by the suprascapular nerve and its function is to rotate the arm outwards. It also stabilizes the scapula-humeral joint.

Teres minor muscle

It is elongated and flattened, and originates from the infraspinatus fossa, near the lower edge of the infraspinatus muscle. It inserts at the lower facet of the greater tubercle of the humerus. Its posterior face relates to the deltoid and the teres major, while the anterior part faces the subscapularis muscle. It is innervated by the axillary nerve, and it externally rotates the arm. Another function is to provide a stabilizing action to the entire joint.

Teres major muscle

It is placed below the teres minor and is also elongated and flattened in shape. It originates from the dorsal aspect of the lower part of the lateral border of the scapula to insert itself at the bottom of the bicipital groove of the humerus. Its posterior part faces the latissimus dorsi and the long head of the triceps, while the anterior part faces the subscapularis, coracobrachialis and other large dorsal muscles. It forms the wall of the axillary cavity together with the latissimus dorsi. Its upper margin, together with the humerus and the teres minor, delimits the triangle of the round muscles. It is innervated by the inferior subscapular nerve, and it adducts, extends and rotates the humerus.

Subscapularis muscle

It originates from the bottom of the subscapular fossa and its bundles converge on the lesser tubercle of the humerus. The anterior part faces the dentate muscle and the vascular and nerve bundle of the axillary region. The posterior face rests on the subscapularis fossa. The insertion tendon adheres posteriorly to the joint capsule. It is innervated by the subscapular nerves, and it adducts and rotates the arm internally.

Arm muscles (Fig. 3.2)

Biceps brachii muscle

It is part of the anterior muscles of the arm and is made up of two heads, the short head and the long head, which converge in a single muscle belly (see Fig. 3.2). The long head originates from the supraglenoid tubercle of the scapula, through a long and cylindrical tendon that inserts into the bicipital groove of the humerus; the tendon becomes fleshy as it exits the bicipital groove and, near the middle third of the arm, joins the short head. The short head originates from the apex of the coracoid process and is brought down to join the long head; from here starts a robust tendon which finds its insertion on the radial tuberosity.

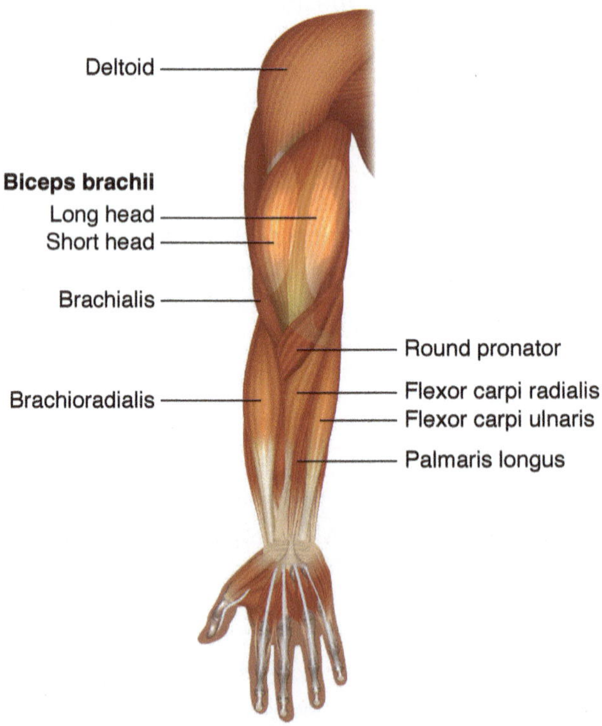

Figure 3.2 Muscles of the arm and forearm.

The biceps brachii muscle lies above the deltoid and the pectoralis major and it borders internally with the anterior brachial. On the side of the biceps muscle, the vein and the brachial artery and, more superficially, the basilic vein travel in two sulci; the cephalic vein runs in the lateral sulcus. It is innervated by the musculocutaneous nerve and its action gives stability to the scapulohumeral joint, keeping the head of the humerus in the glenoid cavity; it also intervenes on the flexion and abduction of the arm in synergy with other muscles.

Coracobrachialis muscle

It is medial and deep in relation to the short head of the biceps. It originates from the apex of the coracoid process of the scapula to insert on the anteromedial face of the humerus. It relates to the deltoid, the pectoralis major, the short head of the biceps, the teres major and the subscapularis.

It is innervated by the musculocutaneous nerve and its action is to flex and adduce the arm.

Brachialis muscle

It is elongated and flattened, and lies beneath the biceps brachii; it originates below the insertion of the deltoid muscle, and moves down to the tuberosity of the ulna (see Fig. 3.2). Anteriorly it is in relationship with the biceps, posteriorly with the humerus and with the elbow joint. Under the action of the musculocutaneous nerve, the forearm is flexed.

Triceps brachii muscle

It is the main posterior muscle of the arm and it consists of three parts: the long, lateral and medial head. The first head arises from the infraglenoid tubercle of the scapula, while the second and third heads from the posterior aspect of the humerus. The three heads converge at the bottom on a sturdy tendon that inserts on the upper and posterior surfaces of the olecranon. The triceps relates to the deltoid, the humerus and the elbow joint. It is innervated by the radial nerve and is the main extensor muscle of the forearm; it also promotes the adduction of the humerus by means of the long head.

Anterior compartment of the forearm (see Fig. 3.2)

It is a group of eight muscles arranged in four layers.

Pronator teres muscle

It is the most lateral muscle of the superficial layer and crosses the upper half of the forearm obliquely, proceeding from top to bottom and from outside to inside. It originates with two bundles, the humeral head and the ulnar head, and ends with a flattened tendon that inserts on the medial part of the lateral aspect of the radius. The median nerve enters the forearm between the two heads of the muscle, while the brachial artery and the radial nerve pass laterally to the muscle. The pronator teres rotates the radius internally and flexes the forearm.

Flexor carpi radialis muscle
It is medial to the pronator teres and the palmaris longus. It originates from the anterior aspect of the epitrochlea, moving downwards to insert on the anterior aspect of the base of the second metacarpal bone. It lies deep lateral to the flector digitorum superficialis. It flexes the hand and the forearm, rotating them internally.

Palmaris longus muscle
It lies between the flexor carpi radialis and the flexor carpi ulnaris, originating from the epitrochlea, and enters the palmar aponeurosis. It is innervated by the median nerve, and it stretches the palmar aponeurosis and flexes the hand.

Flexor carpi ulnaris muscle
It is the innermost of the epitrochlear muscles and is medial to the long palmar. It has two heads: a humeral head and a larger ulnar head. The insertion tendon ends on the pisiform bone, which remains included in its fibers. It is innervated by the ulnar nerve, under whose action it flexes and adducts the hand.

Flexor digitorum superficialis muscle
It forms the second layer of the anterior compartment of the forearm. It originates with a humeral and a radial head, then joined by a tendon arch which is itself the origin of other muscle bundles; dividing into four bellies about halfway up the forearm, it carries, with the four tendons that originate from it, to four fingers (from the second to the fifth finger). The four tendons are not in the same plane. In the fingers, each tendon is wrapped in a mucous sheath and connected to the anterior face of the phalanges. Under the action of the median nerve, it flexes the middle phalanges of the four fingers (excluding the thumb), cooperating with the flexion of the hand on the forearm.

Flexor digitorum profundus muscle
It occupies the third muscle layer together with the flexor pollicis longus muscle. It originates in the anterior and medial surfaces of the ulna and in the medial margin of the radius, and its belly divides into four bundles to which as many insertion tendons belong, which are fixed at the base of the third phalanx of the last four fingers, succeeding, with its own action, to flex them under the control of the median and lateral nerves.

Flexor pollicis longus muscle
It forms the lateral part of the third layer, arises from the anterior surface of the radius and from the coronoid process of the ulna and its tendon is inserted on the volar face of the first phalanx of the thumb. Under the action of the median nerve, it flexes the distal phalanx of the first finger.

Pronator quadratus muscle
It is a square-shaped muscle and it lies deep in the lower anterior part of the forearm. It originates from the anterior surface of the ulna and inserts inferiorly with its bundles into the anterior distal diaphysis of the radius. It rotates the arm medially.

Lateral muscles of the forearm

Brachioradialis muscle

It originates from the lateral margin of the humerus and its belly moves downwards, occupying a superficial position, and continues in a long tendon that inserts into the styloid process of the radius. It is innervated by the radial nerve and it flexes the forearm. It is important for the stability of the elbow joint.

Extensor carpi radialis brevis muscle

It is posterior and lateral to the long radial extensor, it originates from the anterior aspect of the epicondyle and its belly continues in a tendon that runs on the lateral aspect of the radius and then inserts on the dorsal aspect of the third metacarpal bone. It is innervated by the radial nerve and, by contracting, it extends the hand.

Posterior compartment of the forearm

It contains nine muscles united in two layers, which can be further divided into superficial and deep. The superficial muscles all originate from the epicondyle, thus being defined as epicondylar.

Extensor digitorum communis muscle

It is the most lateral of the superficial muscles, originating from the posterior aspect of the epicondyle, the short radial extensor of the carpus and the extensor of the little finger. At the level of the middle of the forearm, the muscle is divided into three bundles: the lateral bundle gives rise to two tendons, and the other bundles to a tendon. The four tendons that are formed in this way insert on the dorsal face of the first phalanx and then divide into three tabs. The median tab attaches to the second phalanx, while the lateral and medial tabs attach to the third phalanx. At the metacarpal level, the four tendons are joined by three oblique bundles, called tendon joints. This muscle extends the medial four digits of the hand and cooperates in the extension of the hand.

Extensor digiti minimi

It is medially to the common extensor of the fingers and, at the level of the fifth metacarpal bone, it merges with the tendon of the extensor digitorum communis of the fingers intended for the little finger. Its contraction determines the extension of the little finger.

Extensor carpi ulnaris muscle

It is medially to the extensor digiti minimi and originates from the epicondyle, the elbow joint and the posterior margin of the ulna. It is brought down medially and, in the lower part of the forearm, continues in a tendon that inserts at the base of the fifth metacarpal bone. It extends and rotates the hand medially.

Anconeus muscle
It is located in the posterosuperior region of the forearm, it originates from the posterior part of the epicondyle and it inserts at the distal part of the ulna. It is innervated by the radial nerve and has little influence on the extension of the forearm.

Supinator muscle
It envelops the upper third of the radius, originates from the epicondyle, the radial ligament of the elbow, and the annular ligament of the radius, and its bundles are inserted into the anterior and lateral surfaces of the radius. It works by rotating the forearm outwards under the control of the radial nerve.

Abductor pollicis longus muscle
It is the most lateral of the deep posterior muscles and originates from the posterior aspect of the ulna, the interosseous membrane, and the posterior aspect of the radius. Its belly continues in a tendon that goes to insert at the base of the first metacarpal bone. It is innervated by the radial nerve and works by abducting the thumb and hand.

Extensor pollicis brevis muscle
It is medially to the long abductor and originates from the posterior aspect of the radius and the interosseous membrane; its belly surrounds the radius along its path. The terminal tendon enters the dorsal aspect of the proximal phalanx of the thumb, which it extends and abducts.

Extensor pollicis longus muscle
It is medially to the long abductor, originates from the posterior aspect of the ulna and the interosseous membrane, and is inserted at the base of the distal phalanx of the thumb, which it extends and abducts.

Extensor indicis muscle
It is the most medial of the deep posterior muscles. It originates from the posterior aspect of the ulna and the interosseous membrane, and its terminal tendon merges with the common extensor tendon of the fingers intended for the index finger, extending it with its contraction.

Muscles of the lower limb

Internal hip muscles

Iliopsoas muscle
It is located in the lumbo iliac region and in the anterior thigh region. It is made up of two distinct portions, the psoas major muscle and the iliacus muscle, which join together to insert into the femur.

The psoas major is fusiform and originates from the lateral surfaces of the bodies of the last thoracic vertebrae, from the first four lumbar vertebrae and from the interposed discs, and from the base of the transverse processes of the first four lumbar vertebrae. It is brought down laterally, passes under the inguinal ligament, and, having reached the thigh, ends by inserting on the lesser trochanter. During its path, it takes an anterosuperior relationship with the diaphragmatic arch, the kidney, the colon, the renal vessels and the inferior vena cava. A mucous bursa is interposed between the sturdy terminal tendon and the fibrous capsule of the hip joint.

The iliacus muscle has a fan shape and originates from the inner margin of the iliac crest, from the two anterior iliac spines, and from the notch between them, the iliac fossa, and from the sacral wing. The bundles that run inferiorly merge, in part, with those of the psoas major muscle. The iliopsoas muscle is innervated by branches from the lumbar plexus and the femoral nerve. By contracting, it flexes the thigh on the pelvis, adducting it and rotating it externally. If it takes a fixed point on the femur, it flexes the trunk and tilts it to its side.

Psoas minor muscle
It is a muscle of modest size, fusiform, anterior to the great psoas. It originates from the lateral faces of the bodies of the last thoracic and first lumbar vertebrae. From here it enters the iliopectineal eminence and the iliac fascia. It stretches the iliac fascia.

External muscles of the hip (Fig. 3.3)

Gluteus maximus muscle
It is the most superficial and, at the same time, most developed muscle in the gluteal region. It originates from the posterior part of the outer margin of the iliac crest, from the posterior gluteal line, from the surface of the hip bone, from the lateral crest of the sacrum and coccyx, and from the fascia of the gluteus medius. These numerous bundles converge towards the linea aspera of the femur, to insert into the gluteal tuberosity. The gluteus maximus lies between the gluteal fascia and the buttock integuments, superficially, and the median gluteus, pyramidal, gemellus, internal obturator, and quadrate of the femur muscles are located deeply. It is innervated by the inferior gluteal nerve, under which it extends and rotates the femur laterally. It contributes to the maintenance of the erect position and to walking, taking a fixed point on the femur.

Gluteus medius muscle
It is a flat, triangular-shaped muscle located under the gluteus maximus. It originates from the hip bone, the outer lip of the iliac crest and the iliac spine. Its muscle bundles converge like a fan and collect in a tendon that inserts on the lateral surface of the greater trochanter. The muscle is covered with a thick sheet of the gluteal fascia, the gluteus maximus and the tensor fascia lata. It is innervated by the superior gluteal nerve and, under its action, the femur is abducted and rotated externally. Taking a fixed point on the femur, it extends and tilts the pelvis laterally.

Gluteus minimus muscle
Also triangular in shape, it originates from the outer surface of the hip bone, anterior to the gluteal line, and from the outer lip of the iliac crest. Its bundles converge

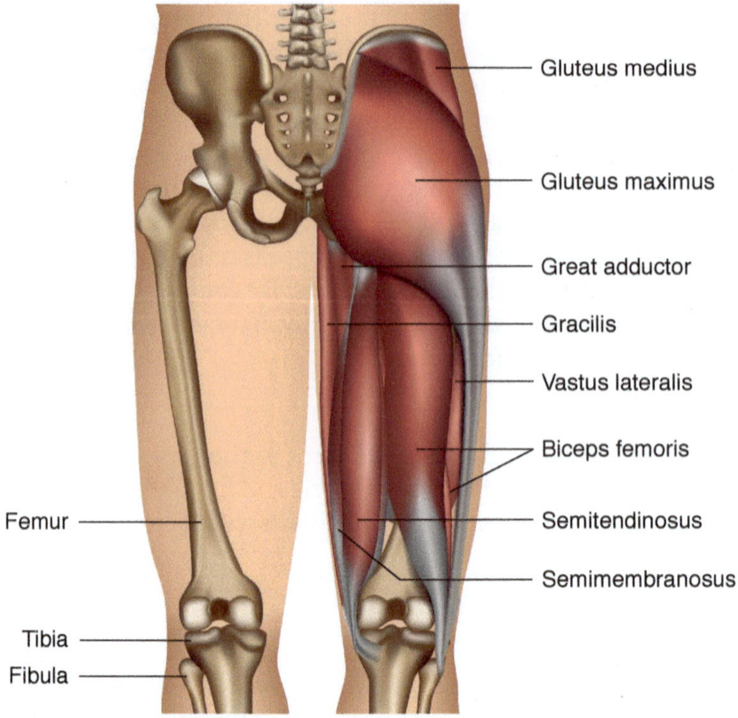

Figure 3.3 External muscles of the hip.

inferiorly, taking insertion on the anterior surface of the greater trochanter of the femur. The muscle is included between the gluteus medius, the iliac wing and the hip joint. It is innervated by the superior gluteal nerve and, by contracting, it abducts and rotates the femur. Taking a fixed point at the femoral level, it tilts the pelvis homolaterally.

Piriformis muscle

It is a flat, pyramidally-shaped muscle, placed partially inside and partially outside the pelvis. It originates from the anterior surface of the sacrum, lateral to the second, third, and fourth sacral fora. It goes laterally and outwards, its bundles proceed outwards through the large ischial foramen and are inserted on the upper end of the greater trochanter. The piriformis muscle divides the large ischial foramen into the suprapiriform and infrapiriform foramina. The anterior surface of the muscle is related to the rectum, while the posterior aspect of the muscle lies against the sacrum. The extra-pelvic part is related to the gluteus maximus and the hip joint. It is innervated by a collateral branch of the sacral plexus. By contracting, it rotates the femur laterally and has a stabilizing action on the coxofemoral joint.

Gemelli muscles
They run horizontally and can be divided into the superior gemellus and the inferior gemellus. The first originates from the outer surface and the lower margin of the ischial spine, and the second from the upper surface of the ischial tuberosity. Both are inserted into the tendon of the internal obturator muscle and, through the latter, into the trochanteric fossa of the femur. They are in proximity with the hip joint, anteriorly, and with the gluteus maximus, posteriorly. They are innervated by the collateral branches of the sacral plexus and they externally rotate the femur and stabilize the hip joint.

Internal obturator muscle
It is located inside and outside of the pelvic cavity and originates from the intrapelvic surface of the obturator membrane and from the contour of the obturator foramen. From here it moves towards the small ischial foramen and then turns laterally to enter the trochanteric fossa of the femur. In its intrapelvic portion, it delimits the ischiorectal fossa. It is innervated by the internal obturator nerve, and it rotates the femur laterally, helping to stabilize the hip joint.

External obturator muscle
It originates from the external contour of the obturator foramen and from the subpubic band; it is brought laterally, up and down, surrounding the coxofemoral joint, before entering the trochanteric fossa of the femur. Anteriorly, to it stand the iliopsoas, the perineum, the great, and the short adductor. It is innervated by the obturator nerve, and it rotates the femur laterally and stabilizes the hip joint.

Quadratus femoris muscle
It is a quadrilateral muscle located between the external surface of the ischial tuberosity and the intertrochanteric crest of the femur. Anteriorly, it is related to the hip joint and the external obturator muscle. The gluteus maximus and the sciatic nerve are located posteriorly. It is innervated by a collateral branch of the sacral plexus and acts by laterally rotating the femur and stabilizing the hip joint.

Anterior thigh muscles (Fig. 3.4)

Tensor fasciae latae muscle
It is a fusiform and superficial muscle placed laterally in the thigh. It originates from the anterior end of the outer lip of the iliac crest, from the iliac spine and from the gluteus medius. Its bundles go downwards, continuing in a long tendon that runs along the thigh for almost all the lower two-thirds, and then inserts into the lateral condyle of the tibia. On its way, the insertion tendon merges with the femoral fascia, forming the iliotibial tract.

The muscular belly is lateral to the sartorius and anterior to the gluteus medius. It is delimited, on the surface, by the subcutaneous layer and, deep, by the gluteus medius and the vastus lateralis. With its action it stretches the fascia lata and abducts the thigh; it also has an extensor action of the leg on the thigh level.

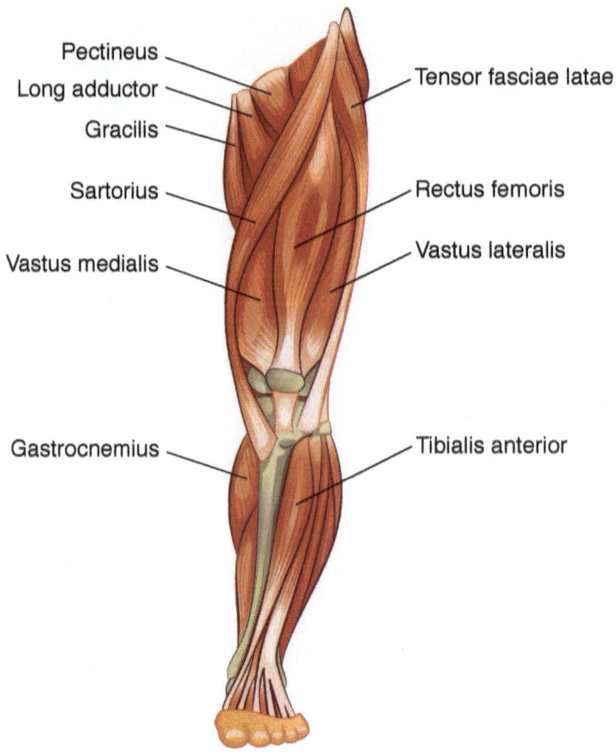

Figure 3.4 Anterior thigh and lower leg muscles.

Sartorius muscle

It occupies a superficial position and looks like an elongated and ribbon-like muscle that crosses the anterior aspect of the thigh obliquely, from the outside to the inside. Its terminal insertion is on the medial side of the knee, on the medial aspect of the tibia. The insertion tendon is common to the gracilis and semitendinosus muscles and, due to its shape, is called "pes anserinus" or "goose foot". Its upper face is superficial and, with the deep one, it comes into contact with the rectus of the femur and the iliopsoas. It delimits the lateral part of the femoral triangle, together with the inguinal ligament, which represents the upper part, and the adductor longus, which represents the medial part. The sartorius is innervated by the femoral nerve and it flexes the leg on the thigh and the thigh on the pelvis. It can abduct and rotate the thigh externally.

Quadriceps femoris muscle

It is the largest muscle in the anterior region of the thigh and, as the name suggests, it is subdivided into four separate muscles (the "heads"): the rectus femoris, the vastus medialis, the vastus lateralis and the vastus intermedius, gathered in a single terminal tendon. The rectus of the femur originates from the anterior iliac spine with a direct tendon and from the highest portion of the acetabulum contour and from the joint capsule with a reflex tendon. The vastus medialis originates from the medial margin of the linea aspera and from the wrinkled line that joins it to the neck of the femur. The vastus lateralis originates from the lateral aspect and anterior border of the greater trochanter, the linea aspera of the femur, and the tendon of the gluteus maximus. The vastus intermedialis, located between the vastus lateralis and the vastus medialis, originates from the margin of the linea aspera and from the anterior and lateral faces of the femur.

The four heads converge at the bottom, maintaining their individuality. At the level of the knee, they are collected in a tendon formed by the overlapping of three laminae, which are almost totally inserted at the level of the patella. Other fibers enter the infraglenoid margin of the tibia, passing above the patella and forming the so-called "quadriceps expansion". The latter is reinforced by two fibrous bands that are carried from the patella to the condyles of the tibia. The deeper bundles of the vastus intermedialis enter the walls of the synovial bursa, constituting the joint muscle of the knee. The quadriceps femoris is innervated by the femoral nerve and, by contracting, it extends the leg. It participates with the rectus femoris in the flexion of the thigh and, with the knee flexed, in the flexion of the pelvis on the thigh.

Posterior thigh muscles (Fig. 3.5)

Biceps femoris muscle

It occupies the posterior and lateral regions of the thigh and originates with two heads: the long head, which arises from the upper part of the ischial tuberosity, and the short head, which arises from the lateral lip of the linea aspera of the femur and from the intermuscular septum.

The two heads converge on the fibular head with a common tendon. Posteriorly, it shares borders with the gluteus maximus, anteriorly, with the adductor magnus, the semimembranosus and the vastus lateralis. It is innervated by the tibial nerve and the peroneal nerve. It contracts by flexing the leg and extending the thigh.

Semitendinosus muscle

It is located superficially in the posterior part of the thigh, in the medial position. It is fleshy in its upper part and tendinous in the lower part. It originates from the ischial tuberosity and descends to the middle part of the thigh to enter the upper part of the medial aspect of the tibia. Posteriorly, it shares borders with the gluteus maximus, anteriorly, with the great abductor and the semimembranosus. It is innervated by the tibial nerve and it flexes and rotates the leg internally, extending the thigh.

Semimembranosus muscle

It lies deep in relation to the semitendinosus and is made up of a tendinous lamina superiorly. It originates from the ischial tuberosity, is carried inferiorly, and, at the level of the knee, its tendon divides into three bundles: a descending one, which is inserted

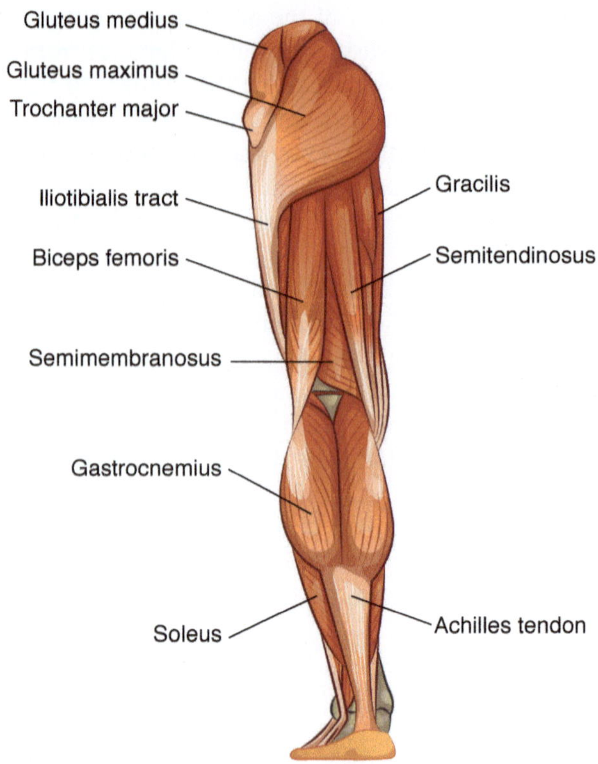

Figure 3.5 Posterior thigh and lower leg muscles.

on the tibial condyle; a recurrent one, which forms the oblique popliteal ligament; an anterior one, which inserts on the medial condyle of the tibia. It is innervated by the tibial nerve and performs an action similar to that of the semitendinosus.

Medial thigh muscles (Fig. 3.6)

Gracilis muscle

It is flattened and ribbon-like and is located medially in the thigh. It originates from the ischiopubic branch, near the symphysis, and then enters the medial aspect of the tibia. Superficially, it is covered by the femoral fascia and it shares borders with the adductor magnus and the adductor longus. It is innervated by the obturator nerve and it adducts the thigh, flexes, and medially rotates the leg.

Pectineus muscle

It is located in the superomedial part of the thigh. It originates from the pubic tubercle of the anterior aspect of the pubis, from the pectin crest and from the pubofemoral ligament. Its bundles, with a lateral course, are inserted distally, on the pectin line of the femur. Superficially, it corresponds to the femoral triangle; deep, it is related to the coxofemoral capsule and with the short adductor. It is innervated by the femoral nerve and, by contracting, it adducts, flexes and rotates the thigh externally.

Adductor longus muscle

It is a flat, triangular-shaped muscle that originates from the upper branch of the pubis, between the tubercle and the symphysis. Its bundles enter the medial branch of the linea aspera of the femur. Its superficial surface is covered by the femoral fascia. Deep, it is related to the sartorius and the vastus medialis. Innervated by the obturator nerve, it adducts and externally rotates the thigh.

Adductor brevis muscle

Triangular in shape, it is deep in relation with the long adductor and superficial in relation to the great adductor. It originates from the superior branch of the pubis and from the ischiopubic branch and is inserted on the harsh line of the femur. Innervated by the obturator nerve, it adducts and externally rotates the thigh.

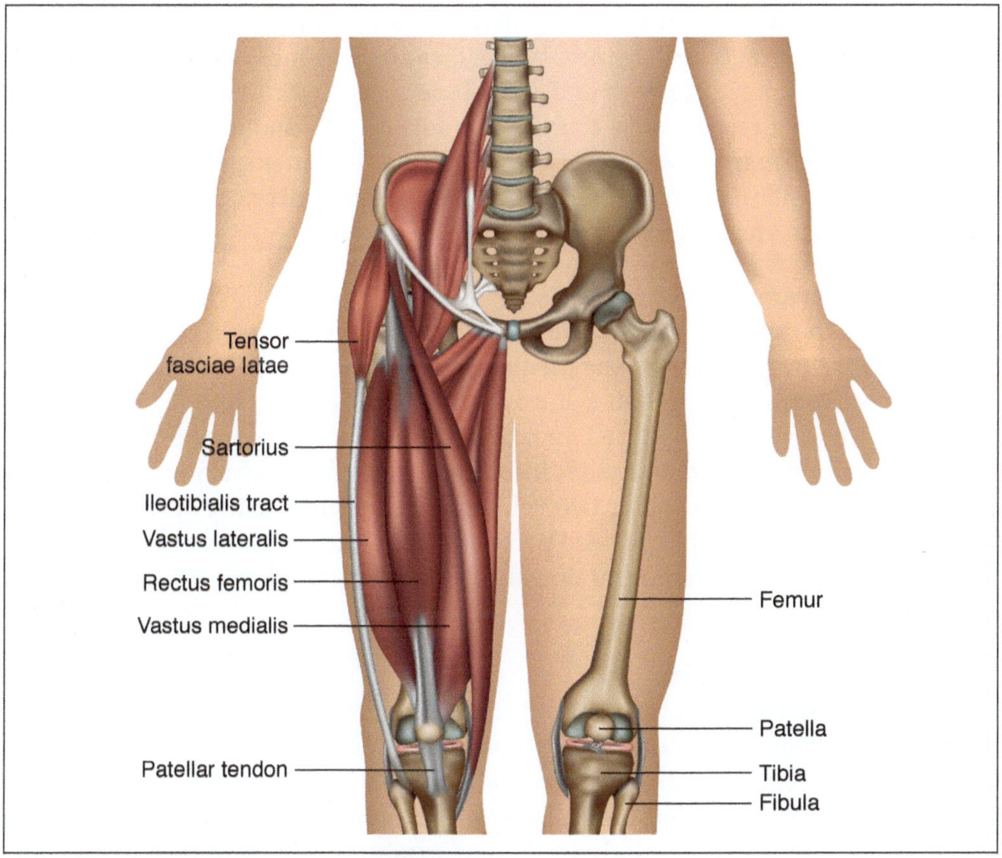

Figure 3.6 Medial muscles of the thigh.

Adductor magnus muscle

It is the deepest compared to the other adductors and also has a triangular shape. It originates from the ischiopubic ramus and the ischial tuberosity. It goes downward and laterally and, having reached the posterior edge of the femur, it ends by inserting on the medial margin of the linea aspera. The insertion of the adductor magnus is interrupted by several orifices, the point of the passage for perforating vessels, including the femoral artery which, at this level, continues into the popliteal artery. It contracts under the control of the obturator and sciatic nerves, adducing and rotating the thigh internally.

Anterior leg muscles (see Fig. 3.4)

They are found in a lodge bounded by the interosseous membrane and the anterior margins of the tibia and fibula.

Tibialis anterior muscle

It is the most medial of the four anterior muscles and originates from the lateral condyle and lateral aspect of the tibia, the interosseous membrane of the leg, the crural fascia and the intermuscular septum. Its bundles are brought down, to enter the tubercle of the first cuneiform bone and at the base of the first metatarsal bone, via the insertion tendon. It relates to the crural fascia superficially and to the tibia medially. Laterally, it relates to the extensor muscles of the toes; the latter separate the insertion tendon from the skin. It is innervated by the deep peroneal nerve, and it causes dorsiflexion, adduction and rotation of the foot.

Extensor digitorum longus muscle

It is lateral to the anterior tibialis muscle. It originates from the lateral condyle and the head of the tibia, and from the medial aspect of the fibula. The muscle bundles run downward, converging into a sturdy tendon that divides into four secondary tendons, each of which is destined for one of the last four toes. In the terminal portion, each secondary tendon divides into three tabs, one of which inserts dorsally to the second phalanx; the other two will attach themselves to the base of the third phalanx. It is innervated by the deep peroneal nerve and, by contracting, it extends the last four toes, contributing to dorsal flexion, abduction, and external rotation of the foot.

Extensor hallucis longus muscle

It originates from the medial aspect of the fibula and from the corresponding portion of the interosseous membrane. It continues in an insertion tendon while running downwards; this tendon is inserted dorsally to the first phalanx and to the base of the second phalanx of the big toe, extending it with its contraction, under the control of the deep peroneal nerve. Similarly to the long extensor of the fingers, it participates in dorsal flexion, abduction, and external rotation of the foot.

Anterior peroneal muscle

It is in an inferolateral position in the front part of the leg, lateral to the long extensor of the fingers, with which it is sometimes fused. It originates from the medial aspect of the fibula and from the interosseous membrane, inserts itself on the dorsal surface of the fifth metatarsal bone, and, by contracting, it abducts and externally rotates the foot.

Lateral leg muscles

Fibularis (peroneus) longus muscle

It is more superficial and longer than the Fibularis (peroneus) brevis muscle. It originates from the head of the fibula and its lateral margin. It is brought vertically downward, inserting its long insertion tendon on the tuberosity of the first metatarsal bone, on the first cuneiform bone, and at the base of the second metatarsal bone. It shares its posterior border with the soleus and the long flexor of the big toe. It is innervated by the superficial peroneal and it abducts and rotates the foot externally. It acts on the arch of the foot, accentuating its curvature.

Fibularis (peroneus) brevis muscle

It is deeper than the previous one. It originates from the lateral aspect of the fibula and from the surrounding intermuscular septa. Its bundles pass through the tendon in which they merge, behind the lateral malleolus, to attach themselves to the dorsal part of the base of the fifth metatarsal. By contracting, it abducts and rotates the foot externally.

Muscles in the posterior compartment of the leg (see Fig. 3.5)

They can be subdivided into superficial and deep compartments.

Triceps surae muscle

It consists of two muscles, the gastrocnemius and the soleus, which, at the bottom, converge in a single tendon: the Achilles tendon. The gastrocnemius is made up of two muscular bellies, the gemelli of the leg. The lateral gemelus originates from the lateral epicondyle of the femur and from the posterior region of the knee joint capsule; the medial gemelus originates from the medial epicondyle and the joint capsule of the knee.

The soleus, placed deep in the gemelli, originates from the head, the dorsal surface and the lateral margin of the fibula. The three muscle heads join in the calcaneal tendon, which inserts on the posterior aspect of the calcaneus. At the level of the knee, the inner edges of the tendons of the gemelli muscles are separated by an open angular space at the top and represent the lower limit of the popliteal fossa. Deep, the gemelli are in contact with the joint capsule, and between them runs the neuro-vascular bundle of the leg, consisting of the popliteal vein and artery, and the tibial nerve. Posteriorly, the soleus is in contact with the gastrocnemius and, anteriorly, with the long flexor of the toes. The triceps surae is innervated by the tibial nerve and, by contracting, it flexes the foot, rotating it internally. It contributes to the flexion of the leg on the thigh.

Plantaris muscle

It is a small muscle, sometimes absent, placed deep in the lateral gemelus. It originates from the lateral ramus of the linea aspera of the femur and from the joint capsule of the knee. The long tendon runs between the gastrocnemius and the soleus, and ends on the medial aspect of the calcaneus. It has an action similar to that of the triceps surae, but less powerful.

Popliteal muscle

It is a flattened muscle, placed under the plantaris and the gemelli. Anteriorly, it is related to the lateral condyle of the femur, with the knee joint and with the upper part of the posterior aspect of the tibia; posteriorly, the plantaris and gastrocnemius muscles, the popliteal vessels and the tibial nerve are placed. With its action, it flexes and rotates the leg inward.

Flexor digitorum longus muscle

It is the most medial muscle of the deep layer and originates from the oblique line and posterior aspect of the tibia and the surrounding intermuscular septa. The muscle bundles converge in a long tendon at the level of the lower third of the leg. The tendon, after passing into the calcaneal groove, crosses the plantar region of the foot and is divided into four terminal tendons which attach themselves to the base of the third terminal phalanx of the last four toes. Each tendon, at the first phalanges, crosses an eyelet formed by the respective tendons of the flexor digitorum brevis muscle. It flexes the last four toes and contributes to the plantar flexion of the foot.

Flexor hallucis longus muscle

It is the most lateral of the muscles of the deep layer. It originates from the lower two-thirds of the posterior surface and lateral margin of the fibula, from the interosseous membrane and from the surrounding intermuscular septa. The bundles end on a long tendon that passes under the medial malleolus and joins the plant region, moving forward and medially, and attaches itself to the base of the distal phalanx of the big toe. The contraction of the FHL (Flexor Hallucis Longus) causes flexion of the other four toes. With its action, it flexes the big toe and contributes to the flexion of the other toes and the plantar flexion of the foot.

Tibialis posterior muscle

It is located deep in relation to the two flexor digitorum longus muscles. It originates from the lower margin of the oblique line and from the posterior aspect of the tibia, from the upper part of the interosseous membrane, from the medial aspect of the fibula, and from the surrounding intermuscular septa. It then continues in an insertion tendon that ends on the scaphoid tubercle. It works by plantarly flexing the foot and participates in the adduction and internal rotation movements of the foot. It also accentuates the curvature of the arch of the foot.

CHAPTER 4

The energy production system

Cellular energy production

Why is oxygen so important? Trying to understand the functions of the cardiopulmonary system in the distribution and extraction of oxygen can help explain the production of energy in the cells, particularly in muscle cells.

The energy exchange currency: the ATP

When a muscle contracts and exerts a force, the energy used to control the contraction comes from a special substance that is present in the cells, known as ATP (adenosine triphosphate). ATP is the body's source of energy, in the same way that gasoline is the energy source of a car engine. The more quickly and effectively the muscle cells produce ATP, the more work these cells will be able to do before they get tired. Even if there is a certain amount of ATP stored in a muscle cell, its availability is limited. This means that muscle cells must continuously produce ATP in order to continue working. Muscle cells feed the ATP reserve using three different biochemical pathways, i.e. different sequences of chemical reactions, described below.

The aerobic and anaerobic energy systems

The term "aerobic" means "with oxygen". The **aerobic energy system** for ATP production is predominant when the cells are supplied with enough oxygen to meet their energy production needs, as occurs, for example, when the muscle is at rest. Most cells, including muscle cells, contain some structures called *mitochondria*. Mitochondria are the sites of aerobic energy production (ATP). The larger the number of mitochondria in a cell, the greater that cell's ability to produce aerobic energy.

The other two energy systems are the primary sources of ATP when cells receive insufficient oxygen to meet their energy needs. In the absence of sufficient oxygen, such as when a muscle cell needs to produce great force very quickly to lift a large weight, the cell switches to the **anaerobic energy system**, which provides a rapidly available source of ATP.

The term "anaerobic" means "without oxygen". The anaerobic production of ATP occurs inside the cells, but outside the mitochondria.

Many cells, such as those of the heart, brain and other organs, have extremely limited anaerobic capacity. Therefore, they must be continuously replenished with oxygen, or otherwise, they die. For example, if a coronary artery (which supplies blood and oxygen to the heart muscle) becomes blocked due to the accumulation of cholesterol deposits, the flow of blood through it will be reduced, causing ischemia. The reduced blood flow can lead to an insufficient oxygen supply to the heart muscle, both during rest and during physical exercise. This often produces a sensation of pain and/or pressure on the chest called *angina pectoris*. If oxygen support fails, such as when a blood clot forms at an arterial occlusion, the area of the heart muscle (myocardium) beyond the block will suffer a myocardial infarction, commonly referred to as a heart attack. If the phenomenon involves a large part of the myocardium, the result is death. In the brain, ischemia can lead to a stroke.

Unlike the heart and the brain, skeletal muscles, such as the triceps and quadriceps, have significant anaerobic capacity. An athlete must know the methods of producing aerobic and anaerobic energy both as a function of the substances used for the production of ATP and as a function of the intensity of the exercise, which finds its extremes in rest and maximum effort. The body uses an extremely complex chemical process to produce ATP. However, even just knowing the basic mechanisms of this process can be of great help to the athlete in the definition and setting of an exercise program. Lipids (fatty acids) and carbohydrates (glucose) are the two substances (substrates) that the body's cells use to produce most of the ATP. Proteins, which are made up of various combinations of amino acids, are not a preferential energy source; in a subject who has a normal diet, proteins play a minor role in energy production. However, when the diet does not provide a sufficient number of calories, the body is able to use the proteins stored in muscle tissues to produce the necessary energy, although this is certainly not an ideal process. At rest, when the cardiopulmonary system is easily able to supply an adequate amount of oxygen to the mitochondria of muscle cells, both fatty acids and glucose are used to produce ATP.

At rest, most of the required ATP is produced aerobically, using both glucose and fatty acids. In fact, at rest, the body produces approximately one calorie per minute. About 50% of this calorie per minute comes from fat, even if the person is not exercising. In a well-trained athlete, fat provides up to 70% of resting caloric expenditure.

When the intensity of exercise increases, the cardiovascular system makes all possible efforts to increase the supply of oxygen to the mitochondria of the muscles that work to produce the necessary amount of ATP aerobically. By continuing to increase the intensity of the exercise, at some point (determined by both the individual's fitness level and their genetic characteristics), the cardiovascular system becomes unable to supply sufficient oxygen to the working muscles, therefore they resort to the anaerobic system to rapidly produce ATP. The exercise intensity at which an adequate supply of oxygen is no longer available is called the **anaerobic threshold** and is reached before maximum effort.

The anaerobic system, however, cannot be used for an extended period of time. The primary source for the anaerobic production of ATP is glucose, which is stored in the muscles and liver as glycogen, a large molecule made up of glucose chains. A second source for ATP production is creatine phosphate (CP), a molecule that can be quickly separated to aid in ATP production. However, as with the ATP reserve in the muscles, there is an extremely limited availability of CP. Research carried out about 20 years ago (Bergstom et al.) showed that, even in a well-trained athlete, the muscles store only the amount of CP and ATP, which together are called phosphagenes, sufficient for 10 seconds of maximum effort.

To recap, as long as a muscle cell is aerobic, it uses both fat and glucose to produce ATP. The aerobic system produces much more ATP than the anaerobic system does, especially since fat gives 9 calories of energy per gram, while glucose and protein give only 4 calories per gram. In addition, the waste products of the aerobic production of ATP are water and carbon dioxide (CO2); both are tolerated fairly well by the body so the aerobic energy production does not cause muscle fatigue. Since water is a waste product of the aerobic production of ATP, it is essential to replace the water that is eliminated by drinking a lot every day. The more you exercise, the more water you need to drink. When an exercised muscle becomes anaerobic it uses glucose (limited to the phosphagen system) to produce ATP.

In any case, the anaerobically produced ATP is not only much less than that produced aerobically for each molecule of substrate used, but **lactic acid** is among the waste products of the anaerobic production of ATP. As the levels of lactic acid and other waste products in the muscle increase, the muscle will be less and less able to carry out continuous contractions. Lactic acid is believed to be the main cause of sudden pain (burning) in a muscle that is being exercised. In addition to forming lactic acid, the muscles send other signals when they can no longer produce the required amount of ATP aerobically. One of these is **hyperventilation**, defined as breathing faster than necessary, which represents the signal that the anaerobic production of ATP is predominant. When sufficient oxygen is not available, the muscle signals the brain to increase breathing rate and depth. However, since the limiting factor is not breathing, but the extraction of oxygen from the muscle, hyperventilation is a futile process.

The chemical process used by the body to produce ATP depends on some organic proteins called **enzymes**. Enzymes are needed to start the chemical reaction that produces ATP, both aerobically and anaerobically. The enzymes that metabolize fat are different from those that metabolize carbohydrates. Also, the enzymes used to metabolize carbohydrates aerobically are different from those used to metabolize carbohydrates anaerobically. Thus, when exercising with an intensity below the anaerobic threshold, the aerobic enzymes that metabolize fat and carbohydrates are dominant in the production of ATP. When exercise is done near the anaerobic threshold, anaerobic enzymes play a dominant role in the production of ATP.

Aerobic training leads to an increase in the capacity of the aerobic system but has little effect on anaerobic enzymes. Therefore, aerobic training significantly increases our ability to burn fat. Anaerobic training, on the other hand, will mainly lead to a functional improvement of the anaerobic enzyme system. All this represents another application of the principle of the specificity of training.

Aerobic capacity

The total ability to consume oxygen at the cellular level is known as **maximum oxygen uptake or maximum VO_2 (VO_2 max)**. This expression represents our maximum aerobic capacity. VO_2 max depends on two factors: (1) the distribution of oxygen through the blood to the working muscles, or cardiac output; (2) the ability to extract oxygen from the blood to distribute it to the capillaries and to use this oxygen in the mitochondria (elements of aerobic energy production that are present in most cells).

Maximum oxygen consumption is represented by the following formula:

$$VO_2 \text{ max} = \text{maximum cardiac output} \bullet \text{maximum oxygen extraction}$$

VO_2 (the volume of consumed oxygen) is measured both in milliliters of oxygen consumed per kilogram of body weight per minute (mL of oxygen/kg/min) and in liters of oxygen consumed per minute (L of oxygen/min).

We can now indicate how much oxygen is used at rest and compare it with a hypothetical maximum aerobic capacity of a subject weighing 70 kg. If your resting heart rate is 60 bpm, the Stroke Volume (SV) unit is 70 mL/beat (remember that heart output = heart rate • stroke volume) and the oxygen extraction is 6 mL of oxygen/100 mL of blood, your resting VO_2 is:

$$VO_2 = 60 \text{ bpm} \bullet 70 \text{ mL/beat} \bullet 6 \text{ mL of oxygen} / 100 \text{ mL of blood}$$

which is equivalent to 252 mL of oxygen/min. Divided by 70 kg, the resting VO_2 is approximately 3.5 mL/kg/min. During maximal exercise, our subject has a heart rate of 180 bpm, a stroke volume of 115 mL/beat, and an oxygen extraction of 15 mL of oxygen/100 mL of blood. Therefore, their VO_2 max is:

$$VO_2 \text{ max} = 180 \text{ bpm} \bullet 115 \text{ mL/beat} \bullet 15 \text{ mL of oxygen} / 100 \text{ mL of blood}$$

which is equivalent to 3105 mL of oxygen/min, or 44.4 mL/kg/min. Although the example refers to a hypothetical subject in average conditions, it clearly illustrates that our body has an enormous ability to increase oxygen consumption; in this example, there was an increase of more than 12.5 times. While the increases in both heart rate and unit volume justify the increase in cardiac output during exercise, the increase in oxygen extraction (also referred to as arteriovenous oxygen difference) is caused by various stimuli.

During exercise, numerous changes occur to make it easier to extract oxygen from the hemoglobin molecules and its subsequent use for the production of aerobic energy in the muscles. These changes include increases in temperature, acidity and the level of CO_2 in the bloodstream.

The resting VO_2 value of 3.5 mL/kg/min is also referred to as a **metabolic equivalent** or 1 MET. Activities are often described in terms of MET; for example, volleyball has a 3-6 MET field, and aerobic dance has a 6-9 MET field. To determine the VO_2 equivalent to a given MET value, just multiply the latter by 3.5. Doctors often prescribe exercises based on the MET value, especially for patients undergoing a cardiac rehabilitation program.

Aerobic training not only induces an increase in VO_2 max but also causes an increase in the percentage of maximum effort at which the anaerobic threshold occurs. In practice, this means that an individual is capable of producing ATP aerobically with an intensity that increases with the level of training. Also, in general, an aerobically trained person can perform more intense activities than an untrained person. The maximum oxygen consumption, like the training heart rate, is influenced by age, hereditary factors and the level of physical fitness. For example, after the age of 30, a slow but progressive loss of aerobic capacity occurs (at the age of 65 it can decrease up to 35%). Some individuals develop considerable aerobic capacity, so they are able to sustain a high-level workout. The greater a person's aerobic fitness, the higher the VO_2 max will be.

Another interesting physiological relationship occurs between oxygen consumption and the amount of calories (kcal) burnt during an exercise. Elementary mathematics teaches us that certain units of measurement can be converted into others. As 12 inches equals a foot and three teaspoons equal a soup spoon, the amount of oxygen spent during an exercise can be converted into the number of calories used in each minute. For example, when a liter of oxygen is used, approximately 5 kcal are burnt. Therefore, a woman who trains aerobically with a heart rate of 135 bpm and who uses an amount of oxygen equal to approximately 20 mL/kg/min (1.16 liters/minute), will consume approximately 5.8 kcal per minute. A man who uses about 1.4 liters of oxygen per minute will consume about 7.0 kcal per minute. Movement physiologists use this energy conversion ratio to calculate the approximate number of calories that are burnt during aerobic activity. Most studies confirm that exercises performed at moderate intensity, within the heart rate training range, will lead to the consumption of 3-6 kcal per minute.

What kind of energy do muscles use?

Muscles perform a job, so they consume energy. This energy is given by a phosphorus compound, the aforementioned ATP. It is produced by a small organ called the mitochondrion, using the sugars that reach the muscle through the blood. The mitochondrion can produce ATP in two different ways: in the first case, it uses oxygen and, consequently, there is aerobic work; in the second case it resorts to anaerobic work, producing lactic acid.

Aerobic work and endurance

As explained above, the muscle uses oxygen to produce ATP through glycogen and fatty acids. Oxygen is transported to the muscles through the blood; this is the reason why, when exerting effort, both the heart rate and the respiratory rate increase. The duration of aerobic work can vary from 1 minute up to 6-7 hours and depends on the motor capacity, called resistance. Aerobic endurance is the ability to produce prolonged moderate effort over time. The amount of ATP required to perform these efforts is what is produced by the oxygen that the cardiovascular system is able to transport to the muscles. Aerobic endurance is more relevant in people who have a higher number of red muscle fibers, which have a higher hemoglobin content.

By aerobic work, we mean a continuous activity, conducted from 60 to 85% of the *maximum heart rate* (which is calculated with the following formula: 220 – age in years), whose duration is not less than 20 minutes and which is carried out at least three times a week. The activities that lend themselves to this type of training are cyclical ones: walking, running, cycling, swimming, canoeing, skiing and cross-country skiing. However, they can also be performed successfully in the gym: (1) with cardio fitness equipment; (2) with aerobic gymnastics in its various expressions (combo, step fitball, etc.); (3) circuit training. All these activities will still have to respect the physiological principles defined for this type of training, which will increase the power of the myocardium, cardiovascular and cardiopulmonary capacity, and weight loss.

Anaerobic resistance

Anaerobic resistance is the ability to produce ATP through the lactic acid cycle, for as long as possible, without the muscle becoming blocked by the excessive presence of the acid itself.

Lactate anaerobic work

In order to bring oxygen to the muscles, heart rate can increase up to about 250 beats per minute. If the effort requires an even greater amount of ATP, this is produced by the mitochondria using lactic acid instead of oxygen. In this case, the duration of the work may vary according to the intensity, since lactic acid is deposited in the muscles, blocking their contraction. Lactacid anaerobic work is typical for medium-high intensity and prolonged activities, such as in athletics (middle distance: 400-800 m) or in bodybuilding, especially in isotensive training cheating forced training and in competitions.

Alactic anaerobic work

This is the definition of the work that muscles carry out when performing high-intensity and short-duration movements. In this case, only the ATP that is present in the muscles at rest is used, which is then regenerated at the end of the work. Alactic anaerobic work is characteristic of speed competitions, jumps, throws, artistic gymnastics, weightlifting and powerlifting.

CHAPTER 5

Muscle hypertrophy

Massimo Spattini and Riccardo Gaspari

When we talk about muscle growth, we are referring to **muscle hypertrophy**, which is nothing more than a physiological and biological event responsible for increasing the volume of all the cells that make up muscle tissue. There are two types of hypertrophy, skeletal muscle hypertrophy and smooth muscle hypertrophy, but clearly, an individual looking for a muscular and lean body will only be interested in the former. The phenomenon of muscle growth can also depend on **hyperplasia**, i.e. the increase in the number of muscle fibers. This is a topic that has sparked much debate among researchers. While muscle fiber hyperplasia is well documented and accepted in animals, few studies have verified it in humans. In this regard, I would like to cite a study carried out through muscle biopsies performed on weightlifting athletes and bodybuilders, which showed that lifters had predominantly fiber hypertrophy, while bodybuilders had a greater number of nuclei, as evidence of the activation of satellite cells which would have led to the inclusion of new cells inside the fiber, a phenomenon known as hyperplasia.

Our desire is to bring as many people as possible closer to training aimed at hypertrophy, which for decades has been labeled as harmful, and we want to make its benefits known to individuals of different ages, morphological characteristics and sex. Weight training, actually, helps prevent sarcopenia, osteoporosis, metabolic syndrome and osteoarthritis. In addition, it plays a positive role in reducing cardiovascular risk, preventing cancer, reducing blood pressure and controlling body weight. It has also shown positive correlations with mood improvement.

In recent years, there has been an increasing discussion about training for **sarcoplasmic hypertrophy** (increase in the volume of the sarcoplasm, the non-contractile component of the muscle), clearly separating it from the hypertrophy of the contractile mass (**myofibrillar hypertrophy**, i.e. number and size of myosin and actin contractile proteins). It is undeniable that two different processes take place inside the cell, and in theory, it is correct to diversify them, but in practice, both adaptations occur simultaneously. Of course, we could stimulate one more than the other, although marginally, but never split them up. Therefore, we can never talk about training aimed exclusively at sarcoplasmic hypertrophy or training aimed exclusively at myofibrillar hypertrophy.

Another important aspect to clarify is the **number of repetitions** to be performed in a workout aimed at muscle hypertrophy. For decades, the concept that has been promoted is that the 6-15 repetition range is the best. In recent years it has been reduced to 8-12 repetitions.

Furthermore, it should not be forgotten that muscle hypertrophy is still related to **strength**, although not proportionally, since an increase in the cross-sectional area of the muscle corresponds to an increase in its potential for producing force. In 2002 Campos et al. have shown how a training program of 4 sets for 3-5 repetitions aimed at increasing maximum strength actually stimulated the same muscle growth as a classic bodybuilding program consisting of 3 sets of 9-11 repetitions.

In this regard, Charles Poliquin, the late guru of training, stated in one of his publications that, having established the existence of a direct correlation between strength and hypertrophy, it must be emphasized that, when it comes to strength, accounting only for the weight lifted is not enough. It is essential to pay attention to the way it is lifted because it is not always true that the increase of a single number (in our case, the kilograms that are lifted) corresponds to an increase in muscle mass; instead when the load is increased thanks to the improvement of the individual's neuromuscular abilities, the lifting is always accompanied by muscle growth. Consequently, everything revolves around the maturation of the motor skills of an athlete, and the execution technique plays a fundamental role in training aimed at muscle hypertrophy.

Before starting a new workout, it is **better to keep the chosen weight** in isometry for a few seconds. If it is not possible to hold the weight in isometry at the beginning of the workout, that load will prove to be too heavy and will inevitably be lifted through the use of cheating (a situation to be avoided).

Strength is and will always remain a topic not to be overlooked in the search for a lean and muscular body. Strength is also a key element for a bodybuilder, despite the fact that recent years have led bodybuilding athletes towards training purely aimed at increasing muscle mass, leaving out this key factor for muscle growth. Let's shed some light on this: for a bodybuilder, strength is crucial not only for muscle volume, but above all for muscle density, a feature highly sought after by athletes, which gives the muscles a rocky, granite appearance. It is undeniable that there are very genetically gifted athletes who are able to reach very important muscle volumes while using low loads and very high repetition sets, but this refers to the elite class of world bodybuilding, composed exclusively of real genetic phenomena.

We are very keen to emphasize that strength training is essential, especially at a young age, in order to lay the foundations for a successful future and enviable sporting longevity. The scientific research carried out to date, combined with individual experiences, leads us to suggest that up to the age of 30-35, **strength training for a healthy subject must be a constant in the training** of every athlete in search of muscular mass growth.

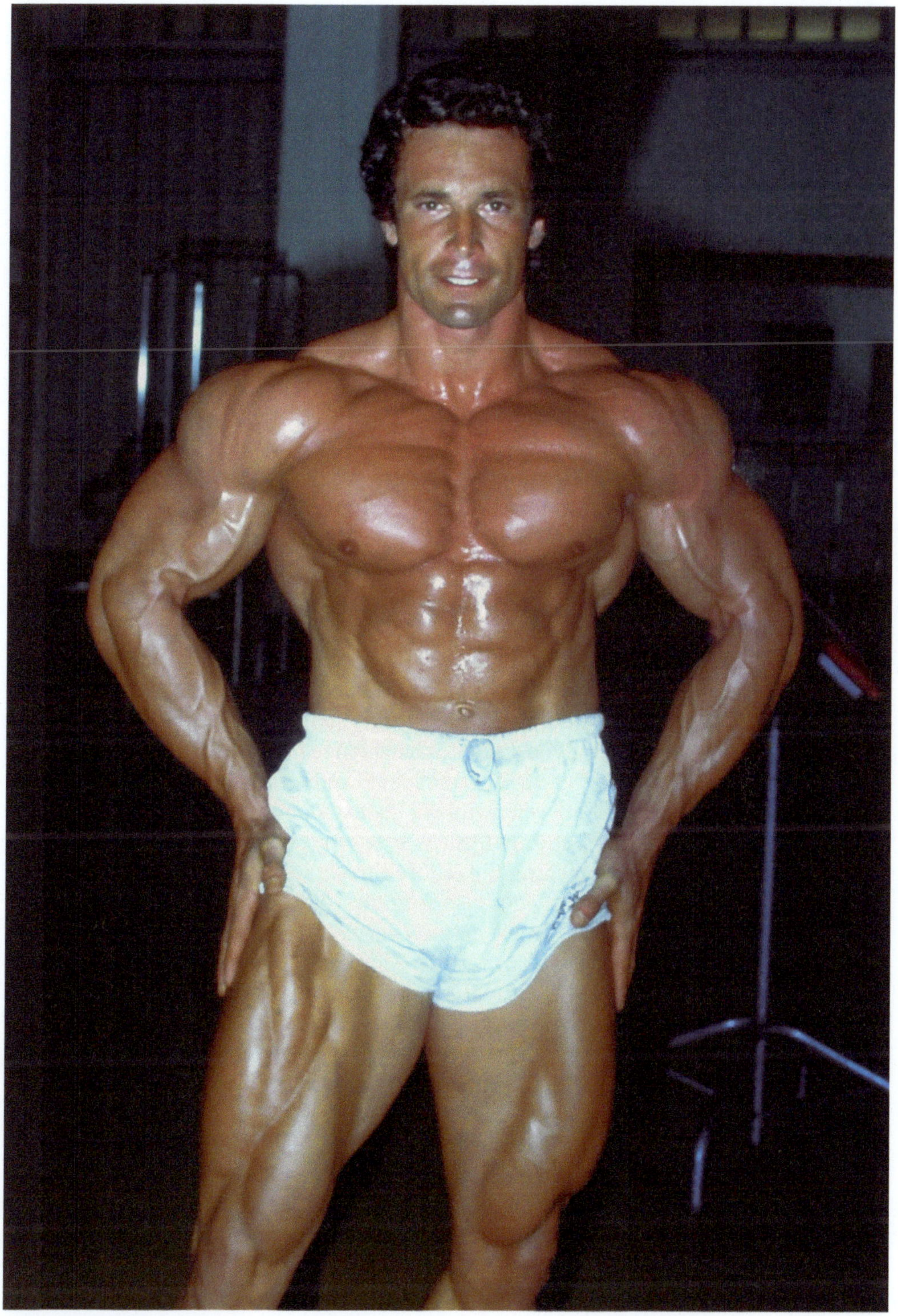

However, although it is true that strength is a very important factor, a research paper by Mitchell et al. that has recently been disclosed to the general public shows that training that leads to muscle failure with just 30% of one's maximum results in the same hypertrophic stimulus at 80% of its maximum; subsequently, several laboratory studies conducted by Schoenfeld et al. confirmed these results.

Studies by Schoenfeld et al. indicate that both low-load training (≤60% 1RM [1 repetition maximum]) and moderate-load training (>60% 1RM) induce significant increases in muscle hypertrophy in well-trained young people. For intellectual and professional honesty, however, it should be emphasized that the sample group of the study that performed the low-load training performed about three times the total volume of the training (sets × number of repetitions) compared to the high-load group.

Similar results were also obtained in a study carried out by Ikezoe which highlighted the importance of performing physical exercise close to muscle failure when using weights in order to maximize muscle hypertrophy results. The authors of the study compared the increases in muscle thickness inherent in the rectus femoris after 8 weeks of training with low loads and higher volumes (30% 1RM, 12 sets × 8 repetitions) in the first sample group with the results obtained from the second sample group, who were trained with higher loads and lower volumes (80% 1RM, 3 sets × 8 reps). Considering that the training volume in the high-load group was significantly lower than that in the low-load group, the degree of muscle thickness achieved after the intervention was almost double in the low-load group. However, it should be noted that, if the sets are not conducted close to muscle failure, it is necessary to reach the minimum intensity threshold (>60% 1RM) to maximize muscle hypertrophy.

This leads us to have unequivocal scientific evidence that shows that the hypertrophic range is more similar to 30-90% of one's maximum, that is to a very wide range of repetitions that oscillates between 3 and 30, instead of between 6 and 15, as instead was hypothesized in the past, and that this is true only in the short term and on the condition that you train by reaching the failure threshold.

This news is really important because it allows us to evaluate truly diversified workouts. Let's not forget that always using a very similar repetition range, such as 8-12, will inevitably lead to a stall in results. Moreover, if we also consider the fact that workloads rarely follow an optimal progression and that, even more often, we use weights that are either too heavy or too light, we will find ourselves wasting time in the gym and getting further and further away from our goals, with the result of being discouraged for not having achieved anything despite all the efforts made.

Resistance training includes three different types of muscle contraction: *concentric*, with the muscle that shortens when we move a weight by lifting or pushing it; *isometric*, when the muscle contracts but the resistance does not move; *eccentric*, with the muscle that contracts and stretches, as when you lower a weight to the ground. Although most bodybuilders focus more on the concentric component, perhaps for the psychological gratification of lifting more weight, recent evidence indicates that the eccentric component plays the most important role in stimulating hypertrophy. This effect is probably due to the more serious damage to the muscle cell induced by this type of contraction, which leads to an adaptive response on the part of the muscle aimed at protecting it from subsequent trauma. It is believed that the mechanisms underlying this response are the inflammatory response, the activation of satellite cells, and "swelling" at the cellular level.

Another important aspect in choosing the ideal or more functional approach to hypertrophy is to consider the **type of muscle fibers** most represented in the specific muscle and in the specific individual. Fast, white type II fibers, i.e. those most responsible for muscle hypertrophy, are the fibers most involved in power sports because they have a predominantly glycolytic metabolism (type IIx) and are able to produce energy by hydrolyzing ATP quickly. They have quick contractions and mainly intervene in efforts that do not exceed 15 seconds but are not particularly resistant to prolonged efforts or a glycolytic-oxidative metabolism (those of type IIa). This makes them defined intermediate compared to slow red fibers with an aerobic oxidative metabolism, which are less prone to hypertrophy. However, there are muscles, especially postural ones, which by their nature and their function must be activated throughout the day, such as the soleus, lumbar muscles, quadriceps, and forearm muscles. In general, intermediate and slow-twitch type I muscle fibers, which have greater resistance, predominate in the muscles. Consequently, it is logical to assume that these muscles are more stressed over a longer time under muscle tension and by a greater number of repetitions, also in terms of hypertrophic response. The demonstration of this hypothesis can be seen in sports such as skating, skiing, or cycling, where we see a remarkable development of the quadriceps in most athletes. This logic can also apply to a set of prolonged squats to exhaustion which, at this point, are not only aimed at aerobic conditioning but also contribute to "swelling the muscles". We have used the term "swell" in a deliberately provocative way, as some are known to criticize bodybuilders as "swollen". However, there is some truth to this criticism, so we must refer to the distinction between functional or myofibrillar hypertrophy and non-functional or sarcoplasmic hypertrophy. By **functional hypertrophy**, we mean an increase in muscle volume due to the increase in the contractile component, i.e. actin and myosin, which corresponds to a significant increase in muscle strength. By **non-functional hypertrophy**, we mean an increase in muscle volume, due to intracellular water retention and an increase in the storage of intra-muscular glycogen and triglycerides, which does not correspond to a proportional increase in strength.

Furthermore, as previously mentioned, there may also be genetic variables, today identifiable with specific genetic tests within everyone's reach, which indicate the predisposition of an individual to a predominantly glycolytic or oxidative muscle metabolism. These tests allow for a more personalized orientation of the planning of training methods through the inclusion of shorter recovery times and sets of 15 or even 20 repetitions, in order to involve the entire spectrum of muscle fibers.

However, the fact remains that, to avoid a stalemate in the results, it is now good practice to periodize and vary the stimuli. In the next few pages, we will see how to proceed in more detail.

MY EXPERIENCE ▸ Riccardo Gaspari

Let's start from the beginning: a young, healthy person with a couple of years of training experience. Until a few years ago I followed a training program that included a week of training aimed at building strength, in a "hypertrophic" context. Trainings were based on exercises such as a 5×5 or a repeated effort with "maintain load" (MC) or "maintain repetitions" (MR) techniques, to be alternated with a week of 12-15 repetitions that would have guaranteed a hypertrophic stimulus and good maintenance of general strength, and would have allowed me to discharge the excessive joint exhaustion that almost everyone experiences with the constant use of heavy loads. During the first week, I used a medium-low volume, hypothetically 9-10 sets for the large muscles and 6-8 sets for the smaller muscles, applying rest pauses of about 2-3 minutes between each sets. The second week, of course, I used a higher volume, about 12-15 training sets for large muscles and 10-12 sets for the smaller muscles. In this case, recoveries were 45-60 seconds.

I kept alternating the "heavy" week with the "light" week, for a total of 8-12 weeks. The body was divided into four workouts per week: the first workout concerned the pectorals, anterior deltoids, buttocks and adductors; the second involved the lats, the posterior deltoids and the trapezius; the third involved the shoulders, biceps and triceps; the last was dedicated to the quadriceps, hamstrings and calves. The abdomen was trained at the end of each session, and I performed three sessions of cardio at 70-75% of the HRmax per week.

This method has given me excellent results, both for myself and for my clients, and it still continues to do so.

However, as with all training programs, including this method, I reached a plateau. From there, an athletically difficult period began for me Guided by the opinions that circulated in the sports world and that were found in the sector magazines, I thought there was nothing left to do but increase the intensity, but unfortunately, it did not work. Let me explain: if I applied techniques such as rest pauses and drop sets, my body catabolized muscle tissue; if I constantly sought to increase the loads, I often found myself injured; if I decreased my training frequency, I ended up training too little and losing muscle. Finally, I decided to focus on volume.

Mainly, I began to increase the training volume of the individual sessions, but this choice also turned out to be a flop: I couldn't recover after so much work, so what else could I do? Fortunately, science never stops and provides excellent answers, always at the forefront, thanks to which I found the correct way to get in the best shape of my life, which today I try to maintain 365 days a year.

MY EXPERIENCE ▸ Massimo Spattini

There are many training methods that can be productive for the increase of muscle mass. We will cover them in this volume, but for now I want to share my personal experience of when I started training with weights.

A philosophy that has long influenced my training plan to increase muscle mass was the belief that, to achieve this goal, I had to lift heavier and heavier weights. I remember the words of my dear friend and my competition opponent, Giovanni Curtarelli, who was my first point of reference in Italy as a physical model to imitate: "Massimo, if you want to get big you have to lift tons".
This belief, however, began to waver when, on my first trips to California on a pilgrimage to Gold's Gym and World Gym, I frequently happened to see athletes with incredible muscle volume who used smaller weights than me. One thing I became famous for was the "firmness" of my muscles, which led many of them to feel them and show surprise and appreciation for this characteristic of mine. Their muscles, on the other hand, were more hypertrophied and rounded, and, when squeezed, they had the consistency of a sponge. Only later did I understand the difference between myofibrillar hypertrophy and sarcoplasmic hypertrophy, which prompted me to review my beliefs and to insert sets with higher repetitions, aimed more at "pumping" than at lifting the load. The load became an instrument and not a purpose.
I had another confirmation of the correctness of this type of training at the seminar I organized in 1985 with Lee Haney at the New Center Gym in Parma, which was the "mecca" of bodybuilding in Italy at the time. At the end of the seminar, since Lee had to train, he told me: "If you want, Massimo, we can train together in the other part of the gym, where I saw the leg equipment, and we can let people watch us while we train". Attending a Mr. Olympia training session seemed very interesting for the participants in the seminar, even though I was a little worried about not being able to handle his workloads. However, I knew I couldn't miss out on this kind of opportunity.
We started with leg extensions and I was worried that there weren't enough plates. In reality, Lee did not manage to use even half of the weight stack, performing the repetitions in a slow and controlled manner, emphasizing the eccentric phase and performing a peak of contraction in the final part of the movement. I imitated his repetition cadence, thinking it was probably just a warm-up exercise. Later we moved on to the press and psychologically prepared myself for the most demanding exercise. Lee started by loading a couple of 20 kg plates per side (I normally started with three plates per side). On the next set I expected it to increase by at least two plates per side, if not more, but instead, he only increased it by one plate. At the third set I thought: "This is it". Instead, Lee only increased the load by one more plate per side, and in the next set he did not increase it at all. At that point I asked him why he used such small weights and he replied: "It's not weightlifting, it's bodybuilding". Then, in the next break, he explained: "You see, Massimo, when I'm traveling, I always prefer to train with loads that I can better control and focus more on muscle isolation to avoid the risk of injury, especially because I don't know the equipment that I am using. However, it is a technique that I often use, alternating it with the use of heavier loads. Fred Hatfield (known as Dr. Squat) squatted with 450 kg, but he had chicken legs: it's not the weight you use, but how you engage the muscle. "
The speech and the example were flawless, and we continued to train in that way for the rest of the session, which consisted of numerous sets of various exercises. At the end of the workout, I was sati-

Continues

Continued

sfied, I felt a noticeable "pump" in my legs and I was not particularly "disintegrated" as I normally was after a "heavy" leg workout; however, the next day, I could hardly walk.

In the last few years, the focus has shifted more to recovery, so training protocols in which the muscles are trained only once a week are adopted more often.
While this approach may work for advanced athletes, who are able to train at a high specific intensity and are also physically endowed with a greater amount of white fiber (today, genetic testing is able to understand this), I believe that, for a beginner who does not yet have the technical and neuromuscular capacity to stimulate the muscle at maximum intensity, the frequency of the stimulus should be greater and that for the first 6 months, if not for the first year, training should take place three times a week.
Next, I suggest switching to muscle training twice a week, thus giving priority to the total training volume. Only when an athlete can be defined as advanced, can the frequency possibly be limited to once a week per muscle, always training at maximum intensity.
Keep in mind that Mr. Olympia Arnold Schwarzenegger, Franco Columbu, Frank Zane, Lee Haney and Ronnie Coleman always trained their muscles at least twice a week (if not more), both in the off-season and in pre-contest periods.
Obviously, these tips are aimed at obtaining maximum result in terms of muscle mass in individuals who can dedicate themselves to training without having to do other heavy work (even if Arnold and Franco, for a certain period, in addition to training, also worked as bricklayers).

CHAPTER 6

Training volume

Massimo Spattini and Riccardo Gaspari

Training volume represents the **amount of work that goes into a single workout**. It is calculated differently based on the sport in question. In endurance-type workouts, volume is represented, for example, by the kilometers traveled, while in Olympic weightlifting it is represented by the tonnage of the weights lifted.

Given the different variants that make up a body-building training session, the parameters mentioned above would not represent a valid formula. In bodybuilding, volume is generally identified by the total amount of work done. Often and willingly, highly trained coaches calculate the training volume of their athletes in different ways: there are those who identify the training volume with the total number of sets performed, those who calculate the duration of the training, those who count the total number of reps and even those, as in weightlifting, who calculate the tonnage. We believe that it is practical to calculate the volume of training based on the number of sets performed per muscle group and in the training unit. Therefore, when we talk about training volume, we refer to the total number of sets performed in a single training session or, if there is a need, more specifically, of the total number of sets performed for a single muscle zone. As a **general rule**, the **total number of sets performed within a workout** is the simplest way to define the training volume.

In the world of bodybuilding and gyms, there has always been a debate between supporters of high-volume training to promote muscle mass gain and supporters of low-volume. The main representatives of these two factions were, on the one hand, Arnold Schwarzenegger, who trained twice a day, 6 days a week, training each muscle group with about 20 sets at least twice a week while, on the other hand, we have Mike Mentzer, who in his latest version of training recommended 2-3 sets per muscle group every 10 days.

These, of course, represent two extremes that, objectively, have produced great results for both athletes. But what is the ideal solution for most people? First of all, we must start from the observation that the fundamental factor capable of producing an adaptation in the organism, which in our case must be hypertrophy, is conditioned by an internal load in the musculoskeletal-endocrine system, which is stimulated by an external load represented by training.

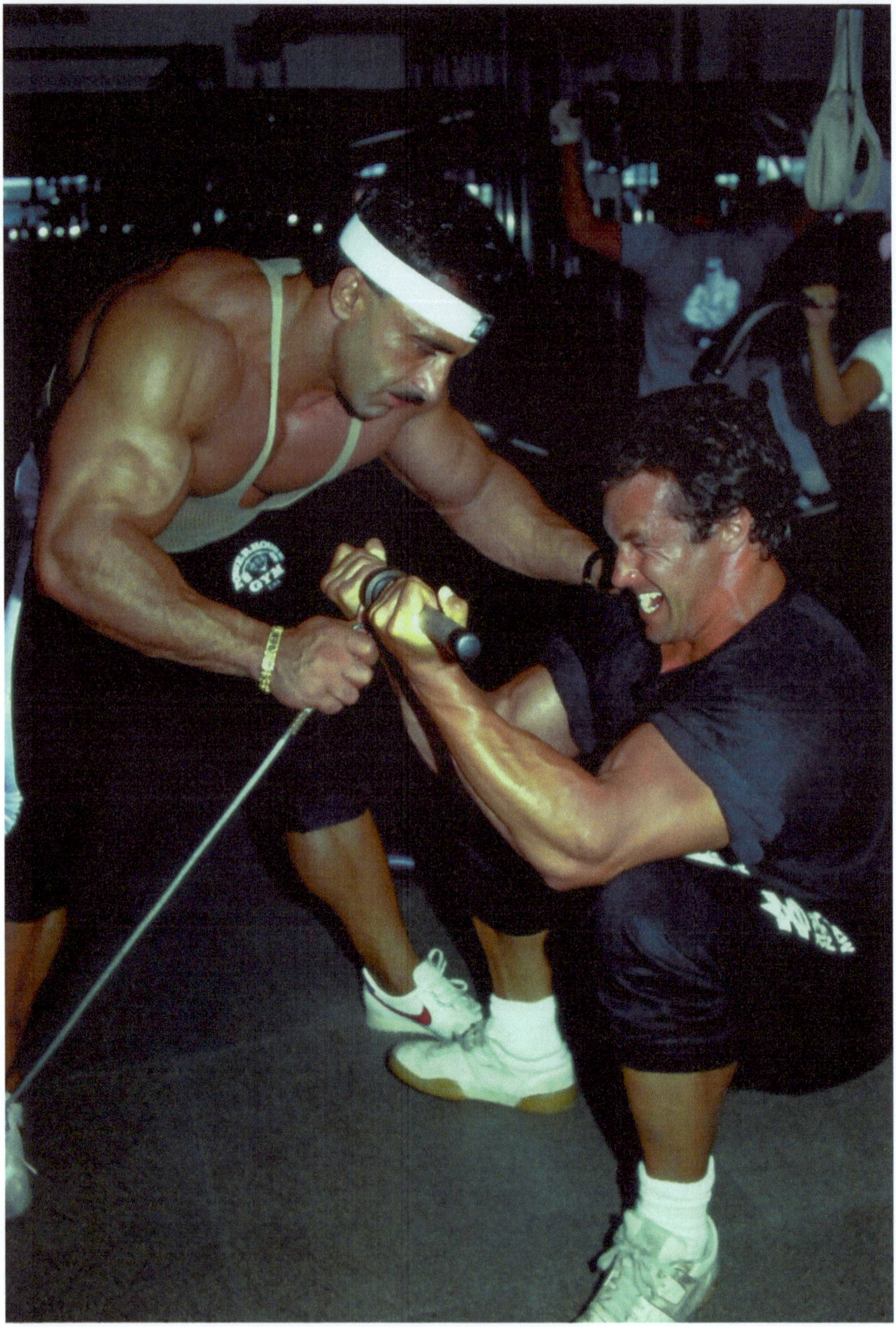

The constituents of the external load are represented by training volume and intensity. Obviously, the more we increase training volume, the more the intensity decreases; vice versa, the more we increase intensity, the more volume decreases, otherwise the training load would be excessive and would lead to overtraining. The problem is finding the balance between these two factors and understanding whether, in order to gain muscle mass, is it better to favor training volume or intensity. Certainly, it is also worth mentioning that thanks to the latest discoveries in genetics, it has been possible to observe that there are individuals with such polymorphisms, that they are predisposed to respond better to high-intensity and low-frequency stimuli; other individuals, on the other hand, respond better to higher volume and more frequent workouts. Today we can access these genetic tests that allow us to better orient ourselves in choosing the most suitable training for us.

In general, however, if the goal is to increase muscle mass, is high volume or high intensity more convenient? The answer likely lies in the middle, even in the specific subjectivity, but this means it is actually more biased towards the high volume of training. Most of the latest research in this area has shown that high-volume workouts are most effective for building muscle mass. Rhea et al. (2003) noted that the total number of sets performed for a specific muscle group is the best indicator of training stress when compared to sets per exercise. Peterson et al. (2004, 2005), analyzed the issue of sets, concluding that multiple sets are better than single sets. One of the **fundamental principles of training** is that the training volume must always be inversely proportional to the intensity: you cannot train intensely for long periods. Consequently, when training volume is high, intensity must be medium. This is because the fundamental factor that produces an adaptation within the organism, which in this case is the increase in hypertrophy, is conditioned by an internal load in the organism on our musculoskeletal-endocrine system, which is stimulated by an external load represented by training. The constituents of the external load are basically represented by the volume and intensity of training which, if poorly balanced, would certainly lead to a plateau of results, if not to injuries and overtraining.

The most important figures in the world and in the history of bodybuilding who give more importance to high-volume training were undoubtedly Arnold Schwarzenegger and Serge Nubret, great champions and top representations of the discipline.

Next, we will talk about training intensity, the fundamental importance of which we absolutely do not intend to diminish, although it has been amply demonstrated that, if the extremes of the training world are represented by high-volume training and high-intensity training, in reality, most people find the greatest benefit from being somewhere in between. The vast majority of the latest scientific research has shown that high-volume workouts are more effective for building muscle mass.

In a meta-analysis conducted by Schoenfeld's laboratory (2016) 15 studies that contrasted high-volume workouts and low-volume workouts were examined, and found a clear dose-response that correlates muscle growth to workout volume, taking into consideration the number of sets per muscle group per week. Running less than

5 sets per week was equivalent to a muscle mass gain of 5.4%; the execution of 5-10 sets, at a gain of 6.6%; from 10 sets upwards there was a gain of 9.8%. Unfortunately, there is currently not enough data in the literature to establish a higher volume level (for example, 15 sets or more).

In another important quantitative meta-analysis (Wolfe et al., 2004), it was observed that, in untrained subjects, single-set or multiple-set protocols produce similar strength gains, while as the training program progresses, multiple sets are more effective than single-sets.

Other studies have established that volume may be more important than intensity to produce muscle anabolism (Burd et al., 2010) and that protein synthesis is better stimulated with 3 sets than with a single set at 70% 1RM (Burd et al., 2010).

Two other meta-analyses conducted by Krieger (2009, 2010) reported a 46% increase in strength and a 40% increase in muscle mass when multiple-set protocols were compared to single-set protocols. Evidence reported in the study conducted by Naclerio et al. (2013) raises the hypothesis that high volumes (3 sets of each exercise for 9 sets per muscle group) are more suitable for increasing strength, while low volumes (1 set of each exercise for 3 sets per muscle group) are more suitable for maintaining strength. However, we do not want to focus only on hypertrophy. We also intend to examine the importance of a good volume of training in a body recomposition program. Kravitz (1996) argues that volume is directly proportional to the energy expenditure of the training, and therefore it is conceivable that high volumes, imposing a greater energy expenditure during exercise, have a favorable effect on the reduction of fat mass. A review by Stone et al. (1991) states that body composition is more influenced and controlled by exercising with weights, training larger muscle groups, and greater total volumes.

According to some research carried out by Børsheim and Bahr (2003), high-volume training could be a variable capable of affecting EPOC (Excess Postexercise Oxygen Consumption), commonly referred to as "afterburn", which represents oxygen consumption and energy expenditure above basal (or pre-exercise) levels occurring in the hours following exercise (in simple words, it expresses the number of calories consumed after the training session). Over the years, several studies (Binzen et al., 2001; Hansen et al., 2005; McCarty, 1995; Poehlman and Melby, 1998) have shown that, during the period in which EPOC occurs, the body initiates recovery and restoration of pre-exercise levels, using additional energy coming mainly from lipids. Moreover, since during the period in which the EPOC extends the energy metabolism shifts to a preferential use of lipids rather than carbohydrates, the EPOC could represent an important component in the reduction of fat mass and for weight management, therefore being perfect for all subjects looking for body recomposition. Volume is generally associated with a greater hormonal response. The research carried out by Mulligan et al. (1996) and by Gotshalk et al. (1997) reported greater hormonal increases, specifically in GH, testosterone and cortisol, given by multiple sets compared to single sets, performed with the same intensity. This was subsequently confirmed by the study carried out by Marx et al.

(2001), who found that even in the long term (6 months), periodic high volume training shows higher levels of testosterone and IGF-1 (Insulin-like Growth Factor) and reduced cortisol levels compared to a HIIT (High-Intensity Interval Training) program. It must be emphasized that the high-volume group also featured greater strength, power, and speed. In 2005, a study conducted by Kraemer and Ratamess showed that weight training aimed at muscle hypertrophy, then performed at moderate intensity (60-80% 1RM), short recovery times between sets (60-90 seconds) and high volumes, caused a greater hormonal response when compared to the more strength-oriented exercises with weights, performed with less volume and at high intensities. Scientific evidence has therefore amply and clearly demonstrated that higher training volumes are more effective in promoting muscle growth. This concept, of course, is a result of the genetics and lifestyle of the individual: there will always be subjects who have a better response to training with low volume and very high intensity, but the science is clear and, for most individuals, volume seems to be the right way to go in order to build more muscle. That being said, don't overdo it, as excessive training can be counterproductive. Excess in the duration and intensity of training can induce negative effects on the production of some important anabolic molecules, such as IGF-1, which is synthesized in the liver under

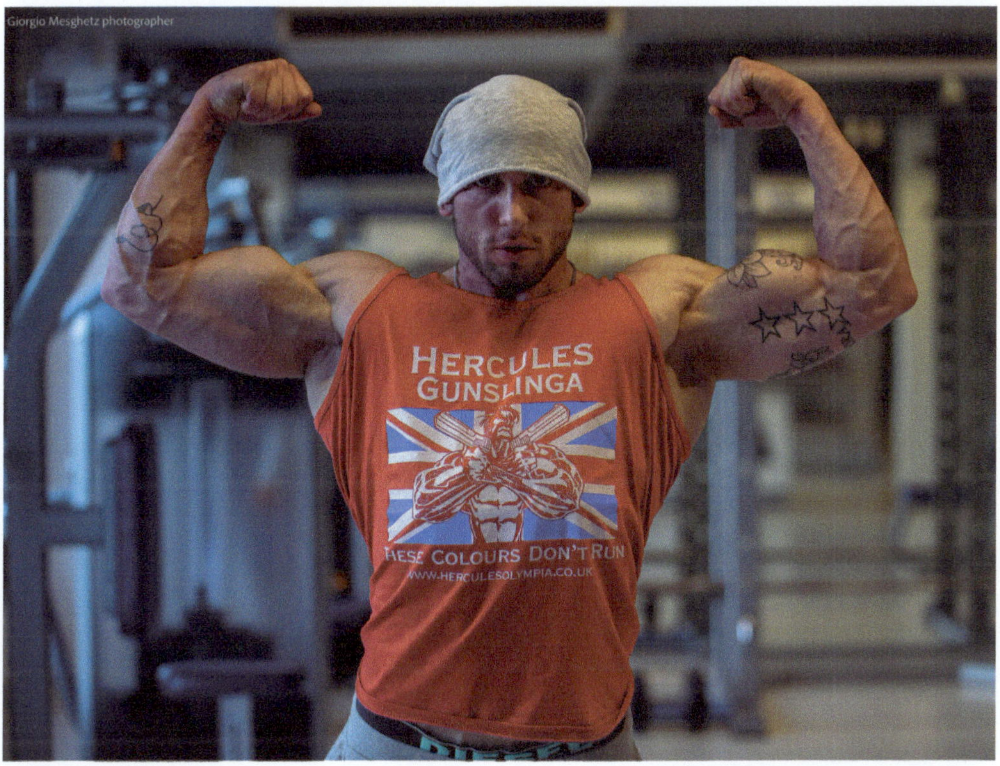

the stimulation of GH (Growth Hormone) and whose main function is to promote protein synthesis in the muscle.
American researchers have found that athletes who increase their energy expenditure by more than 1000 calories per day by practicing prolonged exercise show drastically reduced levels of IGF-1, even in contexts of high-protein and high-calorie diets. This represents an interesting result for all bodybuilders: increasing your protein and caloric intake won't be enough to compensate for the drop in IGF-1 production caused by excessive energy expenditure due to high-intensity and high-volume workouts. Therefore, if you are trying to increase your muscle mass and strength, it is advisable not to perform excessively intense and prolonged workouts and not to overtrain, in order not to compromise muscle anabolism.

MY EXPERIENCE ▸ Riccardo Gaspari

Leaving science aside just for a moment and delving into the world of anecdotes, I want to describe how I have found the right training volume for me, which allowed me to overcome the plateau that I mentioned previously. Like everyone else, I started with training routines aimed at various muscle groups (agonist-antagonist or push-pull, distant muscles or, again, thinking in kinetic chains), and then moved on to training one muscle group per week. Well, if I trained too many muscle groups, the following group did not receive adequate stimulation (i.e. I used all my energy in the first muscle group and I found myself really tired when I had to train the following ones). If at that point I reduced the weights, the stimulus was insufficient to induce growth. If I increased the intensity and added training techniques, the muscles were exhausted (I could not recover enough and the workload was excessive for my body). If I lengthened the recoveries between sets by increasing the loads and lowering the reps, I gained strength but the muscles did not grow and I often got injured. So, I simply decided to choose a pattern that I liked to do (pushing muscles, pulling muscles and legs, the whole body divided into three parts) and from there I started with four workouts per week in rotation: the muscles that I trained on Monday were retrained on Friday. For example, if I was training my chest with 9 sets on Monday and 9 more on Friday, in the end, the weekly training volume was 18 sets for the chest. Then I started to increase the workouts, to get to my current routine, where I do three workouts in a row, rest one day, rerun the three workouts, and so on. For a growth phase, I find that the ideal is to perform the three workouts with 4 sessions per week (maximum 5, but only in cases where the subject has genetic standards higher than the norm), while maintaining a low percentage of fat body and an adequate muscle pumping, together with a 3-day break. A 3-day break is what gives me greater success. Moreover, it is excellent for those who mainly want to burn fat or for those looking for a path to body recomposition. This, however, is only the first step, since my definitive training method includes other features, which we will see later, that allow you to maximize the benefits of weight training and the modulation of training volume.

MY EXPERIENCE ▸ Massimo Spattini

From my first experiences with weights, I have learned the hard way that training more does not always lead to more results. This made me realize that, in order to achieve maximum results in bodybuilding, one must have the utmost understanding of how the human body works, so I enrolled in Medicine. I must say that my medical studies were very useful to me, especially for the notions of physiology, biochemistry and endocrinology, which I was able to apply to nutrition and integration strategies. However, in regard to training methodology, I honestly did not find many "inputs", partially because the knowledge underlying the mechanism of muscle hypertrophy, in those years, was extremely scarce and unproven. As a result, my approach to the weekly amount of training, i.e. volume (number of sets) and frequency (how many times per week the muscle is trained), remained somewhat empirical. Since my idol at the time was Arnold Schwarzenegger, I was fascinated by the high volume of training he recommended: about 20-25 sets per muscle group, training the same muscle groups twice a week or, sometimes, even three. However, the high volume of training, which involved 6 workouts per week, was unsustainable for me and led me to overtraining within 2-3 weeks, which prevented me from sleeping well at night and made me hate the gym.

Anyway, when I was preparing for my first competition, "Notte dei Campioni", in 1984, I continued with the high volume, as I believed that, in the cut phase, this approach was absolutely necessary. I trained three times a day: an early morning aerobics session and two weight training sessions, one at noon and the other at 6 pm. In this way, I trained my whole body in 2 days and then repeated the same routine on the other days, for 6 days a week, thus training all the muscles three times a week, for a minimum of 20 sets per muscle group. The result was quite good: I went to the competition with a level of definition that, in those days, could represent a new standard, and I beat athletes who were bulkier than me but less prepared. Maybe I had lost some muscle mass and, frankly, the preparation had been a real torture. I remember that I would have preferred to fast rather than go to the gym. I was practically a zombie, barely able to train (obviously with a medium-low intensity), eat what my diet allowed me, or sleep or, in any case, lie in bed.

After this preparation, I realized that I had to change something. Thus, I began to study high-intensity training techniques and, in the summer of 1985, I decided to leave for Los Angeles to train with the greatest proponent of this type of technique: Mike Mentzer. After returning to Italy from my summer internship in Venice, California, where I trained several times under the guidance of Mike Mentzer together with my friends and champions (Caleffi and the Zambelli brothers), I followed Mentzer's methods for about 2 months, but then I abandoned them due to very poor results, even seeing a certain regression; so did my friends. This was my first impact from a high intensity, low volume training system. Some of you might think that, perhaps, the lack of results came from incorrect application and insufficient commitment, but you have to take into account that we were already all national athletes and champions. Once, as a challenge, Caleffi and I had managed to do 50 sets for legs "to

Continues

Continued

exhaustion" in a single training session (10 exercises of 5 sets each), so I don't think that four or five sets, even with "a gun pointed at us", could have frightened us too much. Heavy Duty training was a nightmare, as I had to mentally prepare myself to give my all in those few sets, otherwise I would have nullified everything.

As a result, I was focused on looking for super motivations before training: autogenic training, visualization and engaging music. Nevertheless, even when I felt I had really given "everything", I did not feel satisfied, I did not have the impression of having stimulated the muscle sufficiently. And yet, after 2 days my muscles were so sore that I was limited in normal movements of daily life, and this gave me the confirmation of considerable muscular stress. However, when I went back to training the muscle after about a week, when the soreness had disappeared, I had the feeling that I had completely forgotten about the previous training and did not show any supercompensation. The soreness that followed the next workout seemed more like the pain you feel when you resume training after vacation or doing a sport that had been neglected for a long time. And this was nothing to be compared with the kind of muscle soreness you get after a good workout.

However, the experience with Mike Mentzer made me understand how intensity was, in reality, a fundamental factor and in my subsequent preparation for the 1986 Italian Championship, I trained the muscles "only" twice a week, reducing the number of sets to 12-16 per muscle group. In this way, I certainly had more energy and was able to stimulate the muscle with a good load at a great intensity. That year I won the Italian Championship in the heavyweight category, and I think that perhaps I was in the best shape of my career.

My next experience with short and infrequent training took place in 1988, also in Venice, California. I was already the Italian champion, graduated in Medicine and Surgery, and I was already training many athletes: a few hundred scattered throughout Italy, and about twenty of them were at least regional or national champions. They trained in my gym, the legendary New Center Gym in Parma, which at the time was a bit like Gold's Gym in Venice, while Parma was a bit like the "mecca" of bodybuilding in Italy. That year I had to prepare for the "Selections for the World Championship", which was to be held in Parma in October. It was an appointment in which I could not fail, but I was aware that, due to my now numerous commitments, I would not have been able to have the necessary tranquility to prepare myself in the best possible way. Therefore, I decided to leave for Los Angeles 3 months before the competition, to be able to dedicate myself exclusively to my preparation. On the very first day, I met my friend Samir Bannout (Mr. Olympia 1983) in the gym, who was preparing for his comeback at Mr. Olympia. Samir, excited to see me, proposed that I train with him for the entire preparation, as Mr. Olympia would be held in Los Angeles that year 3 weeks before my competition. Training with a Mr. Olympia in preparation for Mr. Olympia, I certainly could not lack motivation, commitment and intensity.

At this point I must tell you that Bannout was an advocate of high-intensity training and a follower of Mike Mentzer's theories, which he had customized: he did not just perform 5 sets per muscle

Continued

group, but sometimes up to 8-10, with pre-exhaustion techniques, and he only trained his muscles once a week.

In fact, in 1985, as I said before, I trained personally with Mike Mentzer and his training consisted of 5 sets per muscle group at very high intensity, with a frequency of twice a week, for a total of 10 sets. So, in reality, it was a high-intensity workout with a decent weekly training volume. Only later did Mentzer intensify the concept of the contrast of intensity to volume and frequency, but I believe this was a marketing operation: it is easier to sell a program by making people believe that they can get better results by training only for 20-30 minutes, 2-3 times a week. Well, during this period of "almost" living with Samir Bannout (we ate together, we worked out together and we took the same supplements), he was improving rapidly, while my progress was extremely slow. I felt I wasn't training enough, I felt the need to train more. At the end of my workout, I was never satisfied with the results, but how can you tell Mr. Olympia that you no longer want to train with him because his training is not going well? So, I continued, hoping that things would improve over time, but that didn't happen. On my return to Parma, when the competition was 3 weeks away, I was clearly behind in preparation: my muscles were not sufficiently prepared and not even "pumped", and the definition was poor. I felt I had to start over: I started training twice a day with about 15-20 sets per muscle group, training all muscles twice a week. Within 3 weeks my body transformed and I was able to reach 90% of my condition (for 100% I needed another 2 weeks). Fortunately, this was enough for me to win the competition by beating all the best Italian heavyweights of that year (Bonaccorsi, Curtarelli, Nocerino, Caminotto, Dall'Amico, Venturi, just to name a few).

Moral of the story: "less is not always more". There are no absolute "dogmas" in training and there is no single way, but everyone must find their own in compliance with the rules of physiology and biochemistry, which have quite wide ranges: finding the right point within them is the key to success. Short, high-intensity workouts are certainly useful for increasing muscle mass and are a good choice for those with time problems. Scientific evidence, however, clearly demonstrates that higher training volumes are more effective in promoting muscle mass gain. Obviously, everything is conditioned by genetics and lifestyles.

CHAPTER 7

Training intensity: subjective or objective variable?

Massimo Spattini and Riccardo Gaspari

We firmly believe that the volume of workouts and their alterations are essential, but for intellectual and professional honesty we cannot fail to mention workout intensity, recognizing its deserved importance. This topic will be treated scientifically, even though its essence is firmly rooted in subjective, rather than mathematical, aspects. To understand the meaning of training intensity, we need to review a brief discussion on the body's energy systems used during our workouts.

As widely discussed and demonstrated in 2004, thanks to the work done by Jones, Round, and De Haan, the main energy systems involved in weight training are anaerobic. **Anaerobic mechanisms** are subdivided into the anaerobic alactacid system (also known as the phosphate, phosphagen, phosphocreatine, or ATP-CP system) and the anaerobic lactacid system (also known as the anaerobic glycolytic system or anaerobic glycolysis). The predominance of one of the two mechanisms is essentially conditioned by two factors, represented by intensity (% 1RM) and duration, the latter recognizable with the parameter of time under tension, or TUT (Time Under Tension), which represents the duration of muscle activity mainly related to the performance of a set.

For very high intensities (80-100% 1RM) and particularly short TUT (up to 10-15 seconds maximum), we refer to **anaerobic alactacid performance**, while for moderate and low intensities (<80% 1RM) and moderate or long TUT (20 seconds or more) the prevailing energy system is **anaerobic lactic acid** (the system used by bodybuilding-style workouts).

The **aerobic system** begins to take on a more important role when intensity is low enough to allow the performance to be prolonged over time, indicatively beyond a TUT of 120 seconds. Also in this case, however, the lactic acid system remains predominant for a good amount of time.

We will not address this subject by delving too deeply into biochemistry, mathematical tables, or exasperated training techniques, but we will provide you with the fundamental definitions of intensity to fully understand its meaning.

In 2006, James Stoppani published a book in which he gave a **definition of intensity** that has become a sort of standard definition of the concept, stating that intensity expresses the degree of physical commitment required by the execution of a given activity in relation to internal load, characterized by a strictly subjective component, and highlighting that it is one of the most important parameters to be established in a progressive overload workout plan.

The really fundamental part of the concept expressed by Stoppani is that intensity is "characterized by a strictly subjective component". To understand how true this is, just note that, etymologically, the term "intensity" derives from the Latin word *tensum*, which means to aim at something, an action that implies a certain mental predisposition in expressing an action by necessarily applying maximum concentration and utmost will.

Scientific literature represents the **concept of intensity** with the following formula:

$$\text{intensity} = \frac{\text{load (kg)} \times \text{repetitions } (n)}{\text{time (T)}}$$

However, this formula expresses only one measurement related to power, while completely excluding the most essential aspect, in our opinion, when it comes to training intensity, or the subjective component of the parameter, which includes concentration, motivation, psychological approach and the athlete's ability to go further.

The two most easily agreed upon definitions regarding the concept of intensity are those given by the late Prof. Emilio They and Massimo Spattini.

Initially, Prof. Emilio They stated that intensity is determined by the number of motor units involved in the unit of time from an angle from 0° to 180° (flexion) or vice versa (extension). His subjective method of calculating intensity was based more on the work method than on the load and led him to state:

> *Having chosen a workload that allows us to complete a certain number of repetitions during a set, consider the extent to which real fatigue has arisen in the number of repetitions performed.*
>
> E. They

A formula for calculating intensity was derived from this:

$$\text{intensity (I)} = \frac{\text{number of missing repetitions (CI)}}{\text{number of performed repetitions}} \times 100$$

Subsequently, Prof. They directed, defined and kept his concept of training intensity for all subsequent years of activity, stating that:

> *The intensity of the bodybuilding effort is the most difficult concept to quantify because it depends only to a small extent on external factors, and very much on the internal, subjective factors of the athlete. Bodybuilding intensity is, at least for me,*

the number of motor units that the athlete manages to engage in a single contraction (isotonic, isometric or negative-eccentric).

E. They

To better understand the concept of intensity, Massimo Spattini states that:

Physiologically, the intensity of the stimulus is essentially characterized by the strength and duration of the individual stimuli and respectively by the work carried out in the unit of time.

M. Spattini

From this statement, Spattini (1990) derived the following formula to **define the intensity** of a bodybuilding workout:

$$\text{intensity} = \frac{\text{number of sets} \times \text{number of repetitions} \times \text{TUT} \times \text{weight}}{\text{time}}$$

TUT is the time to which the active muscle is subjected for the duration of the sets.

To clarify, if you perform a set of bench presses explosively, you may eventually be able to do 10 reps with 100 kg to failure. If, on the other hand, the execution of the repetition was slow and controlled, using 3 seconds in the concentric phase and 5 seconds in the eccentric phase, it would be impossible for you to complete 10 repetitions because this type of execution makes lifting more difficult, thus increasing its intensity. Consequently, in this case, to make the intensity formula more compatible with bodybuilding training, the execution time of the sets must be put in the numerator (i.e. above the fraction line). From what has been explained so far, it is clear that, in addition to training volume, intensity is a really important factor for muscle growth and it is necessary to continuously and progressively raise the level if you want to continue making progress and thus achieving, in strength and mass, the limit of one's physical and genetic potential.

There are tons of ways to **increase the intensity of your workouts**, including but not limited to the overload principle, pyramid sets, drop sets, giant sets, forced reps, cheating, negative reps, rest pause, etc.

That said, intensity is almost exclusively a personal factor and is difficult to measure or calculate through external data or mathematical formulas: only the athlete can really know how far they have gone, and even an expert coach will have only a rough idea of the intensity levels achieved by their athlete. Only those performing the movement will know what percentage of intensity they really worked at. When **planning a workout** after understanding that the concept of intensity is actually very personal, you must never make the mistake of including various training techniques as a decisive intervention to increase the intensity of a workout. To clarify, let's suppose that three sets of leg extensions are included in a workout dedicated to the quadriceps; while the drop set is a brutal and really high-intensity technique, if the athlete does not perform the three sets to the fullest of their abilities, the training cannot be defined as intense.

On the other hand, if an athlete performs three sets of leg extensions of 10 repetitions each, using the maximum load possible, using the maximum effort he is capable of, and trying to push himself beyond his limits with each set, we are faced with a workout carried out at high intensity without the use of particular techniques. This is to demonstrate, once again, how much training intensity is a strictly intimate and personal value of the athlete. It is no coincidence that the definition of the term intensity is "accentuated force of action and/or participation". Training in buffering (without ever reaching exhaustion) will not give the same results in terms of hypertrophy, therefore using a training technique, such as a superset or a compound set, without reaching muscle exhaustion at each station will be less effective. As a matter of fact, most of the very few studies about this have shown that the muscle exhaustion technique produces better results than other techniques. However, it is equally true that this technique can lead more easily to incorrect executions and to a greater need for recovery in order not to overtrain and, consequently, it should be cycled.

Greater effectiveness is due to the fact that the final 2-3 repetitions are the most productive of the entire set, but only if you have reached your limit. The first few repetitions are simply preparation and help build strength. These repetitions are of limited value because their intensity is low and, since the muscle is fresh and strong, they engage fewer muscle fibers.

The number of fibers involved could be increased by performing the movement as fast as possible, but this is not desirable because fast movements when the muscle is not warmed up are dangerous, as a great force is exerted on the tendon moreover, when you perform a fast movement, there is always a tendency to help yourself with whole-body movements, thus not isolating the trained muscle. So, the first few reps should be done slowly and in perfect execution.

The final repetitions are the most productive because their intensity is high. In the last repetitions, you can try lifting the weight as quickly as possible because, since strength has decreased, the weight will be lifted slowly, without the risk of injury.

In his first movie, *Stay Hungry*, Arnold Schwarzenegger says: "You have to burn to grow." Feeling your muscles burning and pushing the reps to their maximum has always been part of an effective bodybuilding workout.

Jeff Willardson, a lecturer at Eastern Illinois University, examined the advantages and disadvantages of the **exhaustion training method**.

Many studies have looked at the optimal number of sets in a program, but few have focused on the effects of exhaustion training on muscle size and strength.

Exhaustion training allows bodybuilders and advanced lifters to overcome the training plateau and move to the next level.

These intense workouts need to be incorporated into short-term cycles to avoid overtraining. Exhaustion training is effective because it recruits more motor units (muscle fibers and related nerves) and stimulates the secretion of anabolic hormones, such as growth hormone (GH), insulin-like growth factor (IGF-1), and testosterone, and increases insulin sensitivity (insulin is a powerful anabolic hormone).

"Training to failure" actually promotes muscle growth, regardless of the load, according to a study by McMaster University and the University of Waterloo, Ontario, Canada. Previously it was believed that a minimum load of 60% of the maximum should be used to have an effect on hypertrophy. Brad Shoenfeld of Lehman College of New York, in a review of the literature (2016), concluded that even high repetitions with a limited load but at exhaustion create metabolic stress that causes the involvement of all muscle fibers.

Furthermore, in this regard, it has been found that post-exercise changes in anabolic hormones are not particularly directly related to the degree of muscle hypertrophy. Expert weightlifters participated in a 10-week training program that involved both high reps with low load and low reps with high load. Both groups trained with exhaustion repetitions on the leg press, bench press, knee extension and shoulder press. On the bench press, strength increased more in the high-load group, but muscle hypertrophy and strength in the other lifts were equal in both groups. This study would demonstrate that training to exhaustion is more important than the total load, which still caused the largest changes in anabolic hormones, to promote muscle hypertrophy over a 2.5-month training period. Obviously, it should not be deduced from this that the hormonal changes that occur during training are not functional in promoting a muscle growth processes.

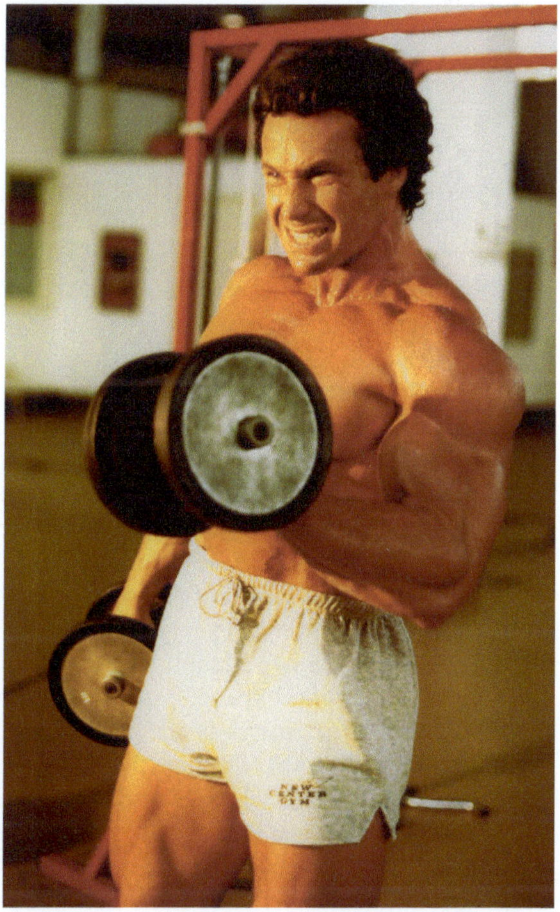

Intense bodybuilding training can cause rapid changes in protein metabolism, with the aim of promoting the repair of any injuries, allowing the body to adapt to stress, eliminating old tissue and producing new muscle proteins to strengthen the fibers. Therefore, if the anabolic processes are favored, muscle growth will be stimulated; on the other hand, atrophy will be stimulated if the catabolic and protein degradation processes are favored.

In beginner bodybuilders, it takes about 6 weeks to observe the first measurable changes in muscle size, since, during training, the degradation processes often exceed those aimed at protein synthesis. What regulates these mechanisms? Hormones are the real protagonists and are able to determine whether muscles will grow or remain as they were even after training.

Some Finnish and American researchers led by Bill Kraemer (2004) have shown that levels of testosterone, free testosterone, cortisol and growth hormone tend to increase significantly following an intense workout with weights, but more experienced athletes are able to further limit the production of the catabolic hormone cortisol; better muscle responses were obtained in the more experienced bodybuilders and in those who performed training programs characterized by repetitions to exhaustion. In conclusion, this study demonstrated that those with the ability and experience to train at supramaximal levels are able to obtain better results thanks to more favorable hormonal stimulation aimed at hypertrophy.

Practical advice

Remember that all sets (super-sets, tri-sets, drop sets, etc.) must be counted as a single set when calculating the training volume; therefore, a chest superset of two exercises, 10 reps each, will be nothing more than a 20-rep set for your muscle group. A fun exercise, yes, but not very useful for hypertrophy, unless, as explained above, you reach exhaustion. Before applying training techniques to increase the intensity of your workouts, make sure you use heavy loads and the correct technique, have an excellent mind-muscle connection, and always reach muscle exhaustion. Furthermore, it should not be forgotten that increasing the loads will not be enough and it is essential to pay attention to the way in which the weights are lifted.

As already mentioned, it is not always true that the increase of a single number (in our case the kilograms on the barbell) corresponds to an increase in strength or muscle mass: on the contrary, you may have overloaded the nervous system. On the other hand, when the load is increased thanks to the improvement of your motor skills, the increase in the weight lifted will always be accompanied by muscle growth. As repeatedly stated by Charles Poliquin, everything revolves around subjectivity, and in this case, the maturation of the motor skills of an athlete revolves around lifting weights. The **technique of execution** plays an absolutely fundamental role in trainings aimed at muscle hypertrophy. When a coach, an athlete or a scholar tells you in simple words that you have to "push" and always push yourself close to your limits, trying to overcome them, they are explaining that you have to train to the maximum of your abilities and, therefore, at the maximum possible intensity. The intensity attainable by an athlete is what really differentiates a champion from a normal person, a professional from an amateur.

It is good to remember that high-intensity workouts take longer to recover from. Some very interesting studies show how the human body is well-prepared to avoid overtraining by intensity; that is why, if an athlete is unable to fully recover after a workout, it is advisable to reduce the number of sets and not the intensity. Therefore, it is generally a mistake to decrease the training loads when an athlete is tired, while it is much more productive to decrease the number of sets performed with that load. The ACSM (American College of Sports Medicine) recommends the use of loads of intensity equal to or greater than 75% of 1RM to maximize hypertrophy and some important scientific papers have established that maximum muscle growth for trained subjects occurs with loads between 80 and 95% of 1RM. This is because, as demonstrated by various studies, such as those carried out by Staron et al. (1990), Hather et al. (1991) and Kosek et al. (2006), loads of this magnitude would be able to recruit all motor units, including IIb fibers, which are the most hypertrophiable and whose maximum recruitment occurs at about 85% of 1RM, as demonstrated by the study by Kenney et al. (2011) and, previously, from the research carried out by Tesch et al. (1998). Recovery times between sets are established on the basis of some parameters, among which intensity seems to be one of the most conditioning. Similar to what happens for the choice of load and, therefore, of intensity, recovery times also affect hormonal and metabolic responses and specific muscle adaptations in the same way. A very interesting study by Jared et al. (2011) delineated the recovery time between sets based on the intensity of load used, arguing that you need to do more than 5 minutes of rest between sets with a load that allows less than 5 maximum repetitions (RM) to exhaustion (>85% 1RM); 3-5 minutes of rest between

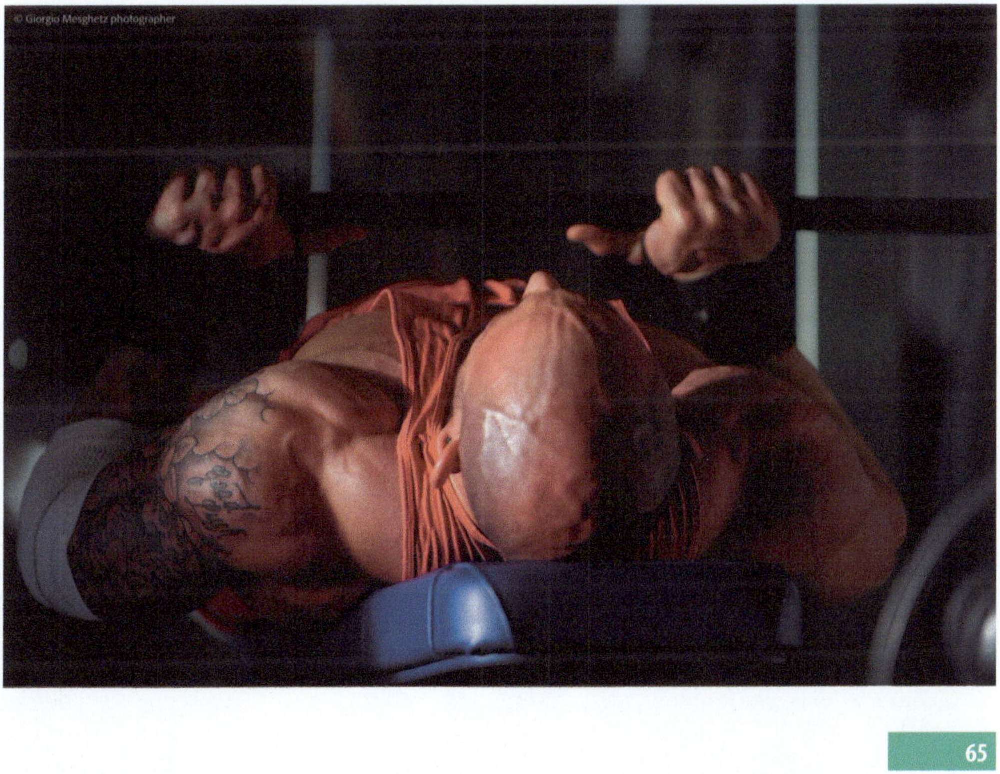

sets with loads that allow between 5 and 7 RM (~85% 1RM); 1-2 minutes of rest between sets with loads that allow between 11 and 13 RM (65-70% 1RM); about 1 minute of rest between sets with loads that allow 13 or more RM (<65% 1RM).

We would like to make it clear how much the concept of intensity is related to the athlete's commitment to performing the movement. In this context we understand the term intensity mainly in relation to the following concept: **give your best in every workout, in every set and during every repetition**; this is what really matters, especially when we know that we will have a "weakness" for the training volume and that we will apply training techniques aimed at further increasing its intensity. At this point, we would not want any confusion about the need to prioritize volume or intensity: the correct interpretation of what has been written so far is that the meeting point between the maximum sustainable intensity within a high-volume workout seems to be the key to obtaining maximum results in terms of hypertrophy. Athletes who, due to genetic characteristics, lifestyles and correct training planning, will be able to do this are those who will obtain the best results in terms of hypertrophy. As we will see later, even workouts not brought to total failure, in the long run, are able to produce better results than "to the death" workouts that are not interspersed with adequate recoveries.

MY EXPERIENCE ▸ Massimo Spattini

In an effort to give a somewhat picturesque definition of high intensity applied to bodybuilding, it seems to me that the idea given in the book *High-Intensity Bodybuilding* by Mike Mentzer could be interpreted as follows: "If you haven't vomited after doing a set of biceps curls with a barbell, do you even know what intense training is? Personally, I think I understood what high-intensity training means when I collapsed to the ground crying for more than 5 minutes after a fateful set of bicep curls, while training under the guidance of Mike Mentzer at Gold's Gym.

Every bodybuilder must know that intensity is a fundamental factor for muscle growth and that the level of intensity of the training must be continuously and progressively raised if one wants to continue making progress and reach the limit of one's own physical and genetic potential in both strength and size.

Principles to apply

There are many ways to increase training intensity: the overload principle, pyramid sets, drop sets, giant sets, forced reps, cheating, negative resistance, training quality, heavy-duty, rest pause and so on. We will now focus on the High-Intensity System. Given that every increase in intensity must correspond to a decrease in the amount of training, in this case there will be a significant reduction in the sets down to only two per muscle group.

Continues

Continued

This system implies the application of some of the principles indicated above, such as cheating and forced and negative repetitions, in order to arrive at total exhaustion of muscular strength and, therefore, to recruit the greatest possible number of muscle fibers.

Unfortunately, many bodybuilders avoid the last two or three final reps in a set, as they believe they are the most dangerous. Actually, the final reps are the healthiest. During this final phase, it is impossible to exert the same force on the tendons as during the initial phase.

However, in the High-Intensity System, increasing intensity with the principle of continuous tension involves lifting the weight in 2 seconds and lowering it in 4, stopping its descent. You need to use a weight for each exercise that allows you to perform between 8 and 12 repetitions with perfect form. At the point where this is no longer possible, two more repetitions are performed with the help of cheating; afterward, the help of a partner is used and two more forced repetitions are performed, and finally, again with the help of a partner, two negative repetitions are performed in which the partner lifts the weight completely and the athlete decelerates the descent holding it for 8 seconds.

It is evident that even one set done in this way is extremely tiring, so you shouldn't perform more than 20 sets for the whole body. A high-intensity set takes about 1 minute to perform perfectly. By taking into consideration 90 seconds of rest after a set or exercise, I estimate that most bodybuilders are able to complete 20 sets in about 50 minutes.

Some research has shown that, after a high-intensity workout, athletes need approximately 48 hours to achieve full recovery.

Many experts have noticed that when large muscles are trained at high intensity, an indirect growth stimulus is triggered, which also affects the other muscles; this appears to be the result of a biochemical reaction affecting the entire body system.

Starting from this concept, since there is a limit to recovery that affects all body functions, it is clear that training every day, in this case, is a mistake. For example, in terms of a stimulus or a training load, not everyone seems to be fully aware of how to intervene in order to increase or decrease it adequately.

This is because the basics are missing; in particular, few people know that the training load is given by intensity, density and volume. High-Intensity Training (HIT) means maintaining a high intensity at each repetition and in all sets, and an impeccable technique and execution quality aimed at total muscle control. Obviously, as there is an inverse relationship between training intensity and training volume, which are the two determining factors of training load, HIT workouts are usually short.

The HIT system takes into account the number of repetitions, the extent of the overload, the muscle tension time (TUT) and the rests. This method is based on the theoretical assumption that an increase in hypertrophy cannot be separated from an increase in strength. Only if you train against progressively higher resistances will you be able to obtain an even greater hypertrophic response.

In reality, if it is true that hypertrophy and strength are strictly dependent on each other, they are not identical in all expressions of the second. For example, training to increase maximal concentric

Continues

Continued

strength does not give the same results, in terms of muscle volume, as performing a workout that emphasizes the eccentric part of the movement, which induces microtrauma at the level of the muscle cell membrane that promotes the release of muscle growth factors which induce hyperplasia.
This is the reason for the different degree of muscular development of a bodybuilder compared to that of a weightlifter: the former is characterized by muscle fibers formed by numerous polynuclear syncytia indicative of hyperplasia starting from the satellite cells; the second, on the other hand, has hypertrophic fibers without the increase in nuclei, indicative of the absence of the phenomenon of hyperplasia. Furthermore, claiming that a workout aimed at increasing hypertrophy must be short does not take into account the fact that one stimulus that promotes the volumetric increase of fibro-cells is the depletion of energy stocks; among these, there are not only phosphates (adenosine triphosphate [ATP] and above all creatine phosphate [CP]) but also glycogen, which is depleted only during high training volumes.
Obviously, with the depletion of phosphates, strength begins to drop significantly, but this is not necessarily a limiting factor for hypertrophy, as demonstrated by pre-exhaustion techniques that use sets composed of multiple exercises; this obviously comes at the expense of strength but induces higher metabolic stress. This brings us to another factor, the production of lactic acid. If the prerequisite for high-intensity workouts is to implement sufficiently long recovery to restore phosphate levels, with shorter breaks, we will instead maximize the production of lactic acid, since the anaerobic lactic acid metabolism takes over after the anaerobic alactic acid metabolism of the phosphates.
Consequently, with longer pauses, also considering the reduced total volume, the chemical-hormonal stimulus for hypertrophy is lacking, i.e. the high levels of lactic acid in the blood, which are responsible for stimulating GH.

MY EXPERIENCE ▸ Riccardo Gaspari

I personally believe that training intensity has been one of the most exploited concepts by the fitness world to try to make more and more profit from it. I say that because I can assert with extreme certainty that there is no athlete in the world, worthy to be called such, no matter what sport discipline, who goes through their training without giving 100% of their abilities (probably also 110%). After decades of experience, I can certainly consider intensity as the degree of (maximum) commitment that the athlete employs in approaching each of their workouts.
As already stated in this chapter, I consider training intensity as an intrinsic characteristic of the athlete, probably the most intimate and personal. However, "in a nutshell", how is intensity applied? Intensity can be applied in very different ways, and they are all correct, because if you give it your all, it always works. That is the secret.

Continues

Continued

My generation grew up with two pillars of bodybuilding, Ronnie Coleman and Jay Cutler: one practically killed himself with loads that would make a powerlifter pale and moved through space with an aggressiveness and malice that not even Mike Tyson had; the other grinded set after set (I've always had a soft spot for Cutler).

How can you say that one used less intensity than the other? Similarly, it is impossible to state this when comparing Lee Haney and Rich Gaspari: the former used a Cutler-style modus operandi, while the latter was more oriented towards heavy loads and explosive training executions. Do we also want to talk about Arnold and Mentzer? Although Mentzer is considered the father of intensity training in bodybuilding, I believe that no one on the face of the earth can claim that there was no extreme intensity in Schwarzenegger's training sets.

Over the years, there has been a great deal of confusion and it has ended with a contrast between the intensity and the volume of training. Even though this may be true, intensity is not just a question of numbers. It is what you put into your training sets, it is your way of interpreting, facing and developing your training session.

In my life, there have been many examples and many masters, but there are four people who have created a well-defined path in my way of interpreting intensity: Sergio Barozzi, Enrico Giacomin, Costantino Polesel and Dr. Luca Silvestrini.

Sergio, a champion, wonderful athlete and truly avant-garde for his time (we are talking about the first striated buttocks shown in Italy, if not in Europe), followed a very linear and absolutely unsaleable training plan for our time; he used the pyramids and the much mistreated (nowadays) 4×10, but he performed every workout to the maximum of his physical ability. The weights had to be heavy and always increased, and the muscles had to lose their contractile capacity; the organism was really brought to exhaustion and, when the workout came to an end, the end was not determined by what was written on a sheet of paper, but by the total depletation of physical abilities. Sergio was "instinctive", but his instinct was guided by experience and rigor.

From Enrico, an exemplary athlete of our years, I learned how to really train a muscle while avoiding incurring injuries. He used many techniques in training (super-sets, stripping, rest pauses, etc.), with an average volume of work and high density, he never used weights out of the ordinary and preferred to slow down the executions, always making everything harder than it really was; each rep squeezed the target muscle hard, never let the muscle group rest, and exhausted it rep after rep, set after set, using a remarkable TUT.

Enrico was and is a "cold and calculating" athlete, and it is this characteristic that allows him to use the maximum intensity possible by channeling it only and exclusively where he wants, avoiding any waste and maximizing the result.

Costantino... what can I tell you about "Costa"? He was an elite athlete on a world scale in the 90s and 2000s, probably among the ten biggest and strongest athletes on the Italian scene and multiple award-winning international champion.

Continues

Continued

Costa is the most brutal I've ever seen during a training session. Believe me, both as a former competitive athlete and as a fitness professional, I have seen hundreds of professional athletes train (from strength athletes to combat athletes, hockey players to rugby players, etc.), but I have never seen anyone train like Costantino. He literally seemed to have an on/off button that turned on at the start of the sets, turning him into a veritable wrecking machine, and turned off at the end of the sets back to the affable big man we all know... but only until the beginning of the next set.

He used very simple and linear, functional training schemes, with medium-high workout volumes, and his intensity was given by the monstrous loads he used and the explosiveness with which he handled them. Also in this case, I think that the results obtained in his career and the validity of his method are indisputable. Even today, I believe that Costa is the only one who, if closed in the Colosseum, would make lions and gladiators pale with his mental attitude.

Finally, let's talk about Luca, Dr. Silvestrini. Luca is the perfect mix of the first three champions, as he is methodical, uses really heavy weights, performs the correct execution and employs some techniques such as drop sets or compound sets, average training volumes, but always leaves an instinctive margin to listen to his body: if he felt good one day, he would add a little more to the volume or increase the weights, or perhaps shorten the rest periods between sets; if, on the other hand, he didn't feel at his best, he adapted the training session by doing a little less or recovering a little more, but always giving his best.

I believe that Luca fully represents the modern approach to training, without ever neglecting the fundamental legacy of the past.

With these examples in mind, I would like to give you four suggestions, one for each athlete, which have greatly helped me improve in both athletic and professional terms.

> *Always try to increase the loads. If the load increases, the body is responding and muscle growth follows; when you feel that you can't take it anymore, keep trying to do a few more repetitions, don't stop when the schedule says so, stop when you really feel you are done. You need intensity.*
>
> Sergio Barozzi

> *You have to train a muscle, not move a weight from point A to point B; concentrate on muscle contraction and burning, never pause during the execution, and never give rest to the muscle, you have to "beat" it continuously, slowly and constantly; drive the repetition from the beginning to the end of the sets as if you were a mechanical piston that runs on oil, and never let the load dominate, as the load must do what you say. It is the means by which we reach our goal, the load shouldn't be the sole purpose. The muscles must be worked and worked on if we want them to give us their maximum.*
> *We must always keep intensity high.*
>
> Enrico M. Giacomin

Continues

Continued

This is an extreme sport and to be able to reach top levels you have to be more extreme than the sport itself; never give up, remember that your brain and your willpower, always give up before your body does, don't listen to them and trust your survival instinct and your body. They will never betray you. You have to give more, if you want to improve, the maximum is not enough, you have to raise the bar and be stronger than the previous day.
The only key is intensity.

Constantine Polesel

Muscles need to work, you must always guarantee them full stroke, maximum extension and maximum contraction; once you have reached a good level of strength, concentrate on muscle contraction, increase the repetitions to avoid the risk of injury, and always maintain impeccable execution that guarantees a high level of intensity: you will see that the loads will increase exponentially.
When the goal is to increase the load and the quality of the movements, it is necessary to recover based on your senses and not train with the nightmare of the stopwatch; being a very demanding job, we must never forget that performance is influenced by our daily life.

Luca Silvestrini

I leave you with these suggestions because they have really helped me find the correct interpretation of intensity, a factor that cannot be enclosed in a text or in a table, but that you must look for in your depths.
From what stated above, you will have noticed how the word "intensity" was mentioned with importance by all four athletes despite the different approaches to training methods, which all gave indisputable results and extremely high athletic levels.
Intensity is the emotional side of bodybuilding, and as with any endeavor, when the going gets tough, the tough get going.

CHAPTER 8

Time Under Tension: the deciding factor

Massimo Spattini and Riccardo Gaspari

The **TUT** (Time Under Tension or Total Time Under Tension [TTUT]) is a **fundamental parameter** for the success of our workouts and represents the time under tension to which the active muscle is subjected during the duration of the exercise; more specifically, it is the time of muscle activity and effort duration from start to finish during an interval set in a weight training program.

The scientific world has only recently recognized and applied the TUT, which was already introduced in the 1990s by Charles Poliquin, Ian King and Massimo Spattini.

The **use** and **manipulation of the TUT** are of great importance, as they allow us to define the substrates used during effort, the hormonal response, the recovery times between sets, and the physiological adaptations produced by a specific training stimulus.

The number of repetitions we perform is nothing more than a reference parameter to the percentage of 1RM, as this is the average time we need to perform a given training set. As we well know, common standards that identify a specific goal in the number of repetitions performed during the sets have been defined in weight training. The number of repetitions is closely related to the percentage of load used in these standards, as are the execution times: with a number of repetitions from 1 to 6 (80-100% 1RM) we stimulate a greater development of maximal strength; 7 to 15 repetitions (65-80% 1RM) will mainly stimulate the development of muscle hypertrophy; over 15 repetitions (<65% 1RM) will essentially improve endurance strength. Understanding this concept is essential to achieve your goals.

The **number of repetitions** should be restricted to well-defined execution times. If the goal of our training is to stimulate hypertrophy, we must perform sets of 8 to 15 repetitions (we believe the ideal range is 8-12, while according to science it is 6-15) which, if performed correctly, i.e. paying attention to the execution method and using the right load, will result in sets of 35 to 45 seconds; science has amply demonstrated that the ideal TUT to have an optimal hypertrophic stimulus is just 40 seconds. Empirically, we have noticed that the average subject takes 40 seconds to perform sets that fall within a range of 10-15 repetitions. Working on the speed of

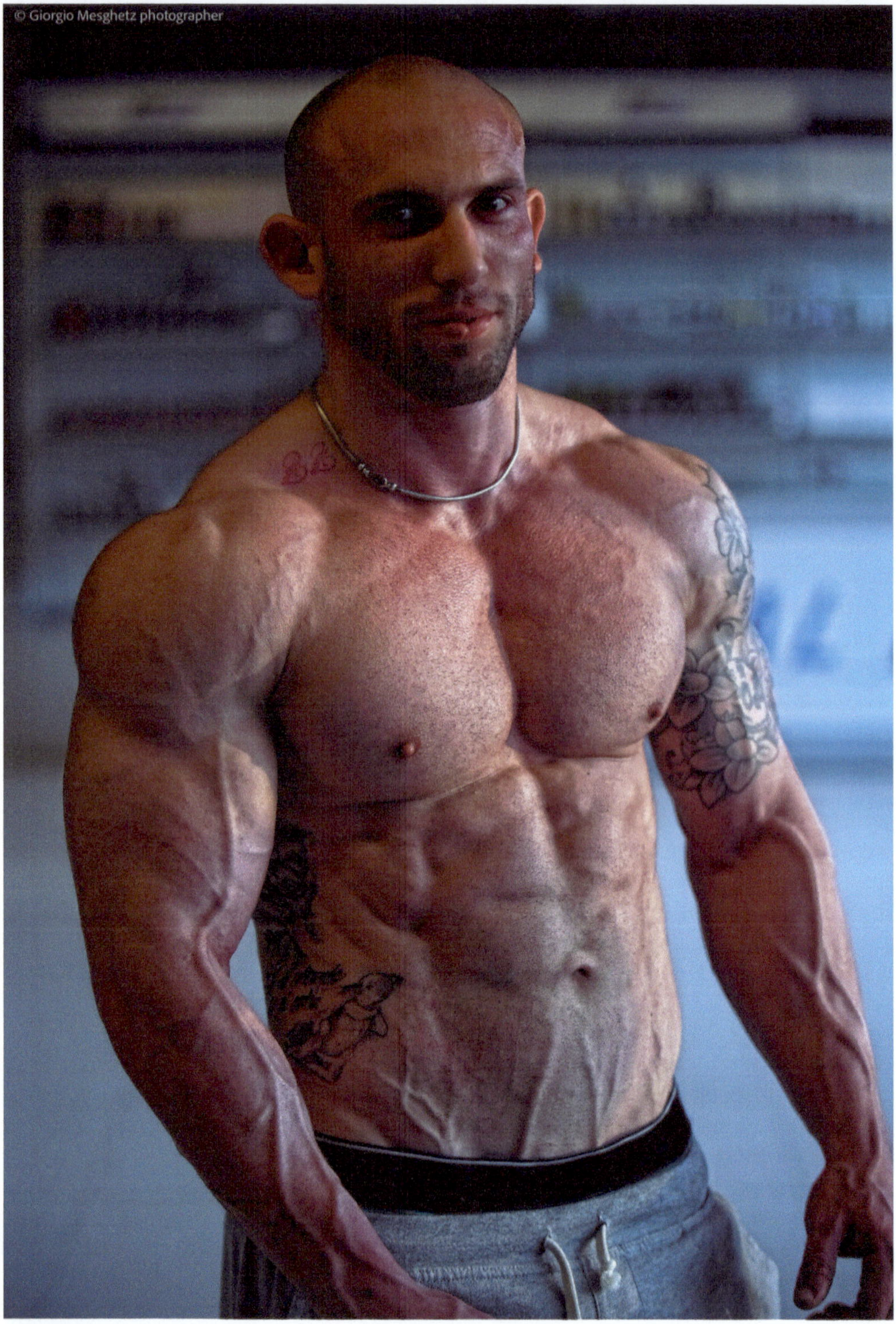
© Giorgio Mesghetz photographer

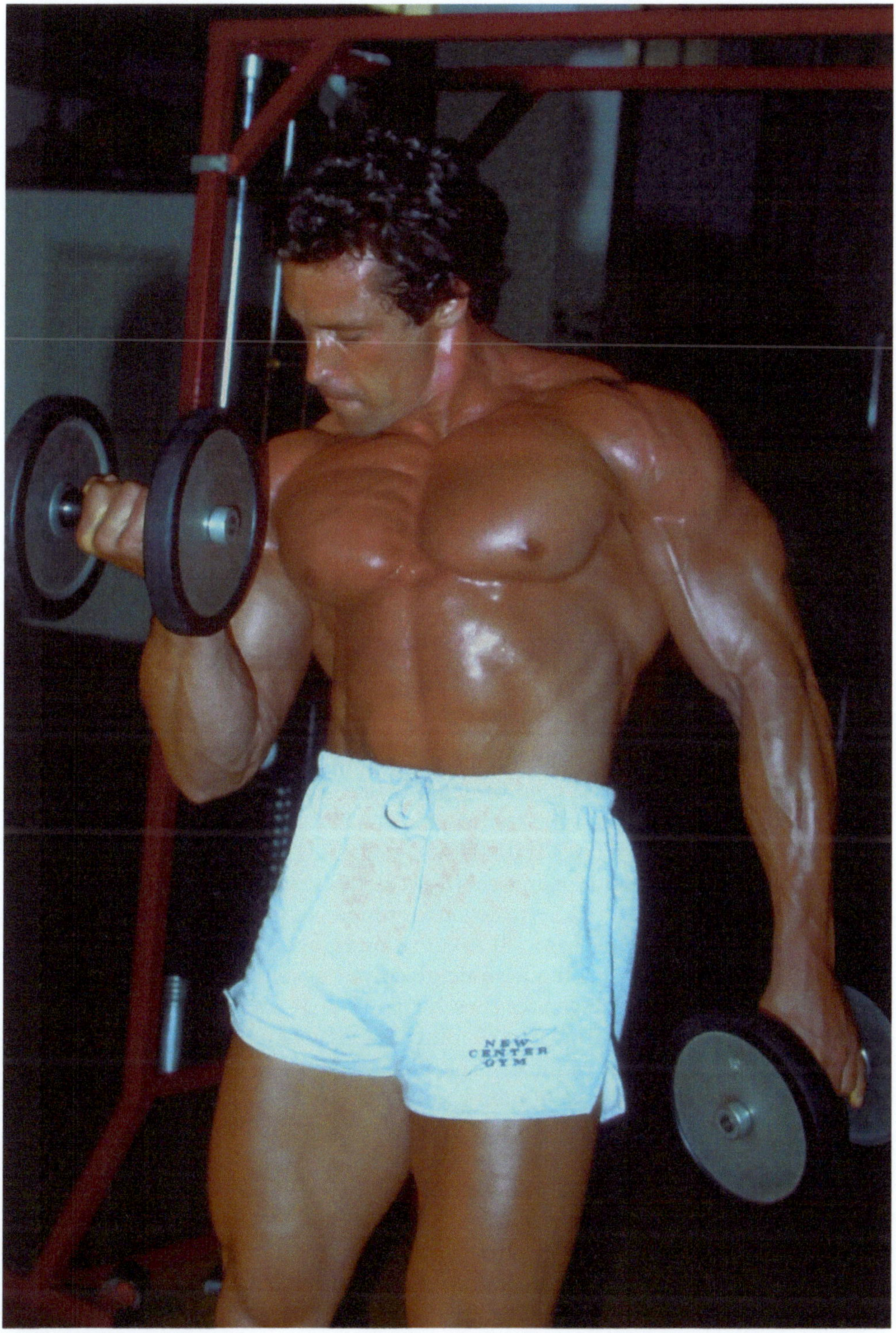
NEW
CENTER
GYM

execution will therefore allow us to achieve our goal with both 8 and 12 repetitions, always making sure we are working with the right percentage of load.

Let's not forget, however, that even working out with a very short TUT (10-15 seconds) and very high intensity (85-90% 1RM) determines the maximum recruitment of IIb fibers (white or fast) with the synergistic intervention of IIa and I fibers, while lower intensities determine a lower recruitment of IIb fibers. We should also keep in mind that bodybuilding (a discipline completely oriented towards the development of hypertrophy) is a practice that weighs heavily on the lactic anaerobic system (best stimulated with the use of 10-12 repetitions). This, however, does not mean that we have to work only with 10-12 repetitions: as we will see later, strength is essential for the construction of new muscle mass. Therefore, the **periodization of the stimuli** and their **progression** become essential in a training system oriented to success.

This demonstrates that our body chooses to use a specific fuel based on the stimulus that is applied to it. For this reason, to allow us to perform an exercise, the body must rely on metabolic mechanisms in charge of producing mechanical energy. Therefore, the type of stimulus is given by various physiological mechanisms, such as the activation of different energy systems, which depends on the relationship between the number of repetitions, the speed of the movements and the intensity of the load used. The intervention of one of the energy systems instead of another is fundamentally determined by the relationship between the intensity of the effort (the load used) and the time under tension. This means that the **duration** and **intensity of an exercise** determine which fuel is used the most and how many and which motor units are recruited to complete the movement.

The three main energy systems for energy supply are represented by the **anaerobic alactic** (or phosphagen) **system**, which provides energy through the use of muscle phosphates such as adenosine triphosphate (ATP) and creatine phosphate (CP) for intense performance (80/85-100% 1RM), with a TUT ranging from 1 to 20 seconds; the **anaerobic lactacid** (or anaerobic glycolytic) **system**, which provides energy mainly through the use of muscle glycogen for moderately intense activities (65-80% 1RM), with a TUT ranging from 20 to 60 seconds; again, the **anaerobic lactacid system** which, together with the **aerobic glycolytic system**, produces energy with the main use of muscle glycogen for those activities that are not very intense (<20% 1RM), with a TUT ranging from 1 to 10 minutes. Obviously, the intensity of the exercise also determines the activation of a specific energy system, and we could evaluate it in terms of the total number of motor units recruited and/or the total number of repetitions to failure, performed within a precise time frame.

Knowing the energy systems also helps us understand how much their activation affects the hormonal production of our body. Lactic acid, through the lactacid anaerobic system, appears to be a by-product of glycolysis. Many scientific publications have reported that with a greater number of repetitions (10-12) and sets, and with short recovery times, we are faced with a significant increase in the production of growth hormone (GH); this factor is closely related to the increasing levels of lactate

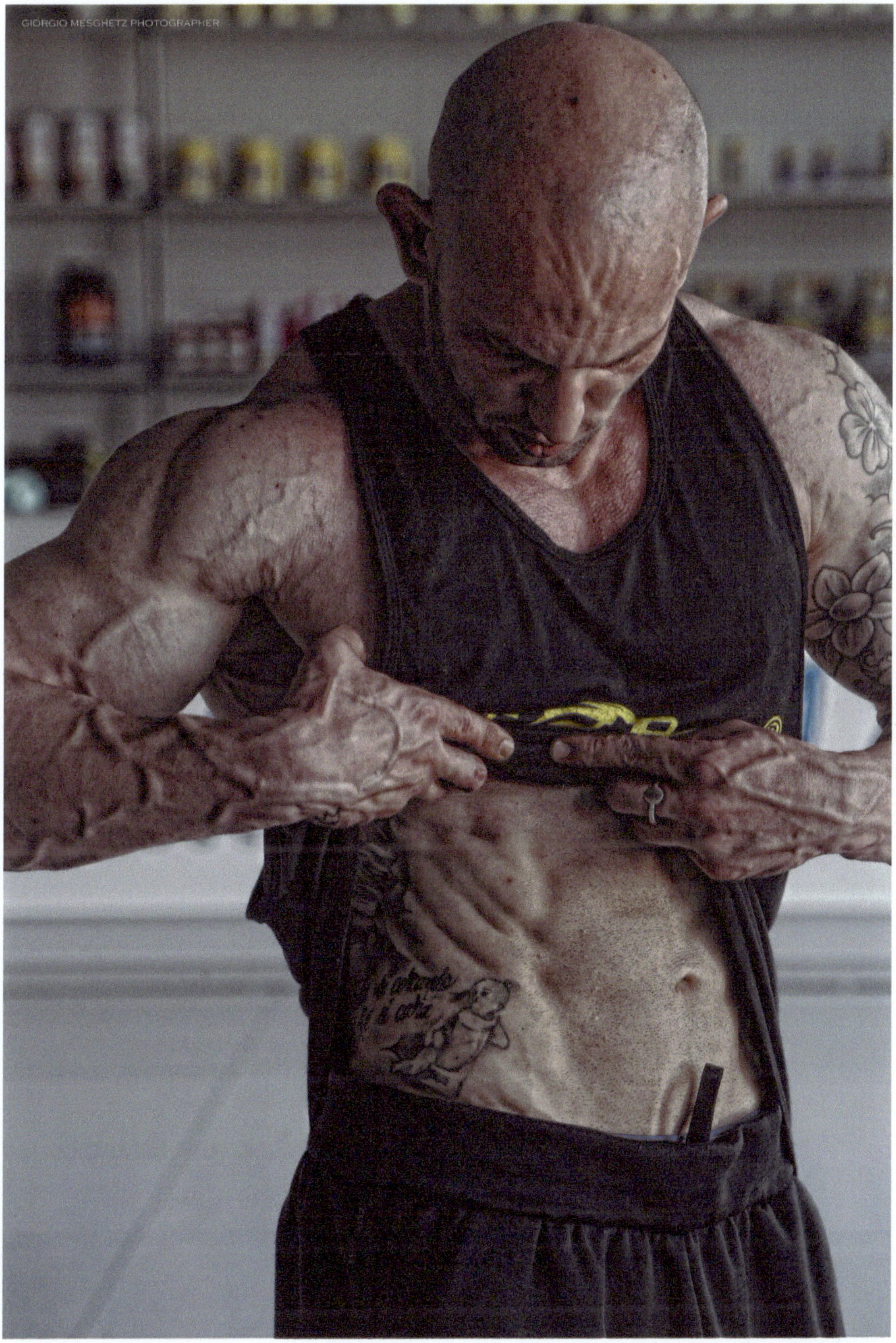
GIORGIO MESGHETZ PHOTOGRAPHER

associated with this type of training. It is therefore clear that, in order to activate the anaerobic lactacid glycolytic system, it is necessary to exert effort for a certain amount of time, using a specific intensity.

On the other hand, if we wanted to stimulate the production of testosterone, we would have to make short and very intense efforts, thus activating the alactic anaerobic system.

In summary, with a **TUT equal to 1-15 seconds**, we will perform a workout of maximum power and strength, with little hypertrophic stimulus (alactic anaerobic system); with a **TUT equal to 20-40 seconds** we will perform a workout aimed at hypertrophy, with little stimulus towards maximal strength (anaerobic lactacid system); with a **TUT equal to 40-60 seconds** we will perform a workout to stimulate hypertrophy and resistance strength (anaerobic lactacid system); with a **TUT >60 seconds** we will perform a training focused on the development of endurance strength (anaerobic lactic acid/aerobic glycolytic system).

It has now been amply demonstrated, both empirically and by science, that to maximize improvements in muscle performance, in particular hypertrophy, a **cyclization of the TUT** is successful and necessary, so as to use different substrates and impose a prevailing activation of different energy systems.

After understanding the importance of acting on the TUT, let's move on to a practical example. When writing a training table, the TUT is often indicated in the last or penultimate column and is defined by four digits. Let's see together how to read and interpret it in practice using the annotation in a training table by Charles Poliquin relating to one of his training methods, called the 4-5% solution:

TUT → 3-1-X-0 → Time Under Tension of each rep*

The first number represents the duration of the eccentric phase (in which we lower the weight); the second number represents the pause time in the phase of maximum stretching; the X represents the duration of the concentric phase (in which we lift the load); the fourth number represents the pause time in the position of maximum contraction.

*Legend: 3 = 3 seconds; 1 = 1 second; X = explosive movement ("explode"); 0 = 0 seconds

CHAPTER 9

Muscle failure: managing it correctly

Riccardo Gaspari

We have seen that performing sets to failure is certainly an effective method to increase the intensity of training. But is it always necessary? **Muscle failure** (or **exhaustion**) is defined as the inability to continue performing further repetitions during a set of weight training and, therefore, muscle activity must be stopped. In practice, muscle failure occurs when the athlete is no longer able to complete the concentric phase of the repetitions during the entire arc of the expected movement (Range of Motion, ROM); this condition indicates the point at which the muscle fibers reach an arrested phase, called ischemic rigor (ischemic stiffness), in which they literally freeze and stiffen due to the depletion of adenosine triphosphate (ATP). Therefore, muscle failure occurs when the neuromuscular system can no longer produce enough force to overcome a specific workload.

Training to failure has been shown to yield significant benefits in terms of **strength gains and hypertrophy** even if it is not essential and certainly not indicated to be maintained over time. Some researchers have recognized muscle failure as a practice conducive to breaking the stall in muscle gains by advanced athletes.

In the context of muscular hypertrophy, important scientific publications have indicated that the maximum development of this specific adaptation is obtained with the use of loads between 80 and 95% of 1RM; other scientific guidelines have established that the optimal repetition range for hypertrophy is between 1 and 12 RM (approximately between 60 and 100% of 1RM). However, even though most guidelines, for years, have established that hypertrophy is maximized with high loads, recent studies are starting to show that even very low-intensity loads (30% 1RM) can cause an increase in protein synthesis and muscle hypertrophy comparable to those obtained with high loads (90% 1RM), provided that these are brought to muscle failure. In this case, the search for muscle exhaustion was fundamental to the purpose.

The study performed by Stowers et al. (1983) found that one set to failure promotes an increase in squat performance, but that three sets of 10 repetitions, including two to failure, cause greater improvement in squat ability.

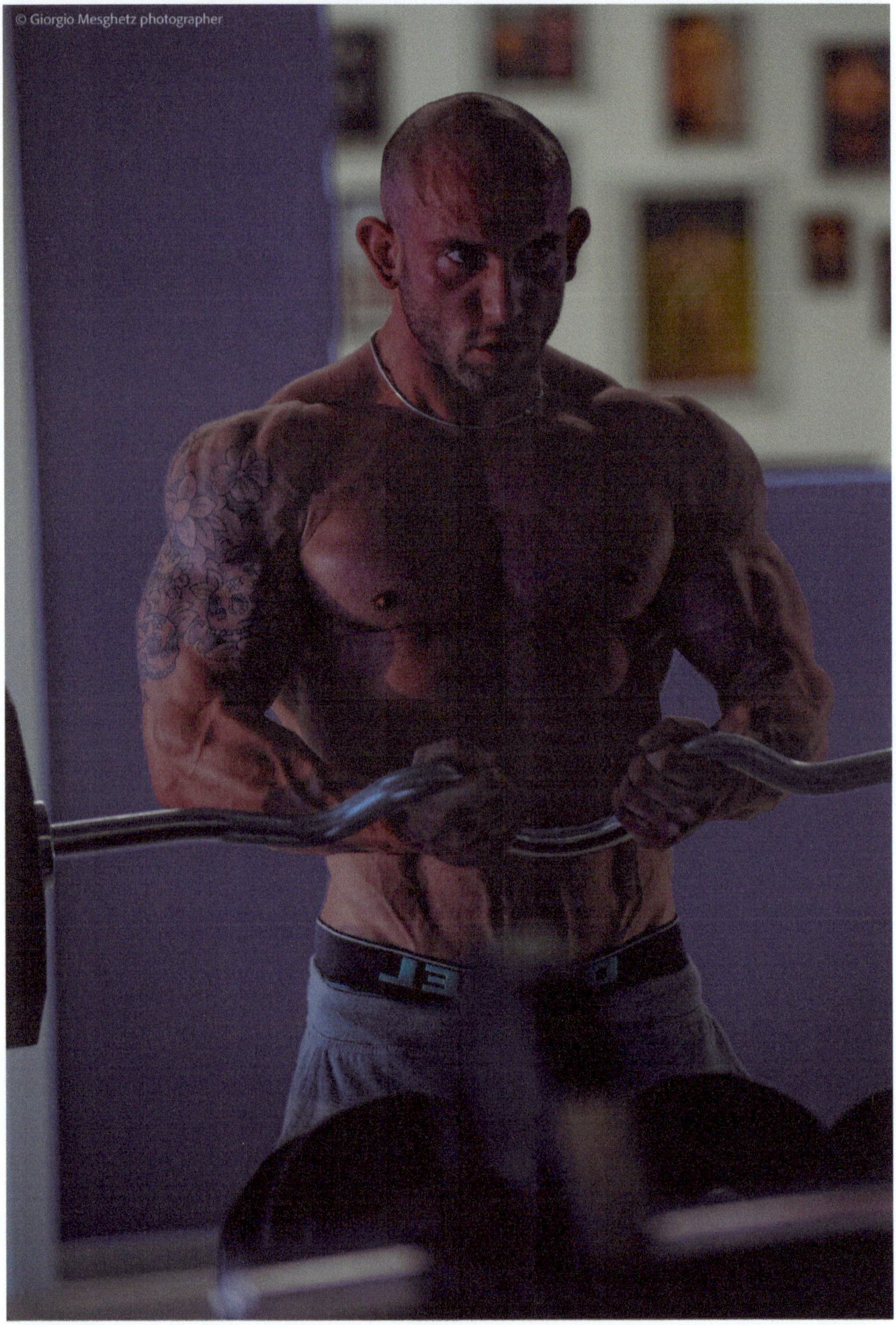
© Giorgio Mesghetz photographer

In 1998, Kraemer et al. conducted a major study in which they examined the effects of a single set of weight training to failure with two multiple-set non-failing protocols, in one repetition maximum (1RM) parallel squat. 43 men were randomly assigned to weight training protocols that emphasized the development of leg and hip strength:

- SS protocol: 1 × 8-12 repetitions to failure
- MS protocol: 3 × 10 repetitions
- MSV protocol: multiple set protocol using varied sets and repetitions

Relative intensity (initial % of 1RM), intensity (average load lifted) and volume of load (load × repetitions) were different between the two groups, based on the comparison of the values measured after 14 weeks. Body mass, body composition and parallel squat repetition maximum were assessed before starting the program and at weeks 5 and 14. The results showed no significant changes in body mass or body composition. 1RM increased significantly in all groups, and between-group differences in 1RM indicated that the MS and MSV protocols had an approximately 50% greater increase than the SS protocol after 14 weeks. The results suggested that multiple sets not performed to failure produced superior gains in the maximum lift in the squat.

Izquierdo et al. (2006) carried out a study to examine hormonal responses in an 11-week weight training program divided into a failure group (group one) and a non-failure group (group two), followed by an identical strength and power protocol lasting 5 weeks, which was assigned to both groups. The subjects included 42 physically active males, randomly divided into two groups. The results demonstrated that 11 weeks of training to failure and no failure resulted in similar gains in maximal strength (1RM), muscle power in the arm and leg extensor muscles, and maximum reps in the squat. Nonetheless, it was observed that after the 5-week period in which a maximum strength and power training program was performed, the non-failure group showed greater increases in strength, power and testosterone levels, and had reduced levels of cortisol, compared to the failure group.

We can conclude by stating that the research shows conflicting results and that, clearly, subjects can positively gain strength and power without always having to undergo the rigorous and acute physical effort associated with muscle failure. Moreover, training to exhaustion is not the only and inexorable way to stimulate muscle hypertrophy, but must necessarily be dosed and alternated, both for safety and for the correct periodization of the stimuli.

CHAPTER 10

Training density, a fundamental but underestimated element

Massimo Spattini and Riccardo Gaspari

Let's start by stating that **muscle density** (the granite aspect of the muscle) is not to be confused with **training density** (the link between effort and recovery within the same training session).

Here density refers to a weight training variable that represents the link between effort and recovery within the same training session.

Contrary to other parameters related to training, such as volume, intensity and frequency, density has not yet been recognized by scientific literature; despite this, its importance in planning a workout remains undoubted.

In our opinion, the best explanation of this important parameter is that provided by the work of Antonio Paoli and Marco Neri, in which they state that density is given by the **ratio between the real duration** (RD), characterized by the time of the session dedicated to the effective execution of the exercise (net of recovery times), and the **total duration** (TD), which represents the time elapsed between the start and the end of the training session.

In the training session (central part), the RD of the tension of a muscle is shorter than the duration of the entire central part of the training session; this difference is essentially determined by the recovery times between one set and another, and from this we understand that the parameter can be influenced by the number of sets performed and by the recovery times. This closely, but indirectly, linked to the intensity load (% 1RM).

$$\text{density (DS)} = \frac{\text{real duration (RD)}}{\text{total duration (TD)}}$$

Reading the Paoli and Neri formula, it is understood that the RD refers to the real duration of the time under effort in the central part of the workout, excluding the recovery times between the sets that are performed before and after the actual session, such as warm-up and cool-down sets. We could therefore say that the RD is the result of the sum of the total Time Under Tension (TUT) of all the exercises in the training session, i.e. the total time in which the muscle is placed under effort.

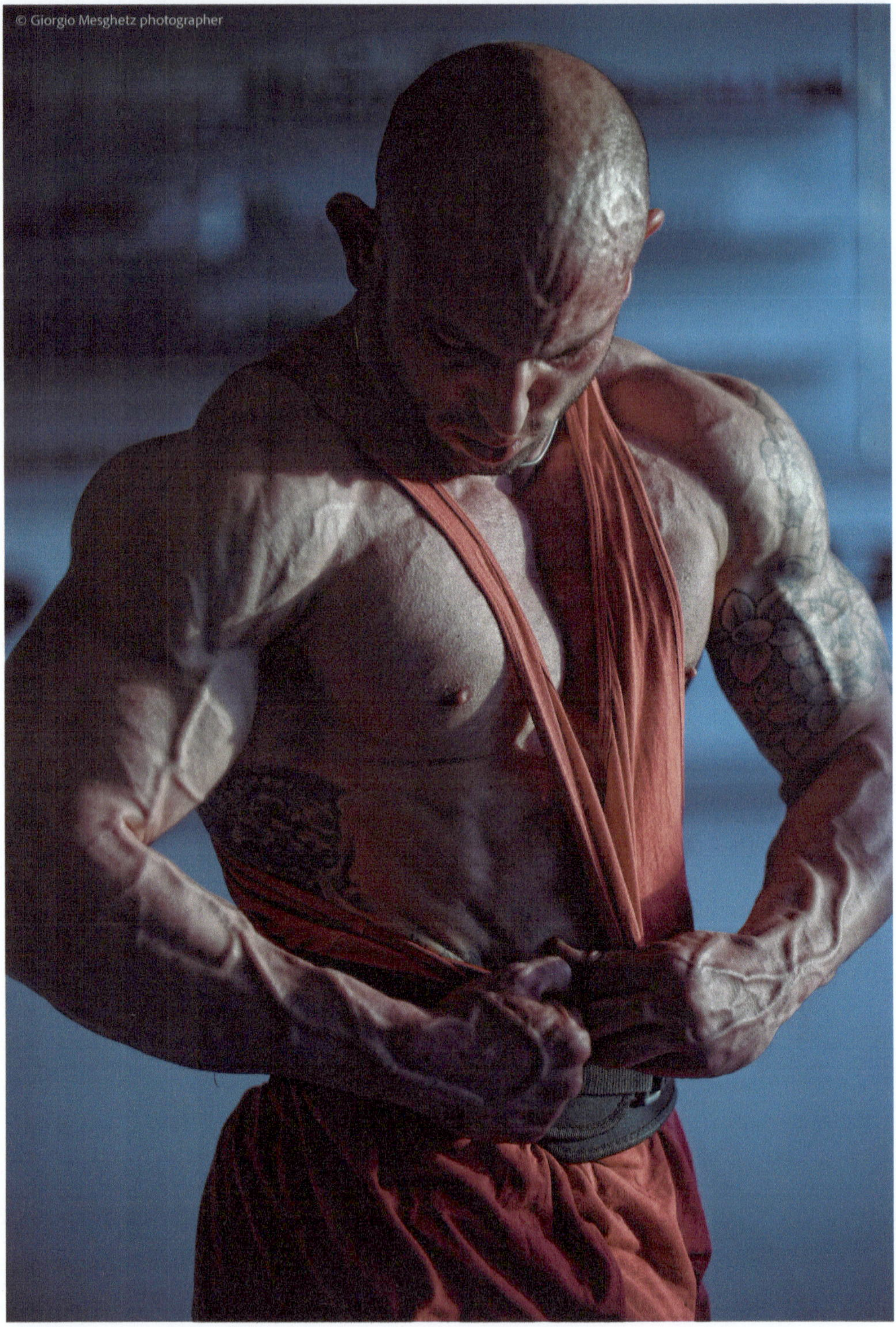
© Giorgio Mesghetz photographer

The DT, on the other hand, refers to the total duration of the central part of the session, including recovery times; therefore, we refer to the sum of the Time Under Tension (TUT) and the recovery times from the beginning to the end of the central part of the workout.

Thanks to the work carried out by Haennel et al. (1991) and Todd et al. (1992), **circuit training** (CT) has been defined as the maximum expression of density, as it consists of a high number of sets, a high number of repetitions, very little or no recovery time and, often, low intensity (the intensity of a circuit is not always low).

Two of the most important benefits of increasing training density are increased caloric expenditure during and after training, and a dramatic increase in GH production. A study carried out by Murphy and Swartzkopf (1992) compared two groups of athletes, subjecting one of them to a standard training and the other to CT. The standard workout included 6 exercises of three sets each, with all sets performed to exhaustion, using a load equal to 80% of 1RM and 120 seconds of rest between sets; the CT was structured in three sets of circuits, 6 exercises, 10-12 repetitions at 50% of 1RM and 30 seconds of rest.

The study reported that, although the total work volume of both programs was similar, circuit weight training elicited a larger Excess Postexercise Oxygen Consumption (EPOC, i.e. the oxygen response following an intense activity, which must satisfy the body's "oxygen debt") compared to the standard weight training program (5 liters and 25 calories versus 2.7 liters and 13.5 calories).

In practice, we have several ways to **increase the density of our training**. The most common techniques are increasing the training volume (through the number of sets and total repetitions), reducing the recovery time between sets, reducing the intensity load (% 1RM) by increasing the number of repetitions, or direct interventions on parameters related to the TUT, such as performing the sets to muscle failure (which would lead to an increase in the TUT) or slowing down the speed of movement (which is also reflected in an extension of the TUT).

The studies performed by Kraemer et al. (1990) and, subsequently, by Smilios et al. (2003) have widely found that training with weights, with the same number of sets, low load intensity, lower recovery times and higher density (given by a reduction in recovery times and an increase in the TUT), produce a higher secretion of GH when compared to weight training at medium or high intensity. From this, we understand that high-density weight training can have a greater impact on caloric expenditure, on the increase in lactate concentrations, on lactic acid tolerance and on the increase in GH and cortisol levels.

In this vein, a recent study by the University of Padua, conducted by Antonio Paoli, Marco Neri, and others, evaluated how two different approaches to weight training determine differences at the metabolic level. The protocols taken into consideration were HIRT (High-Intensity Resistance Training or short but high-intensity weight training - total time 32 minutes) and classic weight training (total time 62 minutes). Seventeen subjects who habitually practiced weight training performed both workouts at different times and were evaluated at rest and 22 hours after the

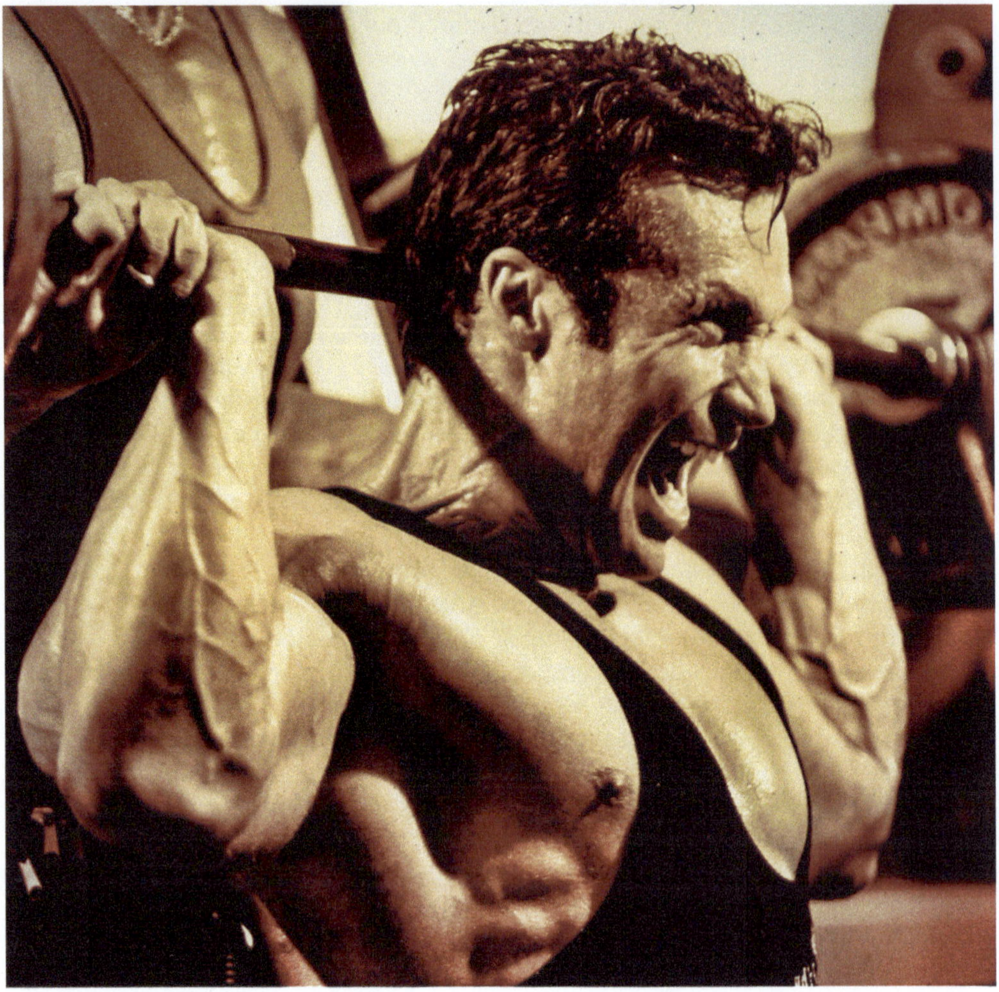

session, measuring Resting Energy Expenditure (REE) and respiratory quotient (RQ), which evaluates what types of metabolites the body is using, mainly fats or carbohydrates. Emerging data suggest that shorter sessions of HIRT may increase post-exercise REE to a greater extent than classic resistance training and may reduce RQ, thereby enhancing fat oxidation. This exercise methodology allows subjects to improve metabolism and, at the same time, muscle mass and strength (as described in other studies). In Western society, where free time and motivation to perform daily physical activity are lacking, this protocol could make a difference in the prevention of **hypokinetic** (from inactivity) **pathologies**: obesity, diabetes, cardiovascular pathologies and tumors.

CHAPTER 11

Recovery times between sets: it's not subjective

Massimo Spattini and Riccardo Gaspari

Recovery time, also called an interval, a pause, a rest period or a rest interval is a fundamental parameter in the study and application of weight training; it is the **rest time** that elapses between training sets and between the various exercises of a training session. The importance of recovery times has been strongly recognized by science but is still too often underestimated in practice; this variable is fundamental in planning and carrying out a workout in the gym, as it plays a fundamental role in acute and chronic responses of a metabolic, hormonal and cardiovascular nature. The main factors on which the recovery time depends are the load used and the relative intensity as a % of 1RM, the training objectives and the energy system to be activated. Keeping in mind that the recovery times between sets must be inversely proportional to the number of repetitions performed (the lower the repetitions, therefore the higher the loads and the intensity, the longer the recovery times will have to be), **three rest periods** are mainly identified: short (30 seconds or less), moderate (60-90 seconds) and long (3 minutes or more); these, in turn, are linked to the objective.

The study carried out by Coburn and Malek (2011) definitively established recovery times based on the training method: this concept has been very clear for many years to all trainers in the sector, but this research, published as educational material for the NSCA, has definitively set the standards. It establishes that with 5 minutes or more of rest between sets, loads greater than 85% of 1RM will be used and fewer than 5 repetitions are to be performed; 3-5 minute breaks will allow for 5-7 repetitions using loads equal to 85% of 1RM; 1-2 minute breaks will allow for 9-13 repetitions using loads equal to 65-70% of 1RM; 1 minute of recovery between sets will instead allow us to exceed 13 repetitions using a load lower than 65% of 1RM; with a 20-30 second break we will be able to perform 20 or more repetitions using a load equal to 40-60% of 1RM.

This is what emerges from the work done by Coburn and Malek, but in practice, fortunately, the possibilities are wider, and it is always preferable to try a load, evaluate it mathematically on the table of maximums and then check it in the gym: never forget to customize each aspect of the training, including recovery. With this

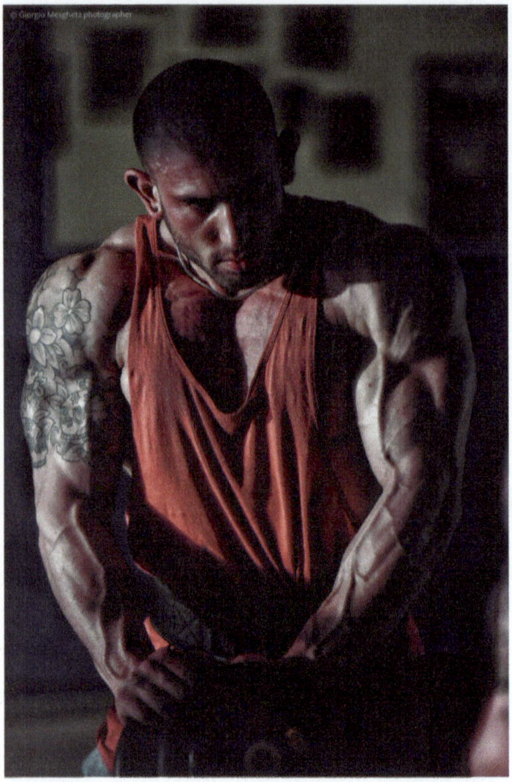

in mind, we can deduce that strength training programs normally envisage recovery times of 3-5 minutes between sets, and that this approach is associated with greater restoration of energy at the muscle cell level, resulting in lower performance degradation in weightlifting. Strength is mainly generated by the contraction of fast white fibers, which use an anaerobic metabolism by initially exploiting the reserves of adenosine triphosphate (ATP) and creatine phosphate (CP). The conversion of ATP to ADP releases the energy needed for muscle contraction and subsequently, CP regenerates ATP by donating its phosphate group to ADP. The time required to restore ATP is approximately 4 minutes.

Hypertrophy is different, as the hypertrophic stimulus is not only linked to the entity of the loads used, which are in any case of great importance, but it also depends very much on a metabolic environmental situation in which the muscle triggers adaptive mechanisms which lead to hypertrophy. As we have seen previously, the substrate of this metabolic environment is the production of lactic acid, which, together with hydrogen ions, favors tissue acidosis, which may lead to localized muscle micro-traumas favoring the release of the growth factors IGF-1 (Insulin-like Growth Factor-1) and MGF (Mechano Growth Factor). These molecules stimulate hypertrophy and possible hyperplasia (an increase in the number of cells) through the activation of satellite cells. Lactic acid is also critical in stimulating testosterone production, even more than GH (Growth Hormone). This creates a post-workout hormonal environment more conducive to muscle growth. A study by Goto et al. (2007) demonstrated that subjects who trained with 30-second breaks had higher GH levels, which were associated with greater muscle volume. This result clearly demonstrates that higher GH levels stimulated by shorter recovery times promote muscle growth.

In a study performed by Villanueva et al. (2015), two groups of subjects underwent high-intensity training with 60-second or 90-second breaks, and the results demonstrated both an increase in testosterone and a marked increase in strength, thus indicating that this recovery time was suitable for both hypertrophy and an increase in strength.

However, the concept that predominates is that longer breaks between sets are more efficient for increasing strength, and shorter breaks are better for stimulating hypertrophy; shorter recovery times have an effect on the increase in the density parameter, increasing muscle pumping and hormonal response; with the increase in the anabolic hormonal response, a more favorable environment could be created for muscle protein synthesis and could increase the activity of satellite cells.

Shorter recovery times between sets increase the accumulation of certain metabolites (lactic acid, H+ ions, inorganic phosphates), and this metabolic stress stimulates muscle growth. Shorter recoveries of 60-90 seconds would therefore induce a greater anabolic response. However, not all studies conducted so far in this regard agree with this statement.

Ahtiainen et al. (2004, 2005) found no significant difference in hypertrophic response between a 2-minute rest and a 5-minute rest in well-trained young athletes. Burish et al. (2009) found a greater increase in arm muscles with resting times of 2.5 minutes compared to the 1-minute rest in untrained young people. Villanueva et al. (2015), on the other hand, found a greater increase in lean mass with 1 minute of rest compared to 4 minutes in untrained elderly people. These discrepancies may be due to the methodological differences of the studies themselves and because hypertrophy was measured mainly with indirect methods.

Recently, Schoenfeld (2016) set up a new study, in collaboration with researchers at the University of Oklahoma, involving well-trained young men who performed a total body routine of 8-12 repetitions of concentric-type exercises to exhaustion (i.e., up to the point where you can lift the weight), performed three times a week for 8 weeks.

The subjects were divided into two groups: one took breaks for 60 seconds, the other for 3 minutes; finally, the increase in mass was measured by ultrasound. The result, of course, was a greater increase in strength demonstrated by increasing the squat and bench press max in the 3-minute rest group, which was not surprising. Contrary to what might be expected, the same group had greater mass gains in the biceps, triceps and quadriceps. The reason is difficult to explain, but it could be due to the increased workload.

The load is calculated with the following formula:

number of sets × number of repetitions × weight used

With longer breaks, you get to use more weight, so the total volume of your workload increases. Furthermore, in this way, as strength increases, the workload also progressively increases, further favoring the increase in muscle mass. Among other things, it is quite logical that one cannot become "big" by lifting "light weights that are always the same".

At this point, putting all the studies together, we can say with some certainty that the **ideal recovery time** between one set and another should be around 90 seconds, in order for the individual to be able to maintain and increase the workload. Does that mean that short breaks of 1 minute or less should be eliminated from hypertrophy training programs? In reality, all training methods, including training routines with shorter breaks, can improve the body's buffer capacity at the muscle level, thus allowing you to perform more repetitions with the same weight, while still increasing the volume of the load; once again, as in the other variables, the key to success, as well as customization, lies in cycling. Regarding short breaks and hormonal response, Boroujerdi and Rahimi (2008) tested the variations in recovery times on 10 trained men (average age 22 years). Subjects performed two weight training protocols, similar in the total volume of work (sets × repetitions × load), but different in the length of breaks between sets (1 minute versus 3 minutes). Both protocols included 5 sets of 10 RM bench presses and squats performed in two separate training sessions. Blood samples were examined before, immediately after, and 1 hour after the protocols to determine blood GH, IGF-1 and lactate concentrations. Post-exercise lactate and GH values were significantly higher compared to pre-exercise levels, but the same increase was not found for IGF-1 concentrations. However, IGF-1 concentrations significantly increased over the course of 1 hour after the workout. Post-exercise serum GH levels and blood lactate concentrations were significantly higher in protocols with short breaks (1 minute) than those with long breaks (3 minutes), although the recovery length did not affect IGF-1 levels. This data suggests that the length of recovery times between sets in weight training greatly influences serum GH levels, so one must consider that short recovery times between sets induce greater acute GH responses than long recovery times. Given that GH is an anabolic hormone, this find-

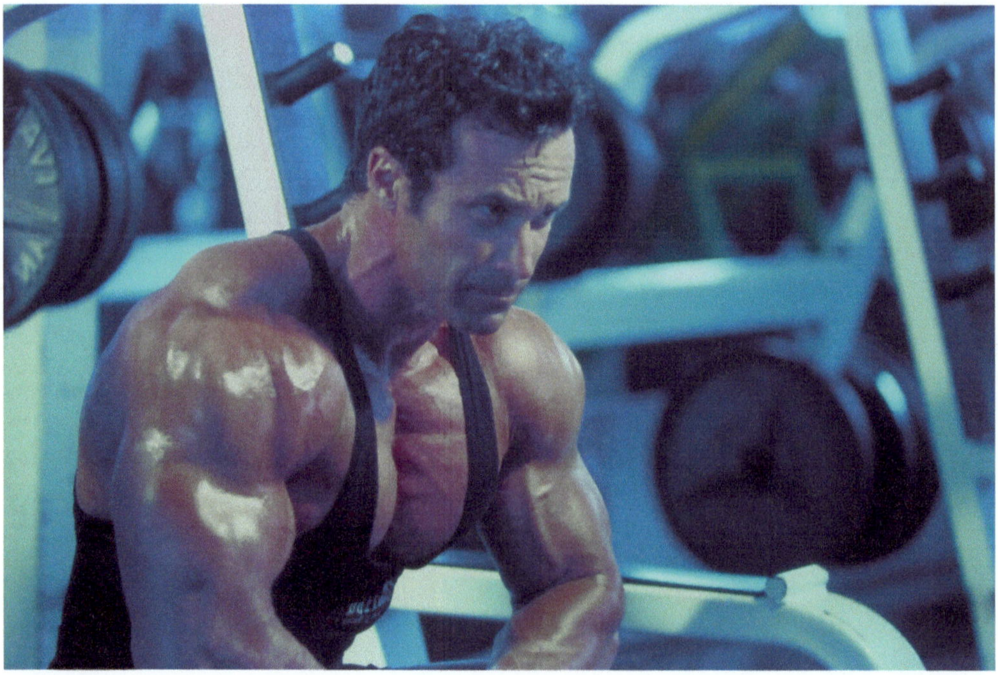

ing could have very important implications in achieving muscle hypertrophy. This was also demonstrated by Kraemer et al. (1990), who compared the hormonal effects of six different weight training protocols on 9 male subjects. The protocols were set up with the same order of exercises, but differed in the number of repetitions, between 5 and 10 RM, and recovery times, between 1 and 3 minutes. Each of these six workouts had a different combination of these two parameters. Among other observations, the authors noted that not all protocols produced the same increase in GH. The highest responses of this hormone were observed in the protocols with more total work, 1-minute rest and 10 RM (roughly correlated with a relative intensity at 75% of 1RM). This research also found that shorter recovery times (1 minute versus 3 minutes) elicited higher acute hormonal responses.

Bottaro et al. (2009) investigated the acute hormonal responses of three different recovery times between sets of lower body weight training. Subjects were divided into three study groups and took 30-, 60-, and 120-second breaks, respectively, between the training sets; the results of the study are perfectly in line with the rest of the research; acute GH responses were higher in the group with 30 seconds of recovery than with 60 or 120 seconds.

In conclusion, the science indicates that **recovery times between sets are an important training variable**, affecting both acute responses and chronic adaptations induced by weight training. In general, bodybuilders prefer fairly short rest periods between sets, about 1-2 minutes on average, while powerlifters often require up to 5 minutes of rest between heavy sets; this is because, as we have seen, shorter recovery times are associated with an increase in the anabolic hormonal response, in particular GH, but also with good stimulation of testosterone (which, however, is optimized with breaks longer than 2 minutes). Several studies have reported a significant correlation of hormone levels with the amount of growth for both type I and type II muscle fibers.

These theoretical concepts can be translated into the daily practice of those who train, and, clearly, the recovery times between sets must also be adapted to the type of exercise performed. In particularly demanding compound multi-joint exercises, such as squats, presses, deadlifts and rowing, a longer recovery is necessary to restore energy, repeat the performance at its best and perform the established number of required repetitions. Vice versa, in single-joint exercises such as leg extensions, good mornings and curls, recovery times can be as short as 1 minute, to better exploit the metabolic effect of the exercise.

CHAPTER 12

Frequency: recovery between workouts

Massimo Spattini

In the previous chapter, we discussed the best length of rest between sets to maximize muscle growth and strength. Now, I would like to talk about the best duration of the break between one workout and another, i.e., the frequency of training. By making a brief excursus into the history of bodybuilding, we note that the first important athletes, such as Steve Reeves, a famous actor in numerous mythological films, used to train the whole body in a single session, three times a week. Later, in the 70s, bodybuilders began to differentiate workouts into "split routines", a system by which the body is divided into two or three parts and only one part is trained in a session; by doing so, the muscles are trained approximately twice a week with 4-6 workouts per week. This was the trend until the late 1980s. Since the 90s, a modified version of split routines began to spread in which a maximum of two muscles were trained at a time and, nowadays, most competitive bodybuilders train by dividing the body into individual muscle groups, training each one once a week; no one trains a muscle group more than twice a week. A recent school of thought offers particularly short and infrequent workouts, conveying the message that training less and less often is the solution.

It is obvious that **the rest between one workout and another affects natural recovery**, which is one of the three variables at the basis of muscle growth, the others being nutrition and training. That means that we can train as hard as we can and follow a perfect diet, but if we don't recover enough, we won't be able to overcompensate and there will be no growth. Actually, there would even be a risk of overtraining and losing some of the results. Recovery between workouts is essential to promote complete recovery, repair functional damage to muscle structures, decrease the risk of injury, recover mentally, and relieve muscle or joint pain caused by working out. Obviously, the amount of rest that we need depends on the type of training, our day job, age, level of physical conditioning and/or how long we have been training, and, last but not least, our genetic factors. In general, practical experience indicates that working out three times a week is ideal for beginners, with at least one day of rest between workouts, and various studies have provided similar indications.

There is also a specific recovery time related to the trained muscle groups. While smaller muscle groups such as the arms and calves can recover in 48 hours, larger muscle groups such as the back and legs need more time. So, a beginner routine might consist of two or at most three total body workouts per week (skipping legs in the midweek workout), or three workouts per week in a split routine, dividing the body into two parts. As training experience increases, it is necessary to increase the stimulus by increasing volume or intensity, using specific techniques. Advanced athletes, compared to beginners, almost always have a higher training volume. While 3-4 sets per muscle group may be sufficient for a beginner, advanced athletes normally perform at least double that, if not triple. This increase in training volume leads to the need to further divide training into several parts, possibly training the biceps with the pectorals and the triceps with back muscles to stimulate the arms several times, bringing the training frequency to four or even six times a week, in such a way that, in any case, at least the minimum 48-hour recovery is maintained between training the same muscle.

Many athletes train several times a day to perform better in competitions. Professional bodybuilders often train in the morning and then do a second workout in the evening. Training twice a day is a "ritual", for example, for soccer players, wrestlers and runners. Yet, the effects of these training programs are not well known. It would seem logical that, if you exercise more, you will make more gains. But is it true? Dr. Ola Ronsen and her collaborators at the Norwegian National Sports Center measured hormonal response after two endurance workouts conducted on the same day. The second workout produced an exaggerated response in the levels of stress hormones, such as adrenaline, norepinephrine, cortisol and growth hormone, while the second training session had a suppressed level of testosterone. These responses suggest that the body may not be able to adequately adjust to these excess workloads. Bodybuilders and other athletes should remember that doing more is not necessarily the best training strategy, nor is doing less. Choosing a program that produces results is ideal, and must be identified on an individual basis.

A mainly concentric type of contraction training allows for muscle recovery over a 48-hour period. High-intensity eccentric training, on the other hand, requires at least 4-5 or more days of recovery, as the muscle micro-lesions induced by this training are greater and require more time to be repaired; DOMS (delayed muscle pain) also lasts longer, so a more prolonged recovery is required to be able to retrain without the limitations induced by pain. For this reason, training schedules have become widespread among advanced athletes in which the muscles are trained only once a week. It could be said that beginner athletes have a lower organic recovery capacity but recover sooner at a muscular level and can train the single muscle groups closer together, while advanced athletes have a higher organic recovery speed, given their training condition but, depending on the specific training intensity, they require a longer recovery time for the individual muscle group. Therefore, the rule according to which beginners recover faster at the muscular level and can train a single muscle even three times a week is likely because their training is normally not at maximum

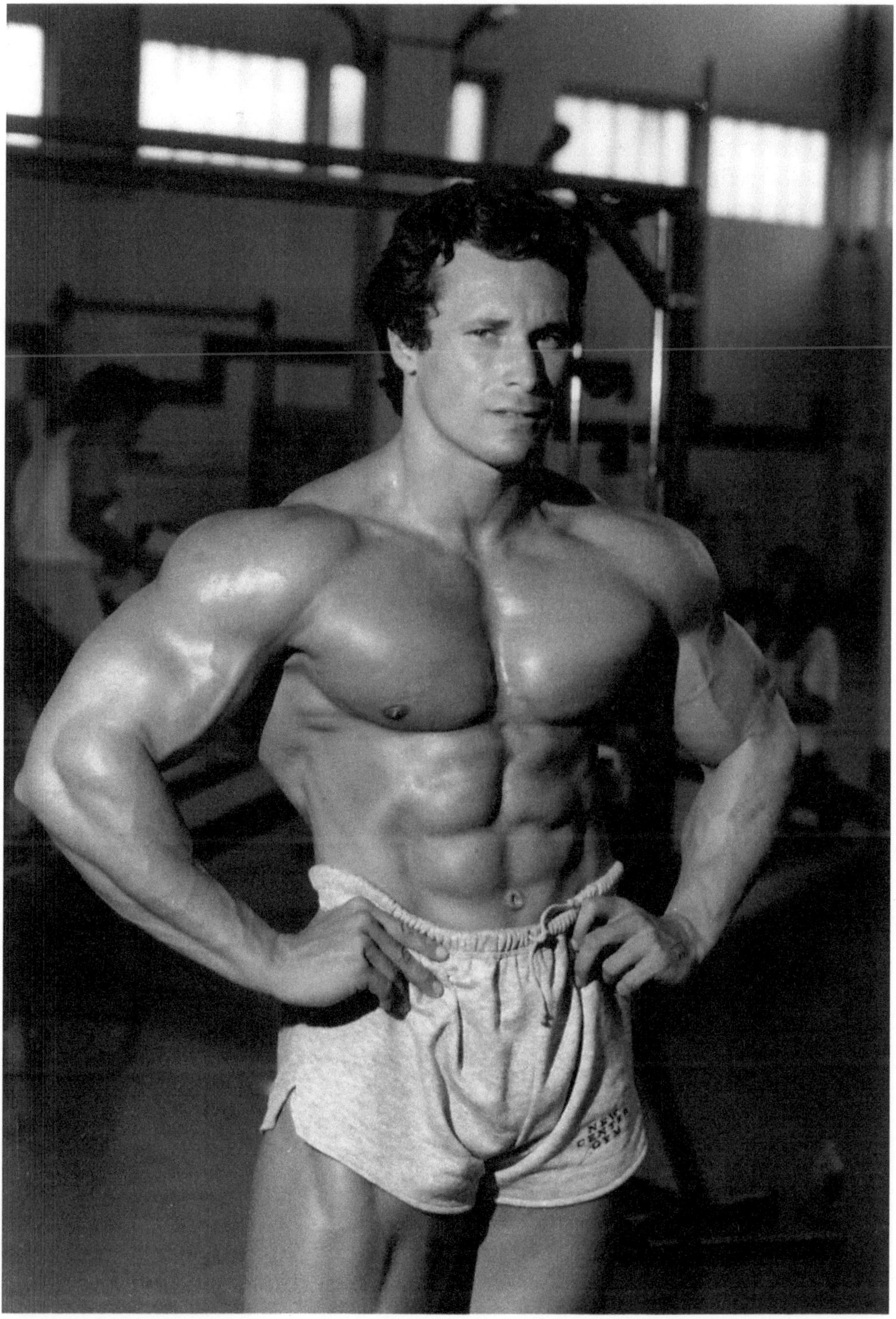

intensity and not even particularly emphasized in the eccentric phase. There is a reason why beginners might benefit from heavy training followed by a long period of rest. You certainly know that the fibers most responsible for strength and hypertrophy are fast-twitch type IIb fibers. In a study by Anderson et al., resistance training combined with substantial rest between workouts was shown to promote the transformation of intermediate type IIa fibers into fast-twitch type IIb fibers. In this experiment, researchers initially verified that the muscle fibers which were exposed to intense weight training had decreased their percentage of fast-twitch fibers from 9% to 2%, but following a long rest, the fast-twitch fibers increased to 18% and, among other things, correlated with a general increase in strength. Since increasing the number of IIb fibers is particularly helpful for beginners to maximize strength and hypertrophy, heavy-weight training followed by an extended recovery period is probably the best strategy; on the contrary, in advanced athletes in whom the conditioning of all types of muscle fibers and angiogenic and sarcoplasmic development is essential, it is advisable to vary the stimulus using techniques that involve lighter weights and a higher training frequency.

Given the obvious importance of training frequency for adaptation, many studies have been conducted in order to establish the best frequency to stimulate hypertrophy, but it doesn't work like that! To date, only one study has compared the results of one set per exercise performed three times a week versus three sets performed on the same day. The result was better in those who performed the exercise three times a week. The limitation of this study is that only three sets per muscle group were performed per week, and this is a workload that does not reflect that of competitive athletes.

Recently, Brad Schoenfeld, one of the leading authorities in the field of training for muscle development, and author of more than 60 published studies, carried out a controlled study in which he compared two routines that included 21 exercises (three exercises per muscle group) targeting major muscle groups in athletes with at least four years of training. Those who performed the split routine trained split muscles three days a week. More precisely: (1) chest and back; (2) legs and calves; (3) shoulders, biceps and triceps. The others followed a routine in which they performed only one multiset exercise per muscle group, but three times a week. The total volume of training remained the same and, therefore, the result would depend solely and exclusively on the variation in training frequency. At the end of the study, the group that achieved the best results was the one that trained three times a week.

This result, which in light of current knowledge may seem surprising, is related to some physiological aspects. Muscle growth is regulated by a balance between protein synthesis and catabolism, and current research indicates that the protein synthesis stimulus remains active for at least 48 hours after training. The body's ability to recover and adapt is important and allows for **supercompensation**, a complex mechanism that includes various biochemical, metabolic and hormonal factors, which allows the body to carry out a subsequent training session in the best possible conditions.

The law of supercompensation commonly requires a recovery time ranging from 48 to 72 hours, leading to higher energy levels that last several hours. However, you lose its positive effect shortly afterwards (the problem is that in bodybuilding, supercompensation concerns both the specific muscular group and the organism, and this makes things more complex).

To sum up, this evidence shows that obtaining the best muscle development requires **muscular training about twice a week**. This can be achieved with a training schedule in which the body is divided into two parts: one day dedicated to the lower part, another day to the upper part, performing four workouts a week; or, with a workout routine that divides the body into three parts: (1) push muscles, i.e. chest, shoulders and triceps; (2), legs and calves; (3) pulley muscles, i.e. lats, rear deltoids and biceps, with an alternation of three training days and one rest day.

Obviously, these considerations are valid for athletes who can devote time to training at an almost professional level, and it is no coincidence that Schoenfeld's study involved college students who were not subject to strenuous or particularly stressful jobs. A study conducted at the School of Medicine and Biomedical Sciences at the State University of New York showed that, in stressful situations, training would further increase insulin resistance, increasing the risks of metabolic syndrome, inflammation and, therefore, premature aging. Sleep is essential for the recovery process, for higher GH production and for a decrease in cortisol levels, as GH exerts a suppressive effect on the production of this substance. The *Experimental Brain Research* journal has published some data showing that lack of sleep compromises postural stability, which is essential for the correct execution of exercises.

Training can be detrimental in case of stress or fatigue. Therefore, it is better to rest or relax to restore energy. For a "normal" person, training must be modulated in a personalized way, taking into account work rhythms and the "stress factor", but despite this, the key concept to take home is that "less is not always more". That would be too convenient!

CHAPTER 13

Training periodization

Riccardo Gaspari

For many years now, periodization has been a much discussed and controversial topic within the bodybuilding circles. In this chapter, we will try to outline its meaning and guidelines according to the dictates of scientific research, the veracity of the method and personal experiences.

Periodizing means systematically varying training parameters and variables within a program designed over the long term to avoid stalemates in progress, injuries, overtraining and excessive stress, with the ultimate aim of ensuring the maximization of gains, recovery, adaptations, and, therefore, results.

The origins of periodized resistance training date back to the 1950s, when a group of sports scientists, athletic trainers and professional coaches from Eastern Europe noticed that, excluding the state of fitness of their athletes (professionals of various disciplines), hard workouts extended over time led to disappointing performance levels.

From this conclusion, the team to adjust volume and intensity parameters, and introduced a real revolution in training planning to maximize the athletic performance of the practitioners, developing cyclically alternating high-volume, low-intensity training phases with high-intensity, low-volume training phases.

However, the real exploit of this methodology occurred between the end of the 60s and the beginning of the 70s, when, following the publication of the first studies, established researchers such as Leonid Matveyev, Nikolaj Ozolin and others recognized periodization as its own scientific concept, expanding its practice to Russia, Romania and Germany. Matveyev and Ozolin presented the concepts of periodization to the rest of the world in 1972 at the Munich Olympics.

Over the years, there have been many periodization proposals, so much so that it has become a predominant method both in the programming of progressive overload training and in other sports disciplines.

It is interesting to note how the **concept of periodization** has received different definitions from authoritative professionals. Dawson (1996) defines it as a sensible, well-planned training approach that leads to maximizing training gains and perfor-

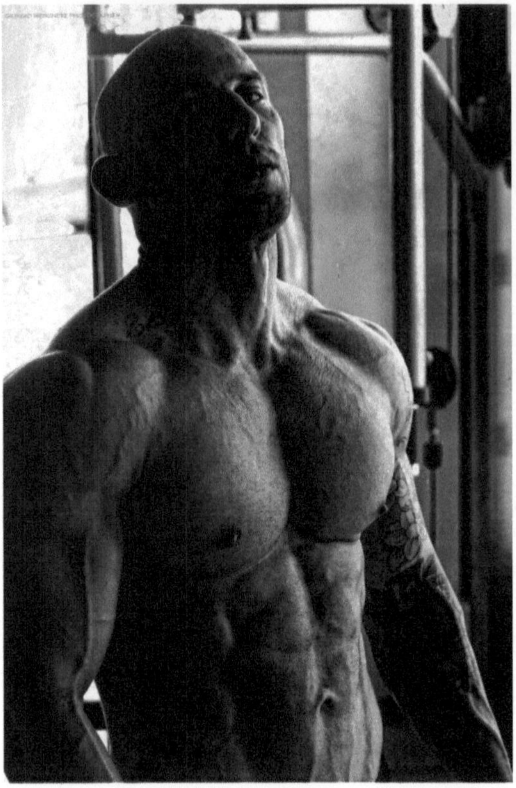

mance improvement. Nadori and Granek (1989) define it as a predetermined sequence of training sessions and competitions. Finally, Issurin (2003) defines the concept of training periodization as the intentional sequence of different training components (long-, medium-, and short-term training cycles and sessions) to achieve the desired state and results from the athlete.

Putting personal considerations aside for a moment, we can see how periodization has always and only been considered an extremely productive methodology, if not even a guarantee of improvement in sports performance.

To better understand this methodology, we must focus, albeit quickly, on the concepts of a training microcycle, mesocycle and macrocycle, which represent the basis on which training periodization is studied.

A **training microcycle** refers to a short training cycle that covers a period of 7-10 days. A **mesocycle** refers to a cycle made up of a series of microcycles and a variable period of time which starts from 2 weeks and usually reaches 8 weeks, although it is not uncommon in some subjective cases or in particular sports disciplines to witness mesocycles lasting 12 weeks, because meoscycles are designed according to the development of a specific phase, either preparation, peak phase or transition, or the period preceding a competition.

As we have seen, periodization derives from the manipulation of volume and intensity parameters in their basics, but currently, the variables that can be manipulated in order to periodize a long-term training program, while maintaining the volume/intensity cornerstone, have expanded dramatically; among these, we must remember the types of contraction (speed of movement), the inability to train to muscle failure and the nutritional state, which add to the number and order of exercises, both total and per muscle group, to the number of sets and repetitions, the type of exercises, the loads used, the frequency of training and recovery times.

Of all the periodization models proposed over the years, science has only recognized four. **Linear** or **traditional periodization** (Kraemer and Fleck, 2007), is a progression of high-volume, low-intensity workouts to achieve lower volume and increase intensity over the various cycles. It should be noted that traditional or linear periodization is the predecessor to the other models, as it was conceived by Russian scientist Leonid Matveyev in the 1950s and until recently was strongly promoted by well-known authors such as Mike Stone and Tudor Bompa (Tabs. 13.1 and 13.2).

The second model is the **non-linear** or **undulating periodization** (Frankel and Kravitz, 2000) (Tab. 13.3), in which the volume and intensity of training are increased and decreased on a regular basis a fixed pattern, but always different from the traditional model. It was created and developed through contributions by training scientists such as Yuri Verkhoshansky and other renowned professionals like Charles Poliquin.

The third model is **reverse linear periodization** (Rhea et al., 2004), which includes an inversion of the parameters of the traditional version, and starts with a low-volume and high-intensity work to progressively arrive at a model of high-volume, low-intensity training.

Table 13.1 Long-term linear periodization model by Lorenz et al.*

Week 4-8	Week 8-12	Week 12-16	Week 16-24
Endurance	***Hypertrophy***	***Strength***	***Power***
3 sets × 15-20 RM	3-4 sets × 10-12 RM	3-4 sets × 6-10 RM	3 sets × 3-5 RM
Total sets: 42	Total sets: 28-32	Total sets: 22-27	Total sets: 21
Rest: 30-45 seconds	Rest: 45-60 seconds	Rest: 2-3 minutes	Rest: 3-5 minutes

* Periodization: Current Review and Suggested Implementation for Athletic Rehabilitation. *Sports Health* 2010.

Table 13.2 Traditional periodization model according to Tudor O. Bompa*

Mesocycle	Sets (volume)	Repetitions	% di 1RM (intensity)
Hypertrophy	3-5	8-12	60-75% (10-20 RM)
Strength	3-5	6-8	80-85% (6-8 RM)
Power	3-5	4-6	85-90% (2-6 RM)
Peak	3-5	2-4	>90% (1-4 RM)

* Periodization: Theory and Methodology of Training. *Human Kinetics* 1999.

Table 13.3 Frankel and Kravitz goal-specific parameter guidelines

Variables	Hypertrophy	Strength	Power	Transition
Sets	1-5	1-5	1-5	1-2
Repetitions	9-12	6-8	1-5	13-20
Weeks	2-3	2-3	2-3	1-2

* Periodization: Latest Studies and Practical Applications. IDEA Personal Trainer 2000;11(1):15-16.

Finally, the fourth model is **block periodization** (Helms et al., 2014), which uses three or four mesocycles that are taken from normal linear periodization.

Of all four types, the only one with flexible programming choice is non-linear undulating periodization, which can be transformed into daily, weekly, scheduled or flexible non-linear periodization.

There is also another form of periodization that was very popular at the time called **overreaching periodization**, a system presented by Stone et al. (1999) which calls for periodic organization of a short-term phase, lasting 1 or 2 microcycles, in which volume or intensity are increased and at the end of which you can return to your normal training program. To better understand this, we need to address the concept of overreaching and, to do so, we need to outline the differences between eustress and distress. **Eustress** represents positive stress that leads our body to a favorable or, in any case, sought-after adaptation (for example, hypertrophic adaptation), while **distress** represents excessive stress to which our body is unable to adapt (instead of adapting, the organism succumbs to this stress, leading us to inevitable overtraining). An example of eustress can be exposing yourself to the sun for tanning in an intelligent way, while exposing yourself to the sun excessively would inevitably lead to sunburn, which represents a clear example of distress; likewise, training intelligently (eustress) will lead to hypertrophy, while training recklessly (distress) will lead to overtraining.

Overreaching is a progressive accumulation of fatigue that precedes overtraining; it is an acute phase of eustress that precedes distress. In this "window", our body begins to give way but, if we use this state intelligently, we can create magic instead of disaster; this time window represents the greatest stimulus of adaptation for our body.

It is at this moment that our body is on the verge of giving in to the accumulation of workload we have subjected it to, but if we include a couple of weeks of deloading, we can guaranteee truly optimal supercompensation. It can be said that each mesocycle should end with the search for overreacing, so as to maximise gains during training deloading days.

We are now ready to discuss the world of practice, in which traditional periodization of bodybuilding training should include the beginning of the macrocycle with a conditioning period, followed by a mesocycle dedicated to strength. Subsequently one would go on to face a mesocycle which calls for the involvement of all the com-

Table 13.4 Comparison between the three periodization models

	Week 1-3	Week 4-6	Week 7-9	Week 10-12	Week 13-15
Linear periodization	3×10	4×6	5×3	6×2	8×1
Non-linear periodization	3×10	4×6	3×8	4×3	4×5
Reverse periodization	8×1	6×2	5×3	4×6	3×10

ponents of the muscle cell (probably at high volume and low intensity), followed by a mesocycle which involves the use of special techniques (certainly at high intensity and low volume), then face a training stage dedicated to the deficient muscle groups, ending with the definition stage, all mixed with targeted unloading periods that have been previously and carefully decided.

I think that in theory, this is all perfect, but in practice things change, and not just by a little. I'm not saying periodization is useless, but I'm arguing that in bodybuilding, unlike most other sports, it doesn't do much.

Unless we are talking about really young athletes who approach bodybuilding, strength training – understood as a real training protocol, such as those followed by weightlifters, pitchers, jumpers, or as those followed in football, basketball, swimming, etc. – has little to do with the results a bodybuilder or fitness model aspires to achieve. In the medium to long term, training with weights guarantees a significant increase in strength: how many of us, at the beginning of our careers, without any basis or criterion, started to bench press 30 kg and after a while found ourselves using 50?

And again, how many times have we done a 3×8 shoulder press with 50 kg, discovering that after a few weeks, instead of 8 repetitions, we were able to do 12? Well, you too have indirectly experienced an increase in strength from the performed program; in the case of young athletes or if you want to particularly increase a load on a muscle area that may be a little lacking, or even just for personal satisfaction, running a program dedicated to strength will be extremely useful. Compared to the result that the mirror, the camera or the competition stage requires, a protocol exclusively dedicated to increasing strength will have contributed very little.

Personally, I find it more appropriate and productive to stop at 6-8 repetitions and reach 4 very rarely (indicatively, no more than three times a year), primarily for hypertrophic intent, and then to stay as far away as possible from the risk of injury.

I exploit this concept a lot, productively, in the classic training sets. Let's take a 4×8 as an example: I like to start with an 8 RM load to muscle failure in the first set and keep it unchanged for all the following three sets; this allows me to have four productive sets. Obviously, from the second to the fourth set, the repetitions will decrease progressively (if I'm able to do 8 reps, the initial load would have been too light) and in the following weeks, you will see that strength will progressively increase.

Before long, you'll find yourself completing all four sets with eight reps using a load that initially only allowed you one set of eight.

At this point, your strength, resilience and workload will have increased, and as you approach four full sets of eight, your intensity will have eased slightly. As you can see, we have already done a sort of periodization that includes the use of intensity, volume, strength and hypertrophy variables, and all in a simple 4×8, without overcomplicating things. Once the four sets of eight have been completed, we increase the load used in the previous workout by 5% and start again with the new 8 RM. Simple and above all, functional.

Another aspect that I can't stand and that I hope none of you can stand anymore is "training for the definition period": there is no such thing as training for definition or training for mass, but rather a diet for one or the other goal. Certainly, some training techniques will help you burn a few more calories or highlight some further details, but most of the results (at least 97%) will always depend on the diet you are following.

As far as muscle groups are concerned, I strongly believe that much more than a mesocycle should be dedicated to them and I find it better to study their training within the entire macrocycle and not just with spot-checks.

Deloading is another aspect that has a discrepancy between theory and practice (except for neophytes). Bodybuilding is a personal activity, in which deciding the deloading periods depends on countless external, internal, physical and psychological variables of the athlete. In twenty years of professional work in the world of fitness as a personal trainer and wellness consultant, and in as many years of weight training, I have noticed that simplicity has guaranteed me the best results. Using too many variables only leads to confusion and loss of control. I think it is better to have a well-defined route and a verifiable path in order to always be able to reach the goal in the best way and as soon as possible, with the smallest margin of error.

My periodization

The two variables maintained in a macrocycle are intensity and volume: as one increases, the other decreases.

A reconditioning period which includes **total body circuit training** lasts 4 weeks, the **first mesocycle** lasts 8 weeks and includes heavy training with a fixed pattern with the mono-frequency pyramid method, in which I increase the overloads. The body is divided into three parts (pushing muscles, pulling muscles and legs) and for the first 4 weeks three workouts per week are performed. In the following 4 weeks, four workouts per week are performed in rotation, approaching a multi-frequency workout. Although training volume is not too high, we are at the beginning of the macrocycle and we are about to face workouts which, by requiring muscle exhaustion with each set and seeking an increase in load, lead us to use significant intensity; consequently, it is inadvisable to immediately attack the body with a multi-frequency scheme, unless you have considerable athletic capacity, also understood as cardiovascular capacity, obviously superior to that obtained by carrying out cardio-fitness.When we talk about mono- or multifrequency in absolute terms, we make a serious mistake, because the study of a long-term training program must always be calibrated, not so much in terms of microcycles, macrocycles or various pre-set periods, but based on the starting point of the athlete we are about to train. They could come from a long period of rest or from the rehabilitation of an injury or they could be in very good shape.

The general principle (slightly different from my proposal, which is my personal approach) that should be applied, basically consists in starting with high-volume mono-frequency in order to be able to develop neuromuscular coordination capacity which, once optimized, will allow you to better deal with an increase in intensity, reducing the number of sets and increasing the loads used. Depending on your needs, the volume or intensity peaks will then be loosened or increased, in case you are looking for rest or an increase in conditioning. I have always done cardio training three times a week for 35-40 minutes in steady state mode, followed by core training on rest days or after weight training. For cardio, I prefer the elliptical cross trainer and the recumbent bike, while for abdominal training I like to alternate crunch exercises both with bodyweight and with added weights (on the machine or with cables), reverse crunches with bodyweight and hanging leg raises. I really like to get to muscle failure with each set of abs training and I much prefer to train with bodyweight rather than with added weights, which I include in my program from time to time anyway. I recommend keeping recovery relatively short, the arc between 30 seconds and one minute is the appropriate when you are unable to train the abdomen with consecutive sessions.

Training volume is relatively low and includes nine training sets divided into three exercises for the chest, back and quadriceps, all performed with a classic 8-6-4 pyramid, eight training sets divided into two exercises for deltoids and hamstrings, where the first exercise is performed with an 8-8-6-4 pyramid and the second with 8-6-4, and finally, biceps, triceps and calves, performed with six training sets divided into

Week 1-2-3-4 Monday: push muscles Wednesday: pull muscles Friday: legs	**Week 5** Monday: push muscles Tuesday: pull muscles Thursday: legs Friday: push muscles
Week 6 Monday: pull muscles Tuesday: legs Thursday: push muscles Friday: pull muscles	**Week 7** Monday: legs Tuesday: push muscles Thursday: pull muscles Friday: legs
Week 8 Monday: push muscles Tuesday: pull muscles Thursday: legs Friday: push muscles	

Note: For beginners, those recovering from a long hiatus, or those unable to recover from volume gains, the pattern of the first 4 weeks can be maintained at this initial stage. If the starting condition leads you to be extremely thin, you can avoid cardio sessions and it is advisable to train the abdomen after weight training.

two exercises, once again trained with an 8-6-4 pyramid. The trapezius and rear deltoids are trained in a single exercise in an 8-6-4 pattern. In order to maximize results and protect yourself from the risk of injury, it is essential to maintain a perfect and controlled execution technique in all sets. Recovery times between sets and exercises are 2 minutes and the abdomen is trained for 15 consecutive minutes.

At the beginning of this program, there are two tricks for starting off on the right foot and using the correct loads: if you are unable to maintain an isometric weight for 20-30 seconds before starting an exercise, this means that the chosen weight is excessive and between the pyramid sets, it is desirable to increase the loads used in the sets by 5%.

At the end of these 8 weeks, I follow a **cross-stimulus training table** (the predecessor of the training that I will present later in this volume) which calls for an increase in volume compared to the previous training: this training includes four sessions a week (I tried five sessions, but the results were clearly lower), alternating one week of heavy loads and reduced volume (so as not to deviate from the work done previously and to create a continuum) with one week of moderate loads with slow and controlled execution. In order to create a constant and productive stimulus, the push-pull-leg model is abandoned and, from a certain point of view, the same goes for multi-frequency training, which distributes the muscle groups in an unconventional way, but with the guarantee of remarkable productivity in terms of results.

The duration of this phase depends on the date in which I must be in top form: I tend to keep it for 12 weeks and sometimes I don't deny that I have also kept it for 16.

Cardio is done three times a week at the end of each workout for 35-40 minutes (never after leg workouts) or, on recovery days, the core is trained to exhaustion at the end of each workout with six sets per day: I change the exercises at each training session.

In the week that I use heavy loads, muscle failure is sought during each set, and I use explosive exercise executions; in the week with higher repetitions, on the other hand, my goal is muscle burning, and all sets are performed in a way that creates continuous, non-stop tension by using 4-5 seconds for both the concentric and eccentric phases of each repetition.

The choice of exercises is almost obligatory: in week A (see the table on the following page) basic exercises with free weights are essential, while in week B (see the following table) isotonic machines, cables and all complementary exercises are ideal. Personally, I have always found it fun and productive to choose exercises following the dictates of POF (Position Of Flexion by S. Holman); this guarantees us excellent muscle stimulation which, combined with a training schedule to be alternated weekly with another training schedule, leads to a perfect mix of motivation (this avoids the drop in enthusiasm that can happen over time with a fixed program) and hypertrophic stimulus (the muscles are really targeted from every possible angle).

The psychological aspect is absolutely not to be underestimated, because, within the guidelines for improving performance, the qualitative variables expressed by motivation, adherence and consent in tackling a training plan represent determining factors for the success of any program. As demonstrated by Stone et al. in 1999, these are psychological factors that greatly influence the quality and quantity of the work done during a training session: the lack of variations (which must, in any case, follow a continuum to ensure a successful path) inevitably leads to boredom and monotony, which will lower the athlete's performance and will lead them away from their goal.

My approach guarantees varying and complementary stimuli and adaptations, which generally result in greater effectiveness of the training program in the long term. Therefore, this mode of periodization offers psychological advantages linked to motivation and adherence in always carrying out workouts at 100%.

But let's turn to the program in practical terms.

To me, this represents "periodization" of training stimuli based on volume, intensity and sports psychology. Anything different and more distributed than what I have tried on myself and on my many clients over the years has produced inferior results. Clearly this is an example that can be easily modified using other training methods, intensity techniques and other parameters (for example, training density), but I decided to faithfully report what worked for me and what continues to work at its best while being able to share a concrete trace.

Monday	**Tuesday**	**Thursday**	**Friday**
Deltoids Biceps Triceps	Dorsal Lumbar Rear deltoids Trapezius	Biceps Anterior deltoid Gluteus Adductor	Quadriceps Hamstrings Calves

Week A		
Back/Pectorals/ Quads	Deltoids/Biceps/ Triceps/Hamstrings/Calves	Lumbar/Posterior deltoids/Trapezius/Anterior deltoid/Glutes/Adductor
12 sets Exercise 1: 8-8-6-4 Exercise 2: 4 × 8* Exercise 3: 4 × 8*	8 sets Exercise 1: 8-8-6-4 Exercise 2: 4 × 8*	4 sets Exercise 1: 8-8-6-4
All rest periods are 2 minutes between exercises and sets		

*In 4×8 exercises, use a load that leads to failure in the first set. In the following sets perform as many repetitions as possible (if the selected load is correct, it will hardly be possible to perform another eight repetitions, the number will certainly be lower) and maintain the load in the following weeks until you manage to close all four sets of eight repetitions with the same load; at this point, increase the load by 5% and start again. The 4×8, therefore, is a 4×8/max/max/max (max always <8) and **not** a 4×8/8/8/8.

Continues

Continued

Week B		
Back/Chest/Quads	Deltoids/Biceps/Triceps/Hamstrings/Calves	Lumbar/Posterior deltoids/Trapezius/Anterior deltoid/Glutes/Adductors
16 sets Exercise 1: 4 × 12 Exercise 2: 4 × 12 Exercise 3: 4 × 12 Exercise 4: 4 × 12	12 sets Exercise 1: 4 × 12 Exercise 2: 4 × 12 Exercise 3: 4 × 12	8 sets Exercise 1: 4 × 12 Exercise 2: 4 × 12
All rest periods are 1 minute between exercises and sets		
In all 4×12 exercises, use a load that leads to muscle failure only in the last set; perform the exercises with slow and controlled execution, maintaining continuous tension, maximum extension and maximum contraction without stopping; focus on finding the maximal muscle burn.		

What about the deload period? I have always included the deload method when I felt the need, either due to physical tiredness or mental tiredness. Believe me, one day there will be many unforeseen events and stressors that will lead you to have to take a few days off from training and I don't think there will ever be more appropriate scheduled deloading than during these periods, in which your body will ask you for it bodybuilding is a truly personal practice and no one will ever be as important for the achievement of your goals as yourself: listen to others, but always listen to yourself!

I would like to reiterate that my assessments are closely related to bodybuilding and not to most other sports, where periodization is truly essential for maximizing the desired sporting performance.

CHAPTER 14

DOMS invalidates "no pain, no gain"

Riccardo Gaspari

One of the most famous bodybuilding slogans is the timeless adage "no pain, no gain", but what does this statement really mean? What pain is this about?

For many years this phrase has been misunderstood, identifying "no pain" as the soreness that is felt in the days following training in a specific muscle group, using the extent of this soreness as a yardstick judgment of the profitability of the workout performed.

Nothing could be more wrong. The "no pain" indicates the amount of sacrifice and determination made in carrying out the workout, the ability to increase the resistance threshold to muscle-burning induced by the performance of the sets, the determination with which one tries to overcome, in each workout, one's limits and the constant challenge with oneself; moreover, it means being on a diet when others can eat anything they want, resting while others go partying and all those things and aspects that distinguish the lifestyle of a bodybuilding athlete from that of "normal" people.

The most serious mistake, however, is to use the muscle soreness of the days following training as a yardstick for judging the effectiveness and productivity of a workout. Let's try to clarify this matter.

This soreness is called **DOMS** (**Delayed Onset Muscle Soreness**, or **delayed onset muscle pain**); DOMS are micro-lacerations that occur to the detriment of the muscle tissue due to overload, especially in the eccentric phase of the movement.

In order to avoid confusion, let's explain that there are two types of muscle soreness induced by exercise: **Acute-Onset Muscle Soreness**, which is the one felt during and/or immediately after anaerobic training (comes with burning sensation) and is directly linked to the excess of lactic acid, typical of lactic anaerobic training (transitional event, since lactic acid is disposed of by the body at the latest within 60 minutes from the end of the activity); and **Delayed-Onset Muscle Soreness** (Fig. 14.1), which is generally perceived in a period of time following anaerobic physical activity, finding its peak between 24 and 48 hours after the end of the activity, and is absolutely not related to the production of lactic acid.

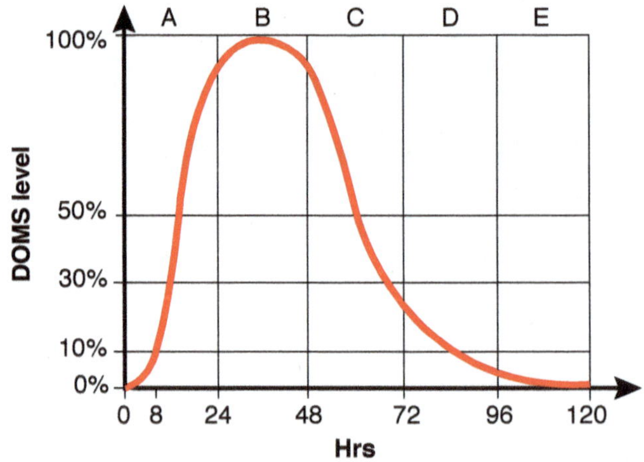

Figure 14.1 The trend of delayed onset muscle soreness. The phases are divided into: (A) onset; (B) exacerbation; (C) decrease; (D) disappearance; (E) full recovery. (Edited from: author A7N8X-Own work_https://commons.wikimedia.org/wiki/File:DOMS.svg).

Once these concepts are understood, it is essential to understand that DOMS cannot be used as indicators to evaluate the quality of the workout performed.

There are two primary theories on DOMS from which subsequent research on the development of DOMS started, Armstrong (1984) and Smith (1991). In 1984, Armstrong proposed his theory on the development of DOMS based on a very large review, stating that the structural proteins of muscle cells and connective tissue are torn and destroyed by high mechanical forces produced by (especially eccentric) training; structural damage to the sarcolemma alters the permeability of cell membranes, allowing an influx of calcium from the interstitial site; at this point, excess amounts of calcium inhibit cellular respiration, decreasing the cell's ability to produce ATP and to remove calcium from within.

Higher calcium levels within the cell activate a calcium-dependent proteolytic enzyme that degrades Z-lines, troponin and tropomyosin, and this progressive postexercise destruction of the sarcolemma allows intracellular components to diffuse into the interstitial space and plasma; these substances attract monocytes by activating mast cells and histocytes in the damaged area. Histamine, quinine and potassium accumulate in the interstitial space due to the activation of phagocytosis and cell necrosis, and these substances, as well as increased edema and temperature, can stimulate pain receptors resulting in DOMS.

In 1991, after understanding that acute inflammation in response to muscle fiber and connective tissue damage caused by eccentric exercise is the primary mechanism involved in the development of DOMS, and that many of the symptoms of acute inflammation, such as pain, swelling and loss of functionality, occur in conjunction with DOMS, Smith proposed his theory regarding the mechanism of development of DOMS, stating that the destruction of the connective tissue and muscle tissue is caused by eccentric exercises; consequently, within a few hours, the blood concentration of neutrophils increases, migrating towards the site of the lesion for several hours following the event; at the same time, the monocytes migrate towards the injured area from 6 to 12 hours after the exercise and the macrophages synthesize E-prostaglandins; at this point, prostaglandins sensitize type III and IV pain afferent neurons and elicit a sensation of pain in response to intramuscular pressure caused by movement and palpation; the combination of increased blood pressure and hypersensitivity produces the sensation of DOMS.

According to a research study done by Dr. Paul Henning in 2013, the evidence for the quality of a training schedule based on DOMS is inconsistent and absolutely not recommendable as a measure of the results produced by training.

In 2010, another research carried out by Flann et al. demonstrated that muscle hypertrophy can occur independently of any symptoms of muscle damage, such as DOMS.

Another study conducted by Schoenfeld and Contrares in 2013 states with absolute certainty that caution must be used in drawing qualitative conclusions, given the poor correlation between DOMS and the extent of EIMD (Exercise-Induced Muscle Damage), i.e. the muscle damage induced from exercise.

Some teams of scientists have studied the factors related to DOMS produced by overload training in depth. They suggested that, presumably, such DOMS derive largely from the laceration of the connective tissue of the muscle and its tendon insertion. In his research, Abraham (1977) noted that the urinary excretion of the amino acid hydroxyproline (a specific byproduct of connective tissue catabolism) was higher in subjects who experienced muscle soreness than in those who did not, and because a significant increase in urinary hydroxyproline levels indicates an increase in both collagen degradation and synthesis, he concluded that more intense training damages the connective tissue, increasing collagen degradation and creating an imbalance in the metabolism of the same molecule. The rate of collagen synthesis increases to compensate for this imbalance.

Furthermore, further research has shown that some muscles are more prone than others to experience DOMS; it seems that there is also a genetic component which, in some individuals, causes the classic persistent pain in the days after the workout, while in other subjects this effect appears to be less significant.

Following the study mentioned above, Schoenfeld stated that high levels of pain should even be considered harmful, because they would correspond to a signal that should not be underestimated, i.e. the overcoming, by the athlete's muscle, of the ability to repair itself; it must also be considered that DOMS, if excessive, can interfere with the ability to train and reduce the will to train itself, compromising training intensity. In recent years, some studies have found that caffeine can help reduce DOMS. According to the study done by Maridakis et al. (2007), if caffeine is taken

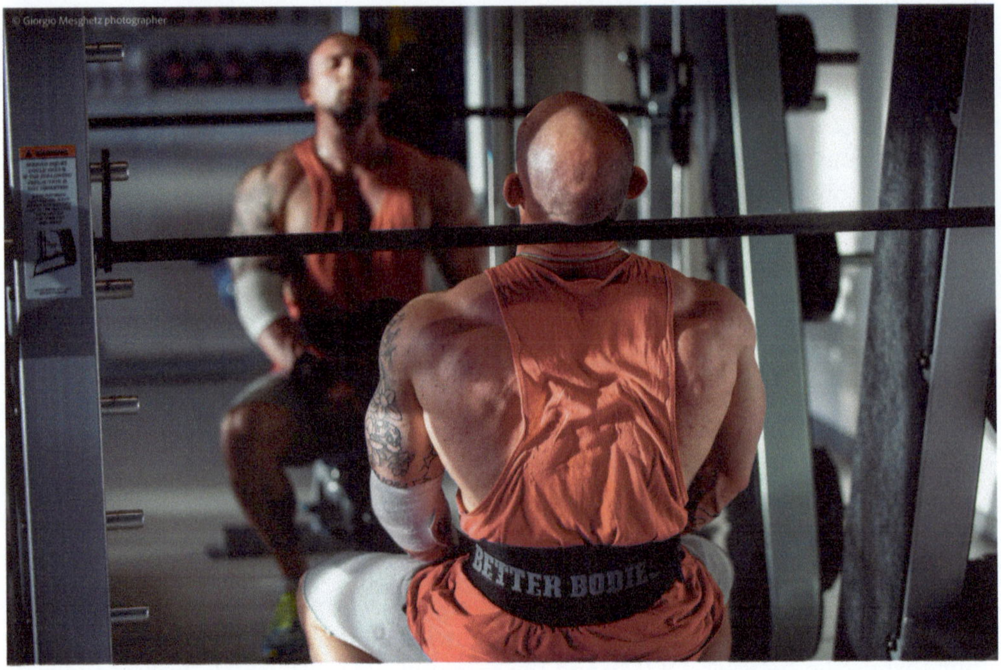

within 24-48 hours of the end of the eccentric activity, in the approximate amount of two cups of coffee, it can produce a significant reduction in pain (even up to 48%) resulting from the eccentric exercise in the following workout. In 2011, Karbaleifar et al. corroborated this thesis, suggesting that athletes can exploit this method to reduce muscle soreness perceived after an acute activity. More recent studies, such as Hurley et al. (2013), demonstrated – again confirming the above – that if 5 mg/kg of caffeine is taken (the equivalent of about three cups of coffee) even one hour before weight training, it can reduce DOMS.

In conclusion, we can say with certainty that using DOMS to evaluate the quality of a workout and the extent of muscle growth is extremely misleading. Based on the above, it is clear that DOMS are not indicators of good or bad training. I would argue that they are not even an index to be accounted for. The only value they can have is to provide an approximate measure of oxidative damage.

Don't waste time studying or tackling training tables based only on the search for extreme DOMS: in my opinion, the old adage "no pain, no gain" has a very different meaning.

CHAPTER 15

The speed of repetitions

Massimo Spattini

Muscles can perform a concentric contraction, thus producing force as they shorten; they can contract statically, thus producing force without performing any movement; alternatively, they can perform an eccentric contraction, thus producing force as they lengthen. The high tension exerted on the muscles during resistance exercises is a crucial element for muscle hypertrophy because it accelerates the entry of amino acids into muscle cells to form new contractile proteins. Furthermore, high tension breaks the muscle fibers, a phenomenon that is the basis of hypertrophy and possible muscle hyperplasia. **Eccentric contraction consists in lengthening the muscle**, therefore in the separation of the insertions, while in concentric contraction there is a shortening of the muscle, resulting in the approximation of the insertions. Based on these assumptions, it should be emphasized that muscles can create more tension by contracting eccentrically rather than concentrically and that, during an eccentric contraction, they develop more tension by contracting rapidly rather than slowly. It is interesting to know that, during a concentric contraction of the muscle, fast contractions produce relatively little force, while the opposite occurs during an eccentric contraction, since fast contractions, in this case, produce much more force.

Many amateur bodybuilders train concentrically and only occasionally eccentrically; moreover, on those few occasions, they perform the sets at low speed.

Before discussing some studies, let us try to understand what isokinetics consists of. **Isokinetics** is a method used in rehabilitation to evaluate and increase the strength and resistance of muscle groups, with which the muscles exert a force at a constant speed. The first study was carried out by a group of Canadian researchers led by Tim Shepstone. They found that fast, isokinetic training for 8 weeks resulted in an increase in the size of the largest (fastest-twitch) fibers and overall muscle strength compared to slow, eccentric training. The speed of contraction, on the other hand, had no effect on the size of the smallest fibers, i.e. the slow-twitch fibers. In a second study, through muscle biopsies taken from subjects after 8 weeks of training, it was found that high-speed isokinetic exercise resulted in greater damage (breaking) to muscle cells. The measurement was made at the level of the sarcomere, the basic contractile unit of the muscle fiber. In conclusion, therefore, we can confirm that muscle damage triggers muscle remodeling, and this results in an increase in muscle mass. If, for example, these findings were applied to training with free weights, high-speed resistance could prove to be a good way to trigger muscle growth. The tension generated in the muscle is the most important factor that triggers hypertrophy. Therefore, as high-speed, eccentric contractions produce more force than any other type of contraction, they promote muscle growth.

Just to make it clear, an **example of an eccentric exercise** in the weight room is the rapid lowering of the weight during a bench press (rapid lowering which always occurs under the control of the pectoral muscles, which remain contracted and control the barbell to avoid hitting the chest) or the dumbbell curl with the lowering part of the movement accelerated initially, as if you were "throwing" the dumbbell, but decelerated thereafter. This mode of execution resembles traditional eccentrics but happens much faster. The awareness of these physiological mechanisms confirmed an intuition that I had already had during the first years of training at Gold's Gym in Venice (California), where, observing many champions (especially Black ones), I had the impression that they "rattled" the weights without controlling them; this had raised great perplexities in me and had suggested that genetics was the most important element. Later, however, observing them more closely, I realized that those athletes actually imparted accelerations both in the concentric and in the eccentric phase. This way, even though it didn't seem like it, the weight was well controlled and held even in the eccentric phase, and not left at the mercy of gravity.

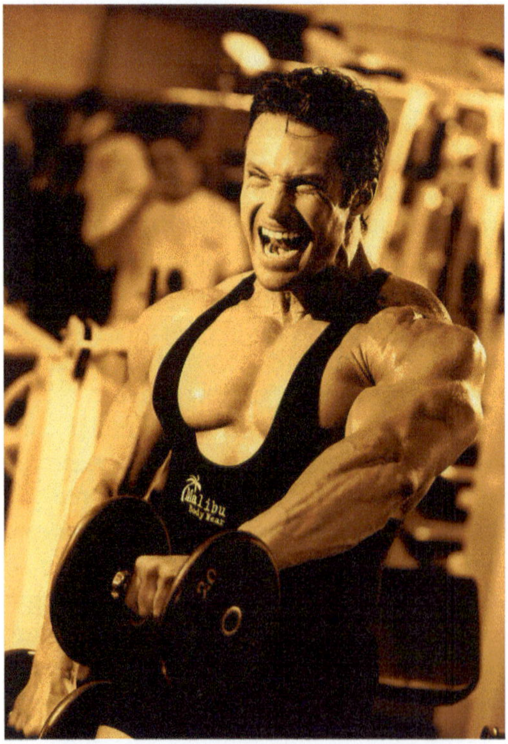

In addition, lifting weights explosively also trains the nervous system to activate muscles quickly and, in addition to promoting strength and power, it burns more calories than slower workouts. A study from Ball State University led by Scott Mezzetti showed that an explosive squat workout consumes about 12% more calories than the same workout done slowly. The researchers concluded that combinations of explosive weightlifting workouts with moderate-intensity exercise could lead to increased metabolic expenditure and promote fat loss. Explosive weight training "turns on the nervous system," which increases strength and the ability to accelerate the lift through greater neuromuscular activation.

Unilateral training is an efficient and alternative training method, which consists of exercising one side of the body at a time. Various studies have confirmed that training one limb individually generates a neuromuscular stimulus that also acts on the contralateral limb. Australian researchers have found that fast one-sided training has a greater effect on the untrained limb than slow training. The unilateral method stimulates the muscles more than using both limbs at the same time, so this method represents a good alternative that could lead to increased sports performance. Unilateral training also increases the strength of the non-active side. If extensions are done with the right knee, the left leg will still have a little training effect, even if it's doing nothing. This fact is very interesting and must be taken into consideration in the event of injuries affecting only one limb.

CHAPTER 16

The lack of basic techniques in bodybuilding

Federico Focherini

In any athletic endeavor, the **basic technique** is essential for success in that sport.

Technique is the path from which one cannot deviate. Every athlete's body has *boundaries* that should not be crossed. Technique is what sets a great champion apart from the average athlete.

You have to be in control of the technique. Mastering the technique is what allows the genetically less gifted athlete to reach goals that seem impossible.

If they lack technique, athletes keep working hard without obtaining results. They perform movements that require great effort but give minimal returns. Athletes who the technique manage to concentrate their strength which ensures maximum returns for effort expended.

How much emphasis should a bodybuilder place on technique?

Bodybuilders often fall into the trap of neglecting their technique and the correct stimulation of their muscles.

Many bodybuilders, or athletes who train with weights aiming to grow their muscle mass, pay little attention to technique in executing their exercises. Proper technique focuses on the actual working of the body's musculature. Athletes erroneously assume that very heavy loads (not lifted perfectly) or a high number of repetitions with low resistance will get them the results they want.

For the growth of muscle volume, many bodybuilders rely on the weight or the number of repetitions, but not on their muscles. Many visualize a goal weight in their minds ("I must manage to" lift it / push it / pull it), while others visualize a *number* of repetitions that needs to be reached and often stop as soon as they reach that number.

Ignoring the importance of muscle development by focusing on more or less reps and heavier or lighter weights

Spurring an athlete to do one more repetition makes no sense if they push or pull without "feeling" it, without contracting the muscle at spasm, i.e. without reaching the muscles limits of the contracting capacity.

In my opinion, this is just a "goodwill gesture" for its own sake. You don't need adrenaline, music that interrupts your focus or "motivational videos" that occupy your mind. In silent focus you have to bring your mind into the muscle. You have to visualize the fibers and communicate with the muscle without allowing any outside influences to interrupt your conversation. Then repeat the process endlessly by increasing the difficulty of the exercise. First, you have *to increase workloads, reduce recovery times, introduce techniques and stress the muscle for increasingly longer periods. And then,* **repeat and repeat and repeat for days, months and years.** It is not a hobby, it is not something you do once in a while to distract yourself. It is a discipline. It is work that will have to be constantly changed and will change you in return.

Real bodybuilding is constantly being subjected to extreme psycho-physical strain. **Bodybuilding is a continuous adaptation to stress!**

In any sport, technique and training to learn it perfectly probably account for 50% of the athletic result. The rest is genetics and athletic improvement. In my opinion, things are much less complicated than we make them.

You need to know how to help the technique guide the muscle in the right direction, **without performing motions that are unnatural for the body.**

Sometimes, in gyms, you see poorly performed exercises and instructors who do not notice their clients' deviation from the technique. They move weights like porters, **pushing and pulling**. That's all. But this is not how bodybuilding works.

Furthermore, it is absurd and ridiculous, in my opinion, to be in an environment where athletes lift weights surrounded by noise and distractions, such as cellphones, headphones or earphones. It is not possible to go under a heavy barbell or create a *mind-muscle connection* while texting on your cellphone, taking a "selfie", checking one of the many social networks while talking with a friend or listening to deafening music. The moment a mind-muscle connection is created, one must have the ability to visualize the trained muscle, control the breathing, listen to the heart, feel the muscles and the arrival of lactic acid, which interrupts the contraction, or understand if an injury may be close.

Silence is essential!

You should not train using adrenaline or the energy boost from your last pre-workout supplement. We need to face the weight with the testosterone capacity of our body, with the contractile capacity of our muscle group, and with our brain which gives the impulse to the nerves and, consequently, to the muscle to contract and lengthen. It is a gesture that is controlled by our mind, it is not a nervous and violent gesture dictated by the athlete's impetus.

Below is a personal observation, which I consider precise and to the point, to explain what weight training for muscle growth means to me.

When I train, I always have the movement of the metronome in mind. For me, it's something obvious and natural, and no one has ever had to explain it to me.

Bodybuilders should internalize and clearly perceive their own body and the rhythms of movement.
*Giovanni Cianti defines it as "***the vital breath of the bodybuilder***".*
I believe that true bodybuilders must feel within themselves the "tick-tock" of the metronome, a bit like Ludwig van Beethoven who, while being completely deaf, had the need to perfectly mark the time inside of himself and asked Mälzel, the inventor of the modern metronome, to create something that would help him compose music, and thus continue to live.
Mälzel built this instrument for him and, although Beethoven had completely lost his hearing, by observing the swing of that upside-down pendulum he was able to regain possession of the tempo of his music, in order to be able to write it again later.
He "felt it inside" and visualized it. It was his, alone, in his silence. This is why I believe that silence and solitude in our minds are necessary in order to establish such a violent and at the same time rhythmic dialogue. I believe there must be a symbiosis but above all, a fusion between the hardness of the movement impressed on the tool, its musical rhythm, and silence in the most absolute isolation.
A scream in the silence.

The basic law is "learn how to do the exercises"!

You need to understand how to get from point A to point B.

How should we move from the starting point to reach a pre-determined and precise goal? This fundamental task is fulfilled by technique, which teaches us movement control. This will lead you step by step through the process that essentially teaches us that technique is all *about domination of the weights through focused muscle contraction.*

When an athlete is performing a heavy exercise of 6-8 reps, they will certainly have their mind engaged with the weight. If, on the other hand, the athlete has to perform sets of 15-20 repetitions, they will concentrate more on the number of repetitions, often without caring much about the performance of the motion itself. Therefore, the lifter is almost always concerned with *how much weight* or *how many repetitions*, not *how to control* the weight during the movement.

Weight is certainly important, but only if it is controlled in the right way. For many months, if not years, the beginner athlete will have to focus on increasing **strength endurance** and **explosive strength**, in order to then be able to train as a bodybuilder.

In other words, the athlete's initial goal is to become strong. At the same time, they will always have to be *in charge* of what they do, of the way they handle the weights. **They will have to become increasingly strong while in complete control of the tools they use. The lifter must master the weight, not the other way around!**

Try to bend your arms, as we do when we do the barbell biceps movement, 8-12 times, quickly. You have no weight in your hand. Can you say that you feel the muscle working and pumping blood? You can't.

Now let's try to perform the same movement, again without the barbell, but performing each repetition very slowly, as if you were underwater; as if you were moving immersed in a liquid even thicker than water.

Stretch your arm throughout the movement and, having reached the apex, contract the biceps for 2 seconds. You are still not holding any weight, but at the end of the repetitions, you will feel the biceps differently than before, more turgid with blood. You'll feel like you've an effort.

In both cases, you didn't have any weight to lift, but the difference was significant. This is the sensation you must feel when you first put the muscle into action, and you must also feel it when you use weights.

The sensation you experienced when moving as if you were in water is your yardstick for measuring efficiency in any exercise. This is the right stimulus, but it is not enough.

Weights should only be the means to work the muscle, a resistance that we apply to the muscle to give it constant tension and stress it, a stimulus amplifier. Of course, we must never consider weight as the goal. The muscle is not intelligent, it has only two abilities: contracting (shortening) and relaxing (lengthening); it cannot read the number of kilos written on the dumbbells and cannot even predict the number of repetitions we have set for ourselves, nor does it count them as we perform them.

The muscle must be given tension for a period of time, it must be stressed, it must be damaged and, possibly, "torn". This is what it understands. It doesn't know what we are thinking, intending or planning. **The muscle is "ignorant"!**

The weight must enhance the sensation without distorting it, without transforming it into something that is not and should not be. The fundamental point is not to exceed the muscles limits and to avoid using weights that are too heavy.

We must always be the ones who command and dominate the weight.

The weights should be as heavy as possible to put maximum stress on the muscle while maintaining the perfect technique

1. The **basic technique** in bodybuilding, as well as in other sports disciplines, represents the foundation. All the other techniques are to be considered *interlocking supplements*, techniques that overlap the basic technique without ever replacing it.
2. The **basic technique** consists of some technical elements that must always be present, in every exercise, for any number of repetitions and for any weight on the machines.

Bodybuilders must perform the exercise as follows:

1. Always push, pull or lift the weight slowly, mastering it and moving it as if it were immersed in a thick liquid.

2. At the top of each rep, you should forcefully contract the chosen muscle.
3. You must avoid cheating, which happens when the execution of the movement cannot be controlled from the start.
4. This is the most difficult aspect: the athlete must not feel dead spots during the movement within the repetition. It must be felt that the movement is led by the opposing muscle or muscles. **If we take the barbell curl as an example, we need to feel the bicep roll up in the upward phase. Once at the top, contract the biceps and, from here, go down by unrolling it. Do not think about lengthening the biceps but think about contracting the opposing triceps.** Do all of this as if you were mentally following your "famous" metronome that marks the movement, always perfect, always the same.
5. I advise the beginner and average athlete that they should use the metronome in certain exercises, to become aware of this beat, this pulsation. A short period will be enough, especially for movements where peak contraction is nearly impossible to achieve, such as squats or shoulder exercises.
6. When I used the metronome, I set the counterweight of the pendulum to the 60-second mark, i.e. one beat per second. Obviously, one can set it to a higher number, but I think this technique, born spontaneously from my need, offers the possibility of making the athlete understand the meaning of moving with the weight as if they were pumping oil in an exact, perfect rhythm, like the pistons of an engine. This way leaves no room for error.
7. **For the muscle, each set that is performed in this way should be like one long rep.** Each movement must be performed and completed in the exact same way, exactly as if the athlete were a machine.

The diversification of work with weights (angle-plane-direction)

This diversification of work was explained to me by Jimmy Pedemonte, a well-known coach and great bodybuilding coach, who drew the exercises and the muscles involved on a sheet of paper. Let me briefly reiterate this concept, expressed in a simple and clear way, exactly as Pedemonte showed it to me.

1. Changing the **angle** is one of the three degrees of diversification. Standing barbell curls, Scott bench preacher curls and dumbbell curls are minimal variations – we basically do the same work over and over again. Doing flat, incline or decline bench presses doesn't mean changing the plane or axis of work, just the angle. **The muscle doesn't know what we're doing. It adapts to the stress that is given to it and I don't think the fibers can tear more or less depending on the change of angle.** At most there may be differences from the point of view of elongation, which is different depending on the angle.
2. Varying the workout **plan** represents the second level of differentiation and stimulation of the work. We have a change of plan when we move from lateral raises to front raises.

3. Change the **sense** of movement. For example, this change occurs when you switch from a biceps exercise, such as the Scott bench preacher curl, to the high cable biceps exercise, in which the biceps oppose the resistance of the pulley from the top down.

It is best to use each of these variations within each training session. An example that I always use for the pectoral muscles is the combination of a push movement, such as a barbell bench press, with a lever movement, such as a fly, and a movement such as the pullover with semi-extended arms and elbows forward. The muscle must be trained in its entirety, following the movements along the axis.

You have to train and get used to the muscle doing what it is meant to do!

CHAPTER 17

Special techniques to increase training intensity

Federico Focherini

In the previous chapter we talked about the importance **of learning the basic techniques of weight training** for building muscle. Once we have learned and perfected this essential technique, we can focus on the second most important thing that is needed to obtain muscle growth: **intensity**.

For me, training intensely means putting maximum effort into the shortest period of time (density), with the maximum possible load, for the highest possible number of repetitions.

In this volume, Massimo Spattini and Riccardo Gaspari explain in detail and scientifically how muscle growth occurs. I will try to explain in simple, succint terms what happens in our muscles when we perform resistance weight training.

Our skeletal muscles are a tissue that continuously adapts to stress and, consequently, to changes. They are composed of several fibers that are activated by different stimuli. Hence the introduction of techniques and training principles of various kinds to recruit the deepest fibers.

Muscle contraction starts from the outermost layers of the muscle. **Our aim is to "tear" the deepest fibers.**

When you train with moderate intensity, the fibers of the outermost layers (those that are easily accessible) begin to give way after consuming their glycogen reserve, therefore their contraction capacity is inhibited. If you continue using appropriate intensity, you prevent the external fibers from recovering, allowing the deeper ones, which are difficult to activate, to be activated.

This is why excessive rest periods between sets allow the outer fibers to regenerate, and we don't want that to happen! Short rest periods stimulate the degenerative repairing process in the layers of deep fibers, causing an acceleration of protein synthesis at those levels and inducing hypertrophy of the muscle cells.

Bodybuilding is an adaptation to stress. As I understand it, it is the most violent, prolonged form of psycho-physical stress on the human body that exists. If you are going to grow lean muscle, *stress will have to adjust to you.* This is the only way that you can make continuous progress.

The following text describes **special techniques**, i.e. tricks that allow you to increase the heaviness of the load, and therefore of the work.

Forced repetitions

We use forced repetitions when we are unable to do another rep at the end of a heavy set. Our training partner applies just enough help on the equipment to allow us to complete another two or three repetitions. These forced repetitions will have to be performed only in the concentric-positive phases. There are many bodybuilders who apply this technique, but only a few apply it at the correct times and in the right ways.

Forced repetitions are a useful way to increase the load and allow for significant muscle growth, taking the muscles beyond the fatigue threshold. The task of forced repetitions consists precisely in "forcing" the muscle fibers to go further, thus receiving a different and more intense stimulus, and forcing the body to react to this trauma. The natural consequence of this stronger and superior stimulus will be a new trend in muscle growth. In this way, we can activate deep fibers that we would never be able to activate on our own.

Three fundamental points of the forced reps

1. **Run out of sets.** Once you have reached task failure, your partner must "force" you to go further, helping you lift the weight for a maximum of 2-4 reps. If you can do more than that, then you did not previously reach task failure, and you should use more weight than you used in normal sets without forced reps.
2. **Getting to this threshold** (i.e., beyond exhaustion) **leads to the possible stress of hard-to-stimulate motor units**, which can greatly contribute to increased muscle growth. However, the frequent use of this technique by a beginner can induce too much stress, possibly overstimulating cortisol and, consequently, causing overtraining. For this reason, a novice athlete should never overuse forced reps.
3. **Help from your partner must be as minimal as possible**: it is you who must try to complete the repetition, and above all the negative eccentric phase will be exclusively your responsibility. I would introduce forced reps once a week per muscle group, applying them during the last two sets of each basic exercise in which you use heavy loads. Alternatively, you can do two or three consecutive workouts with forced reps in a week, alternating two or three no-force workouts.

Negative repetitions (eccentric reps or retro-gravity principle)

Every single repetition has a positive phase, called **concentric**, and a negative phase called eccentric. Let's consider the flat bench press for the chest muscles. In the "push" of the barbell from chest level to complete relaxation we have the positive (concentric) phase; in the "descent" of the weights on the chest, we have the **negative** (eccentric) phase.

The recruited motor unit fibers do harder work, which places greater stress on the muscle fibers. When you reach exhaustion, you can no longer complete the positive portion of the rep, but you can still do at least a few more negative repetitions.

The muscle is able to sustain a greater load during negative repetitions than during positive ones. It is stronger in the negative phase than in the positive phase.

When an athlete performs negative repetitions (also called "negatives") in a set, they always feel pain, which is caused by the *myosin* and *actin* filaments of the muscle rubbing together.

When carried out under electromyography, **flat bench exercises for pectoral muscles**, have shown that, by eliminating the negative phase of muscular work, the subject does not reach the pain thresholds experienced during workouts that also include negative repetitions.

The eccentric work which causes this rubbing of the myosin and actin filaments, with consequent muscle tearing, often causes "delayed" pain (DOMS), i.e., occurring two days after training. In addition to the rupture of the fibers, we have noted various reactions in the muscle belly which is subjected to eccentric tension, such as inflammatory processes and activation of satellite cells.

In addition to the possibility of injury (almost all athletes get injured while they are in the negative phase of movement), there are also biochemical problems, such as disturbances affecting the mechanism of lactic acid disposal.

The principles of negative reps

1. **Negative reps are only introduced towards the end of a set**, when the positive phase has been brought to failure or when you have just finished two or three forced reps.
2. **The number of negatives depends on the ability to hold the weight that is coming down.** Usually there are two or three reps and you try to lower in a time frame of no less than 4-10 seconds, so we can consider 7-8 seconds a fair average. When the athlete has exhausted their capacity and the weight drops in less than 3-4 seconds, we consider the sets and the exercise completed.
3. **This technique should not be used often**, and should be always performed with a partner.

The negatives allow you to activate a greater number of muscle cells because you can hold a load up to 30-40% more than the weight you can lift concentrically. In addition, by performing a few repetitions only in the negative phase of a multi-joint exercise, with a load up to 125% over your maximum, you will be able to activate a greater anabolic stimulus.

This technique is similar to that of forced repetitions and it is advisable to use it just after performing a few forced repetitions with your partner.

These techniques are intended to take the athletes beyond their working capacity with proper techniques (beyond the exhaustion of concentric work capacity). You can overcome this barrier by getting help from someone or by helping yourself.

By the time an athlete runs out of concentric positive force, **eccentric negative force**, and no-motion, or isometric force (all in this order), they have explored every type of force that exists in nature that can be applied to the muscle.

Variable pace training (the importance of tempo in the execution of repetitions)

As we have seen, there is no single way to train and there is absolutely no best workout. Weight training should vary according to the characteristics of the athlete. Our body responds and reacts to training variables: by changing them we force it to implement an adaptation process.

Muscle growth is the result of adapting to ever-changing stress. One of these variables is the speed of execution of the exercise. This element is often missing in the diversification of the training method and is the time in which the muscle remains under the tension of a heavy load. Therefore, speed is the sum of all phases of muscle contraction, *concentric*, *eccentric*, and *isometric*, protracted over time, which stimulate our body. If a set is performed with the maximum possible load, then you will be able to stimulate muscle growth to the maximum. To obtain constant improvements we don't have to continuously increase the weight lifted or decrease the rest period, which will certainly lower our loads, but we should instead increase the stress applied to the muscle.

As the tension time varies during the execution of the exercise, the energy system that we use will vary. Barbell flat bench press × 10 repetitions, performed in the 1-0-1-0 system (i.e. 1 second to go down and 1 second to go up, without pauses in the two moments of lengthening and shortening) **won't be any different** if it is performed with the same weight for the same repetitions in the 4-0-4-0 system (i.e. 4 seconds going down and up, without rest in the two moments of lengthening and shortening). In the first case, an **alactic acid** system is used, while in the second a strong **lactic acid** component intervenes. Therefore, both types of stimuli are effective for muscle hypertrophy and both should be used.

In all of his methods, the great training coach, Charles Poliquin, emphasized the "technique of tempo" that needs to be used during the execution of the movement. According to him, the speed of execution of each exercise is fundamental and **the optimal time during which a muscle must contract during a set, in order to develop maximum muscle mass, should be 20-70 seconds**. Variations can be made within these sets; for example, you can perform a single repetition that lasts 70 seconds or perform 15 repetitions that last a total of 70 seconds. Within this time, you can do fast, medium-slow, and very slow repetitions, and use different loads. Poliquin states that bodybuilders do not necessarily have to perform shorter or longer sets, but that most of their sets should stay within this time frame.

The "time method", first developed by the Australian strength trainer Ian King, taken up by Poliquin, and later included in the training methods of the great Serbian bodybuilder Milos Sarcev, was initially simplified with a formula that is expressed in three figures. The first digit is the portion of the movement in which the weight is lowered (*negative-eccentric*); the second digit is the pause phase (*isometric*); the third digit represents the return movement (*positive-concentric*).

Sarcev developed this formula in four phases: the eccentric phase, the lengthening phase at the bottom of the movement, the concentric phase and the contraction at the top of the movement. In practice, two digits represent the static phases, one of which is for the isometric phase in lengthening and one for that in shortening, and two digits represent the movement phases.

When the athlete has learned to control the equipment at every point of its trajectory, this system of dividing the movement into eccentric, isometric and concentric contractions will come absolutely naturally. Let's take the 3,2,1,0 squat as an example. The number 3 refers to the three seconds it takes for the lifter to squat down, the 2 represents the 2-second pause in the bottom position, the 1 refers to the 1 second the lifter should take to return to the starting point, the 0 is the time in which they remain in an upright position. Sometimes the "X" is also used to indicate very fast concentric movements of less than a second.

Five more possibilities are listed in Table 17.1.

Table 17.1 The duration of each phase of the repetition

Phase	Time (seconds)			
1. Time needed for the negative phase (maximum control of the weight)	2	1	3	0
2. Time needed for the static phase Time needed for stretching (weight control and greater muscle damage)	4	1	2	1
3. Time needed for the positive phase (heavier version due to increasing time of both negative and positive phases)	4	1	3	1
4. Time needed for the static phase (dangerous technique; explosive positive phase not recommended for squats)	2	1	1	1
5. Shortening (the "X" indicates super short movements and is used in explosive exercises such as snatches)	3	0	X	2

In order to obtain an increase in muscle hypertrophy, the speed of execution of weight exercises is the simplest and least used training component of all. **I believe that the attention with which we treat speed within every single repetition is essential to being able to make each of our training sessions maximally intensive.**

Compensatory acceleration training

This is a technique used to stimulate the white, explosive, fast fibers to the maximum. Dr. Fred Hatfield, also known as Dr. Squat, took up this concept in his "compensatory acceleration" system.

The speed at which you train is more important than the weight. In other words, we can increase force by increasing the weight on the machine, or by increasing the acceleration used in lifting the weight. Therefore, the principle of compensatory acceleration lies in the fact that, when lifting submaximal weight, one can compensate for the lack of resistance by accelerating the movement as shown by the following formula:

$$\text{force} = \text{mass} \times \text{acceleration}$$

Thus, the more we accelerate, the more force we put into our movement.

Going back to the world of Bodybuilding, Vince Gironda and his student Larry Scott argued that the best stimulus for muscle growth is one that **"exhausts the most in the least amount of time"**. This means that the best workout is shorter, with the same muscle breakdown.

The goal is, therefore, to speed up stamina, movement and muscle contraction.

Heavy loads + fast movements

This technique consists in focusing on the speed of movement in the concentric-positive portion of every single repetition or during the positive phase of the repetition itself. Instead, the negative-eccentric phase of each repetition must be performed at a moderate speed, with complete control of the machine.

Therefore, it is a matter of organizing an increase in the speed of the repetitions within the sets, for example by dividing the number of repetitions into two parts. Let's take the example of a set with 10 repetitions: mentally divide this set into two parts; the first half will be performed in a normal and concentrated way, with good control of the machine and awareness of the muscular work, while the second half will be sped up.

It is therefore a matter of switching gears and speed when the muscle starts to burn and you are unable to complete the repetitions like before.

Speeding up the movement does not mean that the execution of the movement has to get worse.

Let's take a 45° leg press as an example. If the athlete loses control of the machine as they accelerate the movement, you will start to hear the weights banging (noise of the weights = **no control**) or you will see that the negative phase (when the legs flex) is accelerated, with potentially dangerous kickbacks. The positive phase (when the legs are flexed) is much more difficult to achieve.

This technique is especially recommended in moments of plateaus and should only be used with basic compound exercises, specifically with press/push exercises such as barbell bench presses for the pectorals, military presses for the shoulders, push presses for the triceps, squats and leg presses. However, it is not recommended for a standard deadlift because you would lose the stance and it could be very dangerous. It is also not suitable for pull-ups and rowing movements to train the lats, due to the excessive workload on weaker points, like biceps and forearms. Personally, I believe that methods of increasing acceleration to increase explosive force should only be used in specific, short periods of the year. I prefer "metronome" training in which the three pillars of movement (speed, concentric acceleration and tension) are kept constant and unchanged.

Peak contraction

Peak contraction is a technique in which the weight is held for a few seconds at the moment of maximum contraction until the movement is completed. It is thought to help the athlete better connect the *mind/muscle axis*, activate the exercised muscle more, and enhance muscle details because it creates greater separation between muscle groups.

Many years ago, the great bodybuilder Berry de Mey talked to me about the use of peak contractions: "Often, what you feel while maximally contracting is much more than the results you get". While that may be true, it is also true that all the best bodybuilders use this technique in numerous exercises, as it definitely improves the muscle's aesthetics, which are more accentuated after the fat has disappeared.

Skeletal muscle contains several systems: contractile, vascular and metabolic. Therefore, it is believed that training all three in order to obtain maximum muscle growth is better.

Peak contraction undoubtedly has a profound effect on the contractile system of the muscle. Muscle contraction is the result of a series of coordinated and synchronized intracellular modifications, which lead to the movement of the muscle fiber.

Thanks to electromyographs (the instrument that records the electrical activity of the muscle), we know that the "electrical activity" or the contraction of the muscle, is considerably higher when the muscle is in the most "shortened" position possible. In the "stretched" phase, electrical activity is lower.

The term "peak contraction" refers to the voluntary contraction by the athlete at the apex of the concentric phase of the repetition.

While partial repetitions avoid the movement where there is no more tension, interrupting the movement before reaching the critical point, and cheating bypasses it with a helping impulse, in peak contraction the problem is resolved with the direct contribution of the athlete, who voluntarily contracts his muscles in the movement phase when there is no more muscle tension.

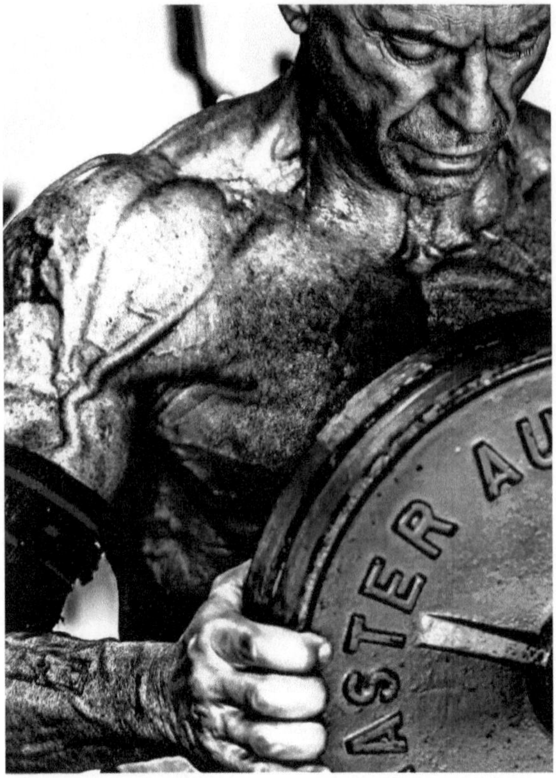

To me, this tehcnique should be included in every set and in every workout, for every muscle group with the exception of squats, for precautionary reasons, and almost all shoulder exercises, in which it is very difficult to achieve the same full contraction that can be achieved with biceps. I consider it to be excellent for quadriceps in leg extensions and for triceps in push-downs (two exercises that I think are very similar), for hamstrings in leg curls, for biceps in preacher curls, for pectorals in cable flyes and press machines, for lats in various types or row and pull-downs, and for abs in leg raises and crunches.

Peak contraction is not a technique in its own right, but rather a fundamental part of a bodybuilder's correct basic technique. In a famous gym in Trento in 1989, I remember seeing Rich Gaspari while he was preparing for Mr. Olympia. He told me that he "religiously" practised this method of peak contraction. I watched him in awe while he practiced. After reaching the top of the movement and starting the contraction, he performed a further contraction before resuming the downward movement of the weight. In doing so, he squeezed and stressed the deepest fibers, enervating the muscle completely.

I believe that athletes should always move the weight by fully controlling it and making sure there is never a drop in muscle tension.

This technique is very useful for achieving desired results and is a fundamental element that needs to be taught to beginners. Beginners always concentrate exclusively on weight and on pace, but the first thing they forget is peak contraction because it requires a huge amount of concentration by their neuromuscular system. We have already mentioned that you should contract for 1 or 2 seconds at the top of the movement (squeeze), much like squeezing a lemon. One variation is to contract for 5 seconds at the top of the movement on the last rep of each set. Peak contraction serves to isolate a muscle and is useful for establishing how that movement should be done in the athlete's mind.

Isometric repetitions

Peak contraction involves strong and decisive static contraction of the muscle. This contraction is part of isometric repetitions.

In isometric repetitions, the muscle produces an "isometric" type of tension that does not change the length of the muscle. Therefore, it is a **"static contraction"** against immovable resistance.

There is a form of isometric training in which the athlete **pushes or pulls the equipment without movement, while in another case they can perform a short movement before getting to a position where the movement stops**.

However, **one cannot train only in isometrics**, especially in pure isometrics, in which there is no movement. Let's take leg extensions for quadriceps as an example. All the repetitions are performed and, at the last one, the legs are brought parallel to the top of the contraction and the quadriceps are kept contracted in peak position for a minimum of 45 seconds and up to a maximum of 60 seconds. This technique is usually performed on the last set of certain exercises. It is an excellent technique both for increasing static and explosive strength and for emphasizing the muscular separation between the vast muscles of the quadriceps.

The most suitable exercises are:

- leg extensions
- trap shrugs
- leg curls
- standing calves
- lat machine for lats
- lateral and front raises
- chest machine
- tricep push-downs
- bicep preacher curls

A bodybuilder who has an established *mind/muscle connection* must always be able to stop the machine at any point of the trajectory of the exercise: in other words, they are "in charge". Blocking the movement in which the machine is blocked in both concentric and eccentric phases can contribute significantly to muscle awareness. **Isometrics** can activate weaker muscles if it is included at the right time in one's workout. However, I believe that the best isometry is one that allows you to perform a movement before reaching the position where you need to stop.

Let's consider the example of an athlete with weak arms, lack of strength and sensitivity, and, consequently, performing low-volume exercises. We go to the power rack and perform **a set of barbell curls with a final isometric contraction**, after having pre-exhausted the muscle with some heavy partial repetitions. We choose a weight that allows us to move from the starting position to the locking stops of the power rack placed at the end of the movement arc.

1. Perform 4 to 6 repetitions in the normal way.

2. When you reach the end of the last concentric repetition, push the barbell against the stops of the power rack for no less than 6 seconds. The stops will be placed at different heights.
3. If this set was successful, you should not be able to do another rep.

First, do the low-range barbell bicep curl (arms extended to 50°), then the medium range (arms extended to 90°), and finally the high range (arms extended to 130°). Thus, it is evident that we have used different placements of the power rack latches. Try doing three sets for each interval. Your biceps workout will be over, and you will certainly be shivering intensely as your nervous system has been hit hard.

For triceps, I recommend **close-grip bench presses** with a low interval (starting from 3 cm above the chest to 10 cm above the chest); therefore, we will have two pairs of stops: the low ones, our starting point, and the high ones, our stopping point. Then you move on to the medium range (starting from 10 cm above the chest to 20 cm above the chest) and then the high range (where you place the fasteners even higher and start at 20 cm above the chest, with the arms fully extended and elbows locked).

Try doing three sets for each interval. You may need to complement your triceps workout with another type of exercise. Perform a different movement in a different plane and at a different angle, such as a French press (decline bench barbell extension) for more repetitions.

These are two examples of **functional isometrics** applied to partial repetition training, excellent to use once every 10-14 days for muscles that do not "unblock". It's a truly exceptional technique, but to be used sparingly at the end of the session, hitting the muscular innervation system decisively.

Partial repetitions

Partial repetitions are a way of ending the exercise to intensify sets when muscle failure has been reached.

Partial repetitions, forced ones, negative ones, up to cheating ones, which I don't consider a technique anyway, are all aimed at a single purpose: to go beyond the muscle exhaustion caused by concentric-eccentric work.

In the same way that forced repetitions aim to overcome the critical point of the movement with the help of a partner, partial repetitions, instead of overcoming the problem of the critical point, circumvent it.

Dead spots, or critical points, are nothing more than points in the movement trajectory where there is no more muscle tension, as the muscle can no longer remain contracted.

So, at the end of the last set of an exercise, when the muscles are exhausted and won't allow us another full rep, I recommend immediately doing a micro-set of about three to four half repetitions, followed by another micro-set of three to four quarter repetitions.

This way, the movement is interrupted, and the range is shortened, stopping immediately before the dead point, i.e. the point without tension (the tension lost by the now exhausted muscle).

There are various exercises in which, at the maximum extension of the limbs, there is no resistance on the muscle in question. If we think about squats, we see that in the peak position, i.e. when the legs are extended, there is absolutely no resistance on the quadriceps. The same thing happens with bench presses when the arms are extended.

The bodybuilder's job is to seek constant tension in the muscle, overcoming or eliminating (when they can't take it anymore) the critical point. How can they do it? The answer is by eliminating the disadvantageous position. Therefore, they will not have to fully extend their legs at the top of the squat, nor their arms in the back kicks, bench presses and curls.

In the 80s, Tom Platz was a great supporter of this system. During training, when he had already reached the end of the sets, he continued until he could not move the weight more than 1 mm. In other words, total muscle failure. I observed the same way of destroying the muscles in Rich Gaspari, when I saw him finish his pectoral training, already exhausted by forced, negative and isometric repetitions, with a set of dumbbell flyes, dying with the range of motion, less and less, until he ran out of movements. But he wasn't finished and, after dropping the dumbbells to the floor, he picked up a lighter pair and continued, again finishing with short movements, starting from the major stretching phase.

When performed correctly, concentrating the effort on the muscles that are being trained with strong contractions, this trick/technique produces excellent results, especially when you're close to a competition.

Isotension

Isotension constitutes the pillar of "basic techniques". It is a crucial point in bodybuilding and is the correct way to maintain a slow and continuous tension of the muscles to maximize the involvement of red fibers. A true bodybuilder should use this way of lifting in every rep of every set of every single exercise.

According to this concept, muscle tension must be activated and maintained throughout the movement and must be as strong as possible in both the positive and negative phases of the movement. The muscle – we repeat – should be squeezed like a lemon from the beginning to the end of the sets.

Being in control of the machine means an absolute absence of leaps and aids of any kind, and this certainly contributes to avoiding trauma and injuries in the tendons and muscles.

Isotension helps to achieve exceptional pumping and consistent vessel occlusion due to the constant contraction of the affected muscle. Contracting to the max reduces blood circulation. Circulation through the muscle is practically eliminated, due to the compression of the blood vessels caused by the contractions of the muscle fibers. There is an absence of blood, and therefore oxygen, in the muscle. **The sets performed in these conditions force the muscle to work in anaerobic conditions.** As soon as the execution of the set ends, we feel an unbearable burning, caused by lactic acid waste and lack of oxygen (*hypoxia*) deriving from the absence of blood.

When we finish the set there will be a huge rush of blood to the part that we trained, called *reactive hyperemia*, which bodybuilders love.

Many years ago in France, Serge Nubret amplified this effect by artificially blocking blood flow through laces and bandages that were removed at the end of the workout. Nowadays, Milos Sarcev applies **isotension** in his techniques and often uses the old trick of the laces, especially with the Japanese bodybuilder Hidetada Yamagishi, who used occlusion bandages for the upper and lower limbs during endless giant sets of exercises.

We will discuss the concepts of hyperemia and blood flow occlusion in more detail later.

Pre-exhaustion

This technique was conceived in the early 1970s by Arthur Jones, the creator of the *Nautilus* asymmetrical cam machines, and was pioneered by great athletes such as Mike Mentzer and Casey Viator.

There are "basic" exercises and "isolation" exercises. The term basic exercises means biarticular exercises in a muscular kinetic chain or multi-joints, which involve multiple muscles during their execution and allow for the use of heavier loads.

The greatest benefit of performing two exercises in pre-fatigue (the first being isolation followed by a basic one) is to eliminate an imbalance between stronger or weaker, and more or less voluminous muscles. Basically, if we perform flyes on a flat bench for the pectorals before moving to the flat bench with barbells, we will tire the pectoral muscles before "terminating" them with a push exercise in which we use the triceps muscles, which are the weak link in this motor chain, but still fresh as they are not used in the first movement. Therefore, we pre-fatigue and warm up the main muscle involved, and then attack it with a substantial weight with the help of auxiliary muscles. Also, doing the isolation move first gives us a big pump and makes us feel more focused on the muscle and, therefore, more willing to lift a heavy load.

The basic concept of pre-fatigue is **to perform a complementary single-joint isolation exercise as the first movement, which begins to fatigue the strongest and largest muscle group** so that when you transition to the basic, multi-joint exercise, **the difference in strength and resistance between strong and weak groups is practically eliminated.**

Below are some examples of the pre-fatigue technique.

Isolation exercises + basic exercises
Chest
Dumbbell flyes + dips or bench press with barbell or dumbbells
Back
Pullover with dumbbell + pullup or lat machine
Shoulders
Lateral raise + shoulder press
Quadriceps
Leg extension + squat or leg press at 45°
Hamstrings
Stiff-legged deadlift + lying leg curl
Biceps
Concentrated dumbbell curl + barbell curl
Triceps
Dumbbell or cable extension + barbell extension or dips

This technique works very well before and closer to competitions and **is one of the ways to create a perfect superset**, which we will see later. There should be no time between the first and second exercises. The execution of the two exercises should be perceived as the execution of a single exercise which contains trajectories that have different directions, and run on different planes and at different angles.

Pumping (pump – saturation training – flushing)

The pumping technique is a system that we all use, sometimes without even knowing it. It is certainly a sensation we always want to achieve and when we don't achieve it, we say that we didn't train as we hoped or that we didn't *feel* the muscle. What actually happens when we use this technique is the influx of the largest possible amount of blood into the affected area. Blood carries the oxygen needed to produce energy for the muscle. Blood carries the amino acids to the muscles, which are needed for muscle growth. Blood "washes away" the lactic acid and other waste substances. The best way to get blood to the muscles is by **flushing**.

In the 1950s, this system began to be practiced with only one set per exercise for each muscle group, but there was no sufficiently intense level of muscular stress for the volume of work and the target was not hit. In other words, it was not possible to build a muscle group with just one set of a single exercise. Back then, people started doing more sets and more exercises, with more than 10 repetitions. It was observed that they could do many more repetitions, but the pumping of blood into the muscle would be less at times. That is always the goal. We need to get to the point where the trained muscle can no longer do anything from being engorged with blood and experiencing the continuous tension and contraction we give it.

I always recommend filling the muscle with blood as quickly as possible. If you have to train multiple muscle groups within a training session, I recommend that you always exercise contiguous muscles, for example, pectorals and shoulders, shoulders and arms (biceps and triceps together), triceps and biceps (in this order), quadriceps and hamstrings, or to follow the *pushing and pulling* method, such as chest, shoulders and triceps one day, lats, traps and biceps another day.

Recently, this system, which was conceived in the early 1970s by the great French athlete Serge Nubret and carried forward by the Serbian athlete Milos Sarcev, has been considerably developed. This amplification and extremization consists in maintaining blood flow for as long as possible in a precise area to facilitate the entry of amino acids, glutamine, creatine, glucose, carnitine and beta-alanine into the muscle. During and after intense weight training, the doors of the muscles are "opened" for 45-60 minutes (depending on the intensity of the training), and during this time every substance you take goes directly to the muscle, transported by blood (anabolic window). Therefore, the only goal in this case is to transport as much blood as possible to the affected muscle and make it stay there!

Milos Sarcev made this observation: in a resting athlete, only 12-15% of the total blood in the body flows to the skeletal muscles. During an intense workout with low recovery times, high work volume, high repetitions (always leading to exhaustion) and large work volume, the athlete can speed up his blood flow by 20 times and get up to 60-70 % blood to muscles. Therefore, his idea is to introduce the nutrients that the muscle needs for growth at that very moment. This produces an "anabolic event" that is impossible to create at any other time of day.

Milos Sarcev applies this concept, called *hyperemia advantage*, through the use of giant sets, which we will see later.

In addition, the **sensation of pumping in the muscles** is imprinted in the brain. The awareness of having filled the muscle more or less completely with blood stimulates the brain to train even better to experience that same sensation again. **This causes a deliberate pursuit of total fullness, of discomfort mixed with pain in every set of exercises for every muscle group.**

Staggered sets

This technique serves to stimulate a weak muscle group in a different way, by "touching or recalling it" while training stronger and larger muscle groups. Typically, you do a basic exercise for one large muscle group and, during your recovery, you attack another smaller group, perhaps previously neglected or in need of volume, with a specific set of exercises. This technique can be applied both when you want to build muscle and in the run-up to a competition. However, it is a technique used to solve the problem of deficient groups.

After one set of flat barbell bench presses for the chest, instead of waiting for the second set, you do one set of an exercise, such as for the calves or other small groups. Between sets for your back, you can train the abdominals, or again, between the sets for the shoulders, you can train the forearms.

While the small group is being trained, the main one starts to recover and this is an obvious advantage.

In the 1970s and 1980s, great athletes like Frank Zane, Roy Callender and Robby Robinson gladly used staggered sets to improve their weaker areas. The volume of Frank Zane's legs was not equal to that of the upper part. Before competitions, he used to do one set of leg exercises interspersed with sets of core exercises, going as far as doing 20 staggered sets per workout. Callender and Robinson used the same technique for their calves, incorporating a calf exercise into each training session. This was all in addition to their "regular" calf workout.

In my opinion, it's a "pleasant" way to attack a muscle that has lagged behind the others, but we don't necessarily mean a specialization of a lagging muscle, as intensity is not high enough. The purpose of this technique is to stimulate and saturate a deficient area with blood on days when it is not trained directly. In other words, it is a quick "booster" for the weaker muscle.

Examples of staggered sets (application: improvement of a weak muscle group)

The program involves training the shoulders, and the lagging group is the biceps. During many pushes or presses with pectoral and shoulder machines, biceps are stretched under the heavy load of the pushes when a full negative eccentric movement is performed. *If you stretch a muscle that has just been pumped from an exercise, you create a stretch of the "fascia", or muscle sheath, consequently increasing hypertrophy.* We'll look at this concept more extensively with Parrillo, Rambod, Hill and Trudel in Chapter 18. By doing so, we won't have to use heavy weights in the barbell curl. Our goal is to induce as much blood flow as possible with minimal effort. Again, the key is to maintain constant muscle tension throughout the movement. The continuous contraction causes an occlusion of the biceps' vessels, with consequent retention of lactic acid and waste substances, immediately followed by a violent rush of blood once the set is over. This will give us a big pump with minimal muscle destruction.

Shoulder exercise: behind-the-head barbell press 5 × 10-12 reps, bicep barbell curl 5 × 10-12 reps

- 5 sets × 10-12 repetitions
  - Barbell press
  - Barbell curl
  - Rest
  - Barbell press
  - Barbell curl
  - Rest
  - Barbell press
  - Barbell curl
  - Rest

  ...and so on!
- 10-12 reps of shoulders and then 10-12 reps of biceps
- 10-12 reps of shoulders and then 10-12 reps of biceps
- 10-12 reps of shoulders and then 10-12 reps of biceps, contracting both in the concentric-positive phase and in the eccentric-negative phase.

Supersets

A superset is the use of two movements, performed back-to-back without pausing, to stimulate opposing muscle groups.

A real superset is applied by performing two exercises in a row for antagonistic muscles. For example, one exercise for the abs (crunch) is followed by one for the erector spinae (hyperextension); one exercise for the biceps (dumbbell curl) is followed by one for the back (pulley push); one exercise for the quads is followed by one for the hamstrings and so on.

A very well-known and common **superset variant** attacks the same muscle from different angles with two different consecutive exercises.

You can create a **superset** by starting with a basic move followed by an isolation move or you can do the exact opposite, i.e. first perform a complementary isolation exercise, such as flat bench presses for the pectorals, followed immediately by flat barbell bench presses. In the latter case, we are in the middle of pre-fatigue, taken up and then "made famous" by my mentor, **Mike Mentzer**.

Below is an example that uses the chest group as a model.

Original supersets

Chest
Incline barbell bench presses
+
Back
Barbell rows

Supersets for the same muscle group

Chest
Flat bench dumbbell flyes
+
Chest
Flat barbell bench presses

Or

Chest
Flat barbell bench presses
+
Chest
Flat bench dumbbell flyes

The **second example of a superset** is Mentzer's pre-fatigue technique.

By training two opposing muscle groups together, nerve impulses increase. This should lead to an increase in the number of fibers called into action, resulting in increased blood flow. In my opinion, this can occur optimally between muscles that are not too large. It is felt less clearly between the pectorals and back or between the quadriceps and hamstrings.

After a superset between small antagonist muscle pairs (for example, biceps and triceps) we obtain higher stimulation of both groups (synergistic effect) and a quick recovery, as the localized blood flow increases, increasing capillarization, which in turn increases the release of oxygen in the blood and the removal of lactic acid. The superset method, especially the one in pre-fatigue, always leads to intense blood flow with a burning sensation, partially due to the accumulation of lactic acid.

It is not true that this technique is valid only in the pre-competition period: supersets can also be used in the muscle-building phase if it is well supported by a correct food plan that is high in protein and carbohydrates. In my opinion, it is an excellent technique for stimulating a muscle from different angles, on different planes, and – sometimes – even in opposite directions, without ever removing tension from the muscle that is being exercised. Therefore, we can "deceive" a muscle as if it were performing a single long set by combining two movements that could even be different from each other, which stimulate it in a way that couldn't be achieved otherwise.

Trisets

A close relative of the superset, a triset, as the name suggests, consists of three exercises performed with practically no rest between each exercise and with normal rest between each triset.

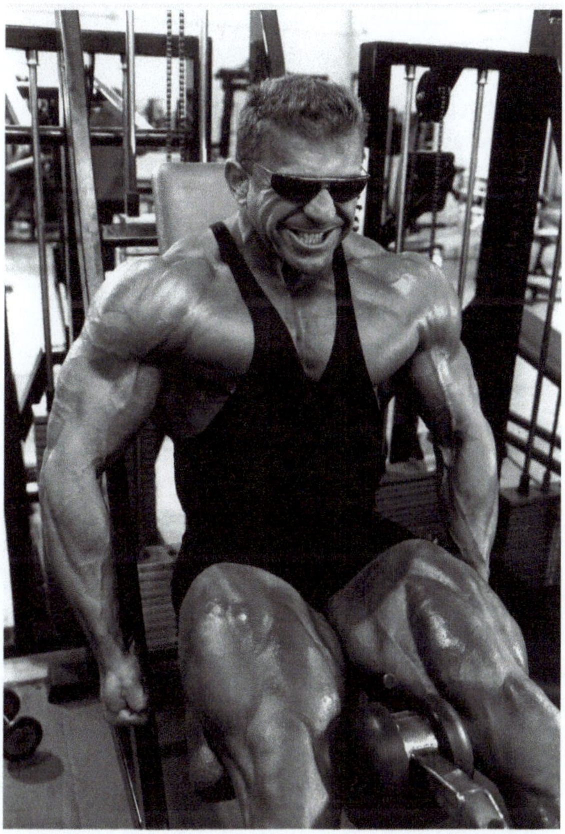

It is certainly a very valid technique when you are closer to a competition.

Trisets can be applied to contiguous and connected muscle groups, such as the shoulders-triceps-biceps group. In this case, the athlete can select three exercises for the same group. Otherwise, they can also take into consideration a more articulated muscular "block", such as the three muscles in the shoulder (anterior, lateral and posterior), which require three different movements, each of which is specific to accurately train a specific part.

In my opinion, another valid **triset is the one for the quadriceps**, which are made up of four muscles that work together. I do not recommend training the quadriceps-hamstring-calf block with trisets. Experienced lifters may find it more beneficial to do a quad-only triset workout, especially before a competition. My greatest degree of muscle separation, resulting in deep thigh splits, was achieved when I "jumped" from the supercharged front squat to the hack squat and, finally, to leg extensions, slaughtering myself with 25-30 repetitions per exercise, while maintaining correct execution and control and contracting to the maximum. Therefore, in this case, the various techniques that we've seen so far are included in every single set (for example, the partial repetitions for front squats or the peak contraction for leg extensions), while maintaining constant tension throughout the arc of the movement, contracting at the top of each rep.

Below are some examples, starting with the shoulder group.

Shoulder triset

1. Shoulder press (anterior deltoid – Basic exercise for the entire shoulder)
2. Lateral raise (lateral deltoid)
3. Dumbbell raise to 90° (posterior deltoid)

Or

1. Barbell front raise
2. Lateral raise
3. 90° raise with crossed cables

Triset for the biceps-triceps-brachioradialis block

1. Seated dumbbell curl (biceps)
2. Lat pushdown (triceps)
3. Reverse grip EZ bar curl (brachialis/brachioradialis)

Or

1. French press (triceps)
2. Barbell curl (biceps)
3. Dumbbell hammer curl (brachialis/brachioradialis)

I don't think these practises should be recommended to beginners, as the execution, concentration and contractile ability can deteriorate when performing so many exercises.

In my opinion, this is an incredibly good technique to train quads 3 months before a competition, such as in the case of an advanced athlete who needs muscle quality, density and separation of the four muscle heads of the anterior thigh.

Triset example (4-5 sets × 15-20 reps)

- Leg extensions
- 45° leg presses
- Squats or front squats

Note: squats are performed at the end to avoid using heavy loads that are harmful to the back or knees. You will already be tired, so it's the right exercise to finish your quadriceps training. You have to be able to make the muscle believe it is performing one endless set with different angles and planes, extending and pushing.
In combination with the right diet, squats can give noticeable splits in the hamstrings and glutes.

Giant sets

Giant sets belong to the family of supersets and trisets, with the difference that in a "classic" superset you perform a set of two exercises in a row (one exercise for a muscle and the other for its antagonist), whereas in a triset you perform three exercises and in a **giant set**, you perform 4-5 exercises for the same muscle group. Thus, it is a circuit of 4-5 exercises performed one after the other, with a very short recovery that allows you to move from one station to another.

You have to make up the necessary time to recover at the end of the fourth or fifth set.

The following is an example for quadriceps to be performed 4 or 5 times.

Giant sets for quadriceps

- Leg extensions × 15
- 45° leg presses × 20
- Squats × 20 (legs apart)
- Hack squats × 15 (narrow stance)
- Walking lunges × 12 per leg

Giant set for the back

Here you start with the hardest exercise performed at the beginning of the giant set.

- Lat machine pull-downs
- T-Bar rows
- Low pulleys
- T-bench dumbbell pull-overs
- Pull-downs on the lat machine, standing with arms outstretched and using the rope

There are two ways to do giant sets: one way starts with heavy basic exercises and proceeds towards isolation exercises, which are less heavy to perform, thus exploiting a favorable energy condition. In the second way, which I prefer based on personal experience, you do the exact opposite, i.e. first you pre-fatigue the muscle where you feel safe and the risk of injuries is low, to then face basic "breaking" exercises (such as squats or hack squats from the first method) towards the end, as you are already tired and therefore do not need to lift a lot to reach the final goal, which is to "destroy" the muscle.

The merit of this technique lies in training muscles from different angles, performing different exercises when energy levels are the same for each of them, and in creating a significant amount of blood flow. This technique is very much loved by Milos Sarcev both for reaching a very high level of hyperemia and because every space of the muscle is filled thanks to the different angles of the movements that are performed one after the other. It is a very valid technique for competitions, especially for large muscle groups.

In my opinion, it is always best to do one or two heavy basic exercises at the beginning of your workout before moving on to the giant set. This way, the muscle will be more congested.

Like the superset and triset, the aim of this technique is to create a single, long muscle contraction made up of different movements, trajectories, angles, senses and planes. This all serves to "upset" the selected muscle and allow it to perform a single job which it would never be able to perform if it were subjected to only one exercise.

Pyramid training

Let's start with **pyramid training** (or "**pyramids**"). It is a weightlifting technique and is one of the most popular methods for gaining muscle mass. Everyone does it without realizing it. There are various types of pyramids. In *intensive pyramids*, typically used by weightlifters to improve maximal strength, repetitions are decreased and the percentage of the load is increased until it reaches 100% of the 1 RM, to then *go down* the pyramid by increasing the number of repetitions again, with a consequent drop in the weight.

Example of an intensive pyramid

- 6 reps with 80% of max load +
- 4 reps with 90% of max load +
- 2 reps with 95% of max load +
- 1 rep with 100% of max load +
- 2 reps with 95% of max load +
- 4 reps with 90% of max load +
- 6 reps with 80% of max load

In a *classic pyramid*, often used by bodybuilders in the muscle-building phase, with gradual concentration and by using heavy loads, you gradually go up from 60% until you reach 80-85% of the maximum load, simultaneously reducing the number of repetitions. Sometimes, when you reach the end of the sets for a certain exercise, you decrease the load and, consequently, increase the repetitions again. This method is used to acidify and saturate the muscle to "finish it".

Example of a classic pyramid

- 10 reps with 60% of max load +
- 8 reps with 70% of max load +
- 6 reps with 80% of max load +
- 6 reps with 80% of max load +
- 6 reps with 80% of max load +
- 8 reps with 70% of max load +
- 10 reps with 60% of max load

Beginners will have to increase a few kgs at a time, and it makes no sense for them to calculate the percentages of maximum loads if they don't have strength and training experience. They can't know their maximal strength because it does not exist yet, as it has never been trained or developed before.

An intermediate or advanced athlete who is already training to the limit must know their ceiling with basic exercises that are performed (such as bench presses, squats, deadlifts, shoulder pushes and barbell rows), on which they will then perform the pyramidal training. This is necessary because later, starting from the ceiling, they can calculate the workloads.

There is another pyramid method that works in the opposite way of the two methods mentioned above, called **reverse pyramid training**. The real pyramids, those frequently used by all athletes, predict a growth in weight with a decrease in the number of repetitions. The reverse pyramid method, on the other hand, is implemented with a progressive decrease in weight and a re-increase in repetitions. Therefore, we start with the heaviest load in the first set at the beginning of the workout when our mental and physical condition is at its maximum.

This example of reverse pyramid is often used before a competition when energy is scarce due to a low-calorie regime, especially in athletes who struggle to maintain muscle mass.

Reverse pyramid training was often used before competitions by the great Lee Labrada.

However, what did we notice in the description of this technique? The athlete has to concentrate on the load being lifted, no matter how: what matters is getting to the pre-set number. This is a commendable goal, but one that is not what a true bodybuilder should seek. Therefore, even during the execution of this technique, it is necessary to squeeze the affected muscle at every single repetition.

The latest technique of this type is ascending **pyramid training**. All bodybuilders around the world, of any level, constantly implement this technique, even without programming or schematizing it, but simply by performing it naturally and spontaneously, both to adapt the muscles to the load and to avoid injuries that could occur if you start with excessive weights. Therefore, there must be a natural adaptation of the muscles to the movement of that exercise, which is implemented by progressively increasing the weight, reaching the repetition limit, often being forced to decrease the number of repetitions in an inversely proportional manner.

This is the limit of this valid and simple technique! Intensity increases relatively. The real increase in intensity within sets should come if, as the load increases, we work hard to complete the same number of repetitions as in the previous set. In that case, we have to accept the compromise of not reaching exhaustion in the first of the four possible sets, to then try to increase the load more and more while maintaining the same repetitions. This is very difficult to do. The moment you fail the last one or two repetitions, you receive the unequivocal signal that your muscle group gives you to make you understand that it is time to stop the exercise, without doing another one by decreasing the repetitions. This is the natural intensity that your nervous system, your contractile capacity, your blood, your lactic acid and your body have established for you.

Stripping / Drop sets / Running the rack

The technique of the descending sets, otherwise called strip sets, drop sets or running the rack, consists in performing a given number of repetitions in succession with progressively decreasing weights. In the following example, imagine you are performing the incline bench dumbbell flyes for the chest.

Example of incline bench dumbbell flyes for the chest
• 3 sets × 8+8+8 reps (stripping method)

The exercise should be performed as follows: grab a pair of dumbbells (for example, 20 kg) and perform 8 repetitions (an advanced athlete should always reach muscle failure; it is better if they can do one or two more repetitions). Put down the dumbbells and grab two other 15-kg dumbbells and do about eight more repetitions. Immediately afterward, take the 10-12 kg dumbbells and perform the last eight repetitions or, even better, aim to reach muscle failure.

I have found that dropping the weight three times is sufficient if each set is taken to exhaustion. More dumbbell changes, in my experience, don't improve much. This is a system that guarantees excellent pumping and is widely used by almost all athletes.

From personal experience, I feel like I can say that the incredible benefit of this technique is found only when **the athlete reaches complete contractile muscle failure, when the lactic acid has irreparably engorged and "seized" the belly of the muscle.**

This technique concludes the training of that muscle, therefore it is performed in the last set of the last exercise of the muscle group. Without meaning to and probably without paying attention to it, when we perform a strip set, we just *go further*, just like when we perform simple cheating or a forced repetition.

We lighten the weight when we can't continue with the initial load, just like when we do it alone or with the help of our training partner through forced repetitions.

Below we see an example for the pectorals in which we combine two basic exercises in an increasing and **classic pyramid** with an exercise in **descending sets**, to acidify the muscle which is now heavily "hit" by the maximum loads.

An example of an increasing and classic pyramid + descending set for the pectorals

1. Barbell bench press: 6 sets × 12-10-8-8-6-6 (weight increase/reps decrease)
2. Incline barbell bench press: 5 sets × 10-8-6-8-10 (classic pyramid)
3. Decline bench dumbbell flyes: 3 sets × 10+10+10 (stripping method)

The technique of the descending sets must not be extended to all muscle groups at the same time. Rather, it must be concentrated on the muscle areas that benefit most from a short but intense workout and on groups with which it is otherwise not possible to achieve the desired pumping. A variant of strip sets, considered practically the same technique, is the **drop set**. The only difference is that in strip sets you don't have any recovery time between one micro-set and another, while in drop sets you only rest for a few seconds, just long enough to breathe and recover.

These techniques of rapid reduction of the weight of the exercise have the great advantage of increasing training density, i.e. more work in a reduced amount of time, and of forcing the muscle to remain under tension longer than in a classic set.

Muscle priority (muscle specialization)

This principle contradicts the *large-to-small* principle, which states you should start by training the largest muscle and then attack the smallest one. Therefore, this new concept should be used by athletes who are no longer beginners. The muscle prioritization technique is a workout building strategy that targets:

1. A specific weak group (this is the most frequent case).
2. A particularly challenging muscle group (legs) or complex group, such as the back (this is the least frequent case).

Using the principle of muscle priority means **training the weak group first, in the context of a workout. The starting point is clear: I train the lagging group first, when I'm full of energy, so that I can train them with maximum effort**, possibly starting with the largest muscle group every time.

Various experiments have been performed on amateur and professional athletes. A classic experiment involved training the upper body in the following order:

- flat bench presses
- pull ups
- barbell shoulder presses
- barbell curls
- tricep push downs

During the experiment, it was observed that the exercises performed at the end of the workout had lower intensity and lighter loads. Instead, the same exercises, done at the beginning of the workout, were performed with more vigor and heavier weights were used. This doesn't mean that, if you have deficient arms, you have to train them before the pectorals and lats, but maybe you can train them alone or with a muscle group that has nothing to do with it, such as the legs.

The same principle can be applied when training a single muscle. **The concept of muscle priority can be used when training a specific muscle group**.

Let's use the shoulders as an example. Usually, you start with a heavy basic pushing movement to fully stress the muscle. Then, you start working the various heads of the deltoid in isolation.

For example, lateral raises for the medial side, front raises for the front, and 90° raises for the back of the muscle. Now, if we notice that the rear part of the deltoid is the weakest and least developed, we can start the isolation exercises from here. The concept is to start "hammering" the weak area when we have all our energy, in order to be able to attack it with 100% of our physical and mental strength.

Let's take the example of an athlete with weak **chest** development. Especially if they train every day, they will not have to include chest training on Friday or Saturday, perhaps after having trained the legs the day before and the back 2 days before.

Now suppose another athlete is deficient in **arm** development. The following sequence may apply to them.

Arm development training

- Monday: **arms**
- Tuesday: **rest**
- Wednesday: legs and calves
- Thursday: chest
- Friday: shoulders
- Saturday: back
- Sunday: **rest**

The day before and the day after arm training, the athlete rests to have maximum energy and time to regenerate the muscle tissue destroyed by training. In addition, on the rest day following the training, the amount of animal protein ingested should increase significantly to aid recovery and growth. Therefore, the athlete and the coach will have to pay attention to preparing a weekly training strategy, always taking into account the athlete's structural and muscular deficiencies.

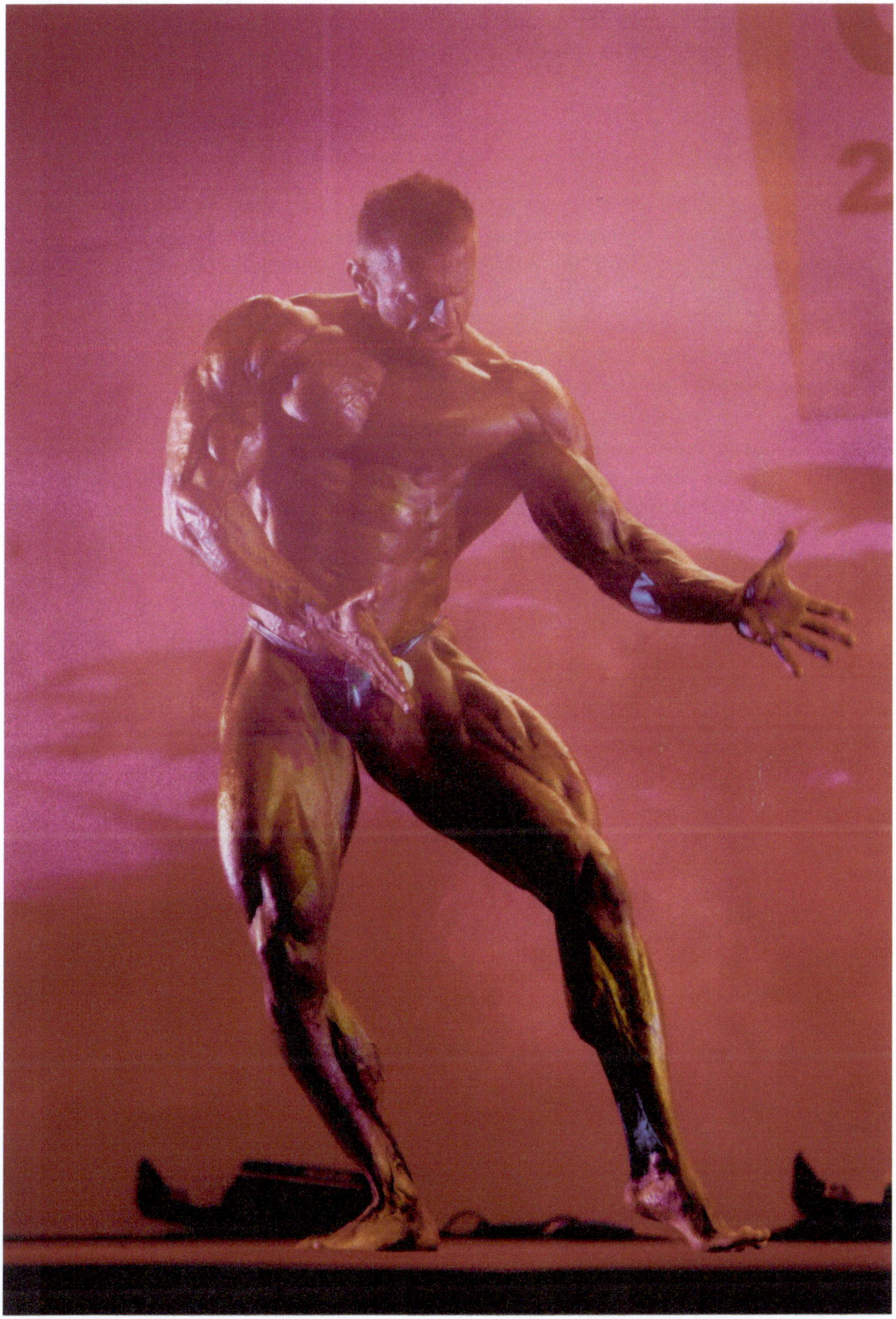

There is no doubt that more could be done to make the most of the principle of muscle priority in advanced athletes, which is what I have structured into the training method that I still follow and which I will cover in Chapters 18 and 21.

Overload

Overload, or overload training, is the foundation of every weight training technique and is the "mother" of all bodybuilding techniques. It is the technique that every beginner must apply to initiate muscle growth, the principle of resistance that must continually adapt to the improvements made by the body. Muscle development must always be forced by putting muscles under ever greater stimuli.

The basic concept of overloading is the principle that the **greater the amount of resistance imposed on the muscle, the bigger the muscle will become**. In theory **this is true, provided that** everything happens by performing the exercise with a perfect execution technique!

After an initial period of growth, many beginner athletes show no further signs of improvement. Often, the cause of this lack of results is due to poor training organization and the fact that the overload principle is not implemented with a progressive systemic approach.

The great Italian coach **Jimmy Pedemonte** has always stated that the biggest problem, in fact, is the lack of technique and organization. He described the situation as follows:

> *Today I do this exercise, next time I do another; today five sets, tomorrow 15, today with a weight, tomorrow with a higher or lower one, it depends on how I feel: a picture of bleak technical collapse.*

I believe that what Pedemonte describes has happened to all of us quite a few times...

The overload system is basically based on the following three principles.

First principle (the original, fundamental one)

- Perform the set for a number of repetitions, for example eight, with a weight that does not allow for an extra repetition.
- Over time the muscle adapts, becoming capable of not only lifting the same load easily, but completing more repetitions. Once you have reached 11-12 repetitions, increase the weight by 2-5 kg (depending on the exercise) and start again from the initial eight repetitions.

This principle was created and developed in the old weightlifting school of the former Soviet Union, spreading throughout the former communist bloc of Eastern European countries.

I always advise beginner athletes to write down every workout, every exercise, set and repetition done, and the weight achieved. This is essential to be able to have references and to continuously monitor your progress.

A heavy weight must never compromise the perfect biomechanical execution of each exercise.

Of course, you can't increase the load on a barbell forever.

The two consequent variations of the overload shown below are logical and natural, they intensify the training session and increase muscle hypertrophy.

Second principle (developed later by American training specialists)

- Increase the number of repetitions, using the same weight.

Third principle (consequent development of intensity and density)

- Reduce recovery time between sets by maintaining the same weight and number of repetitions.

These three methods of overloading **are all limited in time**: as mentioned above, the first principle cannot be applied indefinitely; the same goes for the second principle, in which one progresses by increasing the repetitions and keeping the load constant, and even more so for the third principle, in which the recovery time is progressively reduced.

However, it is still a great training system for beginner athletes, and perhaps the most natural and instinctive for every bodybuilder, including the most advanced ones. We can state that **overloading is the perfect system for beginners, as well as intermediate athletes and advanced athletes**.

CHAPTER 18

Methods and systems

Federico Focherini

In this chapter I will explain detailed methods to structure and organize your workouts, distinguishing between training and recovery days, and in some cases, suggesting the most adequate and suitable nutrition.

Heavy Duty (Mike Mentzer)

In the 1970s, the great Mike Mentzer was urged by Arthur Jones (creator of the *Nautilus* machines) and Casey Viator (famous bodybuilder) to adopt this technique, which became the training basis, if not a real "creed", of thousands of bodybuilders around the world. He started from an empirical observation, quite obvious, if you like, but certainly objective: observing those who support long and resistant activities, prolonged over time, such as marathon runners, is enough to understand that a workout of this type cannot lead to any increase in muscle mass.

The physique of sprinters and other athletes who practice disciplines in which the work intensity is very high is an indication of the proportional value of the intensity, with respect in muscle development.

Mentzer states that the harder an athlete trains, the shorter the workout will be. **The relationship between volume and intensity is inversely proportional.**

Definition of the concept of intensity

Overcoming the obsolete and absolutely erroneous conceptions that interpret intensity as a percentage of the maximum weight lifted, Mentzer rightly argues that, in bodybuilding, **intensity can be defined as the percentage of the athlete's momentary capability to exercise in terms of depletion of muscle reserves**.

The unique concept of muscle growth according to Mentzer

Mentzer identifies the last, almost impossible repetition as the true core of the question, the true nucleus of intensity as the determining factor of growth. His system is based precisely on the concepts discussed up to now, i.e. the absolutely most important rule for growth is that of pushing the muscles up to the **"point of momentary exhaustion" (point of failure)**, the only one able to break the barrier below which there is no muscle growth.

Throughout his life, Mentzer maintained that a single set brought to the maximum limit of the contractile capacity, with the achievement of muscle failure, is enough to trigger the mechanism of muscle growth. Any further effort can lead to overtraining, our worst enemy, so it must be avoided.

Mentzer identified the increase in intensity in these three systems:

1. Gradually increase the weight
2. Reduce the time needed to complete the training session
3. Try to increase the number of sets

What does *point of failure* mean? Mentzer analyzed the three main types of muscular tension, and on this analysis he developed his brilliant theory.

For Mentzer, reaching the last repetition, at best, does not mean having reached the peak of exhaustion of the muscle's contractile capacity (**positive concentric phase**). There are two other levels to be exhausted, i.e. those of static (**isometric**) activity and eccentric activity (**eccentric negative phase**). Only when all three levels have been exhausted, we can say that we have reached total exhaustion.

Therefore, first we will have the exhaustion of the *concentric-positive* phase, then we will have the exhaustion of the *static-isometric* phase, and lastly we will have the exhaustion of the *eccentric-negative* phase.

Each repetition should be performed slowly and with maximum control. Each repetition must last no less than 4 seconds.

Following the principle of pre-exhaustion, i.e. pre-fatigue, a complementary exercise is performed first which prepares the large muscle to be "finished" with the basic exercise, in which the small muscles, not yet involved, come into action.

Between the isolation sets and the basic sets, there should be no rest time.

Example for chest workout
• Dumbbell flyes + dips or incline bench press

A rest period of more than 3 seconds would allow the large muscle (in this case, the pectoral) to restore up to 50% of its contractile capacity.

Use a load with which you can do no more than 6 repetitions with perfect technique; in case you have used a weight that allows you to do 7, continue: **the important thing is not to stop at a pre-set number, but to go on until failure**. Once you have exhausted the ability to lift the bar, immediately continue with two forced repetitions.

Then proceed with 4-5 negative repetitions (the descent of the equipment should last 6-8 seconds). So go on until you get to the point where you will no longer be able to control the equipment. The number of workouts per week must not exceed four.

At the beginning, each workout may last even more than 1 hour, even 1 hour and 20 minutes. Within a couple of weeks, and after having become familiar with this method, you will have to gradually reduce the time, until you get to finish it in about 30 minutes.

This training method is not suitable for everyone and is based on the "explosive" effect of each individual set. Each set is seen by Mentzer as an entire training session. Therefore, a session of 6 sets for a given muscle group is actually made up of 6 very intense mini-workouts. In his sessions, there is always a spasmodic search for performance. By training in this way, it will not only be necessary to deal with muscle and tendon wasting, but above all with the exhaustion of the central nervous system and, consequently, mental exhaustion. Mentzer started taking amphetamines to increase his concentration during training. If he neglected a few repetitions during one of these performances, it would undermine his entire training session. The main problem lies right here: this technique requires an ability to recruit all physical and mental forces and to do it immediately, in one single moment.

But not everyone is capable of such a feat.

Practical example of training with the Heavy Duty technique

Monday and Thursday

Legs and calves
- 1/a) Leg extension (pre-exhaustion) 1 × 8-10 (exhaustion)
- 1/b) 45° leg press 1 × 6 + 2 forced + 3-4-5 negative
- 2) Squat 1 × 6-8 + 2 forced
- 3) Lying leg curl 1 × 8 + 2-3 forced
- 4) Standing calf machine 2-3 × 8-10 + 3-4 forced + 3-4 negative

Chest
- 1/a) Dumbbell flyes (pre-exhaustion) 2 × 8-10 (exhaustion)
- 1/b) Incline chest press (barbell or dumbbells) 2 × 6 + 2 forced + 3-4 negative

Triceps
- 1/a) Push down (pre-exhaustion) 2 × 8-10 (exhaustion)
- 1/b) Dips 2 × 6 + 2-3 forced

Tuesday and Friday

Back
- 1/a) *Nautilus* machine pullover (pre-exhaustion) 2 × 8-10 (exhaustion)
- 1/b) Lat machine forward, narrow grip 2 × 6-8 + 2 forced + 3-4-5 negative
- 2) 1 arm dumbbell row 2 × 8 + 2 forced

Continues

Continued

Tuesday and Friday

Traps
- 1/a) Shrug (pre-exhaustion barbell or dumbbells) 2 × 8-10 (exhaustion)
- 1/b) Chin pull-up 2 × 6-8 + 2-3 forced

Shoulders
- 1/a) Lateral raise (pre-exhaustion) 2 × 8-10 (exhaustion)
- 1/b) Reverse lat pull-down 2 × 6 + 2 forced + 2-3 negative
- 2) Dumbbell raise to 90° 2 × 8 + 2 forced

Biceps
- 1/a) Seated barbell curl/preacher curl/dumbbell curl (pre-exhaustion) 2 × 8-10 (exhaustion)
- 1/b) Pull-up, narrow and reverse grip 2 × 6 + 2 forced + 2 negative

The following information is **particularly important**:
1. The rest period between the pre-fatigue set and the "base" set should be "zero", like a superset.
2. Try to shorten the training time with each session.
3. Start each movement slowly and with full control, without any cheating.
4. Each repetition must be complete.
5. Add weight whenever possible; from the 6 starting reps, you'll reach exhaustion with 9 reps.
6. Each repetition should be performed with maximum control and slowly. Each repetition must last no less than 4 seconds.
7. Don't add more sets.
8. You can change exercises as often as you like.
9. Never train more than four times a week. Usually three workouts will be more than enough once you have mastered the workout.

Frequently, those who train for the first time with this system may feel that they have not done enough, so they add something, modifying this method and distorting it. The same thing happened in 1992 to the two disciples of Mentzer, David Paul (Barbarians Brothers) and Aaron Baker, who gained a lot of body weight, and to Dorian Yates the following year. In 1993, Yates swept away all other competitors by achieving a muscle density that was never seen before. He had followed the dictates of the great Mike for only two weeks, then he had continued to prepare for that year's Olympia by reworking the training, abolishing the supersets and slightly lengthening the frequency compared to the first version of Mentzer's training. Later we will discuss his type of training.

True Heavy Duty is very difficult to do perfectly. Mike Mentzer remains the only one to have invented an example of a logical technique, created by reasoning and observation. **This is the most brilliant of bodybuilding techniques.**

Rest-pause training (Mike Mentzer)

This system was developed in the late 1950s and it wasn't successful until Mike Mentzer took it up and reworked it with it **Heavy Duty System**. This system is great for both strength and the development of muscle hypertrophy.

The original version of Mike Mentzer's Rest-pause training

The original version of the Rest-pause training requires that the athlete, after a good warm-up, performs one or two repetitions with maximum weight. After resting for about ten seconds, they repeat the lift, for a total number that never exceeds three repetitions:

1. Performing one or two reps with maximum weight
2. Rest of about 10-15 seconds
3. Performing one or two extra reps

Mentzer claimed he never performed more than three sets per muscle group, and sometimes he did only two. He reached a total of 7-13 sets per training session only with the Rest Pause technique. Of all the great bodybuilders of all time, only Mentzer's peer, Casey Viator and, later, six-time Mr. Olympia Dorian Yates had the unique ability to destroy a trained muscle in such a short time.

Another version of this technique (the one I have often used in the best moments of my career) involves a different number of repetitions, with the intention of being able to perform twice as many repetitions as the ones performed in the first sets. Let's see it in detail in the following table.

1. Set of 8 very heavy reps to failure
   15-second rest period
2. Set of 4 reps to failure
   15-second rest period
3. Set of 2 very heavy reps to failure
   15-second rest period
4. Very heavy 1-rep set to failure
   15-second rest period
5. Very heavy 1-rep set to failure

In this case you get to perform a much higher number of repetitions than in the first version. It is preferably applied to basic exercises, such as bench press, pull-ups, lat pull-downs, barbell curls, tricep dips, deadlifts, etc. It is best to avoid squats for safety reasons in favor of other quadricep exercises.

Rest Pause is used on one or two exercises per muscle group and on only one muscle group per workout, once a week.

When we talk about Rest Pause, we always start from the physiological law of muscle adaptation to overload.

This is an excellent technique that many athletes use to overcome a moment of stagnation in results.

Mentzer's grand vision was to be able to do twice as many repetitions with a weight compared to a normal athlete.

For this reason, the method has changed and developed, since it was soon understood that two or three repetitions per set are too few to be able to set in motion those physiological processes underlying muscle hypertrophy. In other words, the number of repetitions is too low, which can lead to several problems. First, when doing three to five repetitions for each muscle group, it is easy to get the loads wrong and, therefore, not get any results.

There are very few athletes who possess that very high degree of concentration that would allow them to give their maximum in just three or five repetitions per muscle group.

The **basic error** lies in seeking the "maximum effort" in what one is doing, expecting an equal "maximum result", but this is not the case. In many cases the result of increased muscle volume is not related to an increase in weight.

Interrupted Sets: the evolution of Rest-pause Training according to Filippo Massaroni

Filippo Massaroni, Mr. Universe in 1981, elaborated a development of the classic Rest Pause in the early 1990s which combined perfectly with Dorian Yates's technique (which we will see later) and with stripping in the same training session.

An example of interrupted sets

- Two sets of bench press × 5 reps + 12-second rest + 5 reps + 12-second rest + 3 reps + (12-second rest + 1-2 reps)

You should perform the exercise using a weight that allows you to complete a maximum of 7-8 repetitions, but you should stop at 5 repetitions, rest for 12 seconds, start again for another 5 repetitions, pause again for 12 seconds and so on for the maximum number of sets you can complete. Usually, if you have really used a weight that allows you to do 7-8 repetitions, you shouldn't be able to go beyond 3 sets. For the second set, you should go on for another micro-set and rest for another 12 seconds, to then attempt a lift, or at most two, if you are able to complete them. It is similar to the classic Rest Pause, with more repetitions.

In short, you can do at least 15 repetitions without any help, with a load that would allow you to perform only 7-8.

Very productive! I have followed this principle for many years with some exercises for the chest, biceps, triceps, deltoids and quadriceps, and have recommended it to many athletes with excellent results.

The Rest Pause technique is considered high motor unit recruitment, i.e. a practice that activates motor units to the maximum in order to increase the contractile capacity of the trained muscle.

Single-rep Training (the extremization of Dr. Hatfield's Rest Pause)

This extreme technique can be used on a single basic exercise, once or at most twice a month, to increase muscle density.

Dr. Frederick Hatfield makes a deeper and more specific distinction between two types of strength, **absolute strength** and **maximum strength**.

The difference is that an **absolute load** (as Hatfield calls it) **can only be lifted once without any outside help**. This is the highest force that the neuromuscular system can develop with a voluntary contraction, once in a workout. In **maximum strength**, on the other hand, that maximum force enables the lifting of a very heavy load which can be repeated even more than once during the training session. This is the subtle difference between Hatfield's two concepts.

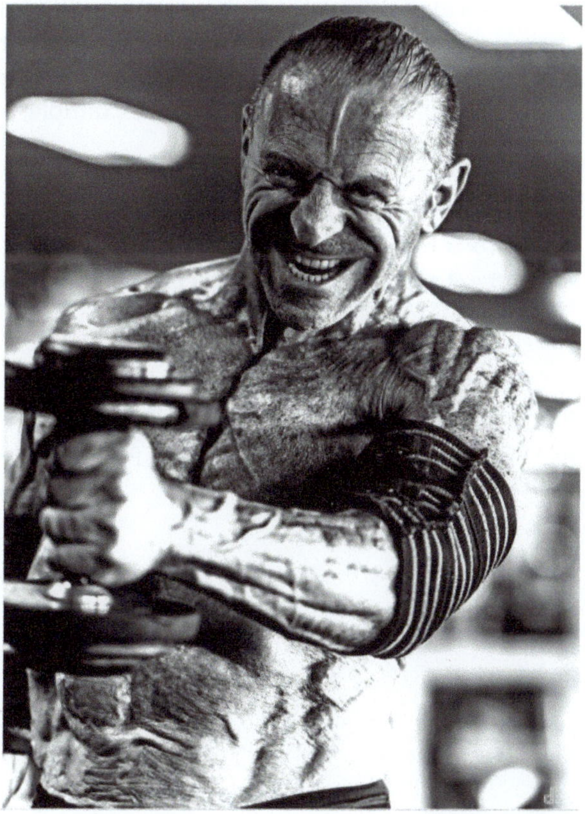

Typically, coaches and athletes simply call the heaviest weight you can lift for a single repetition *maximum strength*. In reality, 100% of the maximum weight that can be lifted is almost never used by bodybuilders, as it does not contribute to an increase in muscle hypertrophy, while it is an excellent way to test one's strength.

Absolute load is one of the most frequent causes of serious injuries in athletes and I advise all bodybuilders to calculate it with pen and paper only, and not to put it into practice.

So, the absolute maximal single lift and the very heavy single lift are two different things.

Hatfield's Single Rep Training protocol consists of training that involves three stages of work in percentage of maximum load, not the absolute one. This means that you can train with a weight as a percentage of a maximum load that would have allowed you to perform 2-3 very heavy repetitions. You therefore train with a manageable load, always 3-4% below the absolute load (too theoretical and dangerous to be put into practice at each session) which would almost inevitably lead to incidents.

Obviously, before starting this scheme, the athlete must be ready and well warmed up.

- 4 sets × 5 reps with 85-88% of the maximum load (*i.e. the very heavy load, not absolute, which we could repeat more than once during the training session*)
- 1 set × 3 reps with 90-92% of the maximum load
- 1 set × 1 repetition with 97% of the maximum load

After 30 seconds of recovery, continue with:

- 1 set × 1 rep with 94%, then 91%, then 87%, then 84% of maximal load, always recovering for 30 seconds between each lift, until you get to perform 8-9 sets

After the first 4 sets of 5 reps, the training turns into a real Rest Pause.
The following table shows a practical example, assuming the athlete is capable of a maximal squat with 140 kg.

- 4 sets × 5 reps with 115-120 kg
- 1 set × 3 reps with 125 kg
- 1 set × 1 repetition with 130-125-120-115-110 kg (30-second rest between sets)

This type of extreme training belongs more to the world of powerlifting than to the world of bodybuilding. Personally, I prefer the old Rest Pause method, developed in various ways, as it is safer, more productive and more adaptable to many basic exercises.

Serge Nubret Training Principles (an extension of the concept of isotension)

Serge Nubret was one of the top bodybuilders in the world between 1972 and 1975, along with Arnold Schwarzenegger, Lou Ferrigno and Frank Zane.

Serge Nubret's three principles are as follows:

1. **Overtraining doesn't exist.** Our body can adapt much more than we think. Serge trained over 2 hours a day, 6 days a week, plus 1 hour of abs every morning as cardio. Before competitions, he even trained 5 hours a day.
2. **The amount of weight to be lifted means nothing.** What matters is how you lift the weight. He always trained in isotension, contracting his muscles as much as possible throughout the range of motion.
3. **Muscles grow best by doing lots of sets and repetitions with little rest time between sets**, because this allows you to get a big pump throughout the workout. Before the competitions, Serge progressively reduced the recovery time between sets by 10-15 seconds every 2 weeks.

As you can see, we are at the antipodes of Mike Mentzer's creed. I would say that his principles are the exact opposite of the concept of having to avoid overtraining at all costs argued by Mentzer.

I met Serge in person, but I didn't have the same luck with Mike and I'm so sorry for that, even though at the beginning of my bodybuilding career I followed his dictates in an orthodox way. I believe that both training philosophies can be valid, but they should always be adapted subjectively to the genetics, ethnicity, morphological structure and neurological abilities of each athlete. Most people don't possess the sharp, defined characteristics of the tough, mesomorphic, nervous, white Caucasian male with fast, explosive muscle fibers to train as Mike professed. A lot of people don't possess slender joints, spongy muscles, slow and resistant muscle fibers and lethargic characters of the black Caribbean male, to be able to train like Serge wanted to. Therefore, I would say that these two great philosophies (as they should actually be called) should be used by all of us, fitting them together and adapting them to our needs and characteristics. I believe that the muscle can respond very well to both of these extreme and diametrically opposed stimuli.

Nubret would do 42 to 72 sets per workout, with 30 seconds of rest between sets for the upper body and 60 seconds for the legs. His arms workout routine consisted of 32 sets for a total of 384 repetitions.

He usually did 6-8 sets of 12 repetitions each and for the first set he used a weight that allowed him to comfortably perform up to 20 repetitions. He never exhausted himself and focused solely on reaching and maintaining tension and blood pumping throughout the workout. This makes it really hard to use heavy weights, as many athletes do just to satisfy their ego. Moreover, **this type of training never stressed the central nervous system, so he could train more often**. In practice, he never wore himself out, but managed to tire only the targeted muscle group.

Nubret was therefore the first one who was able to destroy trained muscles without affecting the central nervous system.

Serge Nubret's workout routine

Monday + Thursday:
quads (20 sets), chest (32 sets)

- Squat: 8 sets of 12 reps
- 45° leg press: 6 sets of 12 reps
- Leg extension: 6 sets of 12 reps
- Barbell bench press: 8 sets of 12 reps
- Flyes on flat bench: 6 sets of 12 reps
- Incline barbell bench press: 6 sets of 12 reps
- Incline bench flyes: 6 sets of 12 reps
- Slightly inclined dumbbell pullover: 6 sets of 12 reps

Tuesday + Friday:
back (26 sets), hamstrings (16 sets)

- Medium-wide grip bar: 6 sets of 12 reps
- Lat machine behind the head: 8 sets of 12 reps
- Frontal pulldown on the lat machine: 6 sets of 12 reps
- Barbell row: 6 sets of 12 reps
- Lying leg curl: 8 sets of 15 reps
- Standing leg curl: 8 sets of 15 reps

Wednesday + Saturday:
shoulders (24 sets), arms (2 × 8 super-sets), calves (16 sets)

- Barbell shoulder press: 6 sets of 12 reps
- Dumbbell front raise: 6 sets of 12 reps
- Barbell upright row: 6 sets of 12 reps
- Low cable lateral raise one hand at a time: 6 sets of 12 reps each arm
- Superset biceps barbell curl with triceps pushdown: 8 sets of 12 reps
- Seated dumbbell curl in superset with tricep dips: 8 sets of 12 reps
- Standing calf raise: 8 sets of 12 reps
- Seated calf raise: 8 sets of 12 reps

Sunday: rest

At each training session you need to add about one hour of abs without rest, performed in the morning on an empty stomach. Alternatively, Nubret forced himself to reach 2,000 repetitions between sit-ups and leg raises. His advice was to do a set only until exhaustion. Next time try to make more. Basically, if an athlete can only do 30 repetitions, he should stop, not do five sets of 30 repetitions. Next time, he should try to do more repetitions in one set. Nubret's was not just a technique, but a real school which many great French and Italian athletes of the 1970s and 1980s followed.

Renowned athletes such as Thierry Pastel, Gerard Buinod, Jacques Neuville, Edward Kawak and Pier Venturato.

The most fascinating and hard thing to believe is that Nubret had been facing all this mountain of work without eating since the previous day. As a matter of fact, he ate **only once a day**, with one long evening meal in which he began with all the red meat he could eat, followed by as many carbohydrates as his stomach could contain, to satiety.

German Volume Training (Rolf Feser, Vince Gironda, Charles Poliquin)

The first version of the method which later took the name of German Volume Training (GVT) appeared over 60 years ago in a California gym. It was called "Vince's Gym" and had been open since 1948. This method was later developed in the mid-1970s, different from the version we know today, by the former East German (GDR) weightlifting team and by the famous coach, Rolf Feser. It was then adapted, developed and made famous by the great Canadian coach Charles Poliquin, in the early 90s. In those years, he immediately rose to the top of the hit parade of training methods, essentially for two reasons. The first is linked to the fame of Charles Poliquin, nicknamed "Strength Sensei" who divulged it; the second, to the elegant mathematical simplicity of its essence, the "10 sets × 10 reps", which had a big impact on our perception. This method was used – and perhaps created – by Vince Gironda in the early days, but it can be argued that 6 × 6 and 8 × 8 were his favorite patterns, for which he later became famous. Vince Gironda, in the 1950s, had started training his students with 10 × 10 for each muscle group; then, over time, he realized that it was too expensive in terms of energy, therefore he halved the number of sets and left the 10 × 10 only for the weak groups, adding a variant of the intensity, i.e. coming to complete the 10 × 10 or 5 × 10 in shortest possible time, only resting 15 seconds between sets.

For many years it has been debated whether the first to adopt this technique was Vince Gironda or the weightlifting coaches of the former East Germany (GDR) directed by Rolf Feser. It has often been argued that the former Communist bloc of Eastern Europe has always been at the forefront of weightlifting techniques, but it seems that some of them have long and constantly consulted the manuals of Bob Hoffman (the father of American weightlifting) and his articles in *Strength & Health* magazine, which he founded.

So what is GVT? It's about 10 sets of 10 repetitions with 60-90-second rests, using 60% of your maximum. It seems easy at first but, in the end, especially the last three sets will be difficult to complete. Poliquin added Antagonistic Pairing to this technique, in which he trained two antagonistic muscles per session, such as chest and back, quadriceps and hamstrings, biceps and triceps, shoulders and back.

He then performed 1 set × 10 reps of the basic exercise for the chest (incline barbell bench press); then rested for 60-75 seconds and did 1 set × 10 reps of the basic exercise for the back (barbell rows), then started over from the first exercise for 10 sets for each exercise. After completing them, he performed two complementary 3 × 10-12 exercises.

Poliquin also added his "science of time", what today everyone calls TUT (Time Under Tension). He taught GVT with an execution in 3-0-2-0 or 4-0-1-0, in which the weight is lowered very slowly and lifted quickly, without pausing in the stretching and contracting phases. So, a set of 10 reps will be 50 seconds of time under tension.

Charles Poliquin therefore renewed the German Volume Training by making these changes of increase in intensity.

The purpose of this method is **to stimulate growth by accumulating a massive muscle fatigue load**. This is due to the high volume of work, the long period under tension and the short recovery time between sets. With this workout you always repeat the same movement for a long time and this neuromuscular stress is really hard to bear in the last sets.

Below is an example of **GVT for beginners**: training protocol set up for 3 training days per week, lasting 5-6 weeks.

A. Chest and back

- Barbell row 10 × 10 reps, 90-second rest (4-0-X-0)
- Pull-up 10 × 10 reps, 90-second rest (4-0-X-0)
- Incline bench flyes 3 × 10-12 reps, 60-second rest (3-0-2-0)
- Barbell row or 1 arm dumbbell row 3 × 10-12 reps, 60-second rest (3-0-2-0)

B. Quadriceps, hamstrings and calves

- Squat 10 × 10 reps, 90-second rest (4-0-2-0)
- Lying leg curl 10 × 10 reps, 90-second rest (4-0-X-0)
- Seated calf machine 5 × 20-25 reps, 60-second rest (2-0-2-0)

C. Arms and shoulders

- Tricep dips 10 × 10 reps, 90-second rest (4-0-X-0)
- Hammer curl with dumbbells 10 × 10 reps, 90-second rest (4-0-X-0)
- Shoulder press with barbell 5 × 10 reps, 60-second rest (2-0-X-0)
- Lateral raise 3 × 10-12 reps, 60-second rest (2-0-X-0)

The **second phase** of the GVT conceived by Charles Poliquin follows a 3-4 week phase in which the reps drop to around 6-8, and the sets are also reduced, therefore 4-6 sets will be performed. Then, the relative intensity percentage (%) is increased from 60% of the maximum load to approximately 67-70% of the maximum load. The goal at this stage is to do 10 sets of 6-8 reps with this load.

Training is always divided into 3 weekly training days.

A. Chest and back

- Incline bench dumbbell press 10 × 6 reps, 90-second rest (5-0-X-0)
- Pull-up 10 × 6 reps, 90-second rest (5-0-X-0)
- Dumbbell flyes on flat bench 3 × 6 reps, 60-second rest (3-0-1-0)
- Barbell row (T-bar) 3 × 6 reps, 60-second rest (3-0-1-0)

B. Quadriceps, hamstrings and calves

- Squat 10 × 6 reps, 90-second rest (5-0-X-0)
- Lying leg curl 10 × 6 reps, 90-second rest (5-0-X-0)
- Standing calf raise 3 × 12-15 reps, 60-second rest (3-0-3-0)

C. Arms and shoulders

- Close-grip barbell press (triceps) 10 × 6 reps, 90-second rest (5-0-X-0)
- Scott bench barbell curl × 6 reps, 90-second rest (5-0-X-0)
- Barbell shoulder press (forward) 3 × 10-12 reps, 60-second rest (3-0-1-0)
- Lateral raise 3 × 10-12 reps, 60-second rest (2-0-X-0)

Poliquin prescribes **5 reps to failure with a load that would allow for 10 reps to failure, equivalent to 75% of the maximum load.** Same training frequency as core training, three workouts per week for 7-8 weeks.

A. Chest and back

- Incline bench barbell press 10 × 5 reps, 100-second rest (4-0-X-0)
- T-bar row 10 × 5 reps, 100-second rest (4-0-X-0)
- Dips 3 × 6-8 reps, 90-second rest (4-0-X-0)
- Pull-up 3 × 6-8 reps, 90-second rest (4-0-X-0)

B. Quadriceps, hamstrings and calves

- Squat 10 × 5 reps, 100-second rest (4-0-X-0)
- Lying leg curl 10 × 5 reps, 100-second rest (4-0-X-0)
- Barbell lunge 3 × 6-8 reps, 90-second rest (3-0-X-0)
- Romanian deadlift 3 × 6-8 reps, 90-second rest (4-0-X-0)

C. Arms and shoulders*

- Incline bench dumbbell curl 10 × 5 reps, 100-second rest (3-0-X-0)
- Close-grip bench press 10 × 5 reps, 100-second rest (3-0-X-0)

Continues

Continued

- Barbell reverse curl 3 × 6-8 reps, 90-second rest (3-0-X-0)
- Seated overhead extension (EZ or 1 dumbbell) 3 × 6-8 reps, 90-second rest (4-0-X-0)

*Poliquin did not consider "direct" shoulder training in this micro-cycle, as he believed it may lead to rotator cuff injuries. Also, the shoulders are indirectly affected when training the chest and back muscles.

Poliquin argued that the classic 10 × 10 workout is critical for the beginner and intermediate athlete. He believed that, after completing these two micro-cycles and following a 2 to 3 week off-load phase, you should increase your intensity by raising the percentage of load used for each exercise. He stated that, after following these training patterns, the athlete must train with higher loads, therefore must perform lower repetitions.

This method was much criticized in the past, as it was considered as an exaggeration of repetitions of the same exercise, with a low load (60% of the maximum) and little rest time between sets.

I applied the 10 × 10 to the barbell bench press, squat, barbell row, and barbell behind-the-head push every time after the competitive season when I returned to training in anticipation of the following season. In my opinion, it was an excellent way to lay the groundwork for a new year of building muscle, and I found it very different and rewarding after all those months of intense, low-calorie workouts.

Most athletes argue that performing 5 × 10 reps of a given exercise is more suitable and has greater effectiveness, since excessive lactic acid production shuts down muscle explosiveness. In any case, I believe it is a very good method for non-advanced athletes who need a durable foundation and I believe that, for large muscle groups, applied to multi-joint exercises, it can build an excellent foundation for young athletes who need to lay a foundation to get hard, real, full and "clean" muscles. I define "clean muscle" as that type of young, separate, thin-skinned musculature, trained for years with fairly heavy loads, always and only with exercises with barbells and dumbbells.

Vince Gironda's system

Vince Anselmo Gironda (1917-1999) was the original "Iron Guru". While Joe Weider claimed to be "the trainer of champions", in reality it was Gironda who had the most followers in the bodybuilding field.

Gironda took Larry Scott from being a 71 kg boy with less than star-studded genetics to winning his first two Mr. Olympias in 1965 and 1966, weighing in at 94 kg. He also worked with Egyptian bodybuilding legend Mohammed "the Sphinx" Makkawy, one of the most plastic bodybuilders of all time. Makkawy was runner-up twice at the Mr. Olympia (1983 and 1984) and won several professional competitions.

These are Vince's two best-known students, but he actually had a team of champions who trained under his tutelage. Among them, we mention Don Howorth (Mr. America 1967) and Rick Wayne (Mr. Universe 1965, 1967, 1969, Mr. World 1967, 1970), who were very popular in those years.

He was also known as the "coach of stars," because when an actor needed to get in shape fast for a role, he would go to Vince. We can mention Burt Reynolds, Denzel Washington, Clint Eastwood, Sean Penn ... he also trained Carl Weathers, the famous Apollo Creed boxer from the movie *Rocky*.

I have always wondered why Gironda, if he was so good, was never as successful as Weider. He never made any noise simply because he wasn't interested in marketing and because he had a very difficult and hard character; he was considered more of an "Underground Guru". What he thought of women, men, actresses and actors, he would tell them to their faces. He certainly didn't know how to sell his image very well. It seems, in fact, that the first time Arnold Schwarzenegger landed in California, he went to Vince's gym and presented himself in a rather arrogant way. He had just won his first NABBA Mr. Universe in London and it was 1967-1968. Gironda said to him: "Well, you look like a fat guy... What are you going to do here?"

I know various anecdotes about Gironda because I was lucky enough to meet Spanish-Argentine Ramon Puig on various occasions, who was his collaborator and the one who followed him continuously cataloging all his teachings. A sort of personal secretary and biographer. Beautiful things that don't happen anymore these days.

In addition to not being the best at public relations, Gironda, with his methods, went against the most famous principles of that time (and also of our time). Some of his ideas were so revolutionary that people weren't ready to accept them. However, the fact remains that no coach besides him, in the history of bodybuilding, has ever brought such a crazy innovation, creative and practical at the same time. I have to admit that Gironda (together with Mike Mentzer) has had a great influence on me and on my essential and spartan way of interpreting the role of the bodybuilder. A distant figure (and perhaps it is better this way) from the interpretation of our days. The more I read his material when I was a "rookie," the more it influenced my way of thinking and training. At first it was only his exercises that piqued my curiosity, but as time went on, I began to absorb more and more of his knowledge and to shape my own by including his theories.

In this chapter, I want to introduce you to some of Gironda's ideas that have had the most profound impact on my training and that of many athletes.

The Gironda system: modern applications

Vince Gironda never liked the classic squat exercise and at "Vince's Gym" there were no racks to perform squats.

I don't agree on this. Indeed, I believe it is an indispensable exercise for an athlete to build not only their legs and buttocks, but also many other stabilizing muscles; moreover, it is a great metabolic and hormonal booster. It wasn't so much the exercise itself that he didn't like, but rather its effectiveness for most beginners.

Basically, he argued that most men have a structure that leads to a better development of the glutes and hips instead of the quadriceps, when using regular squats. For this reason, he recommended avoiding the normal back squat, opting for some variations of the squat such as the front squat, the sissy squat and the frog squat (which we perhaps know better as the ballerina squat).

He also knew that some male bodybuilders have a frame that allows them to perform classic squats without rising the hips and glutes too much (Sergio Oliva was among them). In general, this structure implies a narrow waist and hips, a relatively long torso and short legs. Gironda believed the squat was good for this type of athlete. Instead, he argued that classic back squats were a great exercise for women in order to build more muscular and round glutes.

Gironda was the first to talk about increasing **density** to build muscle mass and lose fat. Actually, he referred to this concept as **intensity**, but that was before this term was used in weight training to determine the load used in training. Therefore, in his writings, when he speaks of training "intensity" he actually refers to the **"density"** of the training, that is, **the amount of work per unit of time**.

Sometimes, using the same terms with different meanings can be misleading. Arthur Jones (the creator of the *Nautilus* machines) referred to **high intensity** as reaching muscle failure; thus, for him, maximal intensity equaled total muscle failure.

The principle of training "density" is probably the most important concept developed by Vince Gironda. He was the first to use the analogy between marathon runners and sprinters to explain this principle. This analogy was taken up and developed by Mike Mentzer in the 1970s. Marathon runners and sprinters are essentially doing the same thing: running. Marathoners do a lot of work over a long period of time, while sprinters do less overall work, but in a much shorter period. The result is that, although the marathon runner performs more total volume, the sprinter, who does more work per unit time (higher density), is the one with the greater muscle mass.

We will have to adapt this logic to our training sessions. We must constantly try to increase the amount of work we do per unit of time. The best Gironda athletes only recovered 10-15 seconds between sets!

Of course, you can't start with such a low recovery, especially if your body is used to 90-120-second rest intervals. We will have to gradually reduce the rest intervals, thereby increasing the training density over time. At the beginning it will be necessary to lower the workloads; then, after some time, the loads will go back to what they were before. Our body and our muscles will therefore have adapted. **The Gironda system is based on the cumulative effect of muscle exhaustion, not on the load itself.** In his training tables, an athlete could reach 6-15 sets per exercise.

Gironda's famous methods: 10 × 10, 8 × 8, 6 × 6, 10-8-6-15 and 15 × 4

When we think of the 10 × 10 method (10 sets of 10 repetitions for one muscle group), we immediately think of Poliquin's German Volume Training. But the fact is that the 10 × 10 pattern comes from none other than Vince Gironda, who already recommended it in the 1950s and 1960s. We've already seen why it's called German Volume Training: the GDR Olympic weightlifting team, coached by Rolf Feser, actually used the 10 × 10 system for their squats, from one point onwards, starting in 1972.

Weightlifting coaches in the former Soviet Union (USSR), Bulgaria, and the GDR of the 1950s and 1960s had read Bob Hoffman's books to gain insight into how their American Olympic weightlifting counterparts trained. Thus, it is possible that the German coaches had also read Gironda's articles and experimented with the 10 × 10 system.

It may be that some people who studied his methods assumed that his 10 × 10 system was influenced by GDR scientists, because in an article in Ironman magazine (March 1976) Gironda advised doing more work per unit of time (increase density), with the following words:

> *Back in 1925 German scientists discovered that to acquire large muscles you must increase the intensity of work done within a given time. That means that it doesn't matter how much work you do. What counts is how fast you do it.*

To tell the truth, Gironda did not claim to be the only creator of the 10 × 10 scheme. Perhaps, both the German coaches and the "Iron Guru" had independently created this method. The fact is that Charles Poliquin made it popular, taking the merits.

No matter how you look at it, **the 10 × 10 system works**. However, Gironda's version was much more challenging than our modern version. As we have seen, the German Volume Training program involves performing 10 sets of 10 repetitions on one exercise per muscle group, resting for 60-90 seconds between sets.

Well, **Gironda's fundamental principle was to try to do more work in less time**. So actually, he recommended using less than 60 seconds of rest. 30 seconds was his baseline, and as mentioned earlier, his best lifters could hit sets with only 15 seconds of rest between sets.

However, while the German version of Volume Training applied the 10 × 10 pattern to each muscle group within a training cycle, **Gironda's 10 × 10 was intended as a period of specialization**: it was only used on one muscle group at a time, which was intended to be given more emphasis in order to achieve a rapid improvement.

Originally, Gironda also used the 10 × 10 system for the whole body, but he quickly found that for most beginners it was too much work to handle. So he decided to use it as a specialization technique: he would use the 10 × 10 pattern for the muscle to specialize and halve the training volume for the other muscle groups.

The 10 × 10 system is perhaps his best known program, but Gironda developed many other equally effective schemes. These training patterns all share a common denominator: **always trying to do more in less time**.

Some of his most effective systems are as follows.

- **8 × 8 system**: similar to 10 × 10, but you perform 8 sets of 8 reps instead of 10 sets of 10 reps, again with minimal rest. This was not a specialty program and it was used for the whole body.
- **6 × 6 system**: the above concept is valid here too, and 6 sets are performed with 6 reps and with minimal rest.
- **10-8-6-15 system**: 4 sets are performed for each exercise (always with minimum rest):
  - *first set* = 10 reps with 50% of the load that will be used for the sets of 6 reps
  - *second set* = 8 reps with 75% of the load that will be used for the sets of 6 reps
  - *third set* = 6 reps with all the weight you can handle for 6 good reps
  - *fourth set* = 15 reps with 35% of the load that was used for the sets of 6 reps

  Again, only one exercise per muscle group is used.
- **15 × 4 system**: 15 sets of 4 reps of one exercise per muscle group are performed, with minimal rest.

Important note: in the 10 × 10, 8 × 8, 6 × 6 and 15 × 4 systems, the same weight should be used for all sets. Hypertrophy will be stimulated by accumulated muscle exhaustion and not by the load itself. If you manage to complete all sets, the load will be increased in the following workout.

Rest intervals should also remain the same throughout the entire exercise. If you decide to rest for 30 seconds between sets, this is the rest interval you will use between all sets.

Gironda's Compound Training

Gironda's **compound sets** are somewhat similar to regular supersets for the same muscle group. In other words, two to four exercises are selected for a given muscle group and performed in succession with minimal rest.

This compound method allows you to keep increasing your training **density** while maintaining its volume and using more exercises for a given muscle group. The main difference between compound sets and supersets is that the rest interval between two exercises in a compound set is longer. With supersets, you have very little rest between the two exercises, but then take a longer rest period between each superset.

The following table illustrates the difference between a traditional supersets and a compound supersets for chest exercises.

Traditional superset

- **A1 (set 1).** Wide-grip bench press to throat: reps, 10-15-second rest
- **A2 (set 1).** Wide chest dips: 8 reps, 90-120-second rest
- **A1 (set 2).** Wide-grip bench press to throat: 8 reps, 10-15-second rest
- **A2 (set 2).** Wide chest dips: 8 reps, 90-120-second rest

---

- **A1 (set 3).** Wide-grip bench press to throat: 8 reps, 10-15-second rest
- **A2 (set 3).** Wide chest dips: 8 reps, 90-120-second rest
- **A1 (set 4).** Wide-grip bench press to throat: 8 reps, 10-15-second rest
- **A2 (set 4).** Wide chest dips: 8 reps, 90-120-second rest

Compound superset

- **A1 (set 1).** Wide-grip bench press up to the throat: 8 reps, 15-30-second rest
- **A2 (set 1).** Wide chest dips: 8 reps, 15-30-second rest
- **A1 (set 2).** Wide-grip bench press up to the throat: 8 reps, 15-30-second rest
- **A2 (set 2).** Wide chest dips: 8 reps, 15-30-second rest
- **A1 (set 3).** Wide-grip bench press up to the throat: 8 reps, 15-30-second rest
- **A2 (set 3).** Wide chest dips: 8 reps, 15-30-second rest
- **A1 (set 4).** Wide-grip bench press up to the throat: 8 reps, 15-30-second rest
- **A2 (set 4).** Wide chest dips: 8 reps, 15-30-second rest

When regular sets are used with the usual 8 × 8, 6 × 6, or 15 × 4 routine, Gironda recommends only one exercise per muscle, for a total of 8, 6 or 15 sets per group. When doing compound sets, you will continue to use the same *total number* of sets (8, 6 or 14, as 15 is an odd number that isn't divisible by 2) per muscle group. So, since you're doing two exercises per muscle group, the number of sets per exercise is half of what you have with your set routines. The example above illustrates a routine consisting of 8 × 8 sets for the chest.

Compound set consisting of four exercises

This is another of Gironda's routines that calls for the use of a compound set for each muscle group. In this case, instead of using a two-exercise compound set, he used a four-exercise one.

He selected exercises that work different parts of a muscle area, so as to attack the muscle from every angle. In his original routine, Gironda recommended only one rotation, but he did it twice a day.

Although, for him, this was the best choice, those who cannot go to the gym twice a day can use two rotations during the same workout.

Here are some examples of compound sets made up of four exercises each.

Chest

- **A1.** Wide-grip throat bench press: 12 reps, 15-30-second rest
- **A2.** Gironda-style dips (wide grip, elbows wide and feet in line with face): 12 reps, 15-30-second rest
- **A3.** Low incline dumbbell bench press (30°): 12 reps, 15-30-second rest
- **A4.** Dumbbell flyes: 12 reps

Back

- **A1.** Low pulley (bringing handle just below the chest): 12 reps, 15-30-second rest
- **A2.** Rope lat pulldown: 12 reps, 15-30-second rest
- **A3.** Incline bench 2-dumbbell row: 12 reps, 15-30-second rest
- **A4.** Hyperextension on horizontal bench (lumbar): 12 reps

Hamstrings

- **A1.** Front squat: 12 reps, 15-30-second rest
- **A2.** Gironda-style leg curl: 12 reps, 15-30-second rest
- **A3.** Leg extension: 12 reps, 15-30-second rest
- **A4.** One-leg standing leg curl: 12 reps

Shoulders

- **A1.** Wide-grip chin pull-up: 12 reps, 15-30-second rest
- **A2.** Seated dumbbell press: 12 reps, 15-30-second rest
- **A3.** Seated dumbbell lateral raise (the back of the dumbbell higher than the front, *as if pouring water on the floor with two bottles*) (note, however, that modern study of biomechanics indicates that this type of exercise places too much stress on the shoulder joint – *Editor's note*): 12 reps, 15-30-second rest
- **A4.** 90° dumbbell raise: 12 reps

Biceps

- **A1.** Wide-grip preacher curl with elbows locked: 12 reps, 15-30-second rest
- **A2.** Barbell drag curl: 12 reps, 15-30-second rest
- **A3.** Incline bench dumbbell curl: 12 reps, 15-30-second rest
- **A4.** Hammer dumbbell curl: 12 reps

Triceps

- **A1.** Barbell pullover and press: 12 reps, 15-30-second rest
- **A2.** French press: 12 reps, 15-30-second rest
- **A3.** Decline dumbbell bench press: 12 reps, 15-30-second rest
- **A4.** Reverse rope extension: 12 reps

It is neither my field nor the subject of this book, and perhaps I shouldn't delve into Gironda's food approach, but I think we can mention it to make the global vision of this "Iron genius" even clearer to the reader. Vince required his athletes and clients in general to eat only fat and protein for 3 or 4 consecutive days, followed by one day of including a large meal containing carbohydrates; subsequently, the cycle would be repeated.

He called this diet the **"Maximum Definition Diet."** It was so effective that Gironda himself, when competing, was considered "too tight" by the standards of the time (which favored a smoother, rounder appearance). However, his maximum definition dietary approach became the preferred diet of several champions, from Larry Scott to Arnold Schwarzenegger, Dave Draper and other stars of the time. At the time it was simply called **"The Meat and Eggs Diet"**... Many, many whole eggs.

Regarding this aspect, Gironda was far ahead. He thought the key to muscle growth was to keep the body in a constant positive nitrogen state. He was absolutely convinced that, as long as there were freely available amino acids in the body, one could not enter a catabolic state, so one would build muscle. Obviously, he was limited by the supplements available at his time, as he had to use dried liver tablets. Despite the rather crude supplement that he used, this method worked very well. Mohammed Makkawy used a lot of it. He advised taking it when you wake up, between breakfast and lunch, between lunch and dinner, and before going to bed.

Gironda's greatest strength was his ability to design exercise variations that perfectly target the desired muscle group. For example, he sensed that for most people, bench presses weren't the best exercise for the chest, as they overstimulate the anterior deltoid and/or triceps rather than the pectorals. So Gironda did something unthinkable at the time (and even today): he practically banned the regular bench press from his gym! None of his students were allowed to perform it in the classical manner. They could only do it with a wide grip, dropping the barbell to the base of the neck, elbows wide and back flat on the bench.

In this way the pectorals are fully stretched and the contraction trajectory is directed according to the orientation of the fibers of these muscles. One wonders why you don't see it done this way more often. Gironda claimed that the bench press was the most ego-boosting exercise for the bodybuilder, who is almost forced to push heavier every time. By doing this movement in the manner indicated by Gironda, you use much less weight than you can use with a normal bench. This is because deltoids and triceps are not put into excessive play. He even dismissed some clients who, in his gym, had asked him how much he bench pressed! He was offended.

It's not clear why, but somehow the bench press has become our proof of manhood. It is therefore difficult to imagine that an exercise that would allow us to move a heavy weight is performed in a way that does not allow us to. In fact, Gironda's version was never successful, and he got very angry about it.

Gironda also popularized several variations of the sissy squat, from the traditional sissy squat to the sissy front squat, to the sissy hack squat (which I find very dangerous). He saw them as a superior way to build quads without involving the hip and glutes muscles. While I disagree with Gironda's anti-squat position, I do agree that variations of the sissy squat can give more separation to the quads.

But Gironda's greatest influence on exercise selection is undoubtedly the preacher curl, which we translate as the preacher curl on the bench, which we mistakenly call the "Larry Scott bench." This bench was first designed by the Easton brothers, owners of Easton Brothers' Gym, who gave Vince Gironda his first instructor job. It was Gironda who continued to use it constantly with his students.

Gironda's greatest student was undoubtedly Larry Scott, which is why the preacher curl is also often called the Scott curl. Gironda taught Scott the correct and perfect execution of the exercises on this bench which, in fact, looks more like a lectern than a bench... Never use the EZ bar, but only and always the straight barbell, with a wide handle, keeping the elbows leaning on the lectern closer than the handle, in order to bring the hands outwards, towards the shoulders, and not towards the inside of the chest. Gironda was able to analyze the exact anatomy and function of each muscle, and then find variations of the exercises to attack it in the most suitable and direct way. He was the Charles Glass of those times.

Gironda invented periodization training. It was he who first mentioned the need for frequent changes in the program design to avoid blocking results. In those days it was customary to keep the training program unchanged. Gironda was misunderstood and, at times, even ridiculed for his **"principle of muscle confusion"**. Perhaps he had chosen a bad name, but he meant that it was necessary to change the structure of the program often if continuous progress in muscle development was to be made.

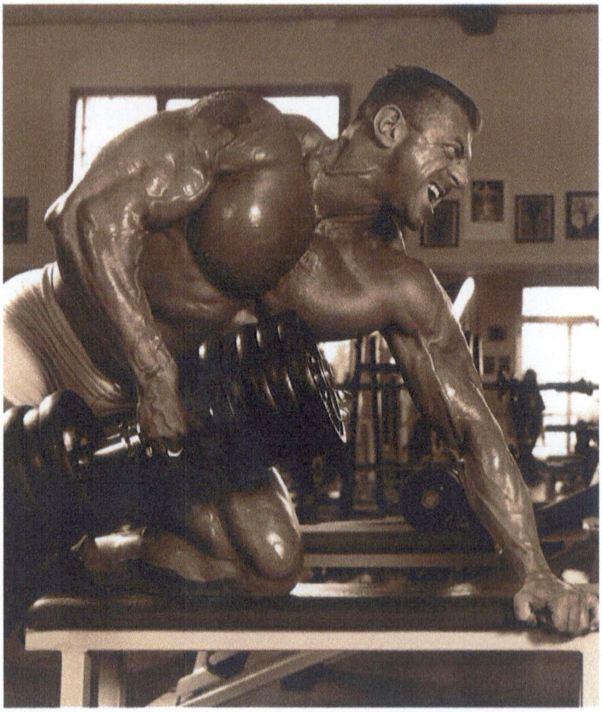

The one exemplified in the following table is a periodic plan based entirely on Gironda's methods. The training cycle lasts 10 weeks, during which you maintain practically the same exercises for the entire cycle. Only the repetitions, sets and rest intervals vary. In fact, it is a very simple program to implement, but it certainly can help build muscle mass and give an initial structure to your training program.

Phase I

Density adaptation (2 weeks)

- Number of exercises per muscle group: 3 for large groups, 2 for small groups
- Sets per exercise: 4
- Number of reps per set: 12
- Rest between sets: 45 seconds for the basic exercise, 30 seconds for the isolation one
- Workout duration: workout must be completed in 50 minutes or less

Workout

- Monday: chest, shoulders, triceps
- Tuesday: back, biceps, forearms
- Wednesday: quadriceps, hamstrings, calves
- Thursday: chest, shoulders, triceps
- Friday: back, biceps, forearms
- Saturday: quadriceps, hamstrings, calves
- Sunday: rest

Phase II

Density buildup (2 weeks)

- Number of exercises per muscle group: 2
- Sets per exercise: 6
- Number of reps per sets: 8
- Rest between sets: 30 seconds
- Workout duration: the workout must be completed in 45 minutes or less

Workout

- Monday: chest, shoulders, triceps
- Tuesday: back, biceps, forearms
- Wednesday: quadriceps, hamstrings, calves
- Thursday: chest, shoulders, triceps
- Friday: back, biceps, forearms
- Saturday: quadriceps, hamstrings, calves
- Sunday: rest

Phase III

Density intensification (2 weeks)

- Number of exercises per muscle group: 2
- Sets per exercise: 8
- Number of reps per set: 6
- Rest between sets: 20 seconds
- Workout duration: the workout should be completed in 40 minutes or less

Continues

Continued

Workout

- Monday: chest, shoulders, triceps
- Tuesday: back, biceps, forearms
- Wednesday: quadriceps, hamstrings, calves
- Thursday: chest, shoulders, triceps
- Friday: back, biceps, forearms
- Saturday: quadriceps, hamstrings, calves
- Sunday: rest

Phase IV

Peak density (2 weeks)

- Number of exercises per muscle group: 1
- Sets per exercise: 12
- Number of reps per set: 4
- Rest between sets: 15 seconds
- Workout duration: the workout should be completed in 30 minutes or less

Workout

- Monday: chest, shoulders, triceps
- Tuesday: back, biceps, forearms
- Wednesday: quadriceps, hamstrings, calves
- Thursday: chest, shoulders, triceps
- Friday: back, biceps, forearms
- Saturday: quadriceps, hamstrings, calves
- Sunday: rest

Phase V

Density deload (2 weeks)

- Number of exercises per muscle group: 2
- Sets per exercise: 3
- Number of reps per set: 10
- Rest between sets: 45 seconds
- Workout duration: the workout must be completed in 45 minutes or less

Workout

- Monday: chest, shoulders, triceps
- Tuesday: rest
- Wednesday: back, biceps, forearms
- Thursday: rest
- Friday: quadriceps, hamstrings, calves
- Saturday: rest
- Sunday: rest

Finally, I would like to remind you that Gironda's original manuals, written in the 1960s and 1970s, are unobtainable or can be purchased at online auctions at very high prices. His most important book, written with Robert Kennedy, founder of *Muscle Mag* magazine, and called *Unleashing the wild physique* (1972), can be purchased on Amazon in the original version at a price of 900.00 USD. This price gives an idea of who Vince Gironda was and what he left for all of us.

Muscle Blasting (Steve Michalik)

Muscle Blasting was a type of training cycle that bodybuilders on the East Coast of the US used in the 1970s to prepare for competitions. Steve Michalik, Mr. USA, Mr. America and Mr. Universe created and popularized this type of training. Steve was a true workout freak taken to the extreme. After winning these three major titles, he became the coach of Mr. USA John Defendis. **"Intensity or insanity"** was his motto which included total muscle destruction during his workouts.

His formula was:

Muscle mass = intensity
(increase in the volume of work and physical effort)
+
insanity (decreased recovery time, acceleration of movement,
combined with increased effort applied to the workload)

There are many variations of his method, but the standard version is that of a cycled system in which you work out in the gym for **9 consecutive days**, then rest for a couple of days. During the cycle you hit each muscle group three times, training every muscle every 3 days. The first three days of workouts are done with light loads at high intensity, and the next three days of workouts are done with heavy loads at low intensity.

On days when you use light loads, you train at high intensity: many exercises (from 8 to 15 per muscle group, depending on the size of the muscle in question) are performed in supersets, trisets and giant sets. The repetitions for each exercise range from 15 to 20, for a total of 30-40 per superset, 45-60 per triset and 60-100 per giant set.

There is no rest time between exercises of multiple sets and you only rest around 20 seconds between one multiple set and another. It is advisable to rest for about ten minutes between one muscle group and another. The tempo of the exercises must be fast, but the movement must always be intentional and controlled. Partial repetitions are acceptable and at some point in your training, you will realize that it is almost impossible not to do them.

On days when heavy weights are used, you train at low intensity: only four exercises, two considered basic and multi-joint, and two complementary isolation exercises. A total of no more than 15 sets of 6-8 repetitions are performed for each muscle group. In this case, the execution of the exercises must be very slow (*4 seconds in the eccentric phase and 2 in the concentric one*), using a few forced and negative repetitions in the last exercise of each muscle group. Rest between sets varies from 60 to 90 seconds depending on the exercise. The loads used must not allow you to go beyond 6-8 repetitions.

I liked Steve Michalik a lot when I was a kid, not necessarily because of his physical characteristics, but because of the fact that he was an anti-hero, the opposite of what American magazines showed at the time. Sadly, Steve was perhaps the first major athlete to wreak havoc on his mind and body through anabolic androgen abuse. His story has always fascinated me, to the point of getting hold of an original version of his manual (moreover, poorly written in a very confusing and aggressive way), many years ago. His book is called *Atomic Fitness* and contains a messy list of all his training absurdities, some of which are really meaningless. I have to admit that I didn't learn much.

Michalik, however, intrigued me because he managed to emerge from a childhood of sexual abuse by his alcoholic father and his time in Southeast Asia during the Vietnam War to earn Three Crowns. His whole life was centered on hallucinatory experiments in training and drugs use that led him to fall ill with liver cancer and eventually total kidney failure. While on dialysis and severely weakened from multiple surgeries, he took his own life in May 2012. It should also be remembered that he spent the last years of his life holding seminars around the USA to explain his mistakes to young people to dissuade them from taking anabolic steroids or doing any other kind of doping, and apologizing for his crazy and aggressive behavior, which had disturbed and offended many people dear to him.

Holistic Training and Breakdowns (Dr. Frederick Hatfield)

Holistic Training

This method was devised by Dr. Frederick Hatfield, nicknamed **Dr. Squat**, an American physician, powerlifting champion, squat record holder and founder of the ISSA (International Sports Science Association) more than 40 years ago.

His method is based on the concept that different fibers respond differently to different forms of stress, so varying the number of repetitions, sets, intensity and frequency will increase muscle mass.

Dr. Hatfield can be considered the first person to document training differentiated parts of the muscle.

In the aforementioned Muscle Blasting system, we saw that training can be radically changed, moving from sessions with heavy loads and good recovery between sets to sessions with lighter loads and without rest. This can certainly stimulate muscle growth.

In his original scheme, Dr. Hatfield proposed three different ratios of intensity and repetition range in order to fully stimulate the muscle. This scheme included sets of 4-6 explosive repetitions, sets of 12-15 rhythmic repetitions and sets of 40 fairly slow and cadenced repetitions. This complicated protocol is called **"ABC training"**. Before going into the details of his protocol, it is necessary to mention the three types of fibers that make up human muscles: fast-twitch, white, type IIb fibers; intermediate-twitch fibers with contraction between fast and slow, type IIa; slow-twitch, red, type I fibers.

Simply put, sets of 4-6 repetitions stimulate white explosive type IIb fibers, sets of 12-15 repetitions stimulate intermediate-twitch type IIa fibers, and sets of 25-40 repetitions stimulate slow-twitch type I fibers.

This method represented the US response to the (very similar) Eastern European training program of that time regarding myofibrillar hypertrophy versus sarcoplasmic hypertrophy.

The key lies in understanding that in order to train the muscle in its entirety and complexity to stimulate growth, all these characteristics must be taken into consideration.

The first part of the muscle to train: "A" (myofibrils make up 20-30% of muscle cell volume)

Many bodybuilders are attracted to the idea of being "crushed" by loads so heavy that they can only perform 4-6 repetitions. On the one hand, this training can lead to injuries and does not create pumps and muscle fullness, but on the other hand, stimulating the growth of myofibrils means causing the muscle a combination of tension, fatigue and damage (understood as tearing of the muscle fibers) which is absolutely necessary to stimulate hypertrophy of the sarcolemma.

Also, by increasing strength with low rep sets, you will be able to increase loads when training with a higher number of repetitions. Therefore, you have more muscle tension and more muscle damage to stimulate growth.

Generally, sets of 4-6 repetitions should be completed in no more than 20 seconds, with a load that corresponds to 80-85% of the maximum load (2-3 seconds in the eccentric-negative phase, rapid explosive concentric positive phase). In this first part of holistic training, the aim is to increase the size of the myofibrils and create muscle density. Rest should be around 3 minutes between sets. This way, 3 to 8 sets can be performed per muscle group.

The fewer repetitions you do (4-6), the more you stimulate the myofibrils.

The second part of the muscle to train: "B" (sarcoplasm makes up 25-30% of muscle cell volume)

If we typically complete the set with a number of repetitions greater than 6-8, we stress the sarcoplasm more, emphasizing hypertrophy. The weight used must remain in a range of 70-80% of the maximum load and each set must last from 40 to 60 seconds. The recovery time between one set and the next should be 1-2 minutes depending on the difficulty of the exercise. Repetitions must remain between 6, 8, 12 and 15 depending on whether we do basic or isolation exercises.

The best repetition range to work with is between 8 and 12. Each repetition should include 3 seconds in the eccentric/negative phase and 2 seconds in the concentric/positive phase.

The third part of the muscle to train: "C" (mitochondria make up 15-26% of muscle cell volume)

This part concerns red, slow-twitch fibers. According to Dr. Hatfield's indications, about 40 repetitions should be completed, but that is often impossible. It later emerged that you can also stimulate these slow-twitch fibers with 20-25 repetitions, reaching 40 repetitions only if you are able to do so. Again, it depends on the muscles in question and the range of exercises. Personally, I think the best choice is to not count the repetitions (our muscles don't know how to count and they don't even know what we intend to do) and to perform a couple of timed sets, working non-stop from a minimum of 1 minute to a maximum of 2 minutes, with a continuous cadenced and rhythmic movement, maintaining uninterrupted and constant tension throughout the execution of the exercise. I recommend isolation movements or machines that simulate basic exercises. However, if basic and multi-joint exercises such as squats are performed, cardiovascular work will inevitably be produced which we don't want to happen. Our only goal is to stimulate red, slow-twitch fibers and the mitochondria.

In my opinion, it is a big, bright and fresh vision of how to train, a high-level practical-scientific combination. It's also easy to set up and organize, but sometimes it can be tricky to match muscle groups following Dr. Squat's rest time guidelines. **He was the first to realize that each muscle group needs a different recovery time**, observing the training schemes that weightlifters of the former Soviet bloc used in their preparations with weights. Therefore, it is a matter of diversified training frequency for each muscle group. This concept was recently taken up by Francesco Currò in his Multiple Frequency System, for which he developed a software that is capable of calculating the optimal time between training and rest for each athlete.

The following was the initial pattern of training frequency given in Dr. Hatfield's 1984 book, *Bodybuilding: A Scientific Approach.*

Training frequency
• **Calves and forearms: every day** • **Abs: every other day** • **Upper back, shoulders, biceps and triceps: twice a week** • **Chest: every 5 days** • **Hamstrings and lower back: every 6 days (train on different days and at a distance from each other)**

If you want to implement it correctly, you have to include every muscle at the right moment in which it should be trained.

Breakdowns

Dr. Hatfield trained eight-time Mr. Olympia Lee Haney as well as Mr. America 1987, Mike Quinn, aka *The black sheep of bodybuilding*. These athletes used a variation of Holistic Training called Breakdowns, which consisted of three exercises per muscle group with three different types of sets for each exercise.

The **first set** is performed with heavy loads that allow the athlete to complete 4 to 6 repetitions. In the second set, the load is reduced by 15-20%, allowing the athlete to perform 10-15 repetitions maximum. In the **third and final set**, the athlete uses half the weight used in the first set and must get to 25-40 repetitions.

The concept is the same as Holistictic Training. The difference lies in the fact that you no longer choose one exercise for "A", one for "B" and another for "C", but in each exercise of the training session you perform a set with each of the techniques. In practice, it is a contraction of the training system.

Example: bench press (pecs)

- **1-2 sets of 4-6 reps (completed in 20 seconds, with a load at 80-85% of maximum load, 2 seconds down, explosive lifting).**
- **3-4 sets of 10-15 reps (completed in 40-60 seconds, with 15-20% lighter weight, 3 seconds down and 2-second lift)**
- **5-6 sets of 25-40 reps (completed in 60-120 seconds, with 50% less weight than the first set, continuous tension without stopping)**

I find this method to be great, simple and functional.

A 2004 Japanese study by Goto, Nagasawa and Yanagisawa, titled *Muscular adaptations to combinations of high and low-intensity resistance exercises*, scientifically confirms what Dr. Squat had achieved empirically with Haney and Quinn: the simple addition of sets with lighter loads at the end of an explosive strength training protocol leads to both a documented increase in muscle volume and an increase in strength.

I repeat: an all-around effective training technique.

Long cycle (Giovanni Cianti and the theory of supercompensation)

The underlying problem in structuring a bodybuilder's training program is the complete utilization of **supercompensation**. A *rebound* represents the moment in which supercompensation's effect is in full play.

The training stimulus would remain only a stimulus if supercompensation wasn't promoted: therefore, results can't be obtained without supercompensation. Diet is also very important because it makes this phenomenon concrete, providing the energetic and muscular means for the beginning of a strong rebound effect. The important thing is to take advantage of the rebound effect through a program that involves planning both training and diet.

The point of training is to increase available energy for muscle contraction during a training session, so as to subject the body to more intense stimulation, which sets in motion an alarm phase and, consequently, the acceleration of protein synthesis, during which the athlete must rest and follow a high-protein diet to regenerate and super-compensate for the proteins destroyed by training. This combination of nutrition and training was carried out by **Giovanni Cianti** and is one of the most ingenious and, at the same time, simplest concepts that exist.

The genius of this insight lies in its simplicity. Just observe basic human nature and its needs, and apply these observations to the daily battle of weight training.

This concept brings us to the only three ways a human muscle can be trained: **power** (nervous breakdown), **high intensity** (ATP/CP depletion) and **pumping** (glycogen depletion and blood saturation).

At first glance, this method may appear similar to Dr. Hatfield's protocol that was discussed above. However, this idea is spread over a program of several days (at least 2 weeks), in which there are more days of active rest than those of Holistic Training. The protocol for maximum activation of the long cycle involves the use of three distinct training programs during a cycle lasting approximately 14 days. Below are the characteristics of the three different types of training.

- Two **power** days, one upper body day followed by a lower body day. **Purpose: training the nerves to transmit maximum impulse to the muscle until nerve failure, not muscle failure.** Five sets of 5-6 repetitions each, 4-minute rest between sets, 1 basic free weight exercise.
- One or two days of total rest combined with a high-protein diet.
- Then we go back to **high intensity**, in which the workout is divided over 4 days. ATP and CP exhaustion, sets should last about ten seconds, all in one breath, do 6 to 10 repetitions, explosive in the concentric phase, controlled but not slow in the eccentric phase; 8-12 repetitions for legs; 3-minute recovery. *We try to avoid the pyramid technique because by increasing the workload and decreasing the repetitions it is not clear how much strength you have in that moment.* Therefore, it is better to choose 8 repetitions for the upper body, then change exercises (approximately after 4-5-6 sets) only when you are no longer able to complete 8 repetitions. Therefore, you must let your body, and not the training program, decide when to stop. After these 4 days of high-intensity, true bodybuilding training, it is advisable to adhere to at least 2-3 days of total "active" rest (on these break days, cardio activity is always an excellent choice), in which the protein intake must be kept very high to *compensate and super-compensate* for the destroyed muscle.
- The third and last type of training, following the 2-3 rest days, is **pumping**, which is also divided into upper and lower parts, including supersets between a complementary and a basic exercise, 20 repetitions, focusing on blood flow in the muscle, 40-50 seconds of recovery between one superset and another.

To start over from the Power phase, muscle pumping has to be followed by two days of regenerative deload.

Training cycles are completely different ways to train muscles, but all necessary and closely connected to each other. **It is a way to *exhaust* the three muscle systems: nerves, energy, and blood!**

In the off-season phase, it is necessary to work more on hyperplasia, i.e. on the increase in the number of muscle cells, but it is also necessary to stimulate the nerves and, consequently, strength, and to supply the muscles with as much blood as possible, also to be able to obtain a good fascial stretching from within.

Cianti sometimes recommends more days of total rest than those listed in the table on the following page, compensating and supercompensating with a very high level of protein.

During heavy-duty pumping days you should maintain a diet of:

- high carbohydrates (70% of caloric intake)
- medium-low proteins
- [many small meals/not high calories]
- low-fat foods
- low-fiber foods

During active rest days, a regimen of:

- high proteins
- moderate fat intake
- [3-4 large meals, 1000-1500 kcal more than on training days]
- low-carb foods
- vegetable fibers

During the 2 days of regenerative deload you should return to a standard diet of:

- moderate to high protein intake
- moderate carbohydrate intake
- low-fat foods
- vegetable fibers

The following table shows how Giovanni Cianti structures his training.

Long cycle structure

Power (depletion of nerve transmission)

1st day: slightly inclined bench

- Dips
- Forward bar or rower
- Shoulder press

2nd day: leg extension (warm up)

- Squat or 45° leg press
- Lying leg curl
- Standing calf raise

Choose 5 × 5 or 4 × 6 or 4 × 8-6-5-4 reps for each exercise, slow downward movement, explosive lifting, always increasing the weight; try to reach exhaustion in the positive/concentric phase.

Day 2-4: rest (30-35 minutes of aerobic exercise only)

Heavy Duty (ATP/CP depletion)

Day 5: chest-biceps
Day 6: legs-calves
Day 7: shoulders-triceps
Day 8: back

- 1st set: rest pause: 6-8 + 1+1+1+1 (or interrupted sets: 5 + 12 seconds + 5 + 12 seconds + 3 + 12 seconds + 1)
- 2nd set: 6 reps alone + 3 forced + 2 negative – 50% (stripping) × exhaustion
- 2-3 exercises per muscle group/2 sets per exercise

Try to go beyond the positive exhaustion of the movement

Day 9-10: rest (30-35 minutes of aerobic exercise only)

Pumping (depletion of glycogen stores)

Day 11: back-biceps
Day 12: chest-triceps
Day 13: legs-calves
Day 14: shoulders-traps

- 3-5 exercises per set/3-5 sets per exercise/12-20 reps

Positive depletion sets, look for maximum saturation, slow and controlled execution in continuous tension.

Regenerative deload (pre-power)

Day 15-16: whole body

- 1-2 exercises × muscle group (isolation exercises)
- 1-2 sets × exercise
- 10-12 easy reps per set

Don't get to muscle exhaustion.

Day 17-18: go back to power training!

Parrillo's technique

John Parrillo was a bodybuilder and powerlifter from Cincinnati, Ohio, before becoming a famous coach and professional bodybuilder. He had the ability to transfer techniques used by powerlifters into the training of bodybuilders, bringing a breath of fresh air in the 1980s with his innovative program.

It is a very complex workout.

The **important and innovative aspect** of this technique lies in the fact that it not only stimulates the muscle by increasing the contractile function but also introduces the **elastic function** of the muscle itself.

A set that Parrillo calls an **"intense set"** is performed after warming up, before starting to train each muscle group. This set is performed with a lighter weight than the one used in the first exercise of the actual workout. Each repetition must be performed very slowly and with isotension. Once you reach the top of the movement, you must contract the muscle in spasm for at least 2-3 seconds.

The athlete must have the ability to maintain full muscle tension throughout the range of motion. Returning to the starting position, one must be warned that the action is conducted exclusively by the antagonist muscle. Do you remember when I talked about performing the barbell curl, in which, in the descending eccentric phase, you would have had to contract the triceps and then go back up by contracting the biceps? Well, it's about emphasizing the negative phase with the antagonist muscle to have maximum tension on the trained muscle.

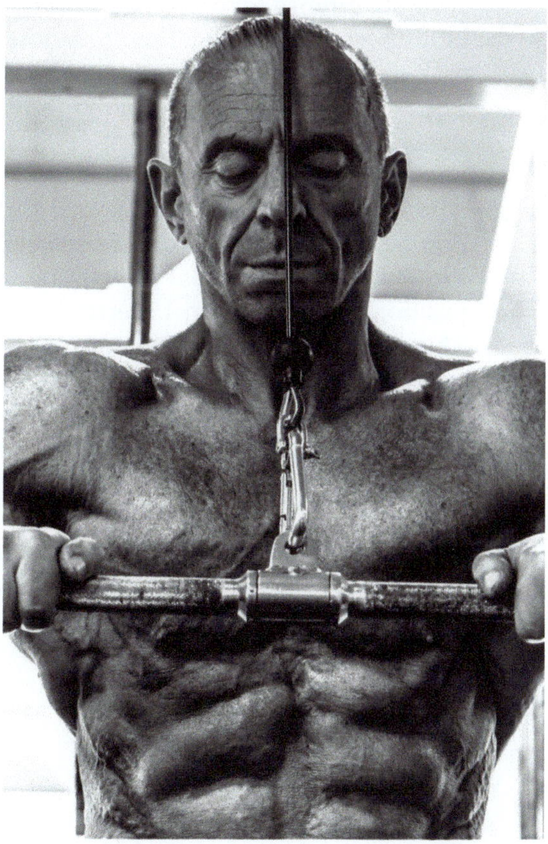

If the movement is performed correctly, after about ten repetitions, the muscle is already well-saturated. From here we move on to the **"pyramid sets"**.

Parrillo recommends performing a number of repetitions that is between 12 and 4. You will perform at least four sets, always adding weight and always decreasing the repetitions: you must get to the last sets, in which you cannot complete more than 3-4 repetitions.

A recovery of 2 to 4 minutes is indicated between each set. It is absolutely not too long, because these recovery minutes will be actively occupied. With this system, you perform a couple of exercises. Only the last sets will have to be brought to complete failure.

After each pyramid set, a **"breakout set"** must be performed. Using a load that allows for execution of high repetitions (15-20) you always reach exhaustion.

And here we are at the real novelty of this system: **"fascial stretching"**. It has nothing to do with usual stretching, instead it is a backbreaking system, suitable only for advanced athletes. It is stretching that affects the muscle that has just been trained and must be performed between sets to "reset" the muscle that has just been "squeezed". It is defined as "fascial" as its purpose is to forcefully stretch and soften the muscle sheath, i.e. the band of connective tissue that contains the muscle belly which is already inflamed and swollen with blood. Thus, the aim is to make the fascia maximally stretched so that the muscle expands maximally within it.

You reach the forced position of maximum stretching alone or with the help of your partner and hold it for 15 seconds. At this point, isometric contractions of the muscle being trained are performed for about ten seconds.

In summary, this is how the Parrillo technique is performed (an example for the pectorals):

1. A **single intense set** of flat bench presses, with a very light barbell, performed as if it were very heavy. Ten ultra-slow repetitions, squeezing your pecs hard each time.
2. The real workout begins with **pyramid sets** (these are four sets × 12-4 repetitions, increasing the weight with each set and only reaching failure on the last one). After each pyramid set, do…
3. … a **set to exhaustion** with a load that allows you to perform 15-20 repetitions, always at the limit of muscle failure.
4. We move on to a **fascial stretching** exercise of the affected muscle, held in position for no less than 15 seconds.
5. This is followed by an isometric bodyweight contraction or a **bodybuilder pose** (in this case, the mandatory side chest pose, pulling to the maximum and repeating the pose at least twice on each side, or the "*most muscular*" type contraction, with the hands joined in front of the abdomen). By posing repeatedly, as soon as the set is finished, the muscle is induced to cramp.

After about 1 minute of rest, you move on to the next set. Let's consider the first set as an example: suppose you load the bench with 70 kg for the barbell bench press, with which you perform 12 repetitions. Immediately after the twelfth repetition, you switch to the *exhaustion sets* with a weight that allows you to perform 15 to 20 repetitions, reaching the inability to move the barbell; this is followed by *fascial stretching*, after which you immediately move on to the pose of the pectorals, then to the *contractions with joined hands.*

You then move on to the second set, increasing the weight (pyramid sets) with 80 kg for 10 repetitions; you move on to the *exhaustion set*, always with a weight that allows you to perform 15 to 20 repetitions, reaching the inability to move the barbell; this is followed by *fascial stretching*, after which you immediately move on to the *pose of the pectorals*, then to the *contractions with joined hands*. Continue to do so for each of the 4 pyramid sets.

This combination of intense training (heavy-light), forced stretching and cramp-prone posing, dramatically increases the elasticity of the muscle sheath. Parrillo's gimmick is brilliant: **saturate the trained muscle with blood and, once it is swollen with blood, forcefully stretch it so that the muscular sheath (fascia) widens.**

It can be said that Parrillo was the first to document this technique, later used by many others, to obtain maximum dilatation of the muscle belly under stress, stretching and expanding the connective tissue of the muscle sheath. The sheath is made up of sheets of connective tissue separated from each other by veils of a lubricant, hyaluronic acid. Its density and thickness can sometimes be the cause of a lack of expansion of the muscle belly. It has been seen that this practice tends to make it more elastic and efficient and it eliminates a large part of the muscle stiffness.

Therefore, the more elastic the fascia, the more the muscle will be able to expand and swell under strain. The pose will, as a result, force the muscle to expand against the newly stretched girdle. Basically, the muscle will find more room to expand.

An example is the shoulders, one of the hardest muscles to stretch. As soon as you complete a set of behind-the-neck barbell presses, hold on to the bar and do a sort of *reverse shoulder stretch*. As soon as you get off the bar, do the back *double biceps* pose, until you reach the deltoid cramp.

Many years before Parrillo, the legendary John Grimek (the first Mr. Universe in the history of bodybuilding) used weights as a means to increase his flexibility/joint mobility.

Fundamental to the development of this system was the use of a "clean" diet, based on many calories/many proteins taken in numerous meals during the day.

Taking a cue from powerlifters, Grimek understood that Power Training + Power Eating would build a lot of muscle, especially in the off-season period. According to Parrillo, the daily calorie intake should reach 6,000 kcal for women and 10,000 kcal for men!

Parrillo introduced the use among bodybuilders of MCT oil (Medium Chain Triglycerides), an oil that our body assimilates almost as if it were a simple carb, that is, it transforms it very quickly into energy. To use it you had to consume four or more tablespoons six times a day, which corresponds to over 2,500 kcal!

Eight-time Ms. Olympia Lenda Murray (who followed Parrillo's lead for a period of her career) used this type of oil in place of carbohydrates during her pre-competition period.

Parrillo's great merit was not only that of having organized training in a practical and simple way that took into account *all the functional characteristics of the muscle*, but also that of having prompted American bodybuilders to introduce *aerobic exercise in the morning on an empty stomach*, in order to activate the metabolism and to keep blood insulin levels low, with the consequent consumption of fatty acids.

FST-7 (Hany Rambod training)

Now that I have finished talking about John Parrillo's brilliant insight, we immediately turn to what I consider to be a major development of his method. Undoubtedly, these methods are part of different historical moments of bodybuilding, but both are very effective.

FST-7 is a training system designed by Hany Rambod, a famous American coach of Iranian origin. Phil Heat and Jay Cutler have been using this technique for years. In recent years, Iranian Hadi Choopan and American Derek Lunsford, along with many others, have also followed his system with enormous success.

"FST" stands for **"Fascia Stretch Training,"** while the number "7" refers to the **seven sets** of the last exercise of the trained muscle group.

The key points of this tecnhique are:

- lengthening of the fascia (sheath), thus creating more space
- satellite cell proliferation
- superior hyperemia after fascial stretching and after the famous final seven sets

There are three types of fascia in the human body, but the type that interests bodybuilders is the deep fascia. It is a dense, fibrous connective tissue that penetrates muscles and surrounds muscles, bones, nerves and blood vessels. The high density of collagen fibers is what gives the deep fascia its strength and integrity. The amount of elastin fibers determines its extensibility and elasticity. In other words, some of us have thicker, sturdier fascia than others. Genetically luckier bodybuilders have thinner fascia and, as a result, their muscular bellies appear bigger and fuller, with that "round" look we all covet. Kenneth "Flex" Wheeler and Phil Heath are two prime examples of individuals with a thin fascia. Their muscles expand easily. Basically, it's easier to inflate a balloon than one of those rubber hot water bottles that Franco Columbu blew up.

Jay Cutler and the late Nasser El-Sonbaty probably had thicker muscle fascia. This, however, did not stop them from building substantially huge muscle mass. Still, the average-level bodybuilder has a thicker fascia than those two champs. In an attempt to expand the fascia and allow growth to occur, some have used junk like *Synthol* or its derivatives (a compound made up of 85% MCT oil, 7.5% anesthetic lidocaine and 7.5% alcohol), injecting it deep into the muscle belly. Others, especially online, have even been led to believe that this is the only solution. Some have even tried to act as though all practitioners use *Synthol* by injecting it topically. *Synthol* and similar substances must be considered foreign bodies, as they are never completely absorbable, they are of dubious origin and of even more dubious sterility and one can never be sure how the body metabolizes them. Among those who have used this product, there have been many cases of serious infections, partial removal of affected muscles and the amputation of necrotic limbs, as well as numerous cases of renal failure. You have to stretch the fascia for optimal growth, but that's not how it's done.

Please, never use it.

In the previous paragraph, we discussed how John Parrillo, in the 1980s, then more recently Dante Trudel of the famous DoggCrapp Training (see below) incorporated rather aggressive stretching during their training sessions. The basic concept, as already mentioned, is that when you perform deep stretching exercises, the fascia covering the muscle belly expands, producing more room for growth.

The FST-7 system is based on stretching the muscle from the inside out to volumize it. This is achieved by reaching the maximum possible pump during a workout.

This method has also been subject to criticism. FST-7 has been said to be a pump-only workout, which is not true. That's just one of its components.

Rambod argues that in order to be stimulated in depth and reach the tearing of the fibers, a muscle must be worked with heavy loads in the range of 6-10 repetitions.

Heavy loads give thickness and density, but not quite that full, rounded look. Similarly, an incredible pump after each session can get you round muscles, but it will never give you extreme muscle volume unless you also train with classic sets and heavy loads. Therefore, you need to focus equally on *maximizing both strength and pump* during the same training session to see the best results. Below is an example FST-7 style biceps workout where you can better understand how to incorporate both types of workouts.

An FST-7 method example

- Alternate dumbbell curl 3-4 × 8-12
- Scott bench curl 3 × 8-12
- EZ-bar barbell curl 7 × 8-12 (30-45 second rest between sets)

In general, it's best not to use a high number of repetitions, as too often you'll feel general fatigue and run out of breath before you hit your maximum muscle pump. And it is better if the load is not excessively heavy, so as not to limit the repetitions to fewer than 8, because at that point form worsens and the auxiliary muscles come into action, "stealing" the correct stimulation from the primary agonist muscle.

You should keep rest **periods fairly short** because after pumping, at that moment of pause, some blood leaves the muscle. **It's like inflating a balloon that has a small leak: even if you inflate it, some air escapes. The secret is to get the pump set after set so that it reaches its maximum size by the last set.** If the rests were too short, you wouldn't have enough energy to perform the seven sets well.

In general, this type of training is too traumatic for larger groups to be applied more than once a week. The soreness tends to linger for a long time, and the microscopic muscle tears, which occur at higher-than-normal rates with FST-7 training, need a little more recovery time than standard training protocols. However, smaller muscle groups (for example, arms and calves) can – and should – be trained twice a week. This way you have twice the opportunity to stretch the fascia to the max in what are often exceptionally difficult parts to build.

Below is an example of a breakdown that shows how you might organize your training.

An example of subdivision with the FST-7 method

- **Day 1:** biceps and triceps, calves
- **Day 2:** legs
- **Day 3:** rest
- **Day 4:** pectorals and triceps
- **Day 5:** back and calves
- **Day 6:** shoulders and biceps
- **Day 7:** rest

This breakdown is suitable for those who aim to build arm muscle. Of course, everyone will focus their workouts on their weakest group, favoring multi-frequency training for smaller muscles.

Some exercises are better suited than others for the seven sets. Multi-joint free weight exercises, such as squats and deadlifts, are usually the worst choice, mainly because they involve so many other muscle groups and are not very good at isolating a particular muscle; secondly, because they require mastery of technique and balance, two qualities we tend to lose when we try to perform multiple sets in a short amount of time.

Machines, on the other hand, are a good choice in many cases because they keep the movement in a fixed plane, thus making it easier to isolate a certain muscle, managing to deposit the largest possible amount of blood in the area.

The following table lists some exercises that lend themselves to this need.

- **Back width:** machine pullover or standing pulldown
- **Back thickness:** rowing machine, low pulley (with a cushion under the buttocks)
- **Chest:** pec deck or chest machine, flyes on the cables
- **Shoulders:** lateral machine raise
- **Quadriceps:** leg extension, 45° leg press
- **Hamstrings:** seated or lying leg curl
- **Biceps:** barbell curl, cable curl
- **Triceps:** rope cable pushdown, cable overhead extension, French press (for advanced athletes)
- **Calves:** standing and seated calf, 45° calf press

The best time for the seven sets is the last exercise of a muscle group. You shouldn't do them first, because it would worsen the performance for the normal heavy sets, which are essential as *they are the ones that allow you to "feel" the pump of the "7" sets.*

Remember that the seven sets must be performed at the conclusion of each muscle group workout; therefore, if you train multiple muscle groups in the same session, you will be doing two or more of these extended pump sets.

Examples of the most classic FST-7s

Back

- Deadlift 4 × 6-8 reps
- T-bar row 4 × 8-10 reps
- Reverse grip lat machine (*with the grip wider than the shoulders*) 4 × 8-12 reps
- Low pulley row or rowing machine 7 × 8-15 reps

Triceps

- Close-grip bench press 3-4 × 8-12 reps
- Dips with weight 3 × 8-12 reps
- French press (forehead barbell extension) 7 × 8-12 reps

Biceps

- Barbell curl 3-4 × 8-12 reps
- Standing dumbbell curl 3 × 8-12 reps
- Cable curl 7 × 8-12 reps

Quadriceps

- Leg extension 3-4 × 8-15 reps
- Squat 4 × 8-12 reps
- Hack squat or 45° leg press 3 × 8-15 reps
- Leg extension or 45° leg press 7 × 8-15 reps

Hamstrings and calves

- Deadlift with straight legs 3-4 × 10-12 reps
- Standing leg curl 4 × 10-12 reps
- Lying leg curl 7 × 8-15 reps
- Standing calf raises 3-4 × 15-20 reps
- Seated calf raises 4 × 15-20 reps
- 45° calf presses 7 × 15-20 reps

Chest

- Incline barbell bench press 3-4 × 8-12 reps
- Incline dumbbell press 3 × 8-12 reps
- Barbell bench press 3 × 8-12 reps
- Pec deck or cable flyes 7 × 8-12 reps

Shoulders

- Seated dumbbell or barbell press 4 × 8-12 reps
- Dumbbell/barbell front raises
- Dumbbell lateral raise 3 × 8 12 reps
- Machine lateral raise 7 × 8-12 reps

In regards to this method, I have to say that ending a muscle group workout with an exceptional pump is something many athletes have been doing automatically for years without ever stopping to consider the fact that they were expanding the fascia or maximizing growth. It has always been done because that's how it's done! Our instinct leads us to do it and we have always seen it done by all the old bodybuilders who trained in our gyms. Personally, I consider it more as a formalization of something that all of us, in various ways, have always done without ever having felt the need to commercialize it as a "method". This is not meant to take anything away from Hany Rambod, whom I consider a great coach.

Dorian Yates' training

I would define this workout as a perfect combination of several techniques, all inserted at the right time. In my opinion, Dorian Yates (awarded six consecutive Mr. Olympia titles) was the greatest bodybuilder of all time, both physically and technically speaking. Yates' program follows a 2:1 pace, i.e. 2 consecutive days and 1 rest day (without considering the days of the week).

Another important aspect is training schedule: he prefers to train in the late morning, around 11 or noon for various reasons, including meal times. At that time of day, Yates is absolutely "full" of glycogen, as he has already eaten two high-carb meals.

The most important aspect to "feeling" his technique well is the **warm-up set**. We will come back to this after more fully explaining what his technique consists of.

A heavy load is chosen for a "basic" exercise, which can be lifted in no more than 6-7 repetitions, maximum 8. This means that, at the sixth or seventh repetition, the athlete is no longer able to perform a single full repetition. Having reached muscle exhaustion, the training partner intervenes, pushing the athlete to perform 3-4 forced repetitions, forcing them to go beyond their natural abilities. Two negative repetitions (8 seconds down) follow. At this point, the athlete just has time to unload the weight by half and (after 15-20 seconds of rest) perform as many repetitions as possible.

According to Yates, this is a single set brought to the limit of the strength and contractile capacity of the muscles!

I feel like adding my thoughts regarding Yates. He helped me with my training for almost 2 years when he had just started winning Olympias, which was the peak of his competitive career.

His neuromuscular contraction was astounding, literally "squeezing" his muscles under heavy weights. His ability to flex a muscle, contract it and slowly release it, feeling the stretched fibers unravel, was a unique, hard, painful and frightening sight to behold. With the utmost concentration, focused on his goal, he attacked it massacring and tearing it apart until it broke, crossing all possible pain thresholds until he pushed them to the limit in each session, deceiving the brain and enduring the unbearable. Truly unmatched!

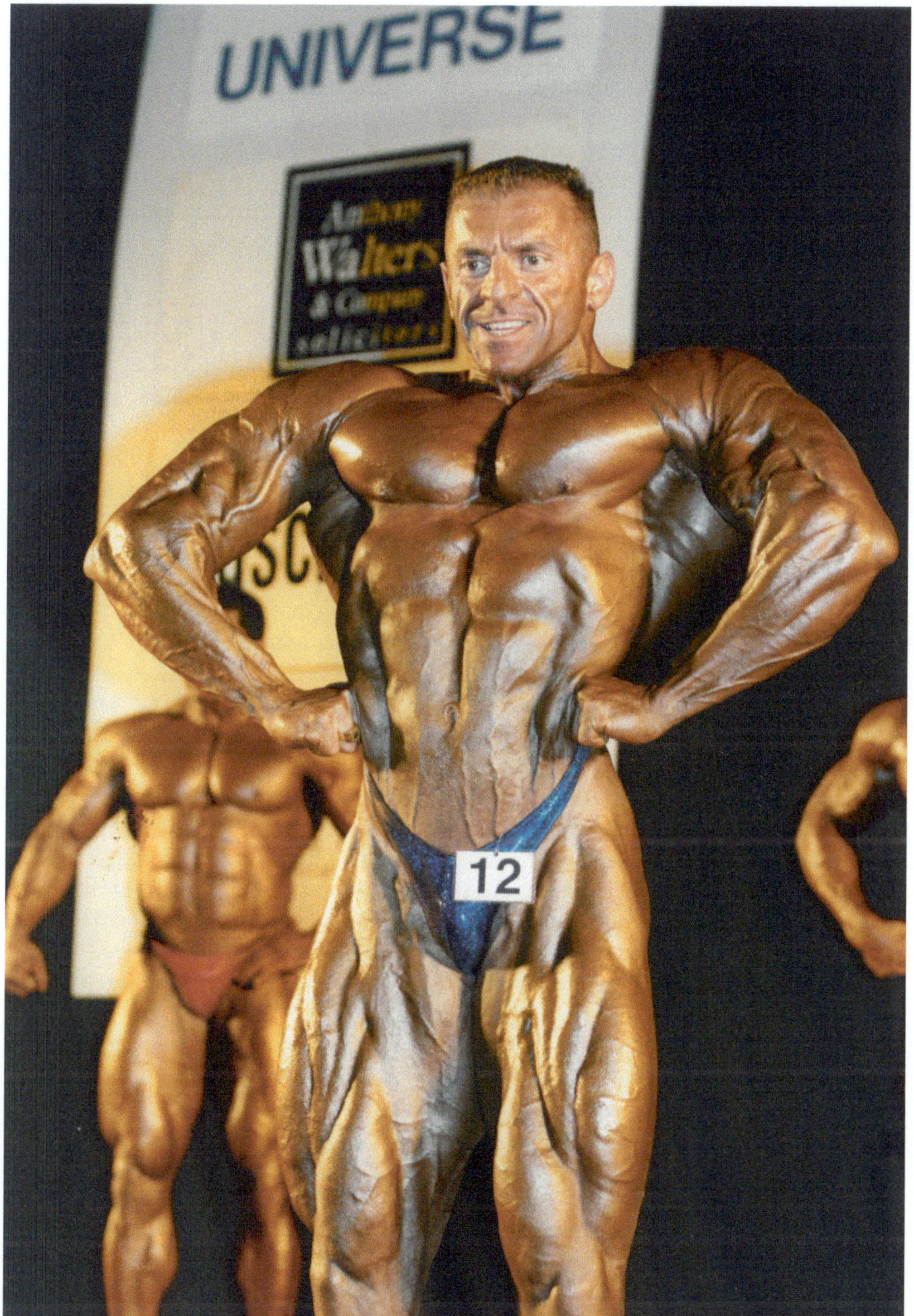
UNIVERSE
12

If performed according to his rules, this system instantly "inflates" the muscle being trained. In addition, it causes a different type of swelling: it is a feeling of fullness combined with muscle cramps. **The muscle, in practice, is immediately "hard" to the touch**.

Therefore, there is a lot of intensity and little volume: from two to four sets. These are Dorian Yates' rules.

Usually, this technique is applied to only one exercise (the first and basic) per group, and on 1-2 groups per workout.

So, we have:

1. 6-7 heavy reps brought to failure.
2. 3-4 forced reps (*with the same amount of weight*).
3. 2 negative reps (*8-second eccentric/negative phase*).
4. 15-20 seconds of rest, during which the weight is reduced by 50%.
5. As many reps as possible with 50% of the starting weight.

This is the set that is repeated two to four times for the main group. **Warming up** is also important. What is **specific warm-up**? Warm-up sets are done using a load that weighs almost the same as the weight used in the first set of the first exercise.

Example: the first exercise consists of flat bench presses, in which the athlete knows they can perform 6-7 repetitions with 120 kg. After a general joint warm-up, there are 2-3 warm-up sets with an increasingly heavier load that reaches 70% of 120 kg or the load to be used in the rest of the workout.

Flyes of light cables should never be part of the last exercise before 6-7 repetitions with 120 kg. In addition to the risk of injury, it is not a correct way to start the actual training, as the initial sets (basically, half of the training) can be "thrown away". This, according to Yates, is the most important motivation for warm-up sets.

Furthermore, if the warm-up sets inadequate in terms of intensity, i.e. if we performed it chatting and joking with our partner (as often happens), or we chose a weight that was too light, then making a mistake in selecting the weight of the initial load, we wouldn't reach muscle failure in 6-7 repetitions, but perhaps after 12 or more. In this way, the effectiveness of the technique is compromised.

The 3-4 forced repetitions become more than 4 that the athlete manages to perform alone.

If warm-up has been performed correctly and the "heavy" set has been exhausted within 6-7 repetitions, it will almost mathematically result in three more forced repetitions with the same weight. Furthermore, the two negative repetitions always imply a very heavy load, which the athlete can no longer control in the positive phase.

So, for it to be a real negative, the load has to be really heavy!

If you have used a very light weight, problems will arise when the time comes to put the weight down and proceed with the 50% downshift. We have seen that it is about cutting the weight by half: the initial 120 kg bench press becomes 60-65 kg, and the initial 150 kg squat becomes 75-80 kg. The right feeling is to feel this heavy load like the one used for the initial 6-7 repetitions.

In the following table, we see a practical example, taken from training the back muscles.

1. Reverse grip lat machine: 1 × 6-7 + 3-4 forced + 2 negative + max reps with 50% of the weight, repeat 4 times (*15-20 seconds rest between small sets, long recovery between sets*)
2. Barbell Row or T-bar row: heavy load 5 × 8 (*or stripping technique*)
3. Low pulley or row (*as in the second exercise*)

We have already mentioned that Yates trained in the late morning, after consuming two high-carb meals. The meal that immediately follows the workout is made up of many complex carbohydrates and animal proteins. After this meal, the protein percentage rises in inverse proportion to the carbohydrates, which will then disappear by the end of the day. *I emphasize this principle, which I blindly believe and which I have always followed and recommended to other athletes who want to build lean muscle mass without gaining fat. In doing so, Yates created an "anabolic event" around training.*

This devastating method of intensity and concentration is present in all aspects of Yates' preparation. Every detail is taken care of to the maximum, nothing is left to chance. This always made him self-confident, to the point of affirming, before winning every Mr. Olympia he participated in, that *it would have been impossible for him not to win, because no one in the world could ever have done the same workouts he subjected himself to in such a maniacally perfect way*, reaching the greatest human limit of physical endurance of extreme pain.

This statement shocked me. I was lucky enough to know him and to be trained by him between 1992 and 1994, and I must say that I consider him to be the greatest bodybuilder of all time because of his intensity and devastating mental attitude. The year he suffered some serious arm injuries, which prevented him from training as he normally would, he decided to officially retire. As a winner.

This time he knew that someone else could have done better than him.

"Y3T" (Neil "Yoda" Hill training)

Neil Hill was a good professional athlete, but he became world-famous for training bodybuilders such as William Bonac and Flex Lewis. Hill had the ingenuity and the ability to and overcome the barrier of injuries caused by heavy-load training, always continuing to train hard. After a lifetime of very heavy sessions, which stressed the joints and connective tissue beyond measure, he began to train cyclically with sessions with lighter loads and higher repetitions, performed in the right place and at the right time, in a very distinct 3-week workout program.

The Yoda 3 Training (Y3T) is "spread" over 9 weeks, which are in turn divided into 3 different weeks. It is recommended to start with a routine of **4 sessions a week**: *2 days on, 1 day off, 2 days on, 2 days off*, and then move on to **five sessions.**

- **Week 1** focuses on basic, compound exercises, with heavy loads and low explosive repetitions in the concentric, slow phase (at least 3 seconds); the eccentric phase includes 6 to 10 repetitions.
- **Week 2** includes a combination of basic multi-joint exercises and complementary isolation exercises with two to three more repetitions than the first week (the **first Y3T**), spending at least 2 seconds in the eccentric/negative phase of the movement. More recently, with the experiences of athletes, it has been seen that the repetitions can also be increased to 16-18.
- **Week 3** of the micro-cycle is based on total muscle exhaustion with lighter loads and high repetitions to maximize muscle volume by also using giant sets. The repetitions, in this week, must go on until total exhaustion and spend a lot of time under tension. Flex Lewis started from a minimum of 20 repetitions up to even 100 in some exercises.

At the end of the third week, the program starts all over again with the second 3-week micro-cycle, using heavier loads for the same number of repetitions. This micro-cycle is repeated three times for a total of 9 weeks. After 9 weeks, if the intensity you sustained was really high, *you absolutely must take 1 full week of total rest from your workouts*, and then start again with a 9-week Y3T cycle.

Y3T can be defined as **three-dimensional** for building very dense muscle fiber. It affects every aspect of the muscle in a short amount of time. After observing and testing this training system, many aspects of it remind me of Fred Hatfield's Holistic Training. This program also hits both the fast and slow fibers hard, violently stretching the fascia, i.e., the sheath that surrounds the muscle belly.

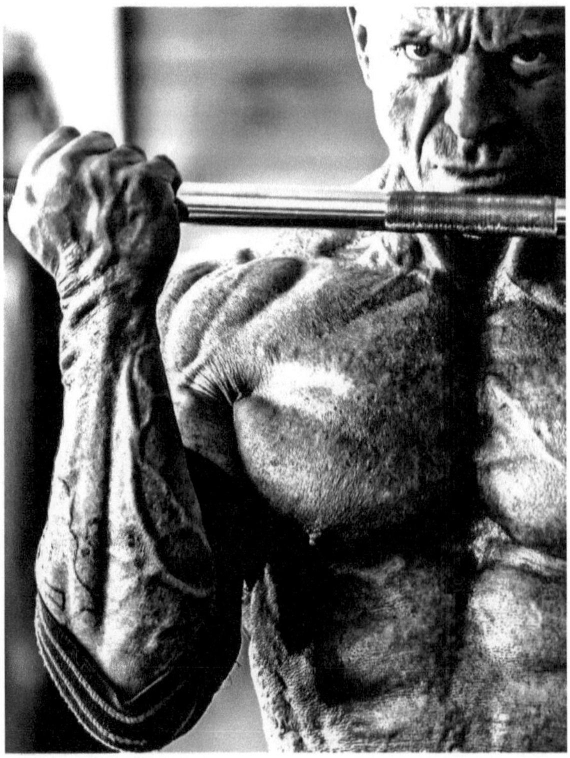

Both Parrillo and Rambod have identified the crucial point of muscle hypertrophy: **expanding the muscle through the forced yielding of the connective tissue that surrounds it.**

We have been witnesses to the continuous development of training methodologies over the years. I call it *development* and not *progress*, since development is the consequent unfolding and evolution of events, in this case of techniques, but it does not necessarily mark the achievement of a clear improvement compared to the previous theory, i.e., progress. In the end, everything always revolves around the same concepts, but some add a piece to the strategy to conquer muscle hypertrophy, often "selling" it well and better than others. Very few have had brilliant insights, which are then scientifically proven.

This cycled system reduces the risk of injury, while maintaining the benefits of lifting loads only using them for a third of the duration of the micro-cycle. Cycling and a week of total rest don't prevent performance injuries as much as overuse injuries, which come from continuous wear and tear of the tendons.

Mountain Dog Training (Push, Pull, Legs system by John Meadows)

John Meadows was a good athlete, both as an amateur and as an IFBB professional, but sadly passed away in 2021 at just 49 years old. Without a doubt, he was an excellent old-fashioned coach and preferred high-intensity and traditional exercises. His characteristic was to break down the body into three different sectors and train them separately from each other with at least one day of rest, to get to train more frequently even for three consecutive days with one day of rest, but always following the *Pushing muscles, Pulling muscles, Legs* protocol.

The following table shows a basic example of Meadows' method.

Basic example of Mountain Dog Training

First week

- Monday: push workout
- Tuesday: rest
- Wednesday: pull workou
- Thursday: rest
- Friday: leg workout
- Saturday: rest
- Sunday: push workout

Second week

- Monday: rest
- Tuesday: pull workout
- Wednesday: rest
- Thursday: leg workout
- Friday: rest
- Saturday: push workout
- Sunday: rest

So, train every other day, alternating the training of *pushing muscles* (*chest, shoulders and triceps*), *pulling* (*back and biceps*) and *legs* (*quads, hamstrings and calves*). If you want to increase the frequency of your training sessions, you can even reach five sessions a week, respecting one day of rest for every three sessions. It will be your decision, based on your ability and your training seniority.

After having mentioned how to organize Mountain Dog Training, the following table shows a more detailed example of the program.

Mountain Dog "Push" Workout		
Exercises	**Sets**	**Repetitions**
Decline dumbbell press	5-6	2 × 20, 2-3 × 3-4, 1 × 6-8*
Incline dumbbell press	3	1 × 10-15, 2 × 6-8
Dips	3	Max reps
Behind-the-neck barbell press	4	8-10
Incline bench Y-raise (low trap and front shoulders)	3	15
Rope triceps pushdown	3	15
Triceps pushdown behind the neck from above	3	15

*Each repetition must be controlled. Max contraction at the top.

Note

You start the cycle with a full pushing motion. The first exercise consists precisely of decline dumbbell presses. Meadows claimed it was the best exercise to activate all the fibers in the pectoralis major. You start with a warm-up set of 20 repetitions, then 2 or 3 heavy sets of 3-4 repetitions and you finish off with a set of 8 repetitions to exhaustion. We move on to the attack of the upper part of the pectoral with incline dumbbell presses. You should vary the angle of the bench according to your body shape. The more the shoulders are hunched forward, the less the bench will have to be inclined. To finish pectoral training, we move on to dips, which is a *great core exercise that, in my opinion, should always be done in its eccentric phase* ***like a reverse shrug for the traps.***

We then move on to the shoulders with the Smith machine barbell press for sets of 8-10 repetitions.

For the lateral and front delts, Meadows favored the slightly inclined bench "Y-raise" to activate the shoulder and lower traps. The workout ended with two triceps exercises with cables. Meadows loved using the rope to be able to maximally contract the triceps during extension. He chose to do the last triceps exercise with the overhead rope because, this way, he was able to fully stretch his triceps, already trained hard by the push exercises performed previously.

Mountain Dog "Pull" Workout		
Exercises	**Sets**	**Reps**
"Meadows row" (a one-handed row performed on the T-bar)	3	8-12
Barbell row	3	8-12
Pull-up	3	8-12
90° raise (*back shoulders*)	3	20-25
Seated dumbbell hammer curl	3	12-15

Note

This day is dedicated to pulling exercises: back, posterior shoulders and biceps. Pulling training begins with the Meadows row. Hold the thick part of the barbell inserted in the bushing of the T-bar (i.e. where the discs are), with a straight overhand grip. Pull the elbow back and up as much as possible and use 10 kg plates to have a wider range of motion, without hitting the ground in the release phase.

From this exercise, we move on to the barbell row. Neutral grip on the barbell, keep the elbow close to the torso, and rotate the shoulder when contracting the muscles. Here too, it is better to use plates that are not too wide so to have a better range of motion.

Now we move on to the bar for forward pull ups. Meadows preferred the band-assisted pull-up, which helped him carry out a spasm contraction in the positive concentric phase.

The next exercise will isolate the rear delts. 90° dumbbell raises with forehead resting on the back of an incline bench. The hand position is with palms facing downwards. Do as many repetitions as you can, to fill the rear deltoids with blood as much as possible.

The last exercise targets the biceps. Meadows went for the dumbbell hammer. It is not true that the hammer exercise only works the brachialis and the brachioradialis since it is also very valid for the biceps itself and can be considered a basic exercise for all the pulling muscles of the arm. This movement can be performed either on the Scott bench, with the elbow resting inside the vertical part of the support, or standing, one dumbbell at a time, not frontally, but nearly rubbing the abdomen against the bench when going up.

Mountain Dog "Legs" Workout		
Exercises	**Sets**	**Reps**
Lying leg curl	3	8*
Spider bar squat (*classic barbell squat with handstands*)	6	2 × 8, 3 × 3, 1 × 6-8
45° leg presses in superset with sissy squat	3	8 + 8
Smith machine split squat (*single leg squat*)	3	8 per leg
Standing calf raises (with 10 seconds of top contraction)	4	8 + 10 second contraction + 8 + 10 seconds + 8

*On the last set, do a double strip of the weight, then partial reps, then finish with 10 seconds of isometric contraction.

Note

The third day of training is entirely dedicated to the lower limbs. Meadows believed that by initiating leg sets with the hamstrings, a lot of blood could be drawn into the back of the thigh. This would improve performance on the basic, heavy exercise which followed, the one targeting the quads.

The first basic multi-joint movement is the spider bar squat. Squats cannot be missing in leg training. According to Meadows, this variation of the squat is more effective, but any type of squat or front squat can work.

After six sets of very heavy squats done to exhaustion, Meadows destroyed his quads with a super-set combination of 45° leg presses and sissy squats with a perfectly straight back or leg extensions in case he didn't have a sissy squat bench.

The final leg exercise is the one-leg Smith machine squat. Basically, from a standing position with a barbell on your shoulders, take a step back and squat 8 times. Then repeat with the other leg.

To complete the entire session, the calves will be trained at the standing calf machine: 8-10 repetitions seeking maximum stretching and maximum movement, alternating with 10 seconds of contraction at the top.

This program can be followed for 6 weeks. As soon as you notice a plateau in your results, you can do one week of intensity deload and then start again. This is certainly a good method to divide workouts in a functional way following the principles of dynamics and kinetic chains. I consider it a valid approach for the off-season period, but as we approach competitions, methods and intensity should definitely change and increase.

DoggCrapp Training (Dante Trudel)

DoggCrapp Training is a training style invented by Dante Trudel in the early 2000s that has found some success among amateur and professional athletes. One of the most famous athletes to practice it was the multi-finalist of Mr. Olympia, David Henry, with whom I had the pleasure of training in 2004 and 2005 at Gold's Gym in Tucson, Arizona. Trudel began studying the common characteristics of professional bodybuilders and discovered that they all had at least three common characteristics: *they all trained as intensely as possible, they all trained one muscle group more than once a week, especially during the competition phase, and they all, more or less, had remarkable characteristics of flexibility.* He drew from these three starting points to organize his simple program, which took its name from his nickname, DoggCrapp, which he had used in a bodybuilding forum in the 90s. It's certainly not a type of workout that a novice lifter can do: you need at least 2 or 3 years of experience under heavy free weights in the gym and you need to understand the concept of intensity before you can dive into it.

The basic principles of this system are: *progressive increase in loads, low volume of work and high intensity, training each muscle more than once a week, use of rest pause, fascial stretching* (since so many famous coaches resumed this practice in their protocols, it means Parrillo was right) *and the introduction of a last infernal set, which he called "The Widowmaker"*, sets which risked leaving your wife widowed.

Trudel observed that a classic bodybuilder typically trained one muscle group 52 times a year, or once a week. However, he thought it was better to train each muscle area 50% more by using one real set, brought "to death" in each session.

The heart of this workout derives once again from a technique by the great Mike Mentzer: the famous **Rest-Pause** This technique, further developed by many coaches, allows you to use a very heavy load, allowing the athlete to perform many more repetitions than would normally be possible.

A concept that, historically, everyone has always agreed on: a heavy load moved many times. Let us consider the example of barbell military presses for the shoulders. After a few warm-up sets, slowly increasing the load, to prepare the joints, load the barbell with a weight with which you can do no more than 8-10 repetitions alone. Do as many as you can until you reach failure.

Put the barbell down and take 10-15 strong "belly" breaths. Oxygen helps the recovery process. Pick up the barbell again and repeat until exhaustion. Put the load down again, breathe deeply 10-15 times, and perform a few repetitions again. In total, you should do between 12 and 15 repetitions.

If you do more than 15 repetitions, remember to increase the weight next time if you repeat that exercise or do a few more repetitions.

Some athletes are able to further intensify the sets by introducing a static repetition in isometrics, for 30-60 seconds, holding the barbell at 90°. Rest-pause cannot be used in all exercises. For safety reasons, it is best not to perform it in basic multi-joint exercises such as squats and deadlifts.

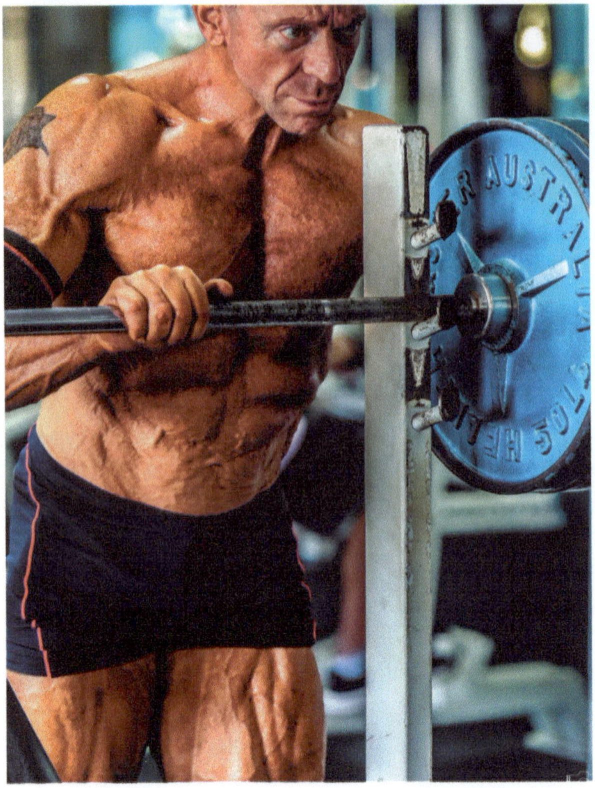

Not all rep ranges fall between 12 and 15. In one devastating set, such as squats, you'll perform about 20 repetitions with maximum weight. The repetitions will also increase during the bicep and tricep rest breaks, and the set will also reach 30 repetitions. If the number of repetitions becomes too high, it does not mean that the sets will be easier. They will always be what Dante Trudel calls "The Widowmaker".

This system is the right combination of a workout to exhaustion with the best frequency.

Those who are about to use this method for the first time are advised to follow the scheme shown in the following table.

First week

- Monday: workout A
- Wednesday: workout B
- Friday: workout A

Second week

- Monday: workout B
- Wednesday: workout A
- Friday: workout B

Each **A workout** consists of working these muscles in the following order:

1. pectorals
2. shoulders
3. triceps
4. back width
5. back thickness

Each **B workout** consists of working these muscles in the following order:

1. biceps
2. forearms
3. calves
4. hamstring
5. quadriceps

It is essential to respect the order in which the muscle groups are trained. Trudel tried changing the sequence of the different groups with various athletes, but without finding any benefits. This, therefore, appears to be the best possible combination.

The hardest and most difficult exercises to complete are done last, so that it is not necessary to conserve energy as if they had been trained first. In fact, after you've completed a heavy set of squats, accompanied by a "Widowmaker" set, the last thing you'll want to do is keep working out.

As for the selection of exercises for each area, you can choose which ones to do, bearing in mind that, for some exercises, it is almost impossible to do a "Widowmaker" set.

Below is a sample of the best exercises to use for each muscle groups.

Pectorals

- Incline barbell/dumbbell press
- Decline barbell/dumbbell press
- Chest machine
- Wide-grip dips

(*Trudel advises against bench press*)

Shoulders

- Seated or standing military press
- Dumbbell press
- Shoulder press

Triceps

- Smith machine reverse grip wide bench
- Smith machine bench press
- Dips

Back width

- Overhead press
- Any type of lat pulldown
- Pullovers

Continues

Continued

Back thickness

- Deadlift
- Straight or reverse grip barbell row
- Back row loading machine

Biceps

- Barbell curl
- Alternate dumbbell curl
- Low cable curl

Forearms

- Hammer curl
- Pinwheel curl (a type of hammer curl in which the dumbbell is brought to the chest)
- Reverse curl
- Forearm push-ups with a barbell

Calves

- Standing calf raises
- Seated calf raises
- Donkey calf raises

(*Perform each repetition by lowering the load in 5 seconds, stay in full stretch for 15 seconds, lift with an explosive concentric movement while remaining on tiptoes in maximum contraction for 2 seconds*)

Hamstrings

- Lying leg curl
- Romanian or stiff-legged deadlift with a curved back
- Glute-ham raise ("dips" from the lat machine)

Quadriceps

- Back squat
- Front squat
- 45° leg press

(*All quad exercises should be performed in one set of 4 to 8 reps, followed by as much recovery time as needed, continuing with a 20-rep Widowmaker of the same exercise*)

After choosing your exercises, use them for workout A; next time change the exercise, and do the same for the third workout, so that each time a workout is different from the previous one. However, try not to change the exercises you have selected from the beginning, at least until you have managed to increase the load, so each exercise remains productive.

Now let's talk about **stretching**.

Trudel, as well as Rambod and Hill, drew from the pioneer of using this technique to increase muscle hypertrophy: John Parrillo.

We have seen that performing fascial or extreme stretching, after having trained the muscle, will allow it to expand more freely within the muscle band in which it is contained. Trudel observed that baby birds stretch their wings in preparation for their first flight.

It has been seen that, after this type of natural and instinctive stretching, the myosin and actin filaments break down, and the size of the muscle cells increases. The stretching recommended by Trudel is based on holding a weight (for example, two heavy dumbbells held in a pectoral stretch position in the push exercise) for a period of time ranging from 60 to 90 seconds.

When performed after the last training set, this stretch is hellish.

The basic concept of DoggCrapp Training is the **adaptation and fast accumulation of muscle mass.**

Athletes who want to follow this practice will have to keep a diary to write down the loads that are used to be able to improve each time and to stop when this no longer happens. The periodization to follow will be based on "blasting", i.e., 12 weeks in which you train aiming to break the previously established records, and on "cruising", i.e., the deload phase, lasting 10-14 days, in which you change the exercises by doing regular sets without reaching muscle exhaustion. If you completed 12 weeks of hell in the best way possible, then you may as well not go to the gym or only do cardio for those 2 weeks.

The purpose of cruising is precisely to let you take a regenerative break. **As far as nutrition is concerned, Trudel never counts the calories, only the animal proteins ingested.** I find this to be a very logical and intelligent indication. I believe it is **the simple and essential principle behind bodybuilding**. Not very commercial and without frills, but realistic and functional.

During the blasting phase, protein intake should be very high, even above 4 g per kg of body weight. This amount will then be dropped by more than 50% during the intensity deload phase.

Do 2-3 warmup sets before starting each exercise. Each rep will consist of one controlled eccentric (negative) and one explosive concentric (positive) movement. Rest between sets for as long as you deem necessary to restart at the maximum. In this way you will use the following techniques:

- **RP (rest pause)**;
- **SS** (straight sets, i.e., sets performed normally);
- **WM** ("Widowmaker").

In **workout A** you will attack the pecs, shoulders, triceps, back width and back thickness, respectively.
In **workout B** you will be targeting your biceps, forearms, calves, hamstrings and quads.

First week

WORKOUT A1

Exercises	Set	Reps
Incline bench barbell press	1	11-15 RP
90° bench dumbbell press	1	15-30 RP
Dips	1	15-20 RP
Lat pulldown	1	15-20 RP
Deadlift	2	5-8 / 9-12 SS

WORKOUT B1

Exercises	Set	Reps
Barbell curl	1	20-30 RP
Hammer curl	1	11-20 SS
Standing calf raises	1	10-12 SS*
Glute-ham raise *(lat machine or hyperextension dips)*	1	15-20 RP
45° leg press	2	4-8 SS + WM

WORKOUT A2

Exercises	Set	Reps
Two-dumbbell flat bench press	1	20-30 RP
Barbell military press	1	11-15 RP
Smith machine – narrow bench press	1	11-15 RP
Lat pulldown	1	15-20 RP
Barbell rows	1	10-12 SS

Second week

WORKOUT B2

Exercises	Set	Reps
Preacher curl (*straight Scott bench*)	1	20-30 RP
Reverse barbell curl	1	11-20 SS
45° leg press	1	10-12 SS
Lying leg curl	1	15-20 RP
Classic squat	2	4-8 SS + WM

WORKOUT A3

Exercises	Set	Reps
Slightly inclined bench press	1	11-15 RP
Military press seated at the Smith machine	1	11-15 RP
EZ bar French press	1	15-30 RP
Reverse bar	1	15-20 RP
T-bar row	1	10-12 SS

WORKOUT B3

Exercises	Set	Reps
Dumbbell curl	1	20-30 RP
Pinwheel curl *(turn the dumbbell towards the chest)*	1	11-20 SS
Seated calves	1	10-12 SS
Hack squat	2	6-10 SS + WM
Romanian Deadlift*	1	10-15 SS

*It will be the only time you do hamstrings after quads. It is preferred to do it this way to avoid stress on the lower back when it comes to performing basic multi-joint movements for the quadriceps.

If you feel tired at the beginning when following this protocol, do not hesitate to take Friday off and do 3 days of total recovery, to then resume fresh the following Monday.

Also, if you are over 40 and prefer to increase the number of repetitions rather than the weights, feel free to reach 15-20 repetitions rather than the usual 10-15.

SST, Sarcoplasm Stimulating Training (Patrick Tuor)

SST is a premium bulking training system developed by former professional bodybuilder Patrick Tuor, who currently trains top Olympian bodybuilders such as Iain Valliere and James Hollingshead, and has trained other professional athletes like Rafael Brandao and Nicolas Vullioud.

The principle on which Tuor's entire theory is based begins with a question that we have to ask ourselves every time we go to the gym: "What can I do to stimulate muscle growth?". The answer lies **in focusing on intensity and never on the workload!**

Classic SST consists of one exercise per muscle group consecutively without pauses and is structured as follows:

- load around 80% of the maximum weight and a set with as many repetitions as possible
- *rest for 15 seconds*
- using the same amount of weight, perform as many repetitions as possible
- *rest another 15 seconds*
- using the same amount of weight, try performing as many repetitions as you can
- reduce the load by 20% and do only one set of maximum repetitions with the *eccentric* (*negative*) phase performed slowly in 5 seconds
- reduce the load by another 20% and do only one set of the maximum number of repetitions with the *concentric* (*positive*) phase performed slowly in 5 seconds
- reduce the load by another 20% and do an *isometric contraction* for as long as possible (*at least 45 seconds*) until failure

This way, you start with a heavier load and end up with a much lighter load, which you'll manage to keep in the final phase of isometrics. You have to push yourself to the max during each micro-set. **If you don't max out and push yourself to the limit, this system won't work.** It's not for novice athletes, but if you want to gain muscle mass and try to do something that deeply tears your muscles, I think it's great. It is also very good for traumatizing muscles that have reached a growth stalemate in advanced athletes with a lot of experience.

Just one set is enough to stimulate all the fibers, deplete the muscles, and trigger significant growth and hypertrophy. Therefore, *you can use this principle either by doing just one set at the beginning or end of your classic workout or you can do the entire workout from start to finish following this system.* Better pumping, higher intensity and more mass. For most athletes, the key to growth is the stimulation of the **sarcoplasm**, the fluid between muscle fibers. This requires long stretch times and short breaks between sets. This produces **sarcoplasmic hypertrophy**, i.e. the expansion not of the myofibrillar tissue, but rather of the fluid within which the myofibrils are immersed. It's a great way to increase muscle volume. To train for strength, on the other hand, it is necessary to build myofibrils, or muscle fibers, which do not necessarily coincide with an increase in volume.

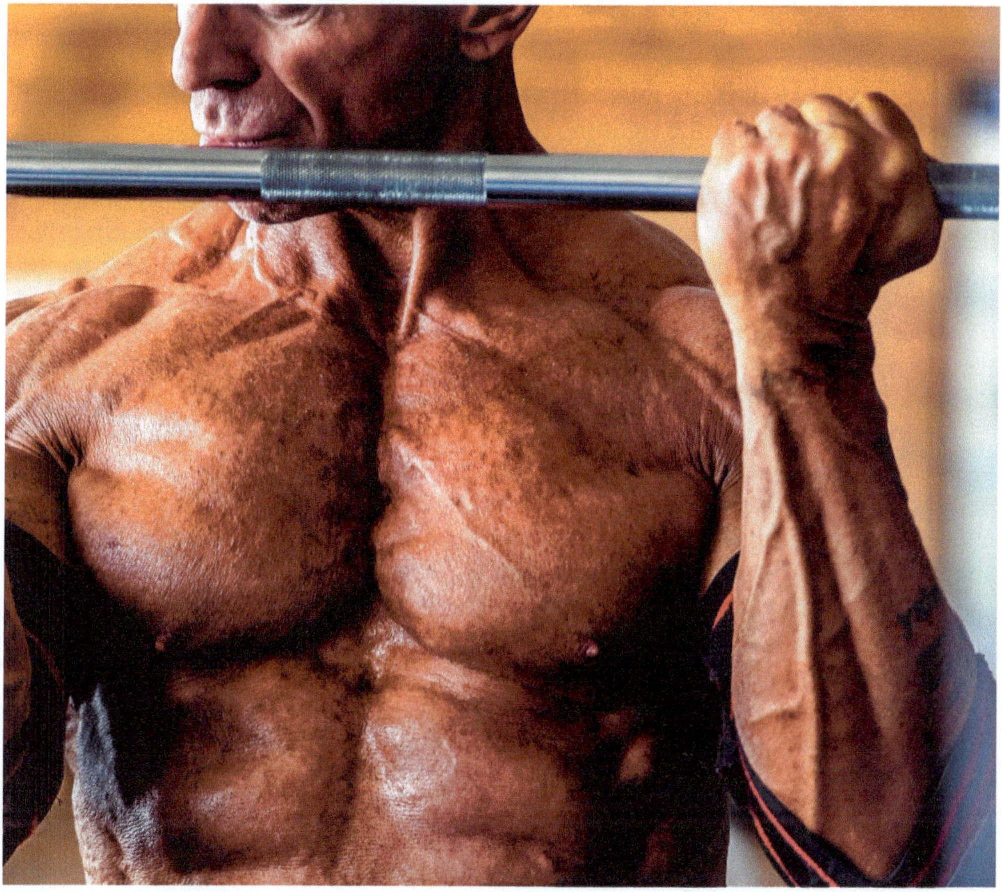

Tuor certainly developed this method considering the experience of Mentzer and Yates (in particular of the latter), keeping an eye on indications from Dr. Squat Frederick Hatfield. In the first three micro-sets of this macro-set, we base ourselves on a very sensible development of rest pause, extending it to more repetitions than those performed by Mike Mentzer.

The macro-set then continues with a *micro-set of Heavy-Duty eccentric negatives*, and then moves on to a micro-set with an emphasis on *concentric positives*, ending with muscle failure in a static contraction that we call *isometric*. In practice, Tuor synthesizes some of the most valid techniques ever, taking the core or essence of the techniques and summarizing them into a single training principle, introducing *stripping* during the sets, while Yates performed it at the end of everything.

Thus, Tuor attacks the muscle with as much force and contraction as possible. The first contraction emphasizes the lengthening of the muscle where the most profitable chemical exchanges take place, where the filaments of myosin and actin rub and tear; the second favors the shortening of the muscle; in the third and last one, the length of the muscle does not change, i.e., it occurs in the absence of movement. Even having reached the end of each micro-set, he always continues with *partial repetitions.* It is therefore a cocktail of the best techniques, each inserted at the right time. Each technique comes into play at the right moment, in sequence.

Dorian Yates had already developed Mentzer's Heavy Duty and Rest-Pause; Tuor goes further, using the third force, that of isometry. In my opinion, the brilliance of his idea was that he was able to combine all these protocols by amalgamating them with the continuous stripping technique, which allows you to complete three rest pauses, an eccentric negative set, a concentric positive set and one in isometrics, interspersed with partial repetitions and managing to do everything in TUT (Time Under Tension), or in a very long time of muscle tension (which we have seen previously), sufficient by itself for hypertrophy.

So, we have everything in one set. The muscle cannot do more than this! **In my opinion, it is an excellent method.**

As for my personal practice, I found it best, after the first 20% drop, to do all the concentric repetitions in 5 seconds and then the eccentric ones in 5 seconds. We are strongest in the downward part of the move, so it should be exploited at the end, not the beginning. This is just my impression and my consideration, but I think it can also be adapted to other athletes. This method requires great intrinsic motivation and a lot of concentration. No repetition can be thrown away and each micro-set must always be performed to muscle failure.

Below is what I consider to be a perfect outline to stimulate muscle growth by following Patrick Tuor's SST principle.

Single set (valid for each basic exercise of each muscle group)

1. Set of 10 reps performed with a weight with which you perform 10 reps maximum. *Rest 20 seconds*
2. Set performed to exhaustion with the same weight. *Rest 20 seconds*
3. Set performed to exhaustion with the same weight. *Rest 20 seconds*
4. Take off 20% of the load and exhaust yourself, 4 seconds down (*eccentric/negative*) and 1 second up (*concentric/positive*). *Rest 20 seconds*
5. Remove another 20% load and exhaust yourself, 4 seconds up (*concentric/positive*) and 1 second down (*eccentric/negative*). *Rest 20 seconds*
6. Take off another 20% of the load and perform an isometric (*static*) contraction held at the point of greatest effort, until exhaustion.

Kaatsu Training (BFR, Blood Flow Restriction Training)

Kaatsu Training is a workout that uses partial restriction of venous blood flow to muscles while maintaining arterial flow.

This technique aims to limit the venous return of blood to the muscles, for a specific amount of time during weight training, using rubber or elastic bands, or with *Kaatsu bands*. Blood flow restriction training involves wrapping a tourniquet or elastic band around your limbs while weight training.

Continued practice of this technique has shown increased muscle growth when light weightlifting is combined with blood flow restriction. Indeed, the continuous muscle swelling caused by the pumping of blood stimulates protein synthesis and prevents the degradation of muscle tissue. Blood = life.

It is not necessary to use Kaatsu bands or other expensive bands to perform BFR. Elastic bands for knees will suffice.

The best approach is to use this technique to "refine" your workout. You should start your heavy hypertrophy training session with your classic training and then finish with several sets of BFR, using *single-joint movements*.

This strategy to stimulate muscle growth can give good results, especially for legs and arms.

BFR is not a new technique: it has been in use for over 20 years in Japan and research on the subject dates back to the 1990s. Despite emerging evidence of its effectiveness, most athletes have only a vague idea of what it entails and how it can be applied within a resistance training program to improve results. In the 1960s and 1970s, Serge Nubret used this system at the end of calf training sessions, placing two elastic bands at the base of the knees and remaining seated for 15 minutes. His goal was to keep the blood in the newly trained muscle area for as long as possible.

In remembrance of Serge Nubret, I'll share an anecdote. In 1987 I was lucky enough to "try" to train with him. He himself told me to do the reflux block in my calves right after I trained them. So, in this case, a resting BFR. I sat, with the laces tightened just below my kneecap, for a total of 15 minutes, completely still.

The next day I couldn't move. Even if I hadn't used the bindings, I believe that the cause of pain mixed with fullness and hardness must have been the fact that I had remained motionless, sitting on a bench, without taking a step. Basically, I prevented the blood from dispersing, forcing it to stagnate in the trained muscle. Serge Nubret, in fact, continually repeated: "Keep the blood in the muscle".

Therefore, blood supply is very important for the life of the muscle!

BFR basics

BFR involves restricting the circulation of blood to the muscle. This is achieved by wrapping a restrictive piece of equipment around the limbs while performing dynamic exercises.

It is important to remember that **the purpose of BFR is to prevent venous return**, not arterial flow into the muscle. So, the laces shouldn't be too tight. In this way,

oxygen-rich blood enters the muscle (flowing in the deeper arteries) **but it cannot escape** (as it returns to the heart in the more superficial veins).

Research on the hypertrophic effects of BFR is very interesting. Clinical studies have shown that the simple restriction of blood flow, twice a day for a duration of 5 minutes each, performed on patients immobilized in bed with a cast on the fractured leg, prevents muscle atrophy.

Walking while restricting blood flow to the legs has been shown to increase muscle strength and size by up to 7 percent. In normal conditions, simply walking definitely would not lead to muscle gain.

However, the real hypertrophic benefits of BFR occur when it is applied with resistance training.

Numerous studies show substantial increases in muscle growth when light weightlifting (20-30% of 1RM) is combined with blood flow restriction. Gains in the initial phase are often equal to those with traditional heavy-weight training, and sometimes even greater.

The exact hypertrophic mechanisms are not fully understood, but metabolic stress is thought to play an important role in the process. Simply put, metabolic stress is the accumulation of training byproducts called metabolites and it is particularly prevalent when training is performed in a state of oxygen starvation (hypoxia), as seen when circulation is restricted. Metabolites implicated in promoting a hypertrophic response include lactate, inorganic phosphate and hydrogen ions. It is hypothesized that these metabolites activate anabolism by speeding up protein synthesis and the activation of satellite cells, key elements that are necessary for muscle growth.

Elastic bands for the knees can be used to obtain good results from this technique. The bands should be long enough to wrap around the limb several times. The brand or type of material really doesn't matter. **Band placement is critical.** You must position it as high as possible on the limbs before training. For the upper arms, the bands should be wrapped as high up as possible on the biceps. For the hamstrings, they should be wrapped just below the crease of the glutes.

If the bands are placed too low, optimal venous occlusion will not be achieved and the beneficial effects of the strategy will be compromised.

The goal should be to secure the bands so that they fit snugly, but not so tightly that they cause excessive discomfort at rest. On a scale from 1 to 10, the pressure should be around a 7. Generally, it takes some practice to accurately quantify the pain-pressure connection, but after a few training sessions, you should have a clearer idea of how much pressure to put in the limb wrap.

However, care must be taken not to wrap it too tightly, or else all circulation to that limb will be cut off. This would increase the perceived effort of the exercise, which would then force you to finish the workout much earlier.

The width of the elastic band must also be taken into consideration. A wide band has been shown to cut off arterial circulation at a lower pressure than a narrower band.

How to integrate BFR into your routine

In the vast majority of studies, BFR was done in isolation as the only training stimulus used during a given research protocol. Training like this may be beneficial for older people or those recovering from injury, but I don't think it's sufficient for advanced athletes. The best results are obtained by integrating this technique into a traditional hypertrophy training program.

As mentioned above, the best approach I've found is to use this as a "finishing" technique. This involves performing a heavy-load hypertrophy protocol (the classic muscle-building workout you've been following) at the beginning of the session, then finishing with several sets of BFRs.

Below you will find the specifications. While BFR can be used with virtually any exercise, it appears to work best with *single-joint movements*, in which only one joint is involved. Biceps push ups, triceps extensions, leg extensions, etc. are all excellent choices. Multi-joint exercises such as squats and presses should always be done at the beginning, in the traditional way. The weights used during BFR should be light. Normally loads equal to 20-30% of 1RM are used for a given exercise, for no less than 20-25 repetitions in the first set.

Subsequently, other sets of the chosen exercise can be performed, keeping rest time at about 30 seconds. Short rest intervals help increase metabolic stress and blood pooling in the muscle. They also reduce the number of repetitions you can perform in the subsequent sets.

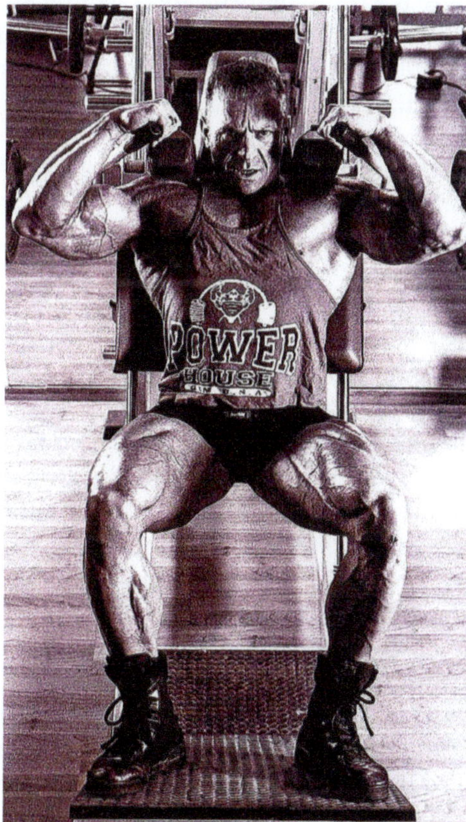

In your final set, assuming you maintain the same weight, you will probably only complete about 8-10 repetitions.

It is also important to keep the limbs continuously tied throughout the exercise. In fact, loosening the bands between sets reduces metabolic stress, inhibiting the growth stimulus. The bands should only be removed after completing the final BFR set. If done correctly and by following the instructions, once the bands are undone, the final pump will be insane. You will see a sudden strong, violent and painful supercompensation of blood, due to the return of oxygen to the muscle. Training in BFR takes place in hypoxia or in the absence of oxygen, therefore it is completely anaerobic. Lactic acid levels will rise, forcing a limit on the muscle's ability to contract. More muscle cells will be activated to ensure that the muscle contracts, ultimately stimulating muscle growth. This lack of oxygen will stimulate the growth of fast-twitch white fibers.

Going to muscle failure in BFR requires a different mindset compared to traditional resistance exercises.

With BFR, the limbs get heavier with each rep. After a certain point, you will get the feeling that they cannot move. This is where mental toughness comes into play. Since the loads are so light, you can force yourself to push through this feeling and pump out a few more repetitions. You have to squeeze until the last possible repetition. Ultimately, this is how you maximize the accumulation of metabolites and, consequently, its anabolic response.

Pro champion Hidetada Yamagishi's training has played a major role in his arm volume gains, where he incorporated BFR into IFBB. Obviously, it must always be considered as a trick to refine arms and legs when the athlete has already completed their heavy training session in the traditional way.

POF Method (Position of Flexion)

POF is a training method created by Steve Holman, editor of *Iron Man* magazine, in 2001. **Holman wanted to make the most of every portion of the range of motion.** So, in his workout routine, he selects three exercises per muscle group, each of them targeting a different range of motion. A POF training routine has three positions in which the muscles can be trained, precisely by diversifying the range of motion, the trajectory and the workout planes:

- **intermediate position**: basic, fundamental exercises that build muscle mass
- **stretching position**: in which the muscle is stretched
- **contracted position**

The POF method increases neuro-efficiency and muscle hypertrophy. The study of this method started from three concepts which I will briefly summarize. According to this theory, there are three fundamental flexion positions with which muscles can be trained: the intermediate one, the stretching one and the contraction one. Analyzing them one by one, we can state that the **intermediate position** is characteristic of *multi-joint exercises* (such as squats, bench presses, deadlifts, etc.), in which intermediate is intended as a movement with which the person who is training does not produce the maximum stretch or maximum contraction resistance on the muscle group.

The **stretching position** is identified as a phase in which maximum muscle stretching is exploited and, therefore, the myotatic reflex (which is precisely stimulated by rapid stretching of the muscle fibers, manifesting itself with an involuntary contraction of the muscle itself), and can be reached with *single-joint exercises* such as dumbbell flyes or the chest machine.

The last position is the one **in contraction**, i.e., of maximum muscle shortening, which uses exercises that allow for strong resistance, even in the position of maximum muscle contraction, given by the external load used for the exercise, such as leg extensions or concentration bicep curls. This last phase of the movement induces the muscle to fill considerably with blood due to the continuous contractions which produce a consistent vascular restriction.

Example of POF Biceps Stretching. Method for the arms (shoulders back)

Biceps routine

Intermediate position

- Barbell or standing dumbbell curl 4 × 8

Stretching

- Dumbbell curl on 60° bench (keep shoulders back) 4 × 10

Contraction

- Concentration curl, spider curl, preacher curl 4 × 12

Triceps Routine

Intermediate position

- Close grip bench press 4 × 8

Stretching

- Dumbbell or behind-the-head EZ bar extension 4 × 10

Contraction

- Push down with a straight bar or with the rope 4 × 12

The aim, therefore, is to hit the trained muscle in three different ways, each of which imposes a different level of contraction and lengthening.

At least **one exercise should be selected for each of these three positions** in order to have a complete workout from all three points of view, in which the muscle is stretched and contracted, and a basic multi-joint exercise in which the maximum is reached in the central part of the movement.

When I train an athlete, I tell them that the specific exercise we are doing is valid for contraction (for example, tricep pushdowns, as indicated above) or only for stretching (for example, pullovers for the back), or it must be performed as if we were rhythmic movement machines that neither reach maximum stretching nor maximum muscle contraction.

I have found that it can only be applied to certain muscle groups and not to the entire body. For some, dealing with an entire program that applies this method becomes very demanding on both a psychological and stress level.

I believe that, in addition to being a method, **it can be considered a logical and necessary device to use and introduce into each session of our training program**. Certainly, it can be combined with any other technique or method that we are using. It is an excellent logical strategy to follow for planning every gym session.

The only real rule is that of carefully choosing the three exercises.

Zone Training (Brian Johnston)

The training concept called Zone Training, or even Stage Training, was created and developed by Canadian coach Brian D. Johnston in the early 1970s and is very effective for maximizing each portion of the movement of a weight-bearing exercise. Simply put, you break the movement of the exercise into two or three parts (repetition trajectory zones) and work these segments separately, focusing on the first segment, then the second, then the third. This concept is based on the simple intuition of dividing the range of motion into at least two distinct areas, the easier area and the less easy one, and then training them one after the other.

But how did Johnston come to this conclusion? He had noticed that in many exercises performed with a full range of motion, total muscle exhaustion is not achieved. Muscle and functional failure occur first and foremost in the most difficult portion of the movement. Both machines and free weight exercises have easier portions of the movement and harder portions of the movement. Brian discovered this type of training quite by accident during a session with a machine of a brand that he had never used.

There are some exercises where there is a lot of tension in the final part of the movement (maximum contraction), but in the initial phase (maximum stretch) there is not enough tension, which makes the part of the movement near the stretched position easier and less effective. On the other hand, there are exercises in which tension is lost in the contraction phase and maximum difficulty is reached in the stretching phase.

Following this intuition, Johnston first performs the most difficult phase of the movement and, once he has reached exhaustion (which normally occurs with a number of mini-repetitions ranging from a minimum of 8 to a maximum of 12) in the trained area, he continues without rest (or introducing a small break of no more than 5 seconds) with the easier area, which, at this point, will also be difficult, as we find ourselves with a muscle that is already considerably pre-fatigued by the work performed previously.

Following this technique will involuntarily increase the repetitions performed and, consequently, contractions during the sets. They will no longer be complete repetitions, but many partial repetitions performed in different segments of the movement trajectory. This results in an increase in blood flow and in the activation of the fibers. The overall intensity of your workout increases and as a result, you will need to lower the number of sets per exercise.

If we divide the workout into two zones, we have sets of 12+12 repetitions, but, if we divide it into three zones, we will use sets of 8+8+8. Johnston suggests this split so that the total of repetitions is 24 in both cases. At the end of this macro-set, you can "finish" the muscle (if it is still possible) by trying to complete one or two repetitions with the full range of motion.

Let's use the **flat bench press** exercise as an example. I have chosen this exercise because it's not as simple and immediate as a barbell curl could be. This way, the execution of this technique will be clear for all the other exercises.

The problem with regular repetitions over a full range of motion is that the leverage changes throughout the motion. When performing a full-motion bench press, you can only use the weight with which you can get through the most difficult point of the movement.

Thus, there is only one point in the exercise where effort is maximal. When you get to the top, more weight could be used because the leverage is better. For this reason, machines with cams were created: to remove that difference in tension on the trained muscle belly. Therefore, the most difficult phase is the one in which, due to the disadvantage of the leverage (or the type of equipment we are using), effort is very high and remains so until a point where the disadvantage of leverage ceases (the load distribution in the machines varies); from that point on, the exercise becomes much easier.

What Johnston was able to demonstrate with Zone Training is that the athlete can be allowed to focus on that specific portion of the movement in the exercise without changing weights.

Quite simply, we do partial repetitions on the hardest portion first, then the medium, then when we're more tired, we'll do partial repetitions on the easier portion of the movement.

For example, with bench presses, we would do 8 repetitions of each segment of the movement (using a controlled motion, with no bounce), 8 repetitions from the chest to a few inches higher, then 8 repetitions in a ROM (Range Of Motion) controlled in the middle of the movement (never straightening and never touching the chest with the barbell) and 8 repetitions from three-quarters of the way to the top in maximum contraction, for a total of 24 repetitions.

For other exercises, it is best to break the movement down into just two phases. For example, in the **standing barbell curl**, the difficult part is lifting the barbell from the position of maximum extension of the arm until 90° between arm and forearm is reached. From that moment on, continuing to lift the bar becomes relatively easier and we get stronger and stronger; however, once the point of maximum difficulty has passed (90° between the ulna/radius and the humerus), resistance gradually decreases, reducing the total impact on our biceps, just when we need it most.

Johnston recommends finishing the sets in no more than 90 seconds in order to mainly involve white and fast fibers. When analyzing this system, what immediately emerges is the large number of mini-repetitions within the sets (from 16 to 24 repetitions); this is not a method with many repetitions, but it should be considered as a system **with a high number of contractions in a single set**.

In this method, Johnston never recommends a specific number of sets to complete in a training session. Each athlete will decide when to end the session for that given muscle once maximum pumping has been reached, a condition which translates into a temporary difficulty in the total contraction of the trained muscle due to muscle swelling caused by blood as a direct consequence of the high number of mini-repetitions.

I consider Zone Training a workout for advanced athletes who are capable of coordinating the nervous system and muscles in an optimal way. If you are a beginner or at an intermediate level, I do not recommend applying these techniques.

I think it's a very interesting technique to supplement your classic training. From my personal experience, I found it to be excellent if performed as a final set of the last exercise to give an incredible pump to the muscle already abused during the session for a superior pumping effect and hardness.

The 10-second method

This method is in total contrast to all Heavy Intensity Training methods, as it does not involve the use of heavy loads at any stage of its development. The method consists in performing 20 to 40 sets of 5-10 exercises per muscle group, using loads that allow for at least 12 repetitions per set with a 10-second rest period between sets.

It isn't a complex training method and it can provide excellent results in a short time, especially in the growth stalemate phases of some muscle groups.

The heart of this method, therefore, lies **in repeating precisely 12 repetitions per set and taking a 10-second break between them**. If the repetitions were reduced to 10 or the rest extended beyond the pre-established 10 seconds, the result would be lower, and the benefits of this technique would be nullified.

The form of execution of each movement must always be perfect, with full concentration and constant isotension, and the movement must be continuous. This allows athletes to concentrate all their efforts on the area that is being traind.

This method is suitable for those who have been training for many years without a partner and for those who have suffered from muscle or tendon injuries. Furthermore, it is indicated for those who have developed a mind-muscle axis which allows them to transmit all the commands of the brain to the muscle belly without compromising the perfect biomechanical execution of the movement. Typically, there are 6 training days a week, with only one day off, and each muscle group should be trained twice a week. Thus, the whole body is divided into 3 days.

This type of training, which may seem easy at first sight, is actually torture. I have personally used it in my latest competitive years, precisely because I had to train alone at unimaginable times and also because of the many injuries I had suffered throughout my competitive career.

In my opinion, it is exceptional, especially before competitions and for older athletes who have a background of years and years of training with very heavy weights.

This method was developed in the 1960s and 170s by Black athletes from the French Antilles who resided in the suburbs of Paris. Serge Nubret, the eldest of them, broke it down and refined it, thus developing this training theory.

Ultra Slow (10-second repeat)

It is a very slow movement, both in the ascent and in the descent phase of the resistance. It is therefore an excellent training technique to increase one's ability to control the equipment. **Each repetition should be performed with constant speed until you can no longer do it. As soon as muscle failure occurs, the athlete instinctively shortens the positive concentric phase**, with the help of a bit of cheating and in any case by reducing the time to lift the weight, trying, as far as possible, **to keep the negative eccentric phase unchanged.**

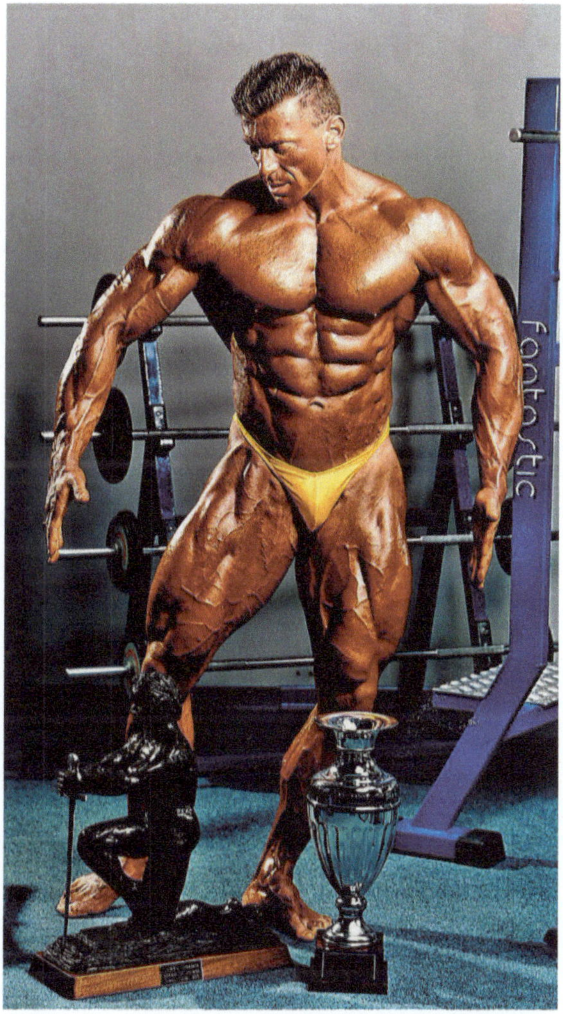

The athlete has total control of the equipment. It could be said that this technique encompasses two other techniques, namely *isotension* and *negatives.*

In the negative phase, the muscles can hold weights that could be even 40-50% heavier than those in the positive phase.

Unlike traditional negatives, given that the positive phase must also be performed very slowly, the weight is not higher than the one usually used; on the contrary, it will be definitely lower.

Usually, two to three sets of 8-10 repetitions are performed.

As mentioned above, the weight must be light, but still give the athlete the clear feeling of lifting a much heavier weight in the final reps of the set. It is an excellent technique for weak muscle groups and can be used once a week for 5-6 consecutive weeks. However, this method must not be used all year round, but rather introduced only at specific times of the year.

This is a useful technique, especially in the early stages of off-season training and whenever there is a need to "feel the muscle" either after following programs that focus on heavy loads (especially pyramid training) or to restore concentration.

The 100 Repetitions Method

The 100 Repetitions Method was developed in the early 1970s for combat sports athletes, wrestlers and American football players. It was later used by Southern California bodybuilders in the early 1980s, as improvements in muscle density and speed were noticed especially when rehabilitating athletes from injuries.

It is a technique too costly in terms of time and energy, which no athlete has ever truly managed to complete in its entirety. In practice, it is too challenging for our brains. I believe that the reason for its effectiveness is still mysterious since no one has ever provided scientific evidence in favor of this workout, which many consider meaningless, but actually this endless torture works (if used for a short period of time) and creates a massive trauma to the muscle, which our body is forced to recover from. This technique was used, tested, customized and modified by a group of Californian bodybuilders in the 1980s, including Tom Touchstone, Diana Dennis and Rory Leidelmeyer.

To perform this technique, it is better to train with machines and not with free weights, in order to perform exclusively isolation exercises, in which a single muscle group is trained.

If you divide your body into 10-12 groups, you can train it all in three workouts, followed by 1 day of rest. This, at least, for the first 2 weeks, after which you can switch to the 2:1 scheme (2 consecutive days of training followed by 1 rest day) or you can continue with the 3:1 scheme.

However, you should finish the total body training in 3-4 days, followed by 1 day of rest. Then you start again.

The goal is to perform 100 repetitions without stopping, possibly using some mental trick in counting the repetitions, dividing the total into 25,25,25,25 or 35,35,30 repetitions.

To begin with, one must choose an appropriate weight, i.e., light enough. Normally, this technique uses a weight that varies between 20 and 30% of that usually used for 10 repetitions: it is advisable to start with a weight that is lighter than the indicated one, rather than heavier. From a psychological point of view, which is of fundamental importance when training with this method, it is necessary to reach the goal, i.e. 100 reps, quickly.

The essential thing is to get to 100 repetitions with good form and with full movements; the weight is less important.

The repetitions should be performed quickly but fully (no half repetitions).

You must be able to perform at least 70 repetitions without interruption. If you stop earlier, you either keep the weight on or you reduce it.

Muscles and exercises

1. Calf: seated or standing calf raises
2. Hamstring: lying leg curl
3. Quadriceps: Leg extension or bodyweight squat (suitable for women who have superior endurance capabilities in their lower limbs)
4. Lumbar: hyperextension
5. Traps: barbell shrug
6. Lateral deltoid: seated lateral raise
7. Chest: chest machine
8. Triceps: push down
9. Biceps: low cable curl
10. Abs: knees to the chest on the incline bench

The scheme shown above was the one followed by Rory Leidelmeyer from 1984 onwards.

- Train each muscle group with isolation exercises, starting with the largest and therefore most challenging group, gradually working your way down to the smallest.
- To build the most effective sequence of exercises for each group, one must consider the *limiting* muscles, i.e. those which, by getting tired earlier, prevent the complete training of the main muscle group. Thus, the triceps is the limiting muscle in pushing exercises, such as bench presses, incline bench presses and shoulder presses (slow back or front with barbells or dumbbells). The back muscles are the limiting muscles of the squat and some rowing exercises.

Therefore, **limiting muscles should be trained last.**

Instead of training the whole body in every session, you should perform the 100s during split routines, as shown below:

- first day: chest-back
- second day: biceps-legs
- third day: shoulders (traps)-triceps
- fourth day: rest

An example of exercise sequence

The first day
("alternating" system: chest + back + chest + back etc.)

1. Incline bench press on the Smith machine
2. Lat machine, wide grip
3. Dumbbell bench press
4. Forward reverse grip lat machine
5. Decline barbell bench press
6. Forward lat machine, with "V" handle
7. Chest machine
8. Low cable

The first day
("orthodox" system: first the whole chest and then the whole back)

1. Incline bench press on the Smith machine
2. Dumbbell push on an incline bench
3. Chest machine
4. Lat machine behind
5. Lat machine forward
6. Forward lat machine with "V" handle
7. Wide handle low pulley, medium handle

Second day

1. Standing barbell curl
2. Biceps on the Scott bench
3. Smith machine squat or 45° leg press
4. Lying leg curl
5. Leg extension
6. Standing leg curl
7. Stiff-legged deadlift
8. Seated calf

Third day

1. Overhead press on the Smith machine
2. Standing lateral raise
3. Raise dumbbells to 90 degrees
4. T-bar row or medium wide grip row
5. Chin pull-up
6. Lying barbell extension
7. Triceps push down

It is recommended not to train with the 100 Reps Method for more than eight weeks.

This should be followed by about 3-4 weeks of "step-through" training, which consists of using weights that can be lifted for a range of 12 to 20 repetitions.

Then, you should continue with 10-12 weeks of "classic" training with heavy loads.

After a sufficiently protracted period of training with 100 repetitions, the athlete's neuromuscular system will be ready and more receptive to the subsequent introduction of heavy loads.

In other words, if I use the 100 Reps Method first, when I go back to using heavy weights, my muscles will respond much better. It is an unbearable trauma for our muscles, which must immediately reverse this violent change of course. This shows that muscles can be traumatized not only by increasingly heavier loads. This useful technique is a bitter medicine which should be taken only for a short period of time.

The Contrast Method (Intra Set Contrast Load, Tempo Contrast, Iso-Dynamic Contrast, Mixed Sets)

Intra Set Contrast Load (Classic Contrast Method)

The Contrast Method is performed using heavy and medium loads in the same set. It is an intra-exercise diversification to increase training intensity.

A typical example is using about 85-90% of your maximum load, doing one rep, reducing it by 10-20%, and doing about 6-10 repetitions. Once you can complete 10 repetitions, increase the weight slightly in the following set. Lifting heavy loads will first stimulate the nervous system and neuromuscular endings, thus activating a large number of muscle fibers. This gives you a *boosting effect*. Using this technique, as soon as you switch to hypertrophy work, you stimulate even more muscle growth.

A variant of the Contrast Method can also be considered to increase the weight during the same sets, and then decrease it. Load the bar with 75% of the weight, then increase it by 10-15% (85-90% of max load), do two or three repetitions, and from there, scale the weight smoothly to execute your drop set. The second load, the one that causes hypertrophy, will feel much lighter, a factor that will allow you to perform many more repetitions than you could have done normally.

1. Do one repetition with a heavy weight (85-90%)
2. Drop the weight quickly (best done by your training partner)
3. Do as many repetitions as you can with the correct technique. You should get tired after 7 to 10 repetitions. If you can go beyond 10 repetitions, you'll need to increase the weight on the next set

This method is great for building muscle. It will also allow you to use heavier weights than usual, resulting in increased strength. You don't need to use more than one exercise to reap the benefits of this training principle. While this method can be used with all exercises, it is best developed with core free-weight exercises such as squats, rows, bench presses, overhead presses and so on.

The basic principle of all stimulation/strengthening methods (applicable to all sports) is that a given weight will feel lighter if a heavier load is lifted first.

By doing so, you are able to reap the benefits of increased neural unit contraction, which allows for more speed, more power, more strength and more hypertrophy stimulation.

Let's consider a squat workout as an example: instead of performing the classic 8-rep sets with 75-80%, you can create a higher training effect by using an inverse pyramid that goes up and then down, like this: 5 × 8 at 75, 80, 85, 80, 75% of maximum load. The final sets will be faster and more explosive than they would be if they were performed with a constantly increased load. This is exactly your goal: to increase your speed and explosiveness. This makes the training session more efficient for reaching explosive power.

Regarding **strength** and **speed** in the squat exercise, instead of doing, for example, 6 sets of 5 repetitions at 85-90% of 1RM, the same reverse pyramid principle can be used, as illustrated in the table below.

An example for increasing strength and speed
• 6 × 5 reps at 85, 90, 95, 90, 85, 80% of max load

Here are two more examples of **how to use intra-exercise changes in load and time** to create a better training effect, more suitable for increasing hypertrophy and strength.

An example in bodybuilding
• Squat: 1 × 5 (up to a maximum of 5 reps), take off up to 40-45% of the load and proceed to a set of 15-20 reps (*you will be able to lift more weight for higher reps*)

An example in bodybuilding
• Squat walkout, an example of Iso-Dynamic Contrast that we will see shortly (load the barbell with 10% more than the maximum, lift it as if you were preparing to perform the classic squat but stand still in a static position without doing any movement for 10 seconds) × 110% of the max, followed by the classic squat × 100% of the max × 1 or 2 reps.

The same principle can be applied to any other fundamental and multi-joint movement or exercise of your choice.

Tempo Contrast

It is a very simple technique, which consists of doing very slow repetitions and repetitions at maximum speed in the same set. For example, you perform two repetitions with a 4,2,4,1 tempo and two repetitions at the maximum possible speed (*x*). The completion of these repetitions is called a "cycle," which concludes with a total of approximately 10-12 repetitions and can be carried out for multiple sets, usually no more than three sets for small muscle groups and four for larger ones, for up to three cycles.

The most common variant involves the use of static holds in peak contraction (maximum contraction at the top of the movement) or alternating different exercises for the corresponding antagonist muscle between the various sets, completing the same number of repetitions and cycles.

Iso-Dynamic Contrast

This technique is a variation of the Contrast Method. It consists in holding a load in an isometric contraction for 30 seconds and immediately after completing between 8 and 10 repetitions, in such a way as to exploit the strengthening/nervous exhaustion obtained from the previous static contraction.

The load used for this mixed set can also be supra-maximal, maintained in a static isometry position for a shorter period (10 seconds), as in the case of the walkout squat, to then perform a variable number of repetitions depending on the objectives, in a way that you can also feel the lightest repetitions (post-tetanic strengthening).

The contraction is maximal when it occurs following a brief *tetanic contraction* (sum of contractions merging into one continuous contraction), so this effect is called *post-tetanic*. **To put it simply, a powerful muscle contraction can be achieved if it is preceded by a strong muscle contraction.**

The Mixed Set

The Mixed Set is a technique that can be considered a variant of the Contrast Method in bodybuilding. I performed it with good muscle hypertrophy effects in 1990-1991, when WABBA world champion, Sauro Calistri, taught it to me during my muscle-building period. It's a simple and immediate idea: alternate a heavy set with a lighter one, with a higher number of repetitions within the same set.

An example of the Mixed Sets

- Flat bench press, 5 sets × 15-8-15-8-15 reps, alternating heavy loads with lighter loads

This causes trauma to the fibers: since the muscle "expects" a type of load and it receives a different one, it has to adapt very quickly and react accordingly.

Usually, Sauro Calistri used this technique in one or at most two basic exercises per muscle group, following it with a heavy basic exercise performed in a classic way and executing it before an exercise that would end with a double and triple weight change. This type of work is very good for the quadriceps.

An example of Mixed Set for the quadriceps

- Squat 4 × 10-12
- **Leg press 45° 4 × 15-8-15-8**
- **Leg extension 5 × 18-10-18-10-18**
- Hack squat 3 × 10 doubles (i.e. 10 reps, drop weight, 10 more reps)
- Hack squat 1 × 10 triples (10 reps, drop weight, 10 reps, another drop, 10 reps)

This is also an example of the Contrast Method. Very simple, his logical and immediate intuition is to create greater intensity within the sets, going to stimulate different types of fibers alternately and forcing the muscle to adapt to different stimuli. Basically, it is a synthetic contraction of Hatfield's Holistic Training.

Our muscles always try to adapt naturally to the stress they are subject to. As we have seen, muscle growth occurs through various paths, but for all these methods, there is a common theme: **to ensure that our muscles** never learn the lesson, so that they search endlessly for a way to fit in, never finding it. **Muscle growth is always due to adaptation to greater and different stress.**

HST, Hypertrophy Specific Training (Bryan Haycock)

The concept on which Bryan Haycock's training philosophy is based can be summarized in light of an experience tested in the laboratory. He says that most of the time you get to muscle exhaustion during a weight exercise is due to a voluntary failure caused by the high volume of work, so it doesn't represent a natural involuntary failure of the muscles.

Involuntary failure is when a muscle no longer responds to a contraction signal tested in the laboratory, under load, while the muscle is subjected to the passage of an electric current. Most athletes reach muscle exhaustion voluntarily, but the electrodes cause muscles to contract even after they reach failure. Haycock uses a low volume of work to bring the muscles to involuntary failure.

The HST method is a combination of a **low volume of work** and **a very high frequency** of structured sessions to stimulate muscle hypertrophy to the maximum, with loads that will gradually increase, accustoming the muscle to working with heavy loads, with the addition of a strategic period of total "deload" which allows for muscle regeneration and prepares the muscles to face the subsequent phase of high intensity and workload with maximum benefit.

This training method is specific for muscle hypertrophy and is based on the following principles.

The mechanical load

Hypertrophy must be induced to increase the size of muscle cells. In addition to causing a laceration of the muscle tissue, this load stimulates other factors widely described in the previous chapters. Thus, the primary stimulus for fiber growth is caused by the load and its movement in the act of lifting and lowering it, not by the effort itself. To better understand this principle, it must be kept in mind that fatigue is not related to the effect of muscle growth.

A load shouldn't tire us out due to its heaviness, but it should be heavy enough to stimulate the muscle tissue. I always remember the saying of eight-time Mr. Olympia, the undefeated Lee Haney: *"Stimulate your muscles, do not annihilate them"*. Instead of reaching training fatigue, one should focus on the *overload* principle. Try to lift a heavier weight than your previous workout.

The high-frequency principle (creating lasting stimuli to optimize growth)

Far from Mentzer's theories (which he approaches due to the progressive increase of the load and the short duration of the sessions), Hancock maintains that, in order for the progressive increase of the load to transform into significant hypertrophy, the stimulus must take place often enough to create a new "environment". Therefore, this has nothing to do with rarefied and very intense workouts, as Mentzer preached. Hancock claims that about 36-48 hours are enough to restore the levels of IGF-1, mRNA, protein synthesis, and prostaglandins. You can train the same muscle again after just 48 hours. In addition to this duration, Hancock considers recovery to be non-regenerative (contrary to many schools of thought). According to him, an athlete finds himself in an anti-catabolism state in which the body tries to fight the loss of muscle. Basically, it would go back to normal, like before you had the growth. Thus, continuous gains and subsequent attempts to avoid losing muscle tissue. Hancock argues that, in this way, a continuous state of hypertrophy cannot occur, but that, at most, anabolism can last 2 days after we stop training, then only a forced balancing and saving of energy sim-

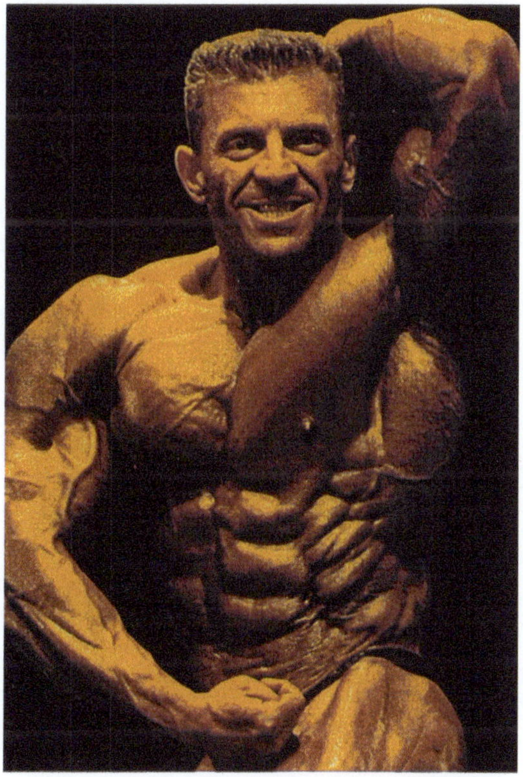

ply begins, without adding anything to muscle growth. This opinion is the opposite of that of Mentzer, Cianti, Massaroni, Yates and Arthur Jones, and very far off from that of many others. So, with this method, you train the same muscle group every 48 hours, i.e., **you train a muscle before it has fully recovered from a structural point of view, without blocking its ability to regenerate**. By doing so, the anabolic activity of the muscle is kept at a high level while trying to slightly anticipate recovery by increasing the load with each workout. According to Hancock, this is the key to continuing to stimulate growth in advanced bodybuilders.

The progressive load

The muscle is not only sensitive to the heaviness of the load itself, but also to variations in the load. Therefore, it is possible to obtain a hypertrophic effect by increasing the load compared to a previous load that was not at the limit of the athlete's abilities. Over time, muscle fibers adapt to slightly higher stress and become increasingly resistant to the destructive effects of the load. This adaptation can take place in as little as 48 hours (Rapid Training Effect) and, as soon as it happens, the hypertrophy process stops. Precisely for this reason, the load used will have to be increased constantly and frequently. This means that if an athlete only increases the load for a specific exercise of the target muscle every 2 weeks, actually he is only maintaining his muscle mass.

Strategic rest from training

What happens when you can no longer scale up your workload? If the athlete has managed to increase muscle volume but is no longer able to increase the load, they will have to take a period of 9-10 days of complete rest to become sensitive again to the stimuli of weight training.

In summary, if you want to apply the principles of hypertrophy, you must:

- train each muscle group three times a week (*every 48 hours*)
- increase the load at each workout
- decrease repetitions every 2 weeks (*I'll explain that shortly*)
- rest (*once you are no longer able to increase training loads*) and then start over

It seems like a simple method or at least one that makes your training program trivial, but it's not. I think it is very difficult to have the physical and mental capacity to face this continuous quest for hypertrophy.

Previously I mentioned the decrease in repetitions after each 2-week block (6 cycles). First, you need to determine the loads for each individual session.

Find your max for 15, 10, and 5 repetitions for each exercise you're going to perform. Your maximum will determine the weight to use for the first training cycle. For the second cycle, you will add 2 to 5 kg depending on the exercise. Each cycle lasts 2 days, so excluding 1 rest day, there will be 3 cycles per week. This method is divided into blocks of 2 weeks each. Thus, one block consists of six cycles. From the first cycle to the sixth and last cycle of the first block, the increase in workloads must go from a minimum of 2 kg (in the first cycle) to a maximum of 10 kg (in the last cycle). Therefore, your last workout at the end of each 2-week block will be done with your heaviest weight.

Let's consider a 2-week block consisting of six training cycles. How do we adjust the loads that we'll use? Find the maximum weight you can do 10 repetitions with on the last (heaviest) cycle and scale up approximately 2-2.5 kg on each cycle, calculating the first one backward. That will be the weight you start this program with. For example, if at the last cycle you used 90 kg × 10 repetitions for a given exercise, the progression from the first cycle will be similar to this progression for 10 repetitions: 79, 81, 83, 85.5, 88, 90 kg.

The repetitions will drop every 2 weeks in the following order: 15 repetitions for the first 2 weeks, 10 repetitions for the next 2 weeks and 5 repetitions for the last 2 weeks. After these last 2 weeks, you can continue to keep the 5 repetitions constant for another 2 weeks, introducing the *negative/eccentric technique* when possible.

If necessary, the workload can always be adjusted at each session, although, it would be best to steadily increase it as scheduled. The truth is that, due to many variations, the calculations made previously do not reflect the actual load that the athlete will then use. Sometimes, in exercises like lateral shoulder raises, you won't be able to increase the load in every session, so you will do it every other workout.

As mentioned above, for the final 2 weeks before the regenerative phase, you will only be using the additional negative/eccentric technique for certain exercises where it can be used. For the other exercises in which this practice is inadvisable, continue these last 2 weeks with your 5 classic repetitions.

There will only be one or two **sets** per exercise. If you train each muscle group every 48 hours, it's no problem if you only do one or two sets per muscle, as long as the frequency and continuous, constant weight gain are ensured.

We said that each muscle group will be trained three times a week. According to Hancock, a load that stimulates hypertrophy must be frequent enough to create a hostile environment for the muscle, to which it inevitably has to adapt. Hancock calls this the "principle of high frequency."

This HST method lasts 6-8 weeks and is followed by 9-10 days of strategic rest, in which you will not train with weights to allow your muscles to regenerate and restart in a better condition than before.

To recap, you'll do 15 repetitions of each exercise during the first 2 weeks (**first block**), where you'll be training each muscle group three times a week. You will only do one or two sets per exercise and one exercise per muscle.

During the following 2 weeks (**second block**) you will increase the weight, reducing the repetitions to 10. In the following 2 weeks (**third block**) you will do the same thing, increasing the load and reducing the repetitions to 5. At the end of this third block, you will do another 2 weeks (**fourth block**) again at 5 repetitions, with the introduction of negative/eccentric techniques. After these four blocks of work, you will carry out a **total training deload**, lasting about 9-10 days, in which you will be able to perform 20 to 40 minutes of fast power walking, uphill, on the treadmill.

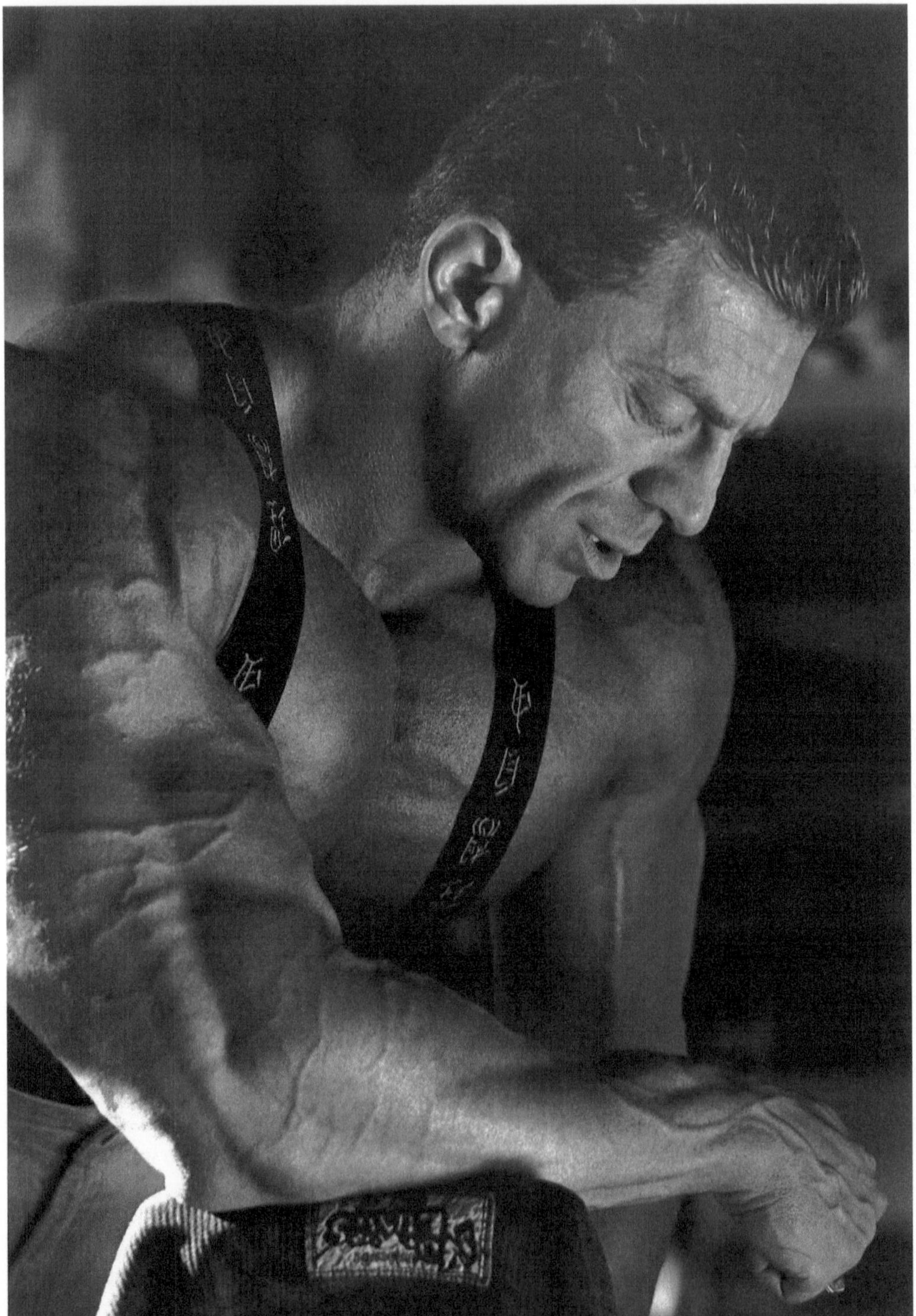

In 1946, the great Bob Hoffmann (York Barbell Company) had already claimed that each muscle should be trained three times a week in order to stimulate growth. Soviet bloc weightlifting coaches drew heavily on his ideas in the 1950s and 1960s. More recently, even Chad Waterbury has supported a very similar theory to that of Hancock's with his HFT (High Frequency Training).

I believe that this principle can be valid if we pay due attention to adapting to the weights to be used. If 15 or 10 or 5 repetitions are a goal, and if you always have to reach muscle failure, the choice of workloads will certainly undergo variations when you are training.

Without a doubt, HST is a method that takes you out of that usual training routine you so frequently find yourself in, with the consequent blocking of any type of muscle growth.

HFT, High-Frequency Training (Chad Waterbury)

Chad Waterbury created this muscle-building weight training program in 2005. He made a big splash in the USA, especially among younger athletes, with various articles and practical tests on athletes, proposing this new idea of physical culture as the new frontier of bodybuilding.

Waterbury claims that training each muscle group more than four times a week is the fastest way to build muscle. That's right, no longer three times a week, as Hancock proposed in his HST, but five times a week.

It's not about the classic workouts that we used to read in magazines or that we see today in the video clips of champions, but often total body workouts with a low volume of work, which vary daily. If you are not used to sustaining these rhythms, it is advisable to start with four sessions for every single muscle per week, and then get to five. If you want to train each group practically every day, it seems appropriate to do only isolation movements.

Waterbury, on the other hand, has his students train with basic/multi-joint and complementary isolation exercises. So, if you plan on training one muscle group for at least five sessions a week, it's imperative that you use as many movement variations as possible. The greater the difference in movement patterns, the less likely you are to overtrain.

It is important to adopt different exercises, angles, planes and directions compared to the previous session. During the week you should alternate basic movements with complementary movements, for each muscle. However, this is only necessary when you train every day, consecutively. If, on the other hand, there is a rest day in between, this is not necessary.

When I learned about this method I was perplexed. It is diametrically opposed to what I would recommend to a young athlete looking to get started in the muscle-building business. If we study Waterbury's methods more carefully, we understand that, in reality, **he pushes his athletes to train only weak muscle groups so many times**, or those that struggle to grow at the same rate as the others. For the other muscles, he recommends following these progressions but stopping "only" at two or three sessions a week. Hence, this method is good for stimulating weaker muscle groups.

It is not recommended to specialize more than three muscle groups at a time. His concept, therefore, is to train deficient muscles **more frequently, not more intensely**. However, I think this method is too much for most athletes.

The following table shows an example of HFT for triceps.

An example of HFT for triceps

- Monday: dips
- Tuesday: French presses on decline bench press with EZ bar
- Wednesday: military presses with top contraction
- Thursday: rest
- Friday: narrow grip barbell presses
- Saturday: push downs with wide grip (*keep your elbows back*)
- Sunday: rest

You can keep doing the same exercises up to 3 weeks before changing the type of movement. It's more than enough to vary the grips in push downs or the angles of the benches, pushes and extensions with the EZ bar, to give a slightly different stimulus to the muscle each time.

Repetitions should be increased progressively during the consecutive days of training. For example, your repetitions will be low on Monday, higher on Tuesday, even higher on Wednesday. How many repetitions should you do? Waterbury argues that they vary according to the athlete's training experience. Starting at five repetitions on Monday for an athlete who has been training for a few years, up to three for a more advanced athlete.

The next day's workout (in this case, Tuesday) should consist of no less than three repetitions more than the first workout (Monday). If you respond well to higher repetitions, feel free to go beyond three repetitions. The third workout (Wednesday) and every workout thereafter follow the same increasing progression of a minimum of three repetitions (if there are no rest days between workouts). If in the second workout you manage to perform more than three repetitions, in the third session you should also be able to complete three more. For example, if you did eight repetitions instead of seven for the second workout, your third consecutive workout should be 11 or more repetitions.

In the example described above, Thursday is a rest day. Then, after a rest day, the rep progression can be started again. You can start from a lower number, if anything increasing by one repetition on the fourth day (Friday), and then increasing again by at least three repetitions on the fifth day (Saturday).

Let's take an athlete with a medium-high training experience as an example. Waterbury does not calculate the work volume based on the number of exercises or number of sets, but evaluates work volume by the set/rep range, which he calls **"Set/Rep Volume"**. For him, every first workout should consist of a total set/rep range of 21-32 repetitions per exercise.

Sometimes Waterbury prefers to start with as few as 24 repetitions. For example, for the triceps exercise, 7-8 sets × 3 repetitions. Thus, the result will be 21 (24) repetitions, which represents the minimum initial phase of the weekly range which will start at 21 and end with the last workout of 32 total repetitions for every single exercise. The fewer the repetitions, the greater the load. The set/rep range increases each day during consecutive workouts.

Second example of HFT for triceps

- Monday: parallel dips 7-8 sets × 3 (21-24)
- Tuesday: French presses on the decline bench press with EZ bar 4 × 6 (24)
- Wednesday: military presses with top contraction 3 × 9 (27)
- Thursday: rest
- Friday: close grip bench presses 6 × 4 (24)
- Saturday: push downs with wide grip 4 × 7 (28) (*keep your elbows back*)
- Sunday: rest

The sets/repetitions range therefore rises with the increase in total repetitions, always in that range between 21 and 32. The key point consists in staying at the minimum limit of the range when doing a few repetitions with high loads and in moving toward the top of the range when doing more repetitions with a lower load.

All other body parts should be trained two to three times a week. It is best to follow a total body workout on days when you are preparing to perform just few sets. For example, if your biceps, back and quadriceps are well-developed, it is best to train them on Wednesday and Saturday, as the number of sets is low on those days. This will allow you to perform a total body workout in no time.

On days when you do many sets (we must remember that these are sessions in which the whole body is trained almost every day) it is better to choose basic/multi-joint exercises that train other muscle groups. For example, still using triceps as an example, we have chosen dips, which also involve the anterior deltoids and pectorals. If you had chosen, for example, an isolation exercise such as the wide grip push-down, for this total body day, you would still need to stimulate both the pecs and shoulders with other exercises. In this regard, Waterbury recommends choosing basic/multi-joint movements also for all other muscle areas of the body that may involve multiple muscle groups. So, always keep exercises like pull ups for the back and biceps, squats for the quads and hamstrings, wide-grip dips for the pecs, and traps. Whenever possible, it would be best to combine and alternate exercises between antagonist muscles. This maintains strength levels that will allow you to recruit more motor units.

This is made possible by reciprocal innervation, a nervous system mechanism that inhibits the antagonist muscles, forcing them to relax during agonist training (pectorals relax when training the upper back; triceps relax when training the biceps). Previously, I talked about this true ability that every bodybuilder should have every time they train with weights. Also, I think it's a great way to build muscle awareness and avoid injuries.

The following table shows a weekly practical example (micro-cycle) of HFT in which triceps are among the muscles that are focused on. It is suitable for athletes with more than 3 years of serious weight training experience.

The set/repetition range (21-32): *there is always an indicative range*, in which the numbers can change, but it is important to follow a constant progression of the number of repetitions.

An example of an HFT micro-cycle

Day 1/Workout no. 1

- Sets: 7-8
- Reps: 3 (always 2 reps fewer than the RM workload)
- Load: 5 reps (85% of 1RM)
- Rest: 45 seconds between alternating exercise pairings
- A1. Dips (chest, triceps, front shoulders)
- A2. Squat (quads, hamstrings and glutes)
- B1. Front barbell press (shoulders)
- B2. Pull-up (back and biceps)

Day 2/Workout no. 2

- Sets: 4
- Reps: 6 (always 2 reps fewer than the RM workload)
- Load: 8 RM
- Rest: 55 seconds
- A1. Romanian deadlift (hamstrings, glutes and lower back)
- A2. Decline bench French press with EZ bar (triceps)
- B1. Hammer dumbbell curl (biceps, brachialis and brachioradialis)
- B2. Bulgarian squat (quads, hamstrings and glutes)
- C1. Dumbbell lateral raise (medial shoulders)
- C2. Reverse crunch (abs)

Day 3/Workout no. 3

- Sets: 3
- Reps: 9 (always 2 reps fewer than the RM workload)
- Load: 11 RM
- Rest: 60 seconds

Continues

Continued

- A1. Military press with top contraction (shoulders and triceps)
- A2. Walking barbell lunge (legs and glutes)
- B1. Standing calf raises (calves)
- B2. Barbell row (back)
- C1. Lying leg curl (hamstrings)
- C2. Barbell curl (biceps)
- D1. Leg raise at the bar (abs)
- D2. Incline bench dumbbell press (chest)

Day 4

- Rest

Day 5/Workout no. 4

- Sets: 6
- Reps: 4 (always 2 reps fewer than the RM workload)
- Load: 6 RM
- Rest: 45 seconds
- A1. Wide grip bar (back and biceps)
- A2. Close grip barbell press (triceps and pecs)
- B1. Front squat with wide feet stance (legs)
- B2. Reverse horizontal hyperextension (lower back and glutes)

Day 6/Workout no. 5

- Sets: 4
- Reps: 7 (always 2 reps fewer than the RM workload)
- Load: RM9
- Rest: 55 seconds
- A1. Good-Mornings with barbell (lower back and hamstrings)
- A2. Flat bench French press (triceps)
- B1. Incline bench dumbbell press (pecs)
- B2. Reverse grip pull-up (back)
- C1. Seated calf raises (calves)
- C2. Reverse crunch (abs)
- D1. Reverse EZ bar curl (biceps and brachialis)
- D2. 90° dumbbell raise (back shoulders)

Day 7

- Rest

Day 8

- Repeat the cycle

According to Waterbury, once you get used to five workouts a week, you can increase your sessions to six by eliminating the midweek rest day. Every 6 weeks you can add another training session up to a maximum of eight weekly sessions, which brings you to two workouts in a day on at least 2 days in the week. However, it is crucial that you leave at least 1 full day of recovery each week.

At first glance it would seem like an approach to weight training that is impossible to put into practice; however, after having examined it more carefully and experienced it becomes more doable, as the time required to complete the sessions is less than an average of 40-45 minutes. Muscle fullness, especially if you are young and very well nourished (and with regards to the daily intake of a high level of carbohydrates), can be considerable.

From the beginning, a bodybuilder may constantly live with a nice feeling of muscle hardness and fullness which, in my opinion does not necessarily correspond to muscle hypertrophy, but rather to chronic inflammation. Later, it turns into a form of stress due to having to train so many times a week, which does not help a young athlete who wants to build new muscle fiber. With this type of training, it is very difficult to reach high levels of intensity, due to the fact that you jump from one muscle group to another in a very short amount of time.

I believe that in order to regenerate muscle tissue and make it stronger, harder and larger in size, it must be trained with the highest possible weight and with maximum repetitions, forcing it to the maximum and putting it under continuous tension for as long as possible. After doing this, I believe the muscle just needs to rest! It is unthinkable to go back to training that muscle the next day and for a whole week.

This can only happen if training intensity is not high. The major defect of this method, in my opinion, lies in the fact that the complete satisfaction of having trained a single muscle area to the maximum is never achieved, as muscle tearing never occurs completely. Therefore, I believe it is a method that should not be used by competitive bodybuilders.

CHAPTER 19

Examples of training programs for beginners and intermediate athletes

Riccardo Gaspari

In this chapter, I'll describe my training program. The body is divided into three training sessions (push muscles, pull muscles and legs) and four training sessions per week, which will be performed following the scheme shown in the tables below.

In the exercises of **Block 1**, you should try to use the maximum possible load and perform explosive movements. The load is equal to 8 RM and 4 RM and muscle exhaustion must be sought at each set (ideal TUT: 2-0-2-0).

In the exercises of **Block 2**, the maximum mind/muscle connection must be sought, with well-controlled execution. It is essential to seek the maximum perception of the elongation and contraction of the target muscle. The load is equal to 12 RM and muscle failure must be sought in the last sets of each exercise, especially in the last two, but without ever losing the emphasis on slow and controlled execution. The ideal TUT would be 4-2-4-2.

Block 3 comes with a combination of giant sets on TUT and circuit training on the target muscles. A correct execution and an ideal TUT of 3-1-3-1 must always be maintained.

Cardio will be managed according to the particular needs of the athlete and cardio sessions will be spread over rest days, except for a short warm-up session.

Three executive solutions are proposed, differentiated from each other by increasing the frequency of training, which in this program represents the means to increase the volume of weekly training. The solutions are aimed at beginner, intermediate and advanced athletes.

Training block 1

Training A1

- 10 minutes of cardio at 60-65% of HRmax
- Bench press 1 × 8 + 2 × 4, 120-second rest
- Flat bench dumbbell flyes 1 × 8 + 2 × 4, 120-second rest
- Chest machine 1 × 8 + 2 × 4, 120-second rest
- Military Press 1 × 8 + 2 × 4, 120-second rest
- Lateral raises 3 × 8, 120-second rest
- Chin ups 1 × 8 + 1 × 4, 120-second rest
- French press 2 × 8, 120-second rest
- Overhead French press (back-of-head extensions) 2 × 8, 120-second rest
- Bilateral kickback 2, kickback 8, 120-second rest
- 10 minutes of cardio at 60-65% of HRmax

Training B1

- Pull-ups 1 × 8 + 2 × 4, 120-second rest
- Dumbbell pullover 1 × 8 + 2 × 4, 120-second rest
- Lat machine pulldown 1 × 8 + 2 × 4, 120-second rest
- Deadlift 1 × 8 + 2 × 4, 120-second rest
- 90° flyes 3 × 8, 120-second rest
- Barbell curls 1 × 8 + 1 × 4, 120-second rest
- Incline bench dumbbell curls 2 × 8, 120-second rest

Training C1

- Concentrated curl 2 × 8, 120-second rest
- 10 minutes of cardio at 60-65% of HRmax
- Squat 1 × 8 + 2 × 4, 120-second rest
- Sissy squat 3 × 8, 120-second rest
- Leg extension 1 × 8 + 2 × 4, 120-second rest
- Stiff leg Deadlift 1 × 8 + 2 × 4, 120-second rest
- Leg curl 1 × 8 + 2 × 4, 120-second rest
- Leg curl with extended toes 2 × 8, 120-second rest
- Donkey calf raises 2 × 8, 120-second rest
- Standing calf raises 2 × 8, 120-second rest

At the end of each workout, always perform 10 consecutive minutes of exercises for the abs, cool down for 10-15 minutes and stretch the trained muscles for 10-15 minutes.

Training block 2

Training A2

- 10 minutes of cardio at 60-65% of HRmax
- Prone chest press or incline bench press 4 × 12, 60-second rest
- Chest machine 4 × 12, 60-second rest
- Cable flyes on incline bench 4 × 12, 60-second rest
- Shoulder press 3 × 12, 60-second rest
- Low cable lateral raises 3 × 12, 60-second rest
- Low cable chest pullups 3 × 12, 60-second rest
- Dumbbell French press 3 × 12, 60-second rest
- Push down with rope behind the head 3 × 12, 60-second rest
- Unilateral push down 3 × 12, 60-second rest
- 10 minutes of cardio at 60-65% of HRmax

Training B2

- Pull-ups 4 × 12, 60-second rest
- Low row 4 × 12, 60-second rest
- Pulley with trazy bar 4 × 12, 60-second rest
- Deadlift 4 × 12, 60-second rest
- 90° flyes 4 × 12, 60-second rest
- Low cable curl 3 × 12, 120-second rest
- Pulley curl 3 × 12, 60-second rest
- Concentrated low cable curl 3× 12, 60-second rest

Training C2

- 10 minutes of cardio at 60-65% of HRmax
- 45° leg presses 4 × 12, 75-second rest
- Bulgarian squat with very high rise 4 × 12, 60-second rest
- Leg extension 4 × 12, 60-second rest
- Stiff leg Deadlift 4 × 12, 60-second rest
- Single low cable leg curl 4 × 12, 60-second rest
- Leg curl extended toes 4 × 12, 45-second rest
- Seated calf raises 4 × 12, 45-second rest
- Standing calf raises 4 × 12, 45-second rest

At the end of each workout, always perform 10 consecutive minutes of exercises for the abs, cool down for 10-15 minutes and stretch the trained muscles for 10-15 minutes.

Training block 3

Training A3

- 10 minutes of cardio at 60-65% of HRmax
- *Giant sets 1 (to be repeated 6 times), rest between giant sets for 60 seconds*: incline bench 15 + incline bench flyes 15 + incline bench cable flyes 15
- *Giant set 2 (to be repeated 5 times), rest between giant sets for 45 seconds*: dumbbell shoulder presses 15 + lateral raises 15 + pull ups 15
- *Giant set 3 (to be repeated 4 times), rest between giant sets for 30 seconds*: French press 15 + push down 15 + kick back 15
- *Circuit 1 to be repeated 4 times with no rest*: chest press 15 + shoulder press 15 + close grip bench press 15 + crunch 30 + cross trainer 2 minutes 55-65% HRmax
- *Circuit 2 to be repeated 4 times with no rest*: prone chest press 15 + lateral raises 15 + French press behind the head to the high cable 15 + crunch 30 + cross trainer 2 minutes at 55-65% of HRmax

Training B3

- 10 minutes of cardio at 60-65% of HRmax
- *Giant set 1 (to be repeated 6 times), rest between giant sets for 60 seconds*: forward lat machine 15 + pullover 15 + lat machine pulldown 15
- *Giant set 2 (to be repeated 5 times), rest between giant sets for 45 seconds*: lat machine behind 15 + pulley 15 + barbell row 15
- *Giant set 3 (to be repeated 4 times), rest between giant sets for 30 seconds*: Scott bench curl 15 + pulley curl 15 + low cable curl 15
- *Circuit 1 to be repeated 4 times with no rest*: forward lat machine with triangle 15 + 90° chest flyes 15 + dumbbell curls 15 + reverse crunch 30 + cross trainer 2 minutes at 55-65% of HRmax
- *Circuit 2 to be repeated 4 times with no rest*: deadlift 15 + dumbbell shrugs 15 + barbell curls 15 + reverse crunches 30 + cross trainer 2 minutes at 55-65% of HRmax

Training C3

- 10 minutes of cardio at 60-65% of HRmax
- *Giant set 1 (to be repeated 6 times), rest between giant sets for 60 seconds*: leg press 45° 15 + stationary lunges 15 + leg extension 15
- *Giant set 2 (to be repeated 5 times), rest between giant sets for 45 seconds*: deadlift with straight legs 15 + killer ham 15 + leg curl 15

Continues

Continued

- *Giant set 3 (to be repeated 4 times), rest between giant sets for 30 seconds*: leg curl extended toes 15 + calf to leg press 15 + calf machine 15
- *Circuit 1 to be repeated 4 times with no rest*: squat 15 + dumbbell leg curl 15 + standing calf raises 15 + V-sit crunches 30 + cross trainer 2 minutes at 55-65% HRmax
- *Circuit 2 to be repeated 4 times with no rest*: 45° leg presses 15 + deadlift with straight legs to the low cable 15 + seated calf raises 15 + crunch 30 + cross trainer 2 minutes at 55-65% of HRmax

At the end of each workout, always perform 10 consecutive minutes of exercises for the abs, 10-15 minutes of cool down and 10-15 minutes of stretching of the trained muscles.

Executive schemes

Below you will find the executive scheme of the training program aimed at **beginner athletes** or anyone who, in any case, is just starting to undertake high-volume training.

	Monday	Tuesday	Wednesday	Thursday	Friday	Saturday	Sunday
Week 1	A1	B1	Cardio	C1	A2	Cardio	Rest
Week 2	B2	C2	Cardio	A3	B3	Cardio	Rest
Week 3	C3	A1	Cardio	B1	C1	Cardio	Rest
Week 4	A2	B2	Cardio	C2	A3	Cardio	Rest
Week 5	B3	C3	Cardio	A1	B1	Cardio	Rest
Week 6	C1	A2	Cardio	B2	C2	Cardio	Rest
Week 7	A3	B3	Cardio	C3	A1	Cardio	Rest
Week 8	B1	C1	Cardio	A2	B2	Cardio	Rest
Week 9	C2	A3	Cardio	B3	C3	Cardio	Rest
Week 10	A1	B1	Cardio	C1	A2	Cardio	Rest
Week 11	B2	C2	Cardio	A3	B3	Cardio	Rest
Week 12	C3	Rest	Rest	Rest	Rest	Rest	Rest

Below is the executive scheme of the training program aimed at **intermediate athletes**, who already know how to move between different and demanding training structures.

	Monday	Tuesday	Wednesday	Thursday	Friday	Saturday	Sunday
Week 1	A1	B1	Cardio	C1	A2	Cardio	B2
Week 2	C2	Cardio	A3	B3	Cardio	C3	A1
Week 3	Rest	B1	C1	Cardio	A2	B2	Rest
Week 4	C2	A3	Cardio	B3	C3	Cardio	A1
Week 5	B1	Cardio	C1	A2	Cardio	B2	C2
Week 6	Rest	A3	B3	Cardio	C3	A1	Rest
Week 7	B1	C1	Cardio	A2	B2	Cardio	C2
Week 8	A3	Cardio	B3	C3	Cardio	A1	B1
Week 9	Rest	C1	A2	Cardio	B2	C2	Rest
Week 10	A3	B3	Cardio	C3	A1	Cardio	B1
Week 11	C1	Cardio	A2	B2	Cardio	C2	A3
Week 12	Rest	B3	C3	Rest	Rest	Rest	Rest

Below is the executive scheme of the training program aimed at **advanced athletes.**

	Monday	Tuesday	Wednesday	Thursday	Friday	Saturday	Sunday
Week 1	A1	B1	C1	Cardio	A2	B2	C2
Week 2	Cardio	A3	B3	C3	Cardio	A1	B1
Week 3	C1	Cardio	A2	B2	C2	Cardio	A3
Week 4	B3	C3	Cardio	A1	B1	C1	Cardio
Week 5	A2	B2	C2	Cardio	A3	B3	C3
Week 6	Cardio	A1	B1	C1	Cardio	A2	B2
Week 7	C2	Cardio	A3	B3	C3	Cardio	A1
Week 8	B1	C1	Cardio	A2	B2	C2	Cardio
Week 9	A3	B3	C3	Cardio	A1	B1	C1
Week 10	Cardio	A2	B2	C2	Cardio	A3	B3
Week 11	C3	Cardio	A1	B1	C1	Cardio	A2
Week 12	B2	C2	Cardio	A3	B3	C3	Cardio

CHAPTER 20

My training program

Riccardo Gaspari

I believe describing the roots of my training program is crucial. The initial concept starts with the training method developed by **Dr. Hatfield**, who studied a program that maximizes hypertrophy. Hatfield proposed a method that was truly revolutionary at the time and focused on stimulating white fibers, red fibers and capillarization for each muscle in a single training session.

The program originally proposed by Hatfield divided the body into two weekly training sessions (A-B) with the goal of performing four training sessions per week (A-B, A-B); subsequently, he proposed a more advanced structure that consisted of three workouts per week (A-B-C) to be completed in rotation of weekly workouts (A-B-C-A; B-C-A-B; C-A-B-C; etc.).

According to his indications, each muscle was stimulated by an average of four exercises. The first exercise was fundamental and performed to improve strength; the second and third exercises were multi-joint and were aimed at hypertrophy, exploiting the anaerobic lactacid metabolism; the fourth and final exercises sought maximum capillarization.

In practice, the **first exercise** involved four sets of 5-6 repetitions with either a constant load or ramping sets, where failure was sought in the last of the four sets; there was a 2-3 minute recovery between sets and the repetition lasted 3 seconds in the eccentric phase and 2 seconds in the concentric phase with no isometric stop; the **second exercise** was performed in three sets of eight repetitions with ascending loading, all brought to failure; an execution consisting of 4 seconds for the negative phase and 2 seconds for the positive phase, with a 90-second rest period between sets; the **third exercise** involved three sets of 10-12 repetitions, also brought to failure, but with decreasing load, with 60 seconds of rest between sets and repetitions with 4-second eccentric phases and 2-second concentric phases, always without stopping; the **fourth exercise** was performed with three sets of 20 repetitions, all brought to failure with slow and controlled execution (continuous tension without stopping) and included 4 seconds for the negative phase and 4 seconds for the positive phase, with a 45-second rest period between sets.

A practical example of the Hatfield method

- Deadlift 4 × 5, 120-180-second rest
- Row with T-bar 3 × 8, 90-second rest
- Pull-ups 3 × 10/12, r60-second rest
- Lat machine 3 × 20, 45-second rest

In my opinion, the unfavorable aspects of the Hatfield method are the use of heavy loads, which led me to injury, sets aimed at capillarization, which burned my muscles, and the beginning with a weekly A-B-A-B, which did not allow time to recover.

The second method that has contributed enormously to my program is undoubtedly the **three-week Y3T training cycle** by Neil Hill, a very famous coach who had some of the best athletes in the world among his clients. The Y3T method is a simple and logical approach to training, which is based on the modulation of stimuli by cyclically periodizing training on intermediate white fibers, red fibers and capillarization. This method consists of three micro-cycles, each lasting 1 week; the total duration of each training cycle, therefore, is 3 weeks, to be repeated 3-4 times.

This training method allows us to give a shock to the muscles and the CNS without being too stressed by the duration of the training sessions, which are relatively short; it also allows the athlete to focus on a single muscle group per session.

The **first week** of the Y3T method involves movements composed of 2-3 training sets with 6-8 repetitions, all brought to failure with a 120-second rest period between sets and explosive execution; in the **second week** there are three compound movements and an isolation exercise, with 2-3 sets per exercise but 8-12 repetitions, with rest periods between sets of 90 seconds and controlled execution; the **third week** includes the use of many techniques aimed at increasing intensity, with a range of repetitions that goes from 40 to 80 for large muscles and from 20 to 30 for small muscles and very short or non-existent breaks.

This method goes far beyond the known schemes and is based, as we have seen, on the rotation of three real distinct micro-cycles, each with a specific purpose; the first is aimed at maximum primary stimulation mainly for strength, the second is dedicated to stimulating hypertrophy and the third is aimed both at the stimulation of hypertrophy, with emphasis on the sarcoplasmic part, and at maximum capillarization.

The aspects of this wonderful method (believe me, it's brilliant) that sent me into a crisis were muscle failure with each repetition, the difficulty of proposing it to my clients given the almost exclusive stimulus aimed at truly advanced athletes, the use of very heavy loads right from the start, which impose considerable stress on the athlete who attempts this method, and the need for a heavily hypocaloric diet to maximize results.

With this method, the body is divided into five workouts per week, which follow the chest, back, legs, shoulders and arms sequence, with 2 days of recovery. Those who want to try the original version should take at least 1 day off during the week (for example, A-B-C-pause-D-E-pause). From my point of view, together with spot reduction, the Y3T method has been both enlightening and revolutionary in the world of weight training.

A practical example of the Y3T method

Week 1

- Bench press 2-3 × 6-8, 120-second rest
- Incline bench press 2-3 × 6-8, 120-second rest
- Dips on parallel bars 2-3 × 6-8, 120-second rest

Week 2

- Incline bench press 2-3 × 8-12, 90-second rest
- Bench press 2-3 × 8-12, 90-second rest
- Flyes 2-3 × 8-12, 90-second rest
- Chest press 2-3 × 8-12, 90-second rest

Week 3

- Incline chest press, 40 repetitions in rest pause (using a load that allows us to perform 15-20 repetitions) in a superset with the pectoral machine, 25 repetitions in rest pause (using a load that initially allows us to perform only 10 repetitions)
- Chest press 1 set with 3 drop sets (for example, 8+8+8 decreasing the load each time by 30%)
- Cable flyes 1 × 25
- Push ups 1 × failure

The third method that has greatly influenced me is **circuit training**. It is often overlooked by male athletes but, if used correctly, offers truly striking results in terms of definition and muscle hardness. Circuit training is a type of resistance training performed in a circuit, i.e. performing multiple sets of exercises with medium-high repetitions, variable intensity, without breaks or with very short breaks between the exercises. The advantages of circuit training are mainly linked to the stimulation of strength, hypertrophy, muscle resistance and aerobic capacity, all in a single training session. This manages to bring the typical benefits of both anaerobic and aerobic training.

Circuit training is a variation of traditional resistance training developed by R.E. Morgan and G.T. Anderson in 1953, at the University of Leeds, England. The term "circuit" refers to the fact that the sets of exercises within the workout are performed consecutively, either without breaks or with very short breaks. As with traditional resistance training, the program can be performed with equipment, strength machines, cables, bands, calisthenics or any combination of them.

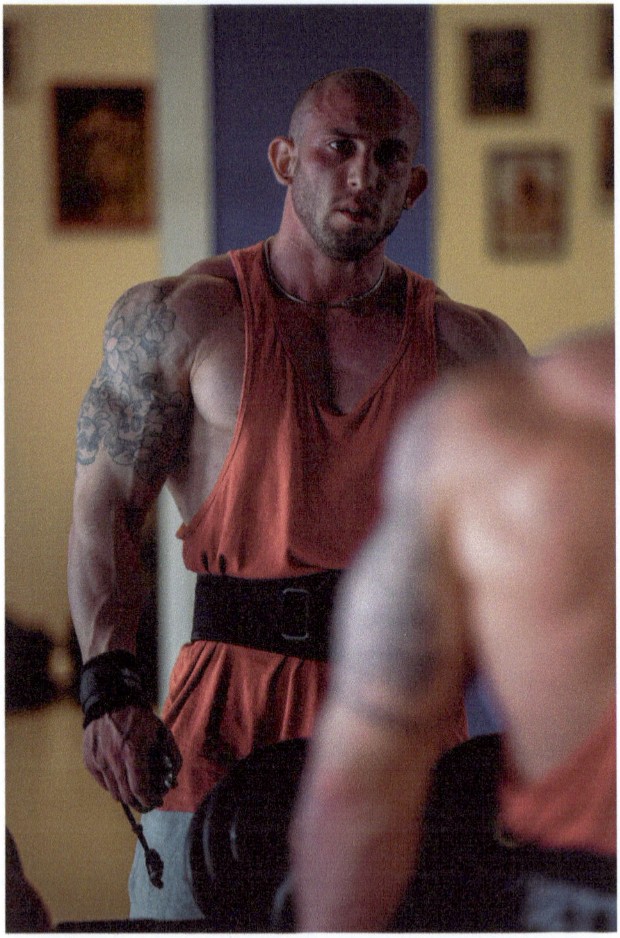

Typically, the number of circuits provided in a circuit training varies from 1 to 5. Generally, circuit training is designed to involve the whole body in a single session (total body mode). For the entire duration of circuit training, heart rate is on average higher than in classic weight training due to very little or no rest intervals. Workouts are faster, take less time and produce greater results.

Circuit training is indicated for people who need a structured program that takes up little time. It is often set up to alternate exercises for the upper and lower body, or by alternating muscle groups.

Circuit training can be considered typical medium-low intensity resistance training to develop muscular endurance and expected loads correspond to about 40-60% of 1RM.

Unlike normal medium-intensity resistance training, which involves recovery times between 60 and 90 seconds, in circuit training intervals are absent or reach a maximum of 30 seconds. This ensures that the aerobic energy system plays a more important role, as the continuous and protracted effort of 60 seconds for over 3-5 minutes allows the increasing intervention of the oxidative metabolism. While, by definition Aerobic Circuit Training (ACT) refers to circuit training interspersed with aerobic machines, traditional circuit training can also be considered a method with an important aerobic component, although it also relies on anaerobic glycolytic metabolism.

Scientific research has extensively investigated the physiological effects and benefits of circuit training. This type of training is generally considered useful for those who want to increase aerobic capacity, duration and muscular resistance. It is also great for improving body recomposition, weight loss, toning and elimination of blemishes like cellulite. It is also indicated for deconditioned people, who have excessive fat accumulation and who need to lose weight, or for heart patients (hypertension, cardiovascular diseases). Studies have also shown an increase in strength, especially in deconditioned subjects. This method has been shown to increase muscle strength by 7 to 32%, while decreasing fat percentage by 0.8 to 2.9%. The same researchers also demonstrated an increase in lean fat mass (or FFM) from 1 to 3.2 kg, without a consequent alteration in body weight. Estimated energy expenditure is about 5-6 kcal per minute for women and 8-9 kcal per minute for men. Traditionally, it has been believed that individuals with cardiovascular disease and hypertension should refrain from resistance training. However, circuit training performed at a moderate intensity (40% of 1RM) in cardiac patients demonstrated a significant increase in strength (13 to 40%) without the occurrence of cardiac or orthopedic complications. Furthermore, circuit training does not appear to elevate resting blood pressure or heart rate and may beneficially lower resting diastolic blood pressure in hypertensive-prone individuals. Available information on the psychological benefits of circuit training points to positive changes in mood, anxiety, depression and aggressiveness.

As far as the choice of exercises is concerned, I prefer to follow the indications of the **POF** (Position Of Flexion) **method** created by Steve Holman; this method is based on the training of a muscle group in **three phases**, an intermediate one, one for lengthening and one for contraction (Tab. 20.1), hitting the target muscle from three different angles, which allow us to train it throughout its range of movement. For this reason, in the United States, this training is also called "3D", because it imposes the stimulus of each muscle from three different angles, and each of these points or positions produces a specific muscle stimulus on the target muscle.

A study carried out by Kawakami (2005) and published in the *International Journal of Sport and Health Science* supports the theses of the POF method, declaring that Holman's theories the scientific results recognize the superiority of using different exercises. It has been clearly demonstrated that different exercises can stimulate different parts of a muscle group, potentially varying their architecture and length.

Table 20.1 The exercises of the Position Of Flexion method (S. Holman, 2001)

Muscles	Intermediate phase	Stretching phase	Contraction phase
Quadriceps	Squats	Sissy squats	Leg extensions
Posterior thighs	Straight leg deadlift	Straight leg deadlift	Leg curls
Calves	Leg curl extended toes	Donkey calf or calf leg presses	Calf raises
Upper abs	Leg lift	Full crunch	Crunches
Lower abs	Leg lift	Full crunch	Leg lift
Upper chest	Incline bench	Incline bench flyes	Incline bench cable flyes
Lower chest	Flat bench press	Flyes on a flat bench	–
Back muscles	Pull-ups or front pull-downs	Pullover with dumbbell	Lat machine pulldowns
Middle back	Pull-ups or behind-the-neck pull-downs	Dumbbell row or close grip cable row	Cable rower with wide grip or rowing with a barbell
Deltoids	Shoulder presses and variants	Incline or cable one-arm lateral raises	Lateral raises or pull to the chin
Biceps	Standing curls	Incline bench curl	Concentration curls
Triceps	French press on flat or close grip bench	Overhead French press	Kickbacks or one arm push downs

The POF method takes into consideration the biomechanical, kinesiological and anatomical principles of skeletal muscles, as well as the interpretation of some scientific results to set up a workout in a more rational and productive way. Different exercises that hit the muscle from various angles, with a different ROM (Range Of Motion), stimulate different bundles or components of a muscle.

A practical example of the POF method

- Pull-ups 2 × 10-12, 90-second rest
- Lat machine 2 × 10-12, 90-second rest
- Dumbbell pullover 2 × 10-12, 90-second rest
- Pulley 2 × 10-12, 90-second rest
- Lat machine pulldown 2 × 10-12, 90-second rest
- Rower 2 × 10-12, 90-second rest

CHAPTER 21

My training program

Federico Focherini

Since I have always had muscle groups that respond worse than others, I have personally prepared and followed a training program for athletes who wish to develop muscles lacking in size the training week.

This is something athletes should do if they want to never stop stimulating muscles that are difficult to develop.

This workout contains almost all of the most fundamental bodybuilding techniques covered in this book and considers the *specialization* of some lagging muscles. In this case, I prepared a training schedule that allowed me to increase the work and growth of two muscle groups, legs and back, with frequent, short extra sessions for other muscles such as calves and shoulders.

An example of my "mosaic"

Day 1: quads and calves

- Leg extension + front squat without ever going up completely (super-set) 4 × 20
- 45° leg presses 4 × 20 (increasing the weight with each set)
- Barbell Walking Lunges 4 × 15 left + 15 right (go all the way down without stopping in between and always push with the back leg)
- 45° leg presses, one leg at a time 4 × 12 (non-stop, *4 seconds down and 1 second up*, keep the foot high and push only with the heel)
- Standing calf raises 3 × 15 reps + 10 alternating stretching (walk) + 15 reps + 10 walk + 15 reps (where repetitions alternate with stretching, without ever getting off the machine)
- Seated calf raises 3 × 20 + 20 + 20 (strip set)

Continues

Continued

Day 2: back (width), shoulders, hamstrings, and glutes

- T-way pullover in super-set with pulldown 5 × 12/max... (pulldown must be performed with a medium grip, elbows forward, straight back, max stretch)
- Lat machine with the triangle-shaped handle grip (same technique as the lat pulldown) in super-set pullover standing on the lat machine with straight arms 4 × 12
- Lat machine behind the neck (kneeling, shoulders to the counterweights) in super-set with barbell press (for the shoulders) behind the neck standing or sitting 4 × 12
- Deadlift with straight legs (curved back and toes on two small plates) in super-set with seated leg curl 4 × 15
- Reverse leg curl* in super-set/leg curl lying 4 × 12

*While kneeling on the lat machine or on the floor, move towards the ground without pushing your glutes back and hold on to your partner's bar, then return to a standing position. It's the opposite of the leg curl!

Day 3: arms

- Barbell curls 5 × 8
- Incline bench dumbbell wide-arm curls (60° dumbbell bench with wide arms) Seated to dumbbell super-set alternating standing dumbbell super-set 4 × 12 (same dumbbells)
- Reverse grip barbell curl 2-3 × 10 + 10 +10 (strip)
- Pullover and press with EZ bar 5 × 8 (what Arnold did for the triceps, a mix between a pullover and a French press!)
- French press in super-set with Californian French press* in super-set with narrow bench 4 × 12 (same bar, same weight)
- Push down with rope 2-3 × 10 + 10 + 10 (strip)

*Go down to your forehead as if you were doing a French press, slide the bar across your face, and, when you're on your chest, push up and squeeze your triceps.

Day 4: chest, middle and front shoulders

- Flat (slightly inclined) bench barbell press 3 × 5 reps + 12-second rest + 5 reps + 12-second rest + 3 reps (+ 12-second rest + 1 rep only in the last set). Use a weight with which you would do 7-8 alone (*it's a development of the rest-pause*)
- Incline barbell presses 1 × 12 (warm-up) 2 × 6 + 3f + 2n – 50% × max (6 reps alone, get to your limit + 3 force with someone to help you go further + 2 negative = 8 seconds down – 50% of weight, continue until failure)
- Dumbbell flyes on a decline bench in super-set with barbell press on decline bench 4 × 12

Continues

Continued

- Flat bench barbell press (slightly inclined) wide grip, bring the barbell to the throat (Smith machine), called "the Cutthroat", *stay 1 second with the barbell on the throat*, in super-set with a pullover, with someone resisting the dumbbell when you lift it 4 × 12
- Super-set dumbbells lateral raise with super-set dumbbell seated Arnold press with thumbs-up lateral raise* 4 × 12
- Front raises on bench 60° in super-set with chin pulls with two plates in rotation** 4 × 12

*With dumbbells or small plates, starting in a cross-hands-on-thighs position, raise the dumbbells to an overhead position with thumbs pointing up.
**This is a 2 dumbbell or kettlebell chin pull, with back rotation of the elbows as if you were about to take off your shirt.

Day 5: quads, hamstrings, calves

- Leg extension + 45° leg press + squat 6 × 20 (triset)
- Deadlift with straight legs + lying leg curl (keep the legs closed and keep the toes forward, unloaded ankle) 4 × 20 (super-set)
- Leg extension 1 × 15 + 15 + 15 + 15 + 15 (strip set)
- Killer quads 3 × 15 (it is the opposite of the leg extension and hamstring exercise of the first day; kneeling on the mat, hands on your chest, letting yourself fall backward keeping your back straight without bringing your glutes back, and return to the straight position)
- Seated calf 4 × 30 (increasing weight with each set and maintaining the same reps)
- Calf press 3 × 10 + 5 seconds + 15 + 10 seconds + 25 + 15 seconds + 15 + 10 seconds + 10 (mega rest pause, after each micro-set rest for 5-10-15-10 seconds)

Day 6: back (thickness) and posterior shoulders

- Classic deadlift 4 × 10 (65% of maximum load) 1-2 weeks/6 × 10/3-4 weeks/8 × 10 from the fifth week onwards
- Barbell row 6 × 8 in super-set with barbell floor presses (pectoral high). *Medium grip, with elbows in front touch the floor and, in a circular motion, bring the barbell above the eyes. maximal contraction*
- Rowing with 2 dumbbells lying on an incline bench in a super-set with a low pulley seated with a cushion under the glutes (in this way you can pull the triangle on your stomach from bottom to top and contract as much as possible) 4 × 12
- Dumbbell or barbell behind-the-neck in super-set with T-bar row 4 × 12/10
- Super-set 90° dumbbell raises with pull the rope at the throat at low pulley row 4 × 12 (keep elbows high and hands low)

Note: Do sit-ups every day, at least 8 sets of 20-25 reps each.

I called this training method a **"mosaic"**: it was my approach to competitions for many years, and it is still the way I train the competitive athletes that I personally coach. I don't think I've discovered anything, but I think it's one of the best ways to train each muscle in the three degrees of distinction and to customize training aimed at the groups that are lacking development: *angle*, *plane*, and *sense*, using many basic exercises with different techniques, combining the training of interlocking muscles, one above the other, one inside the other, recalling and re-training them, giving stress of all kinds at high intensity and with a short recovery time.

The *tempo* of each movement is emphasized, always maintaining muscle tension, with the ultimate goal of reaching the inability to complete a further contraction, not due to exhaustion of the energy source but due to the impossibility of carrying out the last muscle contraction. Your muscles will have to perceive this attack as one long, hard set.

Each joint involved in the training session is conceived and adapted to the muscular and structural flaws of the athlete.

Here we have extended the concept of **muscle priority** to the specialization technique. In this case, the concept of specialization is put into practice using the **muscle priority system**, with the insertion of many techniques altogether, which stimulate the muscle from every angle, without ever leaving it time to "understand" or "learn the lesson".

This way, the body has to adapt and has to adjust and respond to the continuous stimulus.

This training method is very valuable for advanced athletes approaching a competition. I recommend following a pattern of 3 days on and 1 day off training.

CHAPTER 22

My training program

Massimo Spattini

When I was 17 years old I was already a fanatic about pushups, which I thought were the best way to build a muscular physique, and I could do over 100 consecutively. Then, one day, my best friend, upon returning from his holidays by the sea, told me that he had seen a friend of his who, compared to the previous season, had transformed his body because he trained with weights for his sport, which was rowing. My friend then had his uncle, who had a machine shop, make him a barbell with iron discs that had a sufficiently large diameter, which we used to perform chest presses lying on the floor and then we'd slip out from under the bar because we didn't have a bench.

Our gym was his 2.5 × 3.5 m basement and our training consisted of barbell squats, lying barbell floor presses, pull-ups hanging from the water pipe that ran through the corridor of the basement, overhead press, barbell curls and lying barbell extension..

Instead of watching television after dinner, we trained after studying during the day, and repeated the same workout (total body) three times a week. We would have worked out even more, thinking we'd get better results, but our parents prevented us from doing it because they thought it was bad for us, and basically they were right.

When I discovered that another friend of mine, who played rugby for the local team, had a barbell and a pair of dumbbells in his garage, I also started training on Saturday afternoons, telling my mother that I was going for a walk in the city centre. In addition, I found a way to train during PE hours in the school gym, which was equipped with a vertical press and a loadable barbell. I thought that by doing more and more, I would get better results, but that wasn't the case.

However, I didn't realize I was wrong until Emilio They, my first bodybuilding mentor, explained the importance of recovery and made me realize that "the more you train, the better" is a concept that doesn't work. So, since I could use my father's painting studio as a gym, I set up a workout schedule every other day without taking Sunday into account, and most of the time I divided my body into two parts: one day legs-chest and lats, the other day shoulders biceps-triceps, doing three exercises per muscle group.

After a few years, in 1979, since my parents had lent me an apartment that I equipped as a gym with help from some friends, I increased the training volume since I had more equipment and the training frequency, doing up to 5 workouts per week, maintaining shoulder and arm training but dividing the leg-back-chest training into two; one day I trained the legs alone and one day the lats together with the pecs. Calves and abs were trained three times a week.

This division, combined with pyramid training and trying to use the maximum load, was my prevailing approach until I went to Los Angeles (1984) and saw that most athletes divided the various muscle groups into more parts and they didn't necessarily always use high loads, but they worked a lot on muscle contraction. Training in close contact and even as a training partner with the greatest champions of that time revolutionized my training method, although I was always looking for "my training method". I have already talked about my training experience with Mike Mentzer and Samir Bannout, and I had a similar training experience with Lee Labrada as well. I got the chance to train with Lee, including on one of his seminar tours that I organized for him in Italy, during which I accompanied him as an interpreter. On that occasion, I was impressed by his systematic approach and his strict adherence to the training and diet program, despite the fatigue and unfavorable travel schedule. Although Lee was often traveling around the world for seminars and exhibitions, he would always stick to his workouts and meals. Labrada's training method consisted of a high-intensity approach in which he started with the maximum load in the first set and then, in the following ones, he decreased the weight. After all, his explanation was rather convincing: "In the first set the muscle is less tired, so it can give its best; then, if I've given my all, the performance will naturally decline and I'll have to reduce the weight". On its face the reasoning was logical, but there was a small problem: it didn't work that way for me. In my case, after a couple of warm-up sets and as I get close to the training load, if I use a weight (let's say 100 kg on a bench press) that allows me to do 10 repetitions to exhaustion in the first set, after adequate rest, in the second set I do 11 with the same weight, in the third 12 and my performance will start declining in the fourth set.

Evidently, my maximum performance capacity is between the second and third sets, so it's not possible for me to give my best with a single set or even starting out with the maximum weight. It is probably a factor linked to "warming up the muscle", to the adaptation of the elastic components of the muscle, to the higher percentage of intermediate-type, more resistant fibers, or even linked to the biomechanical issues of a joint. Over the years, I've noticed that athletes who practice high-intensity, low-volume training mostly have shorter builds and aren't tall; as a result, their joints are less stressed. Think of the distance required to bench press for an athlete who has relatively short arms versus one who has long arms. This is even more evident in the execution of a squat by an athlete of relatively short stature compared to a volleyball player, who must be very careful when performing this exercise.

In this regard, I want to tell you an anecdote that happened to me while I was training at the World Gym in Venice (Los Angeles). I was training on the outdoor terrace while Lee Priest was training with a 45° press using impressive tonnage. He was known as the "Giant Killer" because of his height of just over 5'2" and arms measuring 21 inches, managing to beat athletes much taller and more imposing than him.

Watching him from a distance, I didn't exactly understand what exercise he was doing, as I had the impression he was training his thighs, but based on the movement of the platform, which was raised by a maximum of 6-8 inches, it seemed he was doing a sort of cheat calf press. Intrigued, I got close enough to see that he was indeed doing leg presses but, given the volume of his quadriceps and hamstrings and the shortness of his limbs, the range of motion was extremely limited, obviously allowing the use of higher loads.

It is no coincidence that all the other athletes presses and who were taller than 5'9" worked out with higher training volumes, which allowed them to perform a higher number of sets, to get to the truly stimulating ones. Some of them include Arnold Schwarzenegger, Lee Haney, Bob Paris, Milos Sarcev, and Berry De Mey.

Among the various training methods that I have taken into consideration and that I have applied to myself, the one that has undoubtedly convinced me the most is Fred Hatfield's system, structured to stimulate all the various muscle fibers and to volumize each structural component of the muscle, from myofibrillar to sarcoplasmic and vascular. I met Dr. Squat in person, who was named after his performance in squats. I contacted him during one of my stays in California and he invited me to his home, where we talked about training for an entire afternoon. His training included an exercise with heavy loads and explosive execution an exercise with moderate loads and slow execution, in continuous tension and one last exercise with higher repetitions with a light load, all for each muscle group and within the same session.

Undoubtedly, this meeting was a source of inspiration for me, because the **concept of a training method that included different techniques of execution of the exercises in order to involve the various muscle fibers** seemed scientifically correct. The only problem in applying his method was that, in the long run, since I trained my muscles twice a week, the use of heavy loads caused me joint overload, and I paid the consequences in inflammation and pain, which compromised the quality of my training.

Consequently, this led me to what then became *my training* method that accompanied me for all the years of my not-so-long competitive career and for the years that followed. Basically, my training was structured like this: 3 training days and 1 rest day, without counting Sunday, or 5 training days a week, resting on Thursday and Sunday but still using a rotational A-B-C subdivision, where on A days I trained the push muscles (pectoral muscles-lateral and front shoulders-triceps), on B days the legs (quadriceps-hamstrings-calves), and on C days the pull muscles (back muscles-trapezius muscles-rear deltoid -biceps). The difference consisted in the fact that I alternated an A-B-C cycle with exercises with heavy loads and explosive execution, with one last exercise performed with high repetitions, to an A-B-C cycle with moderate loads and slow and controlled execution, with the last exercise at superslow speed, that is, with even lighter weights and even slower or very fast "pumping" execution.

This training method allowed for better recovery from a physical, mental and joint point of view. Doing squats with 200 kg was undoubtedly a great stress on the body as a whole and on the joints, but from a mental point of view it was extremely stimulating; moreover, the maximum effort took over only in the last repetitions, when things got tougher. On the other hand, training with more moderate weights undoubtedly allowed me to have greater physical and joint recovery, but it was extremely onerous for my mental concentration because applying the technique of continuous isotension and "muscle isolation" (maintaining maximum tension at any moment of the arc of movement) required considerable mental effort. In practice, after 3 days of training with heavy loads, I really wanted to train with lighter loads and concentrate on the muscle, while after 3 days of slow and concentrated training I really wanted to "lift a few tons", while obviously respecting correct execution.

I strongly believe that a person's success in a certain field is largely linked to being able to try their hand at that field while having fun, and I enjoyed it that way.

Another aspect that characterized my training programs was an execution method that favored form over lifting the weight itself. In the beginning, performing most of the exercises in front of a mirror constituted an aesthetic need for me: bodybuilding is an aesthetic sport and it seemed absurd to me to try performing exercises with execution methods that did not respect a criterion of symmetry, composure and elegance. For this reason, I have always preferred to perform the exercises with a complete ROM of movement: they seemed "cleaner" and more aesthetically pleasing to me; only later did I discover the scientific reason behind it. Furthermore, empirical observations of the various champions while they were training led me to realize that training with full ROM movements led to more harmonious muscle development, with greater separation between the various muscle fibers and a more elongated muscular structure. In the 1980s, the law of all or nothing was valid for muscles: it was thought that the muscle contracted equally in all its parts and, therefore, thinking in terms of exercises for the lower part and for the top of the biceps made no sense. This too was later refuted by electromyography and ultrasound studies, but at the time the shape of a muscle was thought to be due to genetics and muscle insertions and not to the type of exercise nor, much less, to their mode of execution.

This belief was further shaken when I watched my friend and champion Bob Paris, one of the most esteemed "aesthetic" physique of all time in bodybuilding, train with his new training partner. Bob was a maniac about the execution of the exercises and each repetition was performed using the maximum range of motion in an impeccable way. He's the one who taught me to say either out loud or in my head "Stretch" at the point of maximum elongation and "Squeeze" at the point of maximum contraction and shortening during every rep. At first, his training partner was a guy about his height but with a lower muscle volume; he trained with Bob and did his own exercises, perhaps with less weight, and with the same execution method. Watching him, year after year, I saw that he was able to develop his own muscle structure to be similar to Bob's in proportion and shape. At that point, it became difficult for me to think that the type of training and exercises and their execution did not influence the shape of the muscles and that it was only determined genetically.

The advantage of full ROM training, including stimulating hypertrophy, was subsequently demonstrated by a few studies (here I will mention two). The first is a study by Pinto et al. (2012), in which Brazilian researchers had one group perform biceps curls with a range of motion from 0 to 130° (full range) and another group with 50 to 100° (partial range) for 10 weeks. At the end of the study, the full range of motion group achieved twice as many results compared to the partial range group. The second study was conducted by Bloomquist et al. (2013), who also compared two groups: one trained three times a week performing deep squats (from 0 to 120° of knee flexion), while the other performed partial squats from 0 to 60°; both used the same weight percentages of their rep max for that type of exercise (obviously, those who did partial squats used heavier loads). In the end, the increase in lean mass occurred significantly in the deep squat group, while almost no one in the partial squat group had a change in their lean muscle mass.

Another interesting thing is that front thigh cross-sectional augmentation occurred along its entire length in the deep squat group; in the partial squat group, however, it increased only in the uppermost area. This study justified my smile when seeing the bodybuilder on duty in the gym with "chicken legs", who tried his hand at 200 kg squats, going down just a few centimeters.

This is not to say that you should never perform partial range of motion exercises, because Brad Schoenfeld has pointed out that using heavy loads in partial movements results in the ability to later use heavier loads in full range movements, but that this training methodology should possibly be used in a structured training program.

This is the training that I then basically practiced until my victory at the 1986 Italian championship.

Workout A: legs-calves
• Warming up of the muscles in question • Barbell squat 5 × 10/8/6/6/4 • Press or leg extension 4 × 8 (1 week press, 1 week leg extension) • Walking lunges with barbell 3 × 20 • Lying leg curl 4 × 10/12/8/6 • Deadlifts with straight legs 4 × 8 • Seated leg curl 4 × 8 • Standing calf machine 4 × 15 parallel feet • Seated calf 4 × 15 • Stretching of the muscles in question

Workout B: chest-shoulders-triceps
• Warming up of the muscles in question • Bench press 5 × 10/8/6/6/4 • Incline bench press 4 × 10/8/6/6 • Flat bench flyes 4 × 10 • Flyes 4 × 12/10/8/6 • Lateral raises 4 × 8 • Dumbbell front raises 4 × 8 • Dips 3 × max • Lying barbell extensions 4 × 10/12/8/6 • Cable pushdown 3 × 10 • Stretching of the muscles in question

Workout C: back-deltoids-biceps
• Warming up of the muscles in question • Pull-ups 4 × max • Lat machine forward 5 × 10/8/6/6/4 • Pulley 4 × 10/8/6/6 • Dumbbell back raises 4 × 8 • Dumbbell shrugs 4 × 8 • Barbell curl 3 × 10/8/6 • Alternate dumbbell curl 3 × 8 • Concentrated curl 3 × 8 • Stretching of the muscles in question

Continues

Continued

An example of the sequence for 4 workouts per week

- **Monday**: A
- **Tuesday**: B
- **Wednesday**: rest
- **Thursday**: C

A-B-C = heavy loads, explosive execution, rest for 1 minute and 30 seconds, 1-0-2 execution (1 concentric, 0 isometric, 2 eccentric).
The time of 1 second in the concentric phase means a fairly explosive execution which, however, in the last repetitions, will certainly slow down and will exceed 1 second, but the fundamental concept is to try, in this case, to lift the weight quickly.

- **Friday**: A1
- **Saturday**: B1
- **Sunday**: rest
- **Monday**: C1

A1-B1-C1 = moderate loads, slow execution in continuous tension, rest for 1 minute, execution 3-1-3 (3 concentric, 1 isometric, 3 eccentric)

- **Tuesday**: A
- **Wednesday**: rest
- **Thursday**: B
- **Friday**: C
- **Saturday**: A1
- **Sunday**: rest

Note
- *Concentric contraction in isotension*: the muscle shortens developing tension (for example, when you lift a weight trying to maintain the same level of muscle contraction).
- *Isometric contraction*: the muscle contracts without changing its length, therefore without moving the load. For example, when performing a voluntary peak contraction or when performing a partial movement while forcibly maintaining the contraction at the stop moment, especially in exercises in which, if the full range of movement is completed, the weight would weigh on the bone-joint chain without stressing the muscle (like bench press or overhead press).
- *Eccentric or negative contraction*: the muscle lengthens developing tension (e.g., slowly lowering the same weight).

In this micro-cycle, the repetitions per set must always be 10 and some exercises, such as pull-ups, which can hardly be performed with this technique, must be replaced. In fact, several exercises can be substituted bearing in mind that, in the explosive micro-cycle, exercises with free weights are to be preferred, while micro-cycle machines can be used in the continuous isotension microcycle.

Then, when my competitive career ended (although it wasn't a definitive thing because I always left a door open to my return, which never actually happened), I continued to train as if I still had to compete. However, I switched to what I would describe as maintenance training, which no longer involved training my muscles twice a week.

Since then, I've been doing a training program that involves two days of training, one day of rest, two days of training, and two days of rest, subdividing the muscle areas to train them twice every 10 days. Subdividing the muscles takes into account the fact that there are muscles that recover sooner, such as the hamstrings; I spaced out some muscle groups and selected some exercises so that there is some sort of pull for the biceps when I work the lats, for the triceps when I work the pectorals and for the hamstrings when I work the quads.

I normally only use heavy loads in the first exercise for each muscle group and use moderate to light loads for the second and third exercises, always focusing on maintaining a good mind-muscle connection. This way, I attack each muscle group differently.

I perform an explosive execution in the first exercise, with 1 second in the ascent phase and 2 seconds in the descent phase. I do an isotension movement in the second exercise, using a moderate weight, focusing on "feeling" the muscle, creating a good neuromuscular connection, and maintaining maximum tension as I lift the weight in 3 seconds and lower it in 4 seconds. I perform the third exercise with light weights, sometimes alternating a very fast execution or doing the exact opposite with a very slow execution, about 4 seconds in the ascent and 5-6 seconds in the descent.

I don't use the same weights all the time. The load can vary, as it depends on many factors, including my energy level, professional workload, use of machines or free weights, how fast I lift the weight, where I train, and whether I'm traveling or not.

Day 1: chest-deltoids-triceps

- Warming up of the muscles in question
- Bench press 5 × 10/8/6/6/6
- Decline bench press 4 × 10
- Incline bench dumbbell flyes 3 × 15
- Overhead press 5 × 10/8/6/6/6
- Single lateral raises on incline bench 3 × 10
- Dumbbell lateral raises 3 × 15
- Lying barbell extensions 5 × 10/8/6/6/6
- High cable forward pushes 3 × 10
- Pushes down on the cables 3 × 15
- Stretching of the muscles in question

Continues

Continued

Day 2: calves-quads-hamstring

- Warming up of the muscles in question
- Standing calf machine 5 × 20/15/8/8/8
- Donkey calf machine 3 × 15
- Seated calf 3 × 20
- Press 45° 5 × 10/8/6/6/6
- Back lunges at multipower 4 × 10
- Sissy squat 4 × 10
- Leg extension 3 × 15
- Lying leg curl 4 × 10/12/8/6
- Deadlifts with straight legs 4 × 10
- Seated leg curl 3 × 15
- Stretching of the muscles in question

Day 3: lats-posterior deltoids-rear

- Warming up of the muscles in question
- Barbell row 5 × 10/8/6/6/6
- Lat machine forward 4 × 10
- Low pulley 4 × 15
- Hyperextensions 3 × 10
- Seated rear delt raises with dumbbells 3 × 8
- Back raises on incline bench 3 × 10
- Rear delt raises 3 × 15
- Barbell curl 5 × 10/8/6/6/6
- Incline bench dumbbell curls 4 × 10
- High cable curl 3 × 15
- Stretching of the muscles in question

Note

- Abdominals of your choice all three days for 10 minutes at the end of the workout, before stretching.
- In **red**: pyramidal sets, 2 minutes of recovery between one set and another; explosive execution, 2-0-1-0 (2 eccentric, 0 isometric in lengthening, 1 concentric, 0 isometric in shortening).
- In black: moderate loads, slow execution in continuous tension, 1 minute and 30 seconds of rest, with the following execution: 3-1-3-1 (3 eccentric, 1 isometric in lengthening, 3 concentric, 1 isometric in shortening).
- In **green**: low loads, fast execution (pumping), rest for 45 seconds, execution: X-0-X-0 (X eccentric, 0 isometric in lengthening, X eccentric, 0 isometric in shortening. Or a very slow execution with recovery phase of 30 seconds, execution: 5-1-4-1 (5 eccentric, 1 isometric in lengthening, 4 concentric, 1 isometric in shortening).
- *Concentric contraction*: the muscle shortens by developing tension (for example, by lifting a weight).
- *Isometric contraction*: the muscle contracts without changing its length, therefore without shifting the load (for example, by pushing against a wall).
- *Eccentric or negative contraction*: the muscle lengthens by developing tension (for example, by slowly lowering the same weight).

My specialty workout for arms and calves

Double-split routine: the theory

The development capacity for an athlete is obtained by means of appropriate movement stimuli. If stimuli are dosed in such a way that they have a training effect, i.e. contribute to the development, consolidation and maintenance of the training state, this is called a "training load".

In a session, the load initially produces a process of fatigue, due to the consumption of functional power and energy, and this fatigue temporarily lowers the functional capacity of the organism. This constitutes the decisive stimulus for the adaptation processes that occur above all in the recovery phase.

That is, the consumed energy and muscle components are not only reintegrated, but the resulting re-stabilization goes beyond the initial level; this supercompensation represents the basic foundation of improvement.

The adaptation process not only allows athletes to achieve greater results, but also increases their physical and mental load capacity.

If the loads remain unchanged, they are conquered more easily than before and produce a lower training effect.

Stagnation of the load also means stagnation of development capabilities. This applies not only to beginners, but also to more advanced athletes.

The widely held notion that the load can be reduced after considerable muscle development has been achieved must not be accepted.

If you want to progress, you have to systematically increase the load. The components of the load that influence development capacity the most are **quantity** (volume) and **intensity**.

The problem lies in what proportion of the amount and intensity of the training must be changed in the single parts and in the periodic cycle and in which components we should place the center of gravity for lifting of the load.

Double-split routines

Double-split routines (i.e. double and split routines performed within the same day) increase the number of workouts and allow you to increase the load. By limiting training to one or two muscles, in addition to always allowing the load to be increased, it facilitates the increase in intensity, thus allowing the concentration threshold to be kept high, making the training more effective and decreasing the risk of injury, which usually occurs at the end of exhausting and endless workouts.

The recovery processes accelerate as the training state progresses, training frequency can also gradually increase.

Double-split routines obviously also meet this need to increase training frequency.

But let's try to translate all these concepts into practical terms.

Application of the principles

Personally, I've always had problems with the development of my arms and calves. I have always devoted the utmost attention to training these muscle groups, but it was only in 1985, when I switched to double-split routines, that I started getting better results, increasing my arms circumference from 45 to 49 cm (cold) and my calves from 42 to 45 cm, in just two years. My routine was set up as shown in the table below.

Monday

- **Morning**: biceps
- **Afternoon**: calves/pecs

Tuesday

- **Morning**: triceps
- **Afternoon**: back/deltoids

Wednesday

- **Morning**: biceps
- **Afternoon**: calves/thighs

Thursday

- **Morning**: triceps
- **Afternoon**: calves/pecs

Friday

- **Morning**: biceps
- **Afternoon**: back/deltoids

Saturday

- **Morning**: triceps
- **Afternoon**: calves/thighs

This workout allowed me to train my biceps and triceps three times a week, thus increasing my weekly workload; moreover, by training a single muscle in the morning, I have maximum physical and mental energy, and this allows me to maintain excellent concentration and intensity throughout the training. It would be impossible for me to train my arms after training other muscle groups.

If, on the other hand, I gave priority to arms at the beginning of the session, it would be impossible for me to train the trunk muscles effectively afterwards, as the arms, which are involved in every movement for the upper body, would already be tired.

In this way, I have formulated a workout that allows me to easily increase the amount, intensity, and frequency of my training, which are the three fundamental components of the training load.

The same goes for my calves, which I train as often as four times a week.

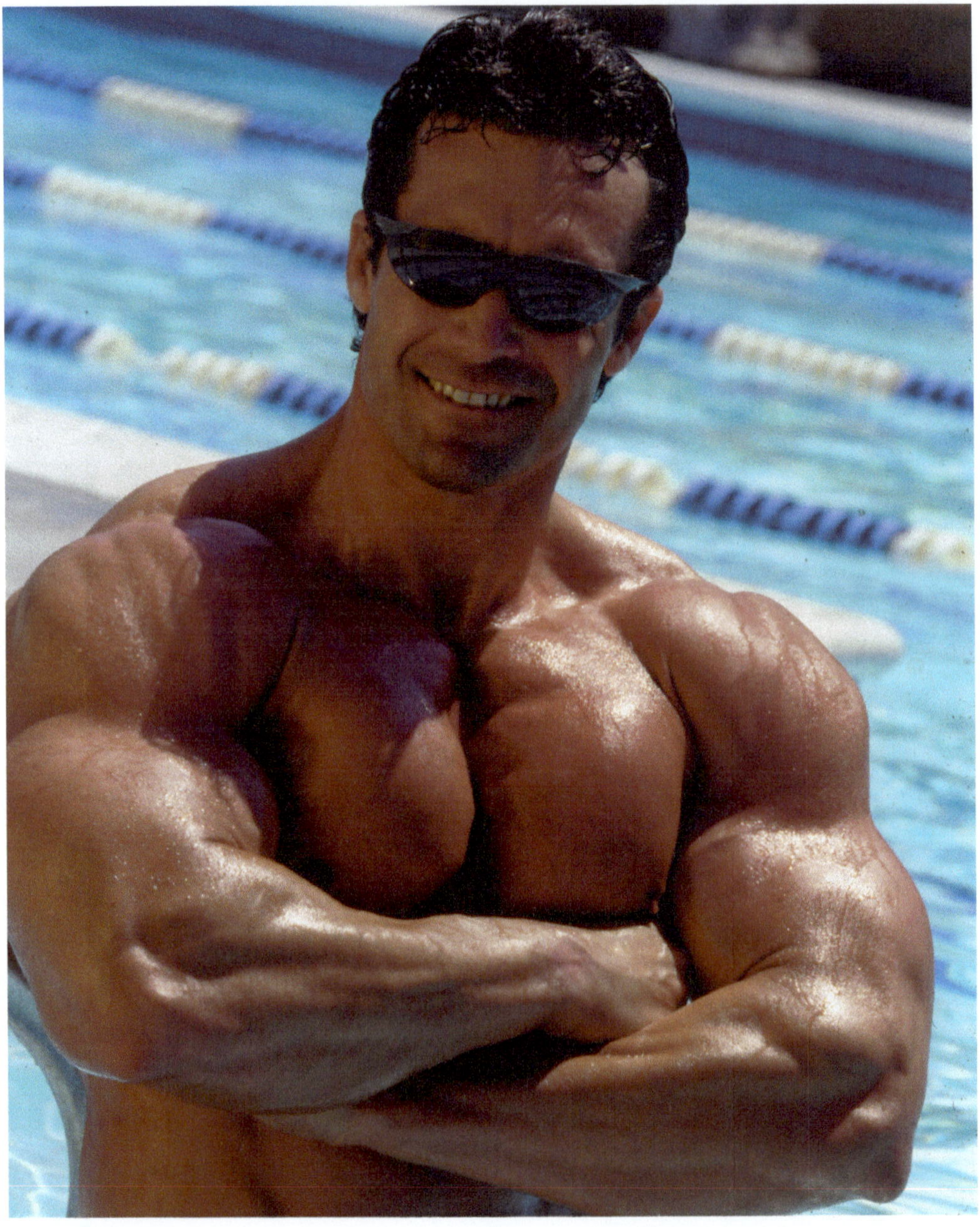

During my first 11 years of training, I developed remarkable resilience, which allows me to maintain my double-split routines year-round.

Albert Beckles, after over 30 years of training, does a complete double-split routine by training all muscles three times a week.

If an athlete with just a few years of training experience approaches a double-split routine, they will inevitably fall into overtraining, with all the imaginable consequences.

To acquire the necessary recovery capacity, it is very important to progressively increase the training load over the years, going from three times a week to 4, then 5 and finally, possibly – and compatibly with the type of work being carried out – even 6 sessions. Obviously, this approach is feasible for a person who can devote the whole day to managing workouts, meals and recovery, i.e. practically a professional athlete or anyone who has the ability to behave like one.

My current training method

At 64 you can no longer train with the same intensity as when you were half this age. The loads "weigh" more and the impact on the joints is greater. If the weight decreases, due in part to joint problems, the volume should be increased to maintain the same workload, but the ability to bear and recover from a high workload also decreases. So, I tried to train one or two muscles every day and it works for me; however, since I often can't train every day due to other commitments, I can hardly train my muscles more than once a week, so I need a higher frequency.

Often, to optimize the time, after an initial **pyramid** exercise where I progressively increase the load with each set, I perform a second exercise with the **stripping** technique until exhaustion and thus end the training for that muscle.

Lately, I happened to train with my friend Ivan Martellato, a bodybuilder, nutritionist, biologist and sports science graduate, who is 30 years old (sometimes, it's stimulating for me to train with younger athletes who push me a little beyond my comfort zone, although sometimes I still push them out of theirs). At one point, as we were preparing to train the biceps and didn't have much time, Ivan said to me: "Let's do reverse stripping".

I asked him: "What is that?" and he replied: "Instead of decreasing the weight, we increase it during the set". Intrigued, I agreed and the first impression was excellent, so much so that I have since then systematically included it in my training routine.

Now let's look in detail at how I do it and try to provide a physiological explanation for it. As you know, normally, stripping involves performing a series with a weight that allows for 6 to 10 repetitions, and, once you reach your limit, you scale the weight just enough to be able to perform another 6-10 repetitions; then scale again for another set, all without pausing, except for the time needed to change the weight.

With this technique, the TUT (Time Under Tension) is particularly prolonged and the production of lactic acid is maximal. On the other hand, in **reverse stripping**, instead of decreasing the weight after each set, it is always increased, practically without a break. How is it possible? Let's get into the details. You start with a weight that allows you to perform 12 repetitions in a slow and controlled manner, in continuous isotension, using 3 seconds in the concentric phase and 3 seconds in the eccentric phase; after that, the weight is increased and, after three quick breaths, 6 repetitions are carried out with the concentric phase of 1 second, with fairly explosive execution, and the controlled eccentric phase is done in 3 seconds; finally, the weight is increased again and 3 explosive repetitions are performed both in the concentric phase and in the eccentric phase, with a negative acceleration. What could the physiological basis of this method be? As for me, I have already specified that I am absolutely not predisposed to immediately starting with a heavy load and techniques such as the reverse pyramid, i.e. doing the first set with the maximum possible weight and then decreasing it on the other sets, do not work well for me because my muscles respond better after a few adaptation sets; so, partially, this method meets my characteristics, starting with a lighter load that prepares my muscle for a heavier load. However, it is one thing to do a set, then rest for 90 seconds, and then increase the load, and it is another thing to increase the load after completing a set to exhaustion without recovering.

What can the reasons for the effectiveness of this method be? The first group of repetitions with moderate weight and slow and controlled execution undoubtedly also recruits the red and intermediate fibers and, involving a TUT of about 70-80 seconds, it already implies a considerable production of lactic acid. It is advisable not to reach complete exhaustion because otherwise the continuation of the exercise would be compromised. In the second group, we find ourselves in a situation of maximum production of lactic acid and the slowed eccentric component further accentuates its production, creating an environment of acidosis at the muscular level which amplifies the lesions at the membrane level of the muscle cell. This occurs above all in the three eccentric repetitions with a negative acceleration, where we use a load that would normally be used in a set that involves an alactic anaerobic energy metabolism. In this case, the movement is performed in a lactic environment, thus creating more muscle micro-lesions, given the combination of the increased weight and the acidic environment. And we know how these micro-lesions are the basis of muscle growth.

In my opinion, this training method includes all three physiological conditions that are needed to stimulate an increase in the protein synthesis rate and muscle mass:

- **muscle damage**, which is directly proportional to the degree of tension generated by the muscle during contraction. Consequently, the heavier the training load (as in the last three repetitions), the greater the degree of muscle damage that is created. Muscle damage at the tissue level is associated with an inflammatory response, responsible for subsequent growth;
- **mechanical tension**: the degree of mechanical tension depends on the tension time produced above all during the eccentric phase of the movement, particularly emphasized in the first two groups of repetitions. Furthermore, it is believed that

global times under tension (TUT) of at least 60-70 seconds are the most suitable to promote muscle hypertrophy;
- **metabolic stress**, generated by insufficient oxygen supply to the muscle tissue associated with anaerobic lactacid type efforts, in this case, prolonged and submaximal, which lead to the complete occlusion of the blood vessels at the muscle level.

But reverse stripping provides another essential advantage: it trains our resilience capacity in a superior way compared to classic stripping and to the rest-pause technique (where once a set of about 8-10 repetitions has been performed, the set is resumed after a rest of only 10-20 seconds).

Resilience (the ability of a material to absorb shock without breaking) is the body's ability to recover from a stressful stimulus of such significance as to activate an adaptive response to stress. Our body sets in motion a stereotyped response aimed at restoring homeostasis. **Resilience is the body's ability to restore homeostasis.**

A set of 70 seconds represents a relevant stress for the organism, and the muscular lactic acid, the accumulation of extracellular potassium in the nervous system, and the scarce reserves of phosphocreatine in the mitochondrion are warning signals. After all this metabolic chaos, reverse stripping not only forces us to immediately do two more sets without rest but also tells us that we must increase the weight, thus generating an awakening of those explosive IIa and IIx fibers. This also recruits the last indispensable phosphocreatine reserves that allow us to give everything we have in those last three repetitions with a decidedly important weight. Reverse stripping trains resilience to make it hormesis (hormesis: what doesn't kill you, makes you stronger), i.e. the body's ability to prepare itself to produce a greater quantity of a substance which, due to the training stimulus, is drastically reduced. In this case, we are talking about creatine and phosphocreatine, the energy currency of exchange of alactic anaerobic metabolism, the one referred to in the last stage of reverse stripping. Adapting our cells to a higher production of phosphocreatine, after the depletion of the same intracellular reserves, allows for hormesis which is expressed in the body's ability to recover from a set sooner, to increase the training density and to increase the weight that is lifted. In a nutshell, this means greater efficiency and greater performance.

This is a high-intensity workout, but it has the advantage that even if the last few repetitions of the set are not many, the load is actually still limited by the repetitions performed in the previous sets. Furthermore, the time dedicated to training is reduced, which is important for me today, on certain days, as even one exercise is sufficient for two sets for a small muscle group and two exercises for the large ones. At least, that's how it is for me, so there is "no excuse" to skip training when I'm late for work.

CHAPTER 23

Female bodybuilding

Valeria Galfano

Modern bodybuilding originated in the United States at the end of the Second World War (1946) and, since then, it has always been considered as not suitable for women.

For too long the weight room has been interpreted as an exclusively male place, designed to forge exaggeratedly hypertrophic muscles and the last stop before competing at Mr. Olympia. Similarly, we have witnessed women nailed to the treadmill or jumping from one stationary bike to the next, for hours on end, afraid of increasing their muscle mass and hoping to obtain some form of an aesthetic result. A result that would be hard to achieve in those conditions!

Gradually, we have learned to accept the change of this trend, and the notion according to which "women must train like men" has become popular, although being only partially true. Unfortunately, this concept, as often happens, has been exaggerated, so much so that today we see women training with very low sets and excessive loads regardless of their physical conformation, their goals and their personal aesthetic taste. Obviously, even under these conditions, the results will hardly reflect the desired ones.

Is there a type of bodybuilding for women?

Physiology

Mesenchymal cells (MSC) are the "jack of all trades" of our body: they are adult stem cells, multipotent, able to replicate and transform into more specialized cells. Mesenchymal stem cells have a regenerative role, they divide cyclically and replace aged or damaged cells. These cells differentiate and, depending on the stimuli they receive from the outside, they can give rise to chondrocytes of cartilage, osteoblasts of bone tissue, adipocytes of adipose tissue, myocytes of skeletal muscle and astrocytes of nervous tissue (Caplan, 1991).

Stem cells are essential for muscle growth; specifically, a particular type of stem cell, which is called a satellite cell.

Muscle tissue is largely composed of long post-mitotic multinucleated fibers. The lifelong maintenance of muscle tissue is mediated by satellite cells, which are found in close proximity to the muscle fibers. Under homeostatic conditions, all satellite cells remain quiescent, but they are always ready to be activated by stimuli such as physical trauma or growth signals. After their activation, satellite cells multiply and differentiate to give rise to progenitor cells, which fuse with each other to restore the integrity and function of the fibers and generate new muscle fibers. This phenomenon is called **hyperplasia** (Dumont et al., 2015). The traumatic event that interests us most is training.

The skeletal muscle (Fig. 23.1) is the most abundant tissue in our body and numerous studies, carried out both on test animals and on human muscle biopsies, have highlighted important differences between male and female muscle tissue, in terms of:

- energy metabolism
- fiber composition
- speed of contraction

Mammalian skeletal muscles are composed of a variety of highly specialized fibers, whose selective recruitment enables them to perform various functional tasks. Furthermore, skeletal muscle fibers can modify their structural and functional properties to perform new tasks or to respond to new conditions (Galfano et al., 2018).

Adaptive muscle fiber changes can occur in response to:

- variations in the neural stimulation pattern;
- load conditions
- availability of substrates
- hormonal signals

The proportion of type I and type II fibers varies from muscle to muscle and changes according to the type and duration of physical activity, age and gender. A person with a sedentary lifestyle has about 40% type I fibers. It has been shown that daily activity of medium intensity increases the proportion of type I fibers by more than 50%. Endurance training increases the percentage of type I fibers in the muscles used during training. On the other hand, resistance training increases the percentage of type II fibers.

In Figure 23.2, we see the histological section of the vastus lateralis muscle. In 2015, more than 3,000 genes that are differently expressed in male and female skeletal muscle were identified. Many human studies are conducted on biopsy fragments of the vastus lateralis muscle due to the relative simplicity of specimen collection. Analysis of biopsies taken from both men and women showed that female muscle contains 35% more type I fibers than male muscle.

In the study analysis (Staron et al., 2000), shown in Table 23.1, the male vastus lateralis was reported to contain 20% type IIx fibers, 46% type IIa fibers, and 34% type I fibers; female muscle contained 23% type IIx fibers, 36% type IIa fibers, and 41% type I fibers. Furthermore, all male fibers have a significantly larger cross-section than female fibers.

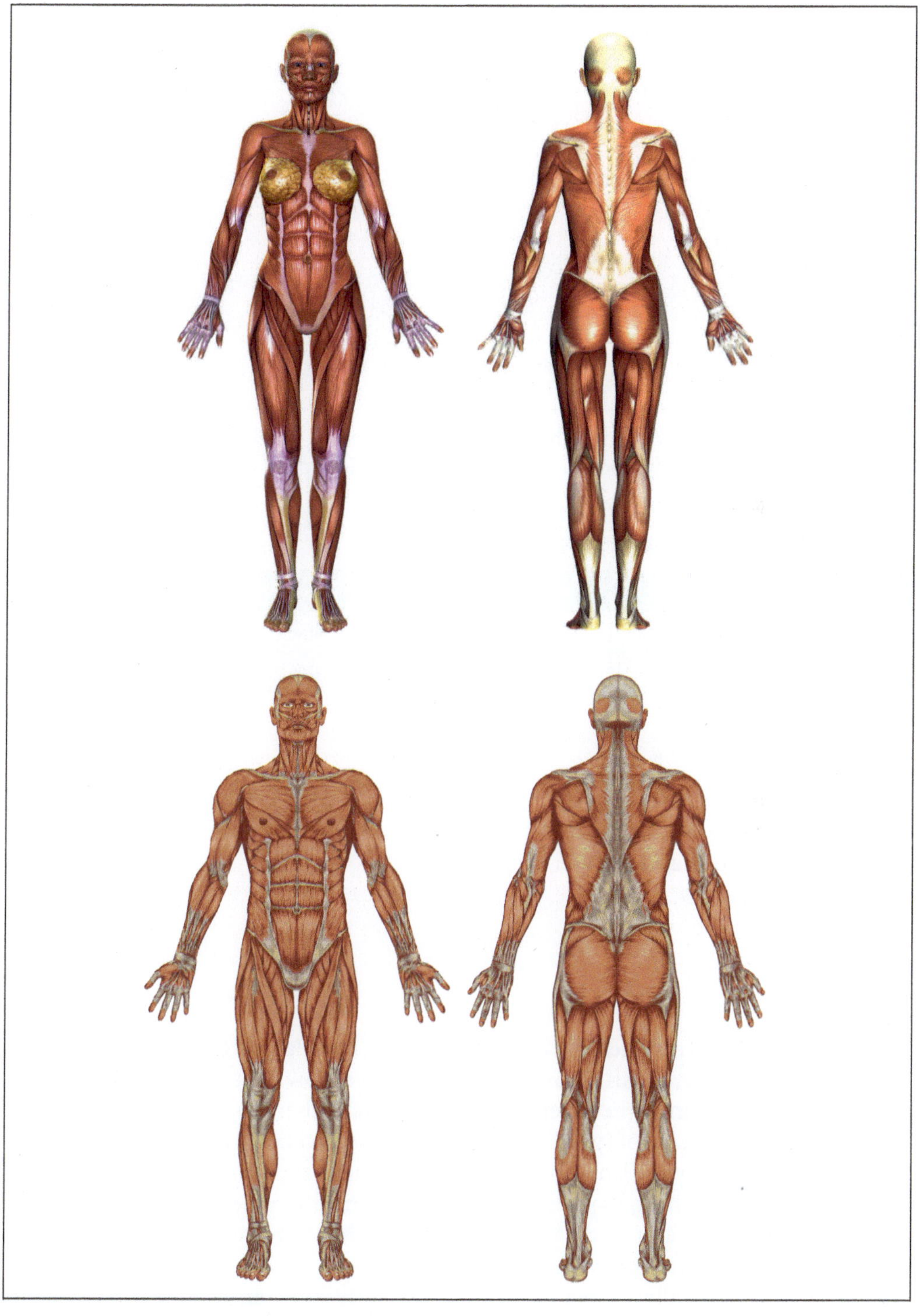

Figure 23.1 Skeletal muscles in the human body.

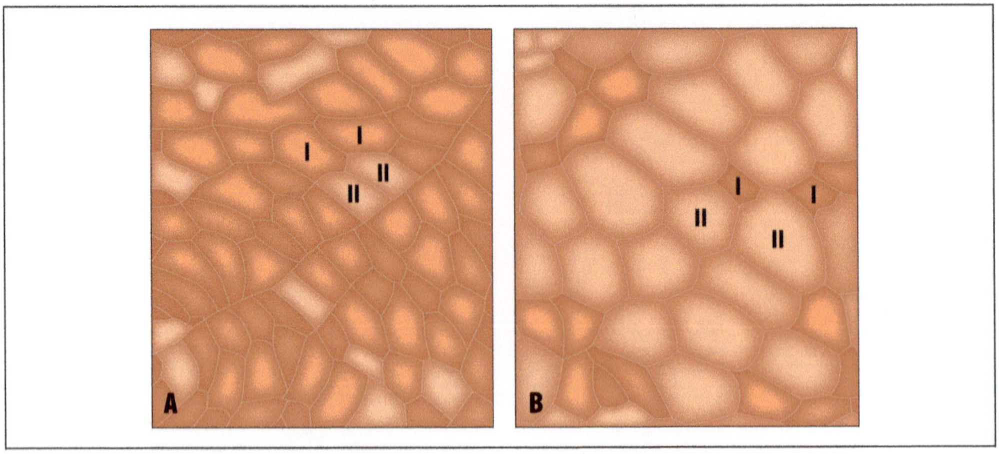

Figure 23.2 Histological section of the vastus lateralis muscle. (**A**) The muscle of a marathon runner; (**B**) The muscle of a bodybuilder. I: type I fibers; II: type II fibers.

Table 23.1 Types of fibers contained in the vastus lateralis muscle

	Type I	Type IIa	Type IIx
Men (> cross-section)	34%	46%	20%
Women (< cross-section)	41%	36%	23%

Hormones and muscle fibers

It seems increasingly evident that hormones influence the different expressions of muscle fibers in men and women. In particular:

- thyroid hormones
- estrogens
- testosterone
- insulin

Tri-iodothyronine (thyroid hormone T3) affects muscle protein expression. Individuals with hypothyroidism show symptoms such as low heart rate, fatigue, muscle weakness, weight gain and conversion of fast muscle fibers to slow ones; thus, they have a higher percentage of type I fibers and a lower percentage of type II fibers. Individuals with hyperthyroidism, on the other hand, have symptoms such as insomnia, fatigue, sensitivity to heat, hyperkinetic heart rhythm alterations and a conversion of slow muscle fibers to fast ones, thus showing a higher percentage of type II muscle fibers and a lower percentage of type I muscle fibers.

Estrogens, especially 17-beta estradiol, certainly have an influence on skeletal muscle tissue. This phenomenon is evidenced by the presence of two different types of estrogen receptors at the level of the muscle fiber (a receptor and b receptor). Their level of expression is independent of gender, but it was found that in trained men, especially in endurance training, their levels are 3 to 5 times higher than in sedentary subjects.

Numerous clinical situations can lead to hypoestrogenism; the most frequent causes can be linked to hypogonadism, hypopituitarism (i.e. reduced pituitary function), anorexia nervosa and menopause. The reduction in estrogen levels is correlated with an increased risk of injury, due to the greater bone fragility induced by osteoporosis, and a reduction in lean body mass.

Estrogens show a protective effect on muscle fibers. These hormones do not appear to have an influence on the conversion of muscle fibers from one type to another, but recent studies have shown that they influence the muscle fiber size, muscle regeneration, contractility and muscle strength; it has been observed that estrogens are able to increase the interaction between actin and myosin.

Testosterone is an androgen hormone associated with increased muscle mass and decreased body fat. Men produce about 50 times more testosterone than women and it is no coincidence that women have higher body fat percentages than males.

The increase in muscle mass appears to be mediated by the increase in the number of satellite cells and by the increase in protein synthesis.

With age, testosterone levels decline, and this deficiency is associated with premature deaths, primarily from cardiovascular diseases, decreased muscle mass and strength, and sexual dysfunction.

Testosterone affects the width of muscle fibers; it was found that male type I fibers are 19% wider, type II fibers are 59% wider, and intermediate type fibers are 66% wider than female fibers. The effects of testosterone deficiency are more noticeable in men than in women; this results in a drop in body mass, a decrease in the diameter of fast-twitch (type II) fibers, and a fast-to-slow fiber conversion.

Insulin is an anabolic hormone with lipogenic action, essential for the regulation of blood sugar levels. Some tissues are defined as insulin-dependent, including skeletal muscle, adipose tissue and cardiac muscle, and they are all united by the presence of GLUT4. This membrane transporter allows glucose to enter cells and is tightly regulated by insulin.

Insulin resistance is a pathological condition in which insulin-dependent cells do not respond adequately to normal circulating levels of insulin. Given the fact that insulin plays a key role in glucose entry into cells, any disturbance in signal transduction is associated with hyperglycemia. This phenomenon is associated with a higher risk of diabetes.

It has been demonstrated that female skeletal muscle is more predisposed to glucose uptake when stimulated by physiological insulin concentrations. Type I fibers, having higher aerobic capacity, have a greater distribution of GLUT4, which makes them more sensitive to insulin than type II fibers. This difference appears to be due to the prevalence of type I muscle fibers in women and contributes to the reduced risk of developing insulin resistance and diabetes compared to men.

Gender-related adipose tissue

Gender-related differences in adipose tissue accumulation are well recognized, with men storing more adipose tissue in the abdominal region and women in the so-called gynoid region (hips and thighs) (Fig. 23.3). Fat is also stored in other tissues, including the liver and skeletal muscle. It has been shown that women accumulate fat mainly within the skeletal muscle and men in the liver, therefore the latter are more predisposed to fatty liver disease.

Fat is stored in the skeletal muscle within lipid droplets, called intramyocellular lipids, which represent an important source of energy for muscles, analogous to muscle glycogen (Beaudry et al., 2019).

Intramyocellular lipid content increases with endurance training and it is higher in athletes than in individuals with a sedentary lifestyle. In obese subjects, the intramyocellular lipid content is higher and it is associated with insulin resistance; on the contrary, athletes show high insulin sensitivity. This phenomenon is called the "athlete's paradox".

Recent evidence suggests that it is not the intramyocellular lipid content per se that correlates with insulin resistance, but rather the location of the droplets within the myocyte. Specifically, insulin-resistant subjects tend to accumulate lipids in type II fibers, while athletes accumulate them in type I fibers, which are mostly represented in female muscle tissue. Furthermore, type I fibers are richer in mitochondria, therefore more likely to use these lipids as an energy substrate through aerobic metabolism. Intramyocellular lipids stored in type II fibers are disposed of with greater difficulty and can obstruct the translocation of GLUT4 towards the plasma membrane; this increases the risk of insulin resistance (Beaudry et al., 2019).

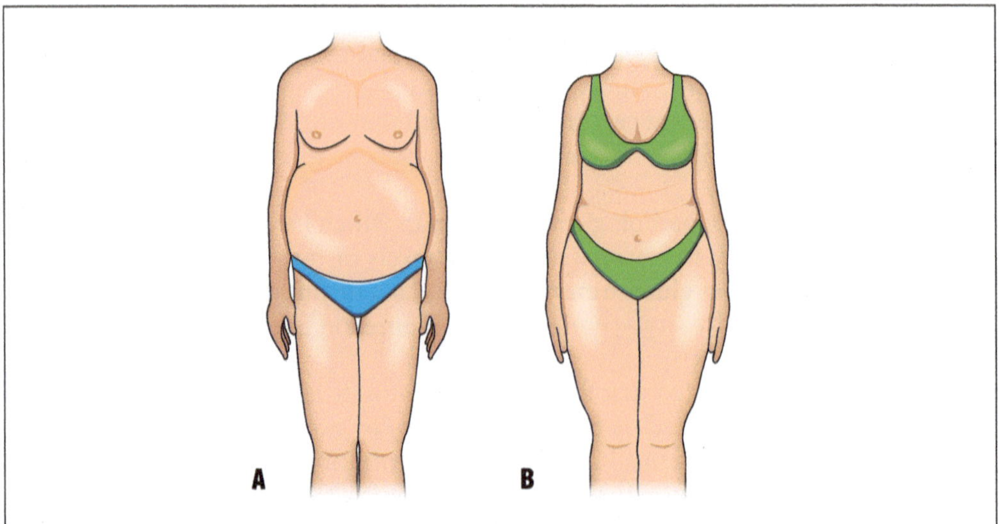

Figure 23.3 The distribution of android (**A**) and gynoid (**B**) fat types.

Women's training

Female muscles fatigue more slowly than male muscles; moreover, women have higher resistance and faster muscle recovery. Men, on the other hand, have faster strength generation and muscle relaxation.

These differences in muscle performance between men and women may be due to the greater number of type I fibers in the latter, which are characterized by aerobic oxidative metabolism and, therefore, by higher resistance. In practical terms, this means that women respond better to exercises with a higher number of repetitions and, in general, to a higher workload, therefore to a greater number of exercises in each training session.

As regards the signs of "cellulite", physical activity plays a preventive role or it can be effective if implemented in the early stages. Physical activity aimed at improving the signs of cellulite must have blood flow stimulation as a prerequisite, and it should avoid an excessive production of lactic acid. You have to pay attention to activities that contrast the physiological venous outflow, such as spinning. On the other hand, anti-gravity sports, such as those performed in the water, are very effective.

As previously mentioned, training represents an inflammatory stimulus that could worsen the blemishes of cellulite, but this does not mean that women cannot train in the weight room. There are different types of training based on women's different body types. Furthermore, it could be very useful to implement some precautions.

For example, at the end of any workout, it is useful to promote venous outflow through the exercise illustrated in Figure 23.4: lie on the floor with your back flat and your legs raised, forming an angle of about 90°, and place your feet on the wall;

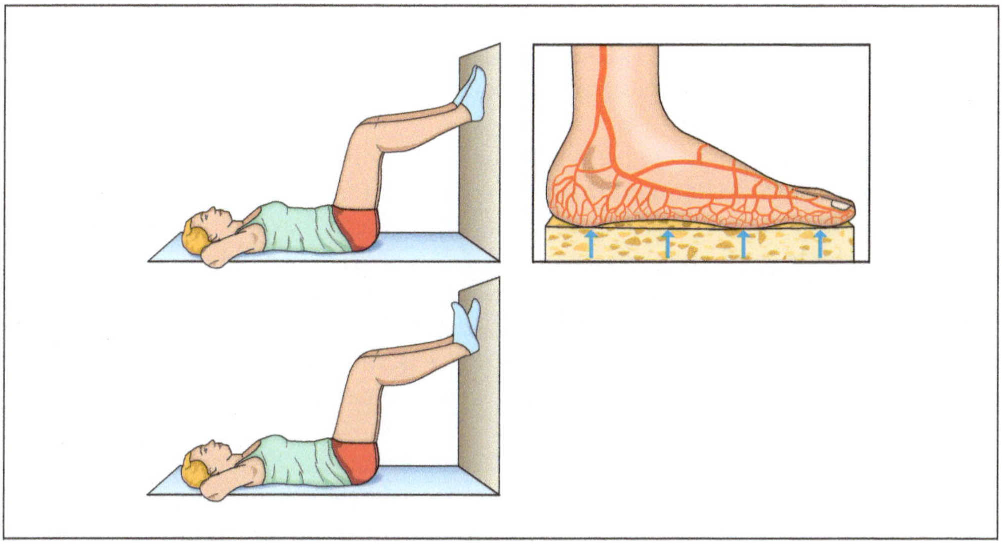

Figure 23.4 An exercise to promote venous outflow (see text).

perform light pushes with your feet, in order to stimulate the plantar venous pump and promote venous return.

As far as aerobic activity is concerned, women respond better to activities of a continuous, regular and intermediate nature, compared to high-intensity and interval training. The differences between male and female fibers also suggest that women, having a higher concentration of red fibers, tend to use lipids as the main energy substrate during a training session, unlike men who mainly use glycogen.

Continuous training is more effective in oxidizing subcutaneous fat, which is precisely where women mostly store fat.

A growing number of studies show that female adipose tissue is more sensitive to lipolytic stimuli than male adipose tissue, when subjected to metabolic stress, such as fasting and physical exercises.

Female bodybuilding categories

In the context of female bodybuilding, women can compete in different categories, which present increasing muscle volume and a gradually decreasing percentage of fat mass:

1. Bikini
2. Figure
3. Fitness
4. Physique
5. Bodybuilding

The **Bikini category** is judged on a number of aesthetic criteria, including a lean and proportionate physique, symmetry, posture and the absence of blemishes. A Bikini woman has a slim waist and firm buttocks. The athletes are divided into height categories and, during the contest, they perform a frontal pose and a back pose. The percentage of fat mass generally possessed by women who compete in the Bikini category is between 10 and 14%.

The **Figure category** is judged on the basis of symmetry, posture and some aesthetic characteristics, including skin tone. In this case, too, the athletes are divided into groups according to their height and, during the contest, they line up and perform a series of quarter turns to the right (front, left side, rear, right side). In this category, the deltoids, the back, the quadriceps and the glutes are of crucial importance in giving the typical "X" shape. A Figure woman has well-developed shoulder and back muscles, a small waist and prominent buttocks and quadriceps. Muscle definition must be appreciable, but obvious muscle lines are not allowed. The percentage of fat mass generally possessed by the Figure woman is between 8 and 12%.

The **Fitness category** can be considered an intermediate category between bodybuilding, dance, gymnastics and martial arts. The competition develops in two steps: the first evaluation is carried out on the basis of the physical condition, similar to the Figures category; next, the athletes present an exercise routine with a backing track that showcases their athletic prowess. The percentage of fat mass generally possessed by the Fitness woman is between 9 and 11%.

The **Physique category** is judged on the basis of athletic fitness that exhibits symmetry, tone, balance and posing ability. The separation of the muscles is well accentuated and lines may be visible, but not excessive. The athletes, always divided into height categories, present a choreographed routine with a musical base and perform some mandatory poses, such as front double biceps, lateral triceps with front leg extended, lateral chest with extended arms, and extended front leg. The percentage of fat mass generally possessed by the Physique woman is between 8 and 10%.

The **Bodybuilding category** is similar to the Physique one; however, female athletes show more muscle volume, more definition and more noticeable lines. For this category, symmetry is a key feature and the athletes are divided into weight classes. The percentage of fat mass possessed by the Bodybuilding woman can sometimes even reach 5%.

Bikini training: my experience on stage

There are different conformations of the female physique, so training must be adapted to the person and never vice versa. Let's begin with the description of a training program for a woman who aims to get on stage and who is probably already in good shape and has a sufficient level of training. If this were not the case, a woman who would like to compete, but is very far from an ideal physical condition, should understand that it is a long journey and that she has to take things step by step and have the patience and perseverance required to bring her results to the stage.

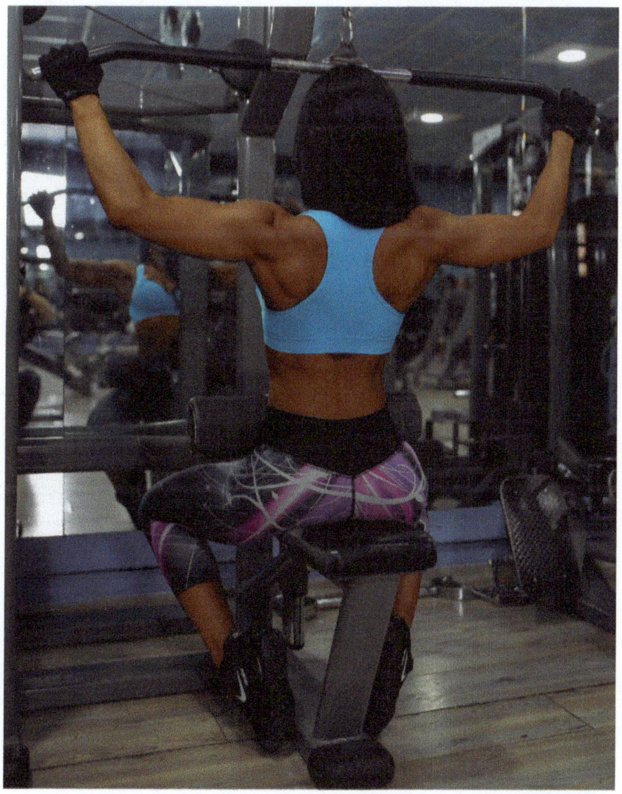

Specifically, I'd like to describe the training path that I followed when preparing for my first competition in 2015.

The macro-cycle defines the amount of time between the start of the preparation and the long-term goal, in this case the competition. The micro-cycle, on the other hand, represents the number of days needed to complete total muscle stimulation.

In my specific case, I completed 4-5 weekly training sessions. The training schedules shown on the following pages have two characteristics in common:

- the high volume of training
- the goal is muscle hypertrophy

Training volume (V = kg × repetitions × sets) represents the amount of work performed in a training unit and is a parameter linked to the duration of the session. In my case, the high training volume is a function that doesn't depend much on heavy loads, but rather on the high number of sets and repetitions for each training session.

Hypertrophy is muscle adaptation that occurs in response to overload. Mechanical load-induced growth may be mediated by an increase in the muscle's length and cross-sectional area. Although skeletal muscle is capable of undergoing longitudinal growth, most studies of mechanical loading models do not lead to significant alterations of the entire muscle length.

The increase in muscle size (Jorgenson et al., 2020) reflects a synthesis process that involves all subcellular structures:

1. Increase in the size of **myofibrils**: this appears to be the result of the increase in actin and myosin filaments.
2. Increased **capillary** count: bodybuilders have twice the number of capillaries per muscle fiber compared to sedentary subjects because training leads to the depletion of energy substrates and to a greater pooling of metabolites, resulting in a higher demand for blood circulation.
3. In addition to providing training with high repetitions and reduced speed of execution, bodybuilding favors the increase in muscle volume and in the number of **mitochondria**.
4. Training also leads to the proliferation of connective tissue cells, thus resulting in a thickening of the **tendons** and **ligaments**.

Myofibrillar hypertrophy occurs via two mechanisms:

1. The activation of satellite cells by growth factors and traumatic stimuli; the cells divide and regenerate the muscle fiber after a workout.
2. The longitudinal segmentation process of muscle fibers, whereby two or more daughter cells derived from a mother cell.

Hyperplasia, or the increase in the number of muscle fibers which has been confirmed in animals, is a subject of controversy in humans and, according to some authors, it is limited to the prenatal and postnatal period; therefore, growth occurs through hypertrophy of existing muscle fibers, either by adding more myofibrils to increase muscle mass or by adding new sarcomeres to the extremities to increase their length (Jorgenson et al., 2020).

Training schedule 1			
Exercises	**Sets**	**Repetitions**	**Recovery**
• SESSION 1			
Legs and glutes			
Barbell squat	4	15	60 seconds
Reverse hack squat	4	15	60 seconds
Leg extension	3	12	45 seconds
Abductor machine	4	25	30 seconds
Leg curl	3	12	45 seconds
Adductor machine	4	25	30 seconds
Rear leg swings at the low cable	3	20	30 seconds
Calves			
Seated calf raises	4	20	45 seconds
• SESSION 2			
Deltoids			
Push up with dumbbells	4	12	45 seconds
Lateral raises with dumbbells	4	12	45 seconds
Hammer front raises with dumbells	3	15	45 seconds
High cable flyes for the rear deltoids	3	15	45 seconds
Triceps			
French press with barbell on a flat bench	3	12	45 seconds
Rope push down	3	12	45 seconds
Kickback with dumbbells	3	15	45 seconds
Abs			
Traditional crunches	3	20	30 seconds

Continues

Continued

• SESSION 3

Back

Lat machine with a wide grip	4	12	45 seconds
Low pulley machine with the triangle	4	12	45 seconds
Vertical rows	3	15	45 seconds
Rowing with dumbbells	3	15	45 seconds

Biceps

Barbell curl	3	12	45 seconds
Hammer curl with the low cable rope	3	12	45 seconds
Concentration bicep curls	3	15	45 seconds

Abs

Reverse crunches	3	15	30 seconds

• SESSION 4

Legs and glutes

Sumo squat with kettlebells	4	15	60 seconds
Dumbbell reverse lunges	3	12	45 seconds
45° press	3	15	60 seconds
Abductor machine	4	25	30 seconds
Half deadlifts with a barbell	4	12	60 seconds
Leg curl	3	12	45 seconds
Adductor machine	4	25	30 seconds

Abs

Traditional crunches	3	20	30 seconds

A noticeable feature of the first training schedule is the high training volume (many sets and many repetitions). The reason is related to the fact that women respond better to a high workload and get tired more slowly than men; moreover, due to the different composition of muscle fibers, we notice very short recovery times. Finally, in this way, a woman obtains a rapid depletion of phosphates, an acidic metabolic environment, and a rapid depletion of muscle glycogen stores. All these conditions favor muscle hypertrophy.

Table 23.2 Macrocycle training phases

Load	Movements	Stimulus
80-85% of the maximum	Fast and explosive	White fibers
70-80% of the maximum	Slow	Red fibers
60% of the maximum	Continuous and slow	Mitochondria, capillaries

During the macro-cycle, it is good to alternate phases in which you train with loads of 80-85% of the maximum with fast and explosive movements, to mainly stimulate the white fibers; loads of 70-80% of the maximum, performed slowly, are used to mainly stimulate the red fibers; loads of 60% of the maximum with continuous and slow movements are used to increase the number and size of the mitochondria and the number of capillaries that surround the muscle fiber (Tab. 23.2).

Training schedule 2			
Exercises	**Sets**	**Repetitions**	**Rest**
• SESSION 1			
Legs and glutes			
Barbell squat	1	15-12-10-8	90 seconds
Bulgarian lunge with dumbbells	3	10	60 seconds
Leg extensions	1	15-12-10-8	90 seconds
Abductor machine	4	25	30 seconds
Multipower glute bridge	1	15-12-10-8	90 seconds
Adductor machine	4	25	30 seconds
Good morning with a barbell	3	10	60 seconds
Calves			
Calf press	3	15	60 seconds

Continues

Continued

• SESSION 2

Deltoids			
Overhead press with the multipower	1	15-12-10-8	90 seconds
Triceps			
French press with dumbbells on a flat bench	1	12-10-8-6	90 seconds
Push down with a rigid shaft	3	10	60 seconds
French press with high cable rope	3	10	60 seconds
Abs			
Crunches with weights	1	20-15-12-10	30 seconds

• SESSION 3

Back			
Lat machine forward with wide grip	1	15-12-10-8	90 seconds
Rowing with a barbell	3	10	60 seconds
Narrow grip reverse lat machine	1	15-12-10-8	90 seconds
Standing pulldown with rigid shaft	3	10	60 seconds
Biceps			
Standing alternating dumbbells	1	12-10-8-6	90 seconds
Dumbbell Hammer Curl	3	10	60 seconds
Scott bench with a curved barbell	3	10	60 seconds
Abs			
Crunches with weights	1	20-15-12-10	30 seconds

Continues

Continued

• SESSION 4			
Legs and glutes			
Sumo squat with kettlebells	1	15-12-10-8	90 seconds
Walking lunges with dumbbells	3	10	60 seconds
Multipower press with back to the floor	1	15-12-10-8	90 seconds
Abductor machine	4	25	30 seconds
Half deadlifts with barbell	1	15-12-10-8	90 seconds
Leg curl	4	10	60 seconds
Adductor machine	4	25	30 seconds
Abs			
Reverse crunches	3	15	30 seconds

In this sheet, we'll describe the pyramid technique, which involves performing a certain number of sets with an ever-increasing load and a progressively decreasing number of repetitions. This technique is important in order to be able to increase the load.

Training schedule 3

Exercises	Sets	Repetitions	Rest
• SESSION 1			
Legs and glutes			
Barbell squat + leg curl	4	10+15	90 seconds
Forward lunges with dumbbells	3	10	60 seconds
Leg extension + half deadlifts with barbell	4	10+15	90 seconds
Abductor machine	4	25	30 seconds
Adductor machine	4	25	30 seconds
Hyperextension bench with plate	4	10	60 seconds
Calves			
Calf press + seated calf	3	10+10	60 seconds

Continues

Continued

• SESSION 2

Deltoids

Shoulder press + lateral raises	4	10+15	90 seconds
Front raises with dumbbells + lateral raises	4	10+15	90 seconds
Pull to the forehead with rope on the high cable setting	4	10	60 seconds

Triceps

French press with barbell + kickback with dumbbells	4	10+15	90 seconds
Push down with rope + kick back with elastic bands	3	10+15	90 seconds

Abs

Traditional crunch + reverse crunch	4	15+10	60 seconds

• SESSION 3

Back

Wide grip forward lat machine + pulley machine	4	10+15	90 seconds
Close grip reverse lat machine + standing pulldown	4	10+15	90 seconds
Single dumbbell row	3	10	60 seconds

Biceps

Barbell curl + low cable rope biceps	4	10+15	90 seconds
Alternating dumbbells + double biceps to high cables	3	10+15	90 seconds

Abs

Traditional crunch + reverse crunch	4	15+10	60 seconds

Continues

Continued

• SESSION 4

Legs and glutes

Sumo squat with kettlebell + glute bridge	4	10+15	90 seconds
45° press + leg curl	4	10+15	90 seconds
Good morning with barbell	3	15	60 seconds
Half deadlifts with barbell	4	15	60 seconds
Abductor machine + adductor machine	4	25+25	60 seconds
Abs			
Crunch on the parallel bars	3	15	30 seconds

Here the workload is even higher and we start to see supersets. It involves performing a set consisting of two exercises performed one after the other. Supersets are performed to maintain high training intensity in a short amount of time. Practically, the training lasts less but is more intense.

Training schedule 4

Exercises	Sets	Repetitions	Rest
• SESSION 1			
Legs and glutes			
Barbell squat	4	8+8	90 seconds
Barbell Jefferson (hack) lunges	3	10	60 seconds
Leg extensions	4	8+8	90 seconds
Abductor machine	4	25	30 seconds
Half deadlifts with dumbbells	4	8+8	90 seconds
Adductor machine	4	25	30 seconds
Gluteus machine	3	10	60 seconds
Calves			
Calf press	3	8+8	60 seconds

Continues

Continued

• SESSION 2

Deltoids

Arnold press	4	8+8	90 seconds
Barbell front raises	3	10	60 seconds
Barbell upright row	4	8+8	90 seconds
Lateral dumbbell flag raises	3	10	60 seconds

Triceps

French press with barbell on the bench at 30°	4	8+8	90 seconds
Push down with a rigid shaft	4	8+8	90 seconds

Abs

Side crunches	3	10	30 seconds

• SESSION 3

Back

Wide-grip forward lat machine	4	8+8	90 seconds
Row with reverse grip barbell	3	10	60 seconds
Narrow grip reverse lat machine	4	8+8	90 seconds
High pulley machine	3	10	60 seconds

Biceps

Biceps together with dumbbell Hammer Curl	4	8+8	90 seconds
Alternating dumbbells on a 45° bench	4	8+8	90 seconds

Abs

Traditional crunches	3	10	30 seconds

Continues

Continued

• SESSION 4

Legs and glutes

Side crunches	3	10	30 seconds
Sumo squat with kettlebells	4	8+8	90 seconds
45° press	3	10	60 seconds
Side lunges with dumbbells	3	10	60 seconds
Multipower glute bridge	4	8+8	90 seconds
Abductor machine	4	25	30 seconds
Half deadlifts with barbells	4	8+8	90 seconds
Adductor machine	4	25	30 seconds

Abs

Traditional crunches	3	15	30 seconds

In this sheet, we see another training technique: stripping. It involves performing the same exercise two or three times, without recovery between the sets, with a decreasing amount of weight (the load must be reduced by about 20%). Stripping is my favorite training technique to promote muscle hypertrophy because it is very complete and involves global stimulation. The first set of reps, performed with a heavy load and speed, will predominantly recruit type II fibers. The second group of repetitions, with a lighter load and speed, will predominantly recruit type I fibers. Finally, the third group, performed with an even lighter load, will stimulate the increase of capillaries and mitochondria.

This technique can often be useful; the aim is to pay particular attention to muscle groups that are deficient compared to the rest. It provides very low-intensity stimulation on days that are not dedicated to the main training of specific muscle groups. The goal is to direct blood flow to the area in question, thus promoting muscle growth. This technique is effective if used for short periods of time (6-8 weeks) and for a few muscle groups at a time. Exceeding these parameters would increase the risk of overtraining.

Training schedule 5			
Exercises	**Sets**	**Repetitions**	**Rest**
• SESSION 1			
Legs and glutes			
Squat with barbell + leg curl + abductor machine	4	10+15+20	120 seconds
Dumbbell reverse lunges	3	10	60 seconds
Leg extension + deadlifts + adductor machine	4	10+15+20	120 seconds
Multipower glute bridge	4	20	60 seconds
Calves			
Calf at multipower	4	15	60 seconds
• SESSION 2			
Deltoids			
Lateral raises + front raises + overhead press	4	10+15+10	120 seconds
Pull to the forehead with rope on the high cable	3	10	60 seconds
Upright row + lateral raises + upper back	4	10+15+10	120 seconds
Triceps			
French press with barbell	4	10	60 seconds
Push down with a rigid shaft	4	10	60 seconds
Kickback with elastic	3	15	60 seconds
Abs			
Crunch machine + traditional crunches + reverse crunches	3	10+15+10	60 seconds

Continues

Continued

• SESSION 3

Back

Forward lat machine + vertical row + pulley machine	4	10+15+10	120 seconds
Pullover with Dumbbell on a flat bench	3	10	60 seconds
Reverse lat machine + pulldown + rowing machine	4	10+15+10	120 seconds

Biceps

Scott bench with dumbbell	4	10	60 seconds
Standing alternating dumbbells	4	10	60 seconds
Biceps with low cable rope	3	15	60 seconds

Abs

Crunch machine + traditional crunches + reverse crunches	3	10+15+10	60 seconds

• SESSION 4

Legs and glutes

Sumo squat + deadlifts + glute bridge	4	10+10+15	120 seconds
Horizontal press + leg curl + abductor machine	4	10+15+20	120 seconds
Half deadlifts with barbell	4	15	60 seconds
Hyperextension bench with plate	4	15	60 seconds

Abs

Crunch on the parallel bars	3	15	30 seconds

Here we see the triset, very similar to the simple superset, made up of three different exercises that are performed in sequence, of which the first and third are generally isolation exercises, while the second is a basic exercise.

Training schedule 6			
Exercises	**Sets**	**Repetitions**	**Rest**
• SESSION 1			
Legs and glutes			
Multipower squat	4	10+5 seconds isometry	90 seconds
Reverse hack squat	4	10+5 seconds isometry	90 seconds
Leg extensions	3	10	60 seconds
Abductor machine	4	25	30 seconds
Standing leg curl	3	10+3 seconds isometry	60 seconds
Adductor machine	4	25	30 seconds
Rear leg swings at the low cable	3	20	30 seconds
Calves			
Seated calf raises	4	10+3 seconds isometry	60 seconds
• SESSION 2			
Deltoids			
Military press with barbell	4	10	90 seconds
Lateral raises with dumbbells	4	10+3 seconds isometry	90 seconds
Front raises with dumbbells	3	10+3 seconds isometry	60 seconds
High cable flyes for rear deltoids	3	15	45 seconds

Continues

Continued

Triceps			
French press with barbell on a flat bench	3	10	60 seconds
Rope push downs	3	10+3 seconds isometry	60 seconds
Kickback with elastic bands	3	15	45 seconds

Abs			
Traditional crunches	3	15+3 seconds isometry	30 seconds

• SESSION 3

Back			
Rowing with barbell	4	10	60 seconds
Pulley machine with triangle	4	10+5 seconds isometry	60 seconds
Vertical rows	3	10+3 seconds isometry	60 seconds
Pulldown with rope	3	15	45 seconds

Biceps			
Barbell curl	3	10+3 seconds isometry	60 seconds
Alternating dumbbells on a 45° bench	3	10	60 seconds
Hammer curl with low cable rope	3	15	45 seconds

Abs			
Reverse crunches	3	15+3 seconds isometry	30 seconds

Continues

Continued

• SESSION 4

Legs and glutes

Sumo squat with kettlebells	4	15+5 seconds isometry	90 seconds
45° press	4	10	60 seconds
Abductor machine	4	25	30 seconds
Multipower glute bridge	4	15+5 seconds isometry	90 seconds
Barbell half deadlifts	3	15	60 seconds
Adductor machine	4	25	30 seconds

Abs

Traditional crunches	3	15+3 seconds isometry	30 seconds

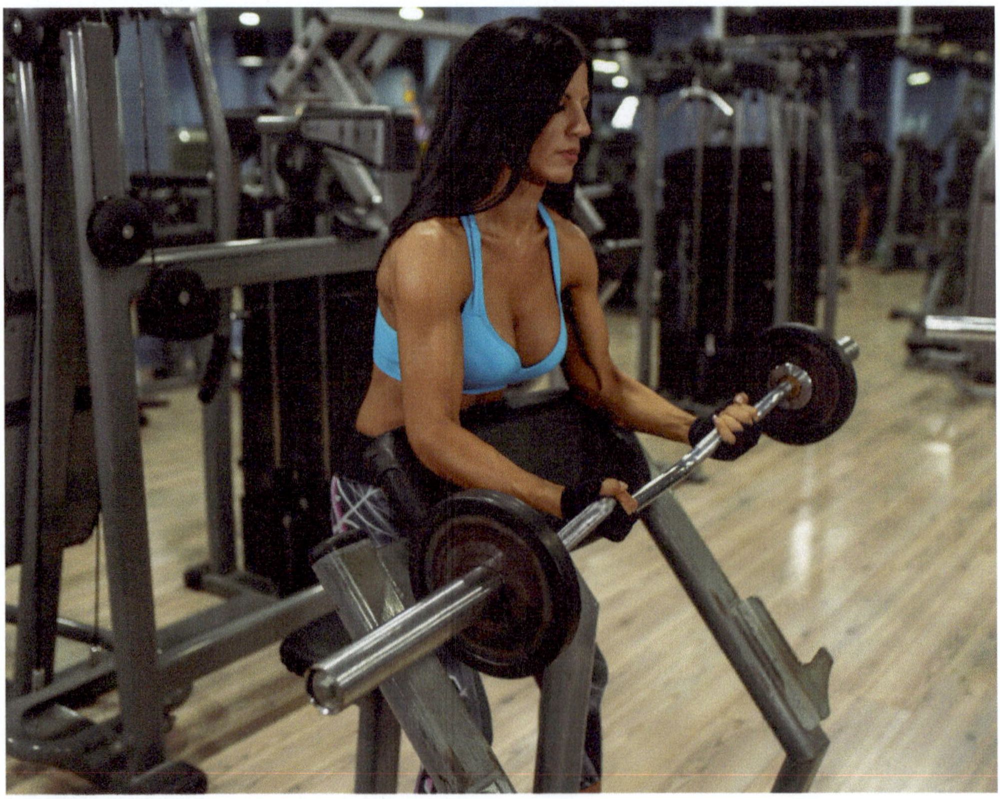

Here we see **isometric training**. This concept entails carrying out a very high volume of training and focusing on the points that, from time to time, are most lacking.

Isometric training is based on static contraction and consists of staying in the muscle contraction position for the time indicated by the exercise. This technique is particularly effective for developing strength, according to some studies, even more than dynamic contractions. This is possible thanks to a progressive recruitment of deeper fibers, as the more superficial ones get tired. In isometrics, the strength of the contraction must always be taken into account. The force developed must be 30% higher than one's maximum (between 40 and 50%). The duration of the contraction can vary from 15 seconds to 2 minutes, depending on the athlete's strength and training level. Recovery ranges from 30 seconds to 3 minutes.

Since isometric exercises cause an increase in blood pressure, it is inadvisable for heart patients and the elderly. Obviously, this is a transient increase in blood pressure, linked to the act of exercise itself, because with constant training there would be a decrease in blood pressure compared to sedentary subjects.

Finally, in the weeks leading up to the competition, we return to light workouts because energy is low and the caloric intake is insufficient to support an overly intense workout. In this phase, a total-body routine is repeated, with very light loads, and cardio is stopped to limit water retention in the lower areas of the body, also because at this point, you should have already reached the ideal fat mass percentage for the competition.

PHA training

Most women have a gynoid-type physical conformation and do not want to reach competitive levels; rather, they just want to find a good balance between health and aesthetic results. What kind of training should these women do?

The optimal training for these women is called PHA, which stands for Peripheral Heart Action. It is particularly suitable for women with circulatory problems or cellulite in the lower limbs. It promotes rapid blood flow to the upper regions of the body, preventing the stagnation of lactic acid and catabolites in the lower regions. Some authors suggest that this training method is particularly interesting for women who have a gynoid phenotype, who tend to accumulate fat in the lower regions of the body, especially in the buttocks and outer thighs, in which the classic anaerobic overload training could aggravate the state of water retention to which they are particularly predisposed (Piras et al., 2015).

PHA is a form of weight training implemented in a circuit training model, with the peculiar characteristic of consecutively stimulating distant muscle groups. In this way, an alternation between exercises for the lower regions and exercises for the upper regions will be created. It is a total-body workout, as all muscle groups are recruited in a single session. It can be modified according to the characteristics of the individual, so it might be more appropriate to focus on some deficient areas and leave out other muscle groups.

A classic PHA workout involves alternating 5-6 different exercises, repeated for 5-6 cycles; each exercise should be performed in 8-20 repetitions; moreover, at each cycle, it is important to try to increase the load. No sets should be brought to muscle failure, but the last cycle should be particularly tiring. A typical workout lasts on average between 30 and 45 minutes, depending on the level of training and the recovery times set between the various cycles (Piras et al., 2015).

PHA combines the circulatory principles of fitness with the muscle hypertrophy of resistance training. The goal is to promote blood flow throughout the body and to avoid localized stagnation of lactic acid and catabolites. These protocols allow you to work at a high heart rate.

PHA determines a lower energy expenditure compared to classic aerobic training; however, it promotes protein synthesis and an increase in muscle mass. This results in an increase in basal metabolic rate and greater efficiency in fat oxidation. Among the benefits of PHA, we can also mention a higher efficiency of the nervous system, which positively affects strength during the execution of the exercises. This benefit can be attributed to the fact that during the breaks while training a certain muscle, an alternative exercise is inserted, which stimulates a different muscle, and this favors a greater expression of strength and a faster recovery of the main muscle.

There is a variant of classic PHA, called **cardio-PHA**, which provides for the insertion of aerobic stations within the circuit. In practical terms, we can say that typical PHA training, or supersets and trisets, is interspersed with short phases of active recovery (about 5 minutes) on aerobic machines, including the stationary bike, the elliptical and the treadmill. The aim is to further improve the aerobic cardiovascular capacity and accentuate the reduction of fat mass.

PHA training was compared to HIIT training on a cycle ergometer. They recruited eighteen men and women, aged 21-27, who were randomly distributed into two groups. After 30 training sessions over the course of 12 weeks, the PHA protocol promoted favorable cardiovascular adaptations, such as the reduction of sympathetic vascular activity and the increase of vagal modulation, resulting in better blood pressure control. Furthermore, PHA training was more conducive to the increase in muscle strength and maximal oxygen consumption compared to the HIIT protocol.

The following table shows an example of training with the PHA technique.

An example of PHA training			
Exercises	**Sets**	**Repetitions**	**Rest**
• SESSION 1			
Kettlebell sumo squat (glutes) + dumbbells lateral raises (shoulders) + standing alternating dumbbells (biceps)	3	10+8+8	120 seconds
Multipower glute bridge (glutes) + dumbbells push-ups (shoulders) + Dumbbell Hammer Curl (biceps)	3	15+8+8	120 seconds
Half deadlifts with barbells (hamstrings) + front raises with plate (shoulders) + traditional crunches (abs)	3	10+10+15	120 seconds
• SESSION 2			
Leg curl (hamstrings) + wide grip forward lat machine (back) + push down with rope (triceps)	3	10+10+15	120 seconds
Lunges forward with dumbbells (legs) + pulley machine with the triangle (back) + French press with barbell on flat bench (triceps)	3	10+15+8	120 seconds
Abductor machine (legs) + narrow-grip reverse lat machine (back) + crunch machine (abs)	3	20+8+20	120 seconds
• SESSION 3			
Barbell squat (legs) + dumbbell front raises (shoulders) + concentration curls (biceps)	3	10+8+8	120 seconds
45° press (glutes) + dumbbells raises at 90° (shoulders) + double biceps at high cables (biceps)	3	15+8+8	120 seconds
Hyperextension bench (hamstrings) + adductor machine (legs) + reverse crunch (abs)	3	15+20+15	120 seconds

Continues

Continued

• SESSION 4

Gluteus machine (glutes) + wide-grip forward lat machine (back) + push forward at the high cable (triceps)	3	15+10+8	120 seconds
Leg extension (legs) + pulldown (back) + standing pulldown with rope (triceps)	3	10+15+8	120 seconds
Low cable rear leg kicks (hamstrings) + seated calf (calves) + side crunch (abs)	3	15+15+10	120 seconds

CHAPTER 24

Bodybuilding for the no longer young

Massimo Spattini

The impact that aging has on the human body extends to a cellular level. The damage accumulated by cells in older muscles is particularly serious because they don't regenerate as easily and, therefore, become weaker, while the mitochondria, which generate energy, decrease in power and number. Weight training can counteract age-related loss of muscle mass by acting directly on type II muscle fibers. Furthermore, the neuromotor stimulus of power training slows down neuronal degeneration related to aging. Weight training promotes the autophagic processes that allow cells to regenerate continuously, helping to maintain the structural integrity of muscle fibers. This type of workout acts on the IGF-1/Akt/mTOR system, a growth factor that stimulates the activation and proliferation of satellite cells and inhibits protein catabolism. Akt and mTOR are two proteins that activate a pathway that stimulates protein synthesis. Israeli scientists (*Journal Sports Science Medicine*, 2007) found that growth factors respond differently in fit older men who undergo intense training than in those who are not in shape. IGF-1 levels increased after a sprint test (Wingate test), contrary to what was observed in unfit older men. **This highlights the importance of training throughout your life.**

Weight training also reduces apoptosis (programmed cell death), which is a key process in aging and loss of muscle mass. Apoptosis is mediated by mitochondria which, with age, become more vulnerable to the aggressiveness of free radicals. A study recently published in *Cell Metabolism*, however, suggests that some types of training can undo certain effects that advanced age causes in our mitochondria. Exercise is good for us, as everyone knows. But scientists have surprisingly little understanding of its cellular impacts and how these might vary based on the activity level and age of a person who does physical exercise. Thus, researchers at the Mayo Clinic in Rochester (Minnesota) have recently conducted an experiment on the cells of 72 healthy but sedentary men and women between 30 and 64 years of age. After establishing baseline measures of their aerobic fitness, blood glucose levels, gene activity, and the mitochondrial health of muscle cells, the volunteers were randomly assigned to a specific exercise regimen.

Some of them trained intensely with weights several times a week; others did short interval training three times a week on stationary bikes (pedaling hard for 4 minutes, resting for 3 minutes, and then repeating this sequence three more times); others cycled at moderate speed for 30 minutes a couple of times a week and lifted light weights on the other days. The control group did not exercise at all. After 12 weeks, the same laboratory tests were carried out. Overall, all exercise groups experienced improvements in their fitness level and improved their ability to regulate blood sugar levels. There were also some unsurprising differences: gains in muscle mass and strength were greater for those who exercised only with weights, while interval training had a stronger effect on endurance. The most unexpected results were found in the muscle cells biopsy. Among the younger subjects who underwent interval training, activity levels changed in 274 genes, compared to 170 genes in those who trained more moderately and 74 genes in those who lifted weights. Among the older subjects, nearly 400 genes began working differently, compared to 33 genes in the participants who used weights and only 19 in the moderate exercisers. Many of these genes, especially those found in the cells of interval trainers, are thought to affect the mitochondria's ability to produce energy for muscle cells; subjects who did interval training showed an increase in the number and health of their mitochondria, with the impact being particularly distinct among the older participants who used the stationary bike. It appears that the decline in the cellular health of the muscle associated with aging was "corrected" with exercise, especially when intensity was vigorous, says Dr. Sreekumaran Nair, Professor of Medicine and Endocrinologist at the Mayo Clinic, and senior author of the study. As a matter of fact, cells of older participants responded to strenuous exercise more than cells of younger participants.

In a study conducted by the Faculty of Science at the University of Queensland, Australia, 100 people (37 men and 63 women, with an average age of 87) performed weight training at a relatively high intensity; the study showed an average 113% increase in the strength of the tested individuals, an 11.8% increase in the average speed of execution of the movements, a 2.7% increase in the cross-section of the thighs and a 24.4% increase in speed when climbing the stairs.

Brazilian scientists compared training done at normal speed to power training; the increase in power was 34% higher in the group that performed exercises with a higher concentric speed and the increase in mass and strength was also significantly higher. It can therefore be confidently stated that **strength training is the best way to increase muscle mass in older adults**.

Another study, conducted by McMaster University and the Buck Institute for Research on Aging in California, showed that after undergoing resistance training (with weights) for a specific muscle group, twice a week for a six-month period, the overall strength of the participants experienced a 36% increase. A really important fact that emerged from this study is that, of the 596 genes taken into consideration, 179 showed an age-related inversion, thus highlighting a great antiaging response.

Another study that supports this thesis was conducted by the Washington University School of Medicine and demonstrated that **resistance training** can increase the degree of muscle protein synthesis in men aged 76 and over, **increasing both hypertrophic response and strength.**

The prevailing indications of resistance training to develop strength and muscle mass in older adults involve the use of loads ranging from 60% to 90% of 1RM, i.e. the maximum load that allows you to perform a single repetition. However, in some cases, especially at the beginning if you are a novice, you can use considerably lower loads, corresponding to only 30% of the maximum load. This allows you to better learn the execution technique, to improve the perception of the work on the muscle, and to verify any limitations due to joint problems or strength deficits in certain angles of the range of movement. To determine the load, it is advised not to use maximal tests and use indirect methods instead, such as the Brzycki equation [1RM theoretical = load lifted / [1.0278 – (0.0278 × repetitions performed)]. Normally, a training volume that is considered functional in terms of increasing hypertrophy and strength is one or two exercises for each muscle group, performed in three sets, for 8-15 repetitions, 2-3 times a week, while even once a week may be sufficient for maintenance. Obviously, these criteria are largely subjective and depend on the training level and experience. If an individual has always been a bodybuilder, the necessary training volume will certainly be higher for an already hypertrophic muscle that is accustomed to certain stimuli. It is obvious that, for those who have been training since they were young, it is easier to obtain good results, which sooner or later will lead to a plateau, likely around 40 years of age, due to the fact that progress cannot be made indefinitely. Conversely, if a person starts exercising in their 40s, they will have much more room for improvement, even up to the age of 50. In a study published in the *Journal of Strength Conditioning Research* (2009), Joshua Lowndess and his co-workers found that there was no difference in muscle strength and muscle mass in individuals aged between 18 to 39, who performed a 12-week weight training program.

This begs the question of whether training volume should be decreased or increased over the years. There are different aspects to consider, which lead us to as many answers. Over the years, in addition to a decrease in the volume of type II fibers, precisely those recruited in explosive efforts, the number of satellite cells responsible for the post-traumatic regeneration of muscle fibers following intense training also decreases. Obviously, this leads to a loss of strength, which is further amplified by a denervation process due to a reduction of spinal motoneurons, which mainly affects the fast-twitch (FT) nerve fibers.

To overcome this phenomenon and limit the loss of strength, the body implements a reinnervation process on the slow-twitch (ST) nerve fibers. This change in innervation leads to a change in the functionality of the innervated muscle cells so that the white type II (fast) fibers progressively take on aspects more typical of the red type I fibers, which are more prone to resistance training. We have already said that the ideal training volume cannot be an absolute value because it is a function of the percentage of white, red, or intermediate fibers of a person.

If a person has many white fibers, which are the ones that experience hypertrophy more easily, they will obtain optimal results especially with particularly intense and not necessarily prolonged workouts; conversely, those who have more red fibers will have to increase the frequency and the volume of their training at the expense of intensity to better exploit the potential of red fibers, which are more resistant. Therefore, elderly bodybuilders find themselves with a fiber profile that is more shifted towards red or intermediate fibers, despite their initial condition. Consequently, in terms of hypertrophy, they respond better to a workout that mainly uses these types of fibers. However, it is equally true that strength training that acts specifically on type II muscle fibers can effectively limit the denervation we have previously mentioned. Therefore, to make training complete, strength training should be introduced to individuals around 40 years of age, an age that is considered to be the threshold of an important change. However, to comfort those who are over 40, a 65-year-old who is in shape can have levels of strength and muscle mass that are comparable (I would even say much higher) to those of a 40-year-old who does not engage in physical activity (Negro et al., 2016). The current position statement from the American College of Sports Medicine states that weight training, when designed with appropriate intensity and volume, can produce gains in muscle mass and strength comparable to the levels that can be achieved in younger individuals. Evans and Rosemberg of Tuft University (USA) administered an 8-week weight training program to nursing home residents ranging from 87 to 96 years of age, which resulted in a tripling of strength and a 10% increase in muscle mass. **Most of the loss of muscle mass that occurs with aging is preventable and even reversible.**

Although many studies have proven the benefits of resistance training in the elderly, less research has focused specifically on the frail elderly. Frailty is a syndrome that meets three or more of the following five phenotypes: weakness, as measured by low grip strength, slowness (slow walking speed), low levels of physical activity, low energy or self-reported exhaustion and unintentional weight loss.

Fiatarone et al. indicated that physically frail elderly men and women improved leg muscle strength by 220% after a 10-week strength training program (three sets of eight repetitions at 80% of 1RM, three times a week). Serra-Rexach et al. found a 17% increase in strength during leg presses of ninety-year-old people after 8 weeks of progressive strength training with lighter loads (two or three sets of 8 to 10 repetitions at 30% of 1RM in the initial phase, and up to 70% of 1RM at the end of the intervention).

Lustosa et al. found significant improvements in leg muscle power at 70% of 1RM, three times a week. Although more research is needed, higher intensity exercises seem to produce greater results.

Sullivan et al. found greater improvements in the muscle strength of frail elderly participants after a 12-week progressive intensity strength training program (starting at 20% and ending at 80% of 1RM) compared with a continuous lower intensity program (20% of 1RM for the entire 12-week period).

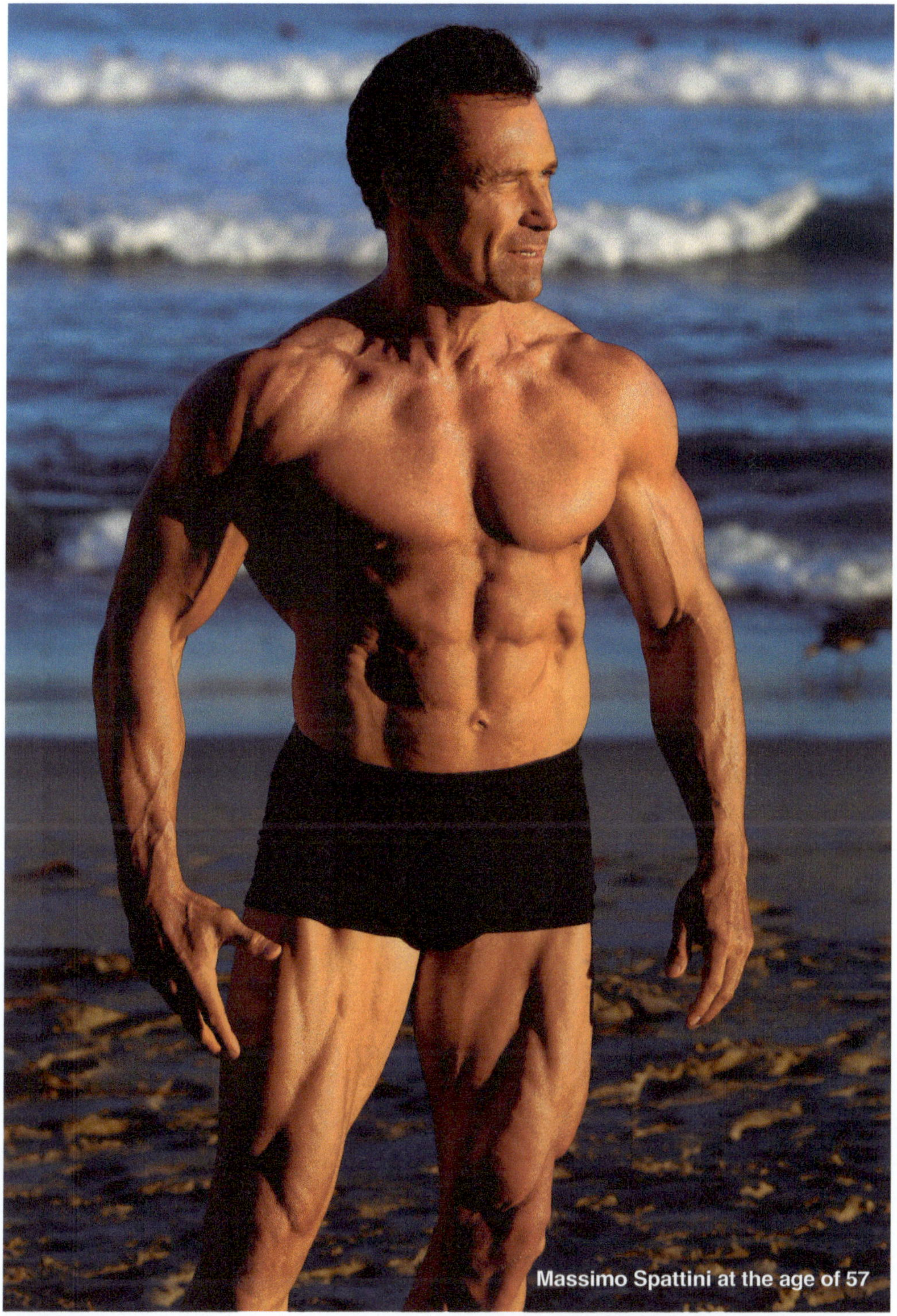

Massimo Spattini at the age of 57

The American College of Sports Medicine recommends a program that includes a range of exercises (strength, endurance, flexibility and balance) to maintain physical fitness in the elderly. Villareal et al. studied the effects of such a program on physical fitness in frail and obese older adults for 3 months and found beneficial effects on muscle mass and physical function.

Another ability of the body that decreases with age is undoubtedly that of recovery: lower ability to recover from an injury, lower ability to recover from a sleepless night, lower ability to recover from heavy and prolonged training, etc. This would argue in favor of a decrease in the training load (load = volume × intensity) and in frequency, except that, with age, the hypertrophic muscle responds to a decrease in training. Consequently, to obtain the same anabolic response in the elderly, we must increase the number of meals and the amount of protein intake, and training must also be more frequent and it must have a greater volume. Obviously, this greater frequency must take into account the need to limit the production of cortisol which, with age, tends to increase; therefore, if possible, workouts should not exceed 45 minutes, favoring shorter breaks that allow you to reach an adequate training intensity without using heavy loads, that are hard on joints, which are often already compromised, and of the body in general. Therefore, bodybuilders over the age of 50-60 can obtain better results with a fractional routine, that they can follow almost every day without reaching muscle failure and while concentrating on muscle control, which by that age should have been mastered. Among other things, this type of training also considers the increase in cardiovascular risk after a certain age: training with a lower percentage of load reduces the risks associated with lifting weights (weight training guidelines for individuals who have suffered a heart attack indicate not to use loads greater than 50% of the maximum).

Weight training increases capillary density in both young and older adults, according to a recent study conducted by Lex Verdijk of Maastricht University Medical Center in the Netherlands. These researchers evaluated capillary density in both young (mean age: 26) and elderly (mean age: 72) healthy male subjects before and after a 12-week training program. Training increased the size of fast (type II) fibers, although they were smaller in older subjects. Capillary density in slow and fast fibers increased in older subjects over the period of 12 weeks. Weight training is an effective way to improve circulation in older men. Capillaries are tiny blood vessels that exchange oxygen, carbon dioxide, water, nutrients and waste products between cells. A good function of the capillaries is essential for metabolic health, physical and sexual performance, and longevity.

People who are no longer young can easily have, or be predisposed to, cardiovascular problems, and intense training with weights, generating a sharp rise in blood pressure, can be problematic.

Sandro Da Silva and collaborators at the Federal University of Viçosa, Brazil, found that bilateral exercises put more stress on the cardiovascular system than unilateral training. The subjects that participated in the study performed three sets of 10 repetitions of biceps curls, knee extensions and a forward bent row, both unilaterally and bilaterally. Systolic blood pressure and stress on the heart were greater during bilateral training for both bicep flexions and knee extensions, whereas there were no pressure differences in the bent row. Bilateral training poses a slightly greater cardiovascular "challenge" compared to unilateral training, so the latter may be a preferential choice for people with hypertension. Resistance exercise (RE) can reduce many risk factors of cardiovascular diseases (CVD). The associations of RE with CVD and other causes of death were analyzed in a study that involved 12,591 participants (mean age: 47) who received at least two clinical examinations. During a follow-up period between 5.4 and 10.5 years, compared with no RE, RE performed once, twice or three times a week was associated with an approximately 40-70% reduction in the risk of total CVD, independent of the aerobic exercises. However, there was no significant risk reduction with a weekly RE longer than 60 minutes.

Indeed, until recently, weight training for patients with cardiovascular diseases such as hypertension was discouraged due to the hemodynamic response observed during isometric (static) exercises. However, it has been shown that weight training is not a purely isometric exercise and a different hemodynamic response has also been found in patients with heart disease. For this reason, weight training studies have been conducted in selected groups of patients with coronary heart disease. The results of these studies, in this small group of patients, have shown that this kind of activity is safe and beneficial in terms of improving the patient's functional capacity. **Resistance training may also favorably influence risk factors of coronary heart disease.** Based on the reviewed studies, we can make recommendations for weight training in patients with coronary heart disease. There is still a restriction in patients who are asymptomatic or only mildly symptomatic; training should be initiated only after a preparation period with aerobic training if the individual is not already fit, doing single-limb exercises and a maximum load that does not exceed 60% of 1RM. Subjects should record their heart rate (avoiding exceeding the critical threshold which corresponds to the appearance of altered electrocardiographic tracing) and their response to the exercise program, and they should adhere to a periodic re-evaluation of the exercise structure.

Additionally, **weight training in older people may be more effective than aerobic training.** This is not so much due to the calories burnt during training which, given the same dedicated time, could easily be higher with aerobic training, but due to the fact that weight training helps counteract the loss of muscle mass which occurs after the age of 40. Since each lost kg of muscle mass corresponds to a decrease in the basal metabolic rate of about 25 kcal, the older a person gets, the more easily they gain weight (without considering hormonal variations such as insulin resistance, the drop in GH, testosterone, DHEA, etc.) for the same caloric intake. This process can largely be stopped by training with weights and by adopting a high-protein diet; moreover, if you train hard, consume enough protein and still have an acceptable hormonal condition, you can even build muscles from scratch, a result that aerobic exercise absolutely cannot achieve. In a study involving 10,000 adults between the ages of 40 and 75 (*Harvard Gazette*, 2014), who were monitored for 12 years, waist circumference was measured as an indicator of body composition, and the subjects were divided into those who did at least 30 minutes of aerobics per day and those who did at least 20 minutes of weight training per day. At the end of the 12 years, there was an average increase in waist circumference of 6.6 cm, but in weight lifters, this increase was 3 cm less. Obviously, this does not mean that aerobic training is not important, due to its effect on the cardiovascular system, but that weight training is more effective for reducing visceral fat, especially in the elderly. In conclusion, we can state that in middle-aged people, in terms of body composition control and the effect on fat oxidation mechanisms, the best result is obtained by **combining aerobic and anaerobic activities**, thus increasing the mitochondrial biogenesis.

CHAPTER 25

Abs workouts

Massimo Spattini

Fortunately, seeing exercises such as sit-ups and straight leg raises for abs performed in the gym is becoming increasingly rare. These exercises, which have been considered the basis of abs training for years, are not specific to these muscles; they do not fulfill the fundamental task of a muscle, which is bringing two bones closer to each other. The rectus abdominis inserts at the level of the xiphoid process of the sternum and pubic bone. Consequently, its function is to bring these two bones together by contracting. If we examine sit-ups or leg raises, we see that this does not happen: the distance between the two bones remains the same, i.e. the distance between the sternum and the pubic bone does not change.

Instead, the muscle that performs the function of bringing the two bone heads on which it is inserted closer together in sit-ups and leg raises is the iliopsoas, which is inserted at the level of the lumbar vertebrae and the femur (hip). Indeed, in sit-ups and leg raises, the lowest part of the spine and the femurs are brought closer to each other. The iliopsoas is the muscle involved in this movement; the abs contract only for a synergistic intervention in an isometric way, avoiding the rotation of the pelvis. In the long run, these exercises can cause excessive stress on the lumbar spine, which causes the common back pain we have all been predisposed to since humans decided to stand up straight. This, however, does not mean that we are destined to suffer from disabling back pain, but that we must understand our body and its muscular kinetic chains in order to maintain the right balance of tone between the abdominal and lumbar muscles and to avoid imbalances which would undoubtedly result in pain. Lower back muscles are naturally hypertonic. Conversely, the muscles of the abdominal wall tend to be hypotonic, therefore, it is very important to strengthen them in order to achieve good balance. But sit-ups and straight leg lifts are not the ideal solutions because they can lead to overworking the iliopsoas, which is a hip flexor muscle that is inserted into the last part of the rachis. In reality, the necessary movement for the complete contraction of the abdominals involves the convergence of the xiphoid apophysis of the sternum to the pubis. This, for example, is obtained with various movements that can involve

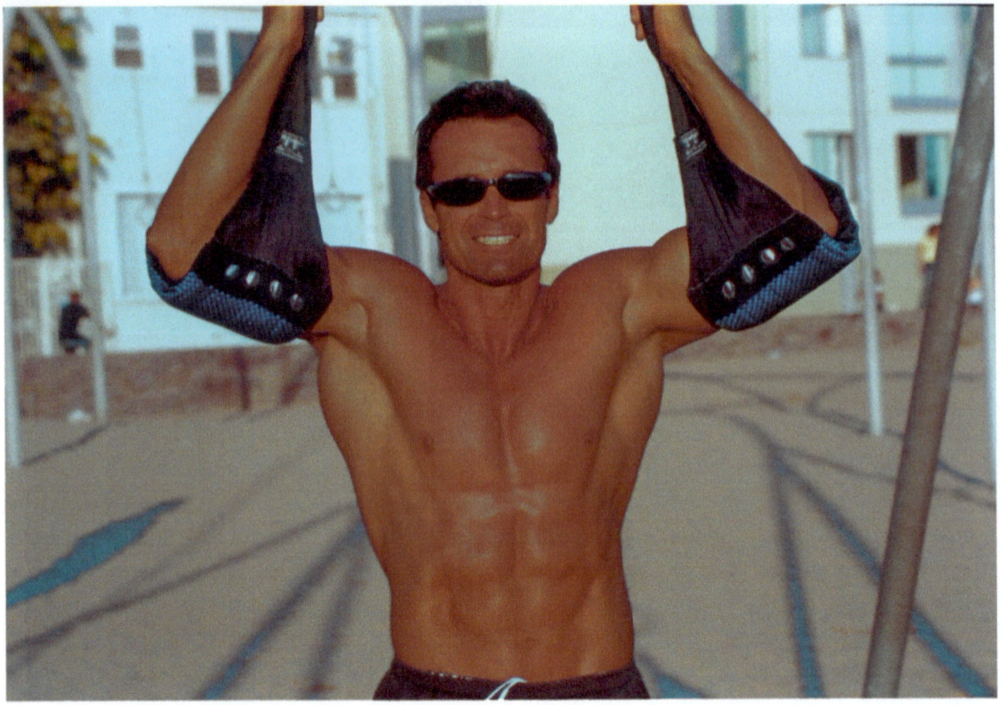

lifting the pelvis by exploiting the force of gravity, being suspended from a bar, or, even better, using the *Ab Origional*, which avoids isometric contraction of the back muscles. Since they are connected by various aponeurotic sheaths (the connective elastic sheaths that wrap around the muscles and create an indirect connection between one muscle and another, as if we were wearing a diving suit) to the lower trunk muscles, they can't be fully stretched, a condition that is essential for subsequent optimal contraction.

If you don't have a pull-up bar in your gym (the pull-up bar, the squat rack and the deadlift platform seem to have given way to the various machines in fitness gyms), you can perform the same hip lift exercise while being suspended with extended arms on the parallel bars. These exercises, without a doubt, are not easy for a beginner because you need to have good control of your abdominal muscles. To perform this exercise correctly, you need to stretch the muscles as much as possible by letting the lower part of the body "slide down", and then "recover" by only contracting the abdominals.

In short, it is necessary to visualize the distance between the xiphoid apophysis of the sternum and the pubic symphysis (the area where our genital organs are located). In the relaxation phase, it is necessary to increase the distance to the maximum and in the contraction phase, it is necessary to try to reduce the distance to the minimum, contracting only the abdominals, keeping the whole body straight, with the legs in line with the trunk. Once you have gained confidence with these exercises, you can increase the intensity and the overload by using weights that can be placed at the ends of the legs.

Personally, I haven't done sit-ups and straight leg raises in more than 30 years. In 1985, I decided to participate in a powerlifting competition with other athletes from my gym, "New Center Gym". Since I had just finished preparing for a bodybuilding competition, I was quite debilitated and, moreover, I had absolutely no specific preparation for powerlifting; however, since my maxes (bench press 175 kg, deadlift 250 kg, squat 230 kg) were sufficient for me to support my team, I agreed to participate. Unfortunately, during the 230 kg squat, I leaned forward and due to the distraction of the two assistants, I found myself in the "good morning" position with 230 kg on my neck. Not able to get up from that position and in order to avoid the "guillotine" effect of the barbell on my neck if I fell forward and I used all my strength to push the barbell away with my arms. I don't know how much pressure was applied to my fifth lumbar vertebra after this effort. All I know is that it caused me a major strain to my lumbar muscles. Not being happy with that, as the team needed points after this injury, I deadlifted 220 kg, just to make them feel safer. Boasting is something that you do when you are young, but it is then paid for throughout your life. Since then, I have not been able to perform sit-ups or straight-legged lifts, and my repertoire of abdominal exercises has been limited to crunches, both in suspension and lying on the floor or on a bench.

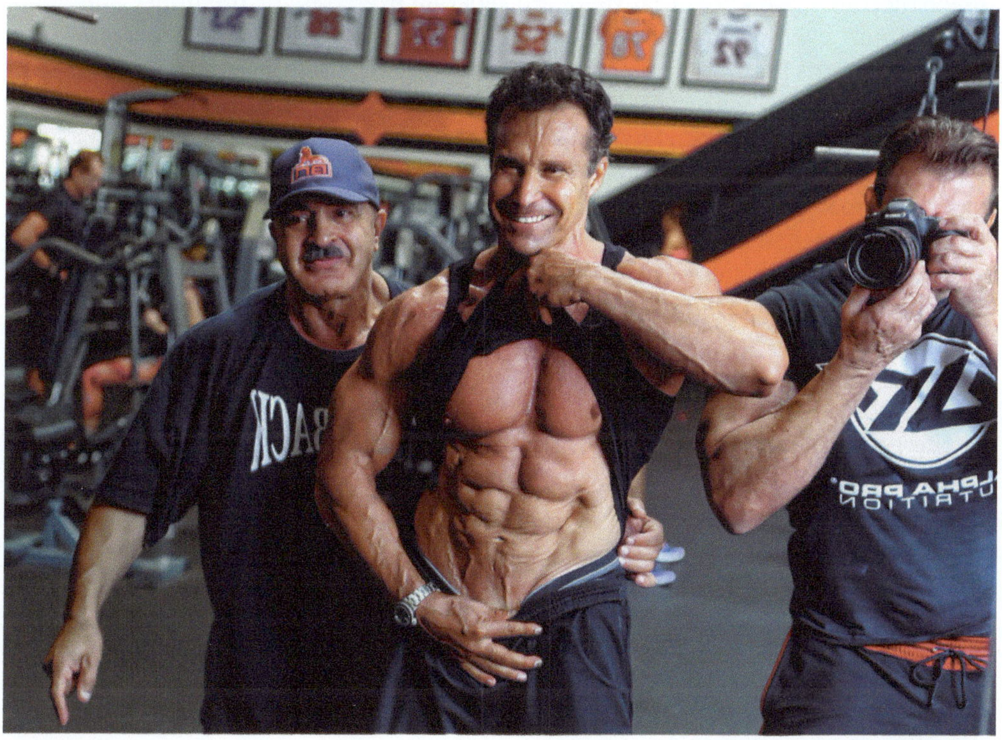

Crunches are a partial movement and practically correspond only to the initial third of the movement of the sit-up; if this exercise is performed, which is almost always the case in gyms, by lying down with your back on the floor, there is no pre-stretching phase, which is essential to obtain the maximum benefits from the contraction of the abs. To remedy this problem, one solution is doing crunches on the Swiss ball. Since the surface of the ball is curved, the upper part of the chest, following the contraction of the abs, flexes forward approaching the pubis and this is the correct movement for which the abs are intended.

To verify the real superiority of Swiss ball crunches compared to flat surface crunches, some researchers examined 8 men with an average age of about 23 and compared the two exercises. The results of the study were published in *Physical Therapy* and they highlighted the advantage of crunches on the Swiss ball. The electrodes of an electromyograph (EMG), a device that records the intensity of muscle contraction, were applied to the abdominal muscles of the athletes. Results showed that the maximum voluntary contraction of the rectus abdominis during flat surface crunches was 21%, with an oblique involvement of 5%. In contrast, during Swiss ball crunch, the intensity of electrical activity averaged 35%, with the external oblique activation reaching 10%.

If the greater activation of the rectus abdominis is explained by the wider range of motion, that of the obliques is explained by the greater intervention of these muscles in stabilizing the chest in a dynamic equilibrium on a spherical surface.

Furthermore, we know that there are separate exercises for the upper and lower abs in almost every gym. Obviously, the definition is anatomically incorrect, as the rectus abdominis is a single muscle that starts from the xiphoid apophysis of the sternum and is inserted with the distal portion at the level of the pubic symphysis, but from a functional point of view, the concept is not that incorrect. Let's discuss why. No matter what kind of abs exercises you are doing, you will tend to always train both the upper and lower rectus abdominis, including the obliques. So, while it is not entirely possible to isolate one specific part of a muscle, it is certainly possible to emphasize its involvement over another. Depending on the choice of exercises, when greater control is achieved over the abdominal region and the exercise is performed correctly, it is possible to have a greater activation of a certain portion, for example, of the lower region. In this regard, it is worth taking some time to discuss the anatomy of the abdomen.

The rectus abdominis is not a group of independent muscles, but rather a long muscular sheath that starts from the sternum and continues all the way down to the pelvis, at the level of the symphysis pubis. Moreover, it is separated by tendons, which are fibrous structures of connective tissue that compartmentalize the abs into segments, resulting in what we refer to as a "six-pack". The interesting aspect is that the upper and lower parts of the muscle are innervated by intercostal nerves which, in turn, branch into collateral branches of various types, thus allowing a selective activation mechanism. This implies that, from an anatomical point of view, there is at least a rationale for the preferential activation of different parts of the rectus abdominis. In other words, the rectus abdominis functions as a semi-independent unit, which can be selectively activated depending on the choice of exercise. To activate the lower part of the abs it is necessary to dynamically perform a posterior pelvic tilt in which the pelvis is pulled upwards, i.e. towards the navel. This movement, which can be achieved in exercises such as reverse crunches and knee-to-chin raises, causes a greater shortening of the lower region, thus stimulating the "lower abs" more than the "upper abs".

Maximizing lower abdominal engagement can be challenging because the pelvis has a very limited range of motion, and if you are not careful with your execution, your hip flexors will tend to dominate during the exercise. Regarding the importance of optimal execution, Sarti et al. (1996) carried out a study in which participants were divided into two groups. One group had a "high level of physical activity", training seriously for at least an hour and a half, 3 days a week for 3 years, while the other group with a "low level of physical activity" did not have to follow the same criteria. Both groups had to perform exercises such as crunches targeting the upper abdomen, and reverse crunches targeting the "lower abs".

Electromyography (EMG) was used to monitor the results, which measured muscle activity in the lower and upper abdominal regions, while execution was monitored by fitness professionals. Subsequently, the groups were divided into "correct" and "incorrect" performers, based on the participants' ability to perform the exercises correctly. In this case, the correct execution of the reverse crunch was dependent on the subject, as it was determined by their ability to implement the posterior pelvic tilt. At the end of the study, it was found that only the participants of the first group, i.e. the individuals who were subjected to a "high level of physical activity", were able to effectively activate their "lower abs". At this point, the following question arises: does greater activation of the lower abdominal area also correspond to greater muscle development? While there are conflicting opinions, research seems to indicate that increased activation is actually associated with hypertrophy.

Another question can also be posed: can the activation of a certain area be associated with targeted fat loss? There are conflicting opinions on this as well, but recent research demonstrates a decrease in the subcutaneous fold, which is indicative of a greater decrease of subcutaneous fat in the areas overlying the muscles that are affected by exercise, probably due to the thermal and vasodilator effect and/or the major catecholaminergic stimulus. Despite this, the extent to which increased activation promotes muscle hypertrophy and targeted fat loss is not well understood, but when it comes to areas that are difficult to develop and define, such as "lower abs", any viable strategy can be considered valid.

CHAPTER 26

Stretching

Massimo Spattini

Joint pain can deprive people of life's simplest pleasures, such as maintaining an upright position, walking, gardening or chasing a tennis ball on the court. Not only can difficulties be encountered even in basic movements that are necessary to get through the day, such as getting into the car or going down the stairs, but obviously, pain can also significantly affect weight training aimed at building muscle.

The most common causes of joint pain include arthritis, tendinopathies, previous injuries, tension due to certain repetitive movements, posture problems and aging. While it is common to try to avoid movements that cause pain, in reality, limiting them completely can weaken the muscles, making joint pain only worse.

Physical activity, or more precisely, the correct execution of targeted exercises, can represent a lasting strategy to suppress pain, in areas such as the ankles, knees, hips or shoulders. For some people, performing these exercises could help delay future surgeries, and the right routine should involve pairing targeted joint workouts with a simple, short walk. Although the type of training must be highly personalized and established on the basis of the characteristics of the person and the problem, I believe that the simple stretching tips listed below can be useful for any kind of training.

1. **Pay attention to the warm-up**. Muscles stretch more easily when they are warmed up. For this reason, doing warm-up exercises, taking a hot shower or bath, or even entering the sauna for a while, could be a good practice before any workout.
2. **Stretch, but avoid pain**. Stretch only to the point of mild tension and never to the point of pain. If a stretch hurts, it is better to slowly return to the starting position and, if necessary, carefully try again. With time and practice, flexibility will improve.
3. **Breathe properly**. Controlling your breathing while stretching and concentrating as much as possible on the movement you are performing is important. Correct breathing is important because adequate oxygenation reduces the state of tension.

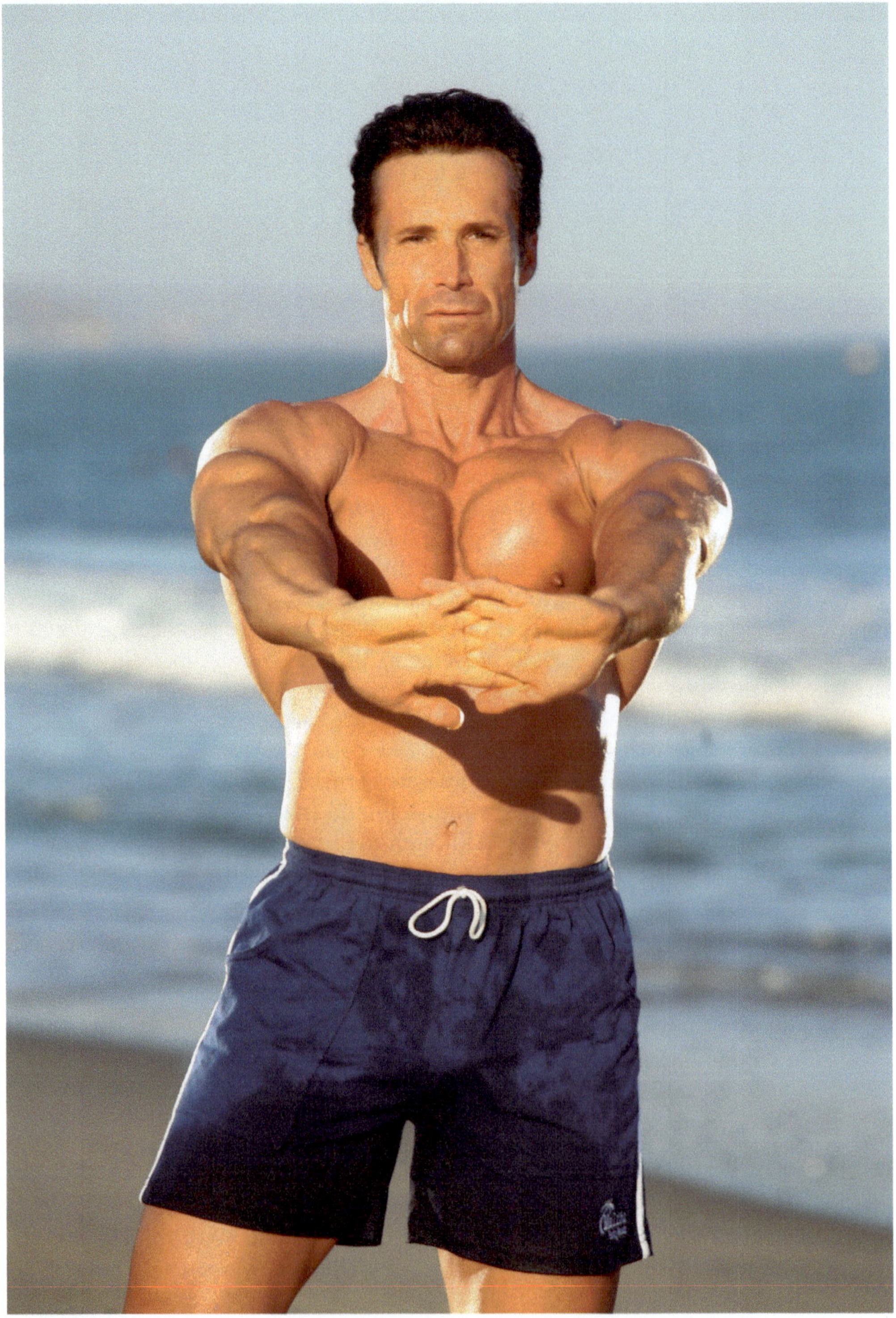

4. **Increase the frequency of stretching sessions.** When stretching is performed more frequently, even several times a day, it is possible to obtain excellent improvements in the muscles and tendons to prevent joint trauma, improve movement capacity, increase benefit on the cardio-circulatory and respiratory systems and, finally, increase benefit for the nervous system by reducing physical stress.
5. **Stretching before or after weight training?** Most training researchers think that stretching at the beginning of the session reduces muscle performance, with a consequent reduction in strength and in the level of hypertrophy-inducing stimuli (Bosco, Cacchi); the causes are not well understood, but they seem to be due to neurogenic and/or metabolic factors. Greek researchers found that muscle power decreases in direct proportion to the time that the muscle lengthens. By stretching for 30 seconds, isometric strength drops by approximately 9%, while with 60 seconds of stretching it drops by 16%. In any case, a Japanese study showed that muscle strength is recovered after 10 minutes. Additionally, stretching increases the range of motion for 30 minutes. Consequently, static stretching could be used as an effective warm-up 10 minutes prior to the performance, followed immediately by general warm-up exercises.
6. **Is stretching after training really beneficial?** According to some people, it promotes the cool-down and recovery phases, reducing post-workout muscle soreness (DOMS) (Shobert, Weineck, Fucci). According to others, it makes no difference (McGlyn, Laughlin, Rowe). Consequently, the best solution is probably to stretch at a distance from a weight training session, unless you perform workouts in which partial movements prevail over those with the maximum range of motion, which exploit a pre-stretching condition that could be considered a form of stretching; in this case, stretching performed after training can prevent muscle shortening.
7. **The importance of stretching for post-workout pain relief.** Given the recent findings regarding the negative effects of stretching on performance and the inconsistent evidence on its role in reducing the risk of injuries, stretching has taken a back seat among athletes. In reality, especially in sports with a significant eccentric component, such as bodybuilding, stretching can decrease DOMS. Thai researchers have shown that after an 8-week stretching program, there was a clear reduction in muscle pain following intense eccentric-type exercises.

CHAPTER 27

Are cardio and weights like cats and dogs?

Massimo Spattini

Resistance training immediately followed by cardiovascular exercise has become standard practice for maximizing muscle mass and reducing body fat.

Despite the popular use of this approach, it is quite evident that the body responds very differently to both modalities of training, especially at molecular and cellular levels. Not only are the molecular and cellular reactions different in response to the two different types of training, but they can also be antagonistic to each other.

Let's look at this concept in more detail.

In general, resistance training increases muscle cell size by activating the mTOR enzyme, which stimulates protein synthesis and, therefore, muscle growth. On the other hand, cardiovascular endurance training reduces the number of fat cells by activating the AMPK enzyme, which increases fatty acid oxidation, ultimately leading to a reduction in body fat.

AMPK activation has been shown to directly shut down mTOR-activated muscle protein synthesis, thereby inhibiting muscle growth. Consequently, it can be argued that performing cardio immediately after lifting weights may not be the best training sequence for optimal muscle growth, since the AMPK activation favored by the final cardio would counteract the action of mTOR in response to the anaerobic work, affecting muscle growth negatively.

In light of this, it can be stated that mTOR function is typically maximized immediately after weightlifting, and this means that the simultaneous activation of AMPK induced by cardio training would significantly deplete mTOR activity and muscle growth.

A study by Willis and Slentz (2012) showed that a considerable part of the weight loss achieved with aerobic activity is actually a loss of muscle mass.

Furthermore, a study by Mournier et al. went even further, clearly demonstrating the negative influence of cardiovascular training at the muscle-level, due to its ability to activate AMPK and directly deactivate mTOR-driven muscle growth. In this study, mice exposed to mechanical muscle overload had increased mTOR activation, while mice that had the *AMPK* gene removed (preventing AMPK function) had an even greater level of mTOR activation in response to an identical amount of mechanical stress.

Therefore, according to this study, since the removal of the AMPK function improves muscle growth potential, targeted removal of endurance training and, therefore, AMPK function after weight training should also support an increase in muscle capacity and muscle growth.

However, in regard to pre-weight training cardio, it appears that performing a standard cardiovascular workout before resistance training does not impair muscle growth.

Since cardiovascular exercise-induced AMPK activation lasts only about 1 hour post-exercise performing weight training during the hour after cardiovascular work should theoretically completely prevent the simultaneous activation of AMPK and mTOR, as well as the muscle loss that results from the concurrent activation of these two enzymes.

To confirm this hypothesis, a study by Ogasawara and Sato (2014) examined the different levels of mTOR activity achieved during cardio training before or after weightlifting. As expected, the researchers found that cardio exercise performed after

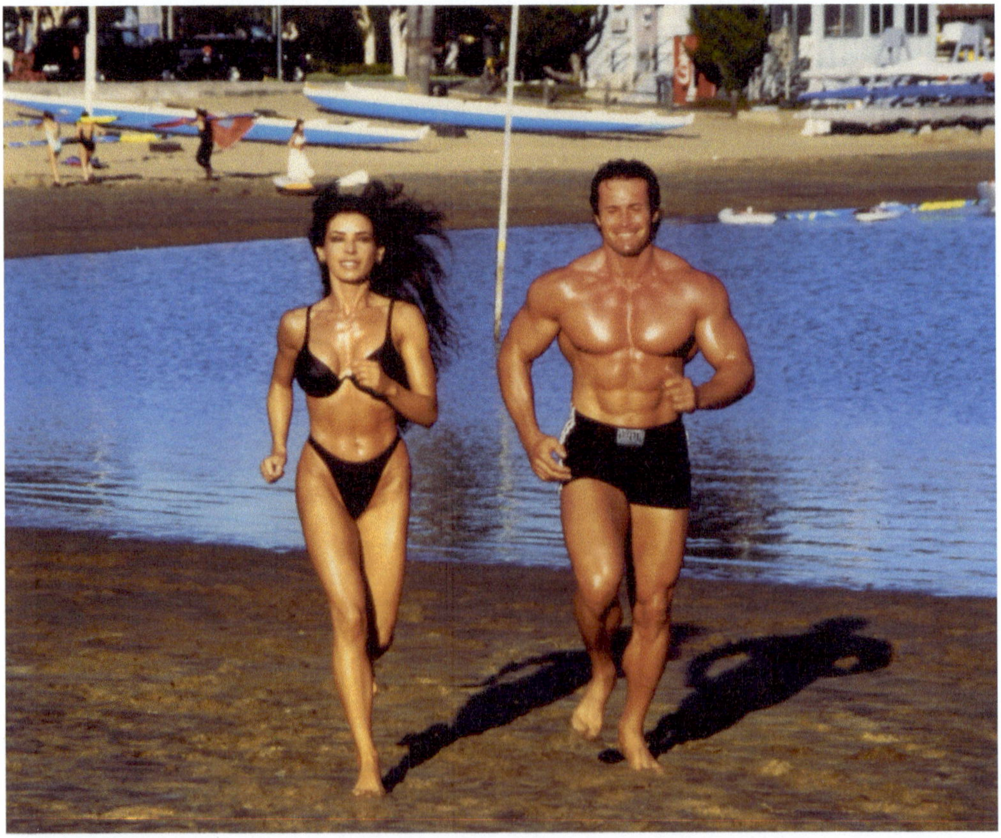

anaerobic resistance training resulted in increased AMPK activity that directly weakened mTOR function and muscle protein anabolism.

However, the opposite order of exercises resulted in AMPK activation for only 1 hour after the end of the cardio work. Because the subsequent resistance training lasted 1 hour, the authors of this study concluded that AMPK activation does not coincide with the mTOR activation by anaerobic resistance training. It is obvious that, in this case, prolonged aerobic training must be avoided, otherwise it would lead to a drop in energy, which would negatively affect the subsequent weight training session.

In conclusion, this training sequence resulted in a higher level of mTOR function, providing a more anabolic environment conducive to muscle growth.

David Pearson of Ball State University in Muncie (Indiana) has shown that, if resistance training is done in the morning and aerobic training in the evening, 7 hours apart, especially if a meal rich in carbohydrates and proteins is consumed after weight training, recovery will be complete and the benefits of adaptation to both types of exercise can be reaped.

In terms of hormonal levels, we can say that standard weight training provides a stimulus that increases one of the most important hormones for muscle building, testosterone.

Conversely, prolonged cardiovascular exercise generally suppresses the level of circulating testosterone (particularly free bioactive testosterone), which probably reduces muscle growth. Furthermore, in order to promote greater energy recovery, considerable energy consumption triggers the inhibition of energy-consuming metabolic processes such as muscle protein synthesis.

Combining cardiovascular exercise with resistance training still reduces testosterone levels, regardless of the order of training. However, the depletion of testosterone from cardio is short-lived and can apparently still promote sizable strength gains, especially when cardio is done before weightlifting.

This effect was demonstrated in a study by Schumann et al. (2014) who examined the acute response on testosterone levels of combined cardio and weight training in two independent groups performing cardio training first or last. The results showed that the group who did cardio first had relatively lower testosterone levels compared to the group who did resistance training at the end. However, lower testosterone levels did not correlate with strength development, as the group that did cardio first actually showed better strength gains, with a 17% increase in 1RM (repetition max) in leg presses, compared to the group that did cardio last, who improved their rep max by only 13%.

These findings indicate that although cardio-vascular training depletes the potent muscle-building hormone testosterone, cardio done at the beginning of the training session is apparently better at promoting mass gain and strength. This is likely due to increased mTOR-driven muscle growth.

Conversely, if we adopt a type of cardiovascular training that we can only partially define as aerobic, such as HIIT, which consists of performing repetitions of about 1 minute at 80-90% of maximum capacity interspersed with recovery periods of about

1 minute at 40-50%, for a total of about 10-15 minutes, we will have a testosterone boost. This type of training, combined with weight training, increases insulin sensitivity, increasing the entry of glucose into the cells, thus increasing energy levels and stimulating protein synthesis.

Finally, the definitive study regarding the compatibility of strength training with endurance training was reported by Kraemer et al. (1995). In this study, healthy male adults were divided into several groups: those who performed endurance training only, those who performed power training only, and those who combined the two workouts. The study showed that, although the group that performed the combined training had improved the parameters of both capacities (power and endurance), the improvements were not at the same level as those obtained by focusing on only one type of training.

Transferring these findings to bodybuilding would suggest that combining power training with endurance training is not a winning strategy. However, for those who train solely for maintenance and for general well-being, combined training may offer moderate benefits for both cardiovascular and muscular capacity.

Moral of the story: aerobics and weights are a bit like cats and dogs. As a matter of fact, Schwarzenegger, referring to a rule that should be adopted in the bulking phase, said: "If you run, make sure you walk; if you walk, stop; if you are still, sit down; if you are sitting, if you can, lie down and if you are lying down, see if you can sleep".

While today this concept seems partially outdated, much like cats and dogs, if combined in the right way, aerobics and weights can also get along.

CHAPTER 28

Cardio management to burn fat more efficiently

Massimo Spattini and Riccardo Gaspari

When it comes to body recomposition or training programs aimed at improving health and/or sports performance, unless you start from an excellent physical condition, combined cardio-weight training is essential. We do not only lose weight because we burn calories by exercising, but also because performing physical activities stimulates our metabolism, increasing the production of certain hormones that allow us to burn a greater amount of body fat throughout the rest of the day. It should also not be forgotten that, metabolically speaking, the physical activity carried out in resistance training (weight training) guarantees better responses compared to aerobic activity alone, and this translates into an increase in muscle mass which corresponds to a metabolic increase, automatically leading to burning a higher amount of fat while at rest.

Contrary to this statement, if during a calorie restriction process our choice was oriented towards exclusively aerobic training sessions, we would find ourselves in a condition in which a significant amount of muscle tissue would be burned in addition to fat, and we would inevitably find ourselves with a slower metabolism.

Not paying attention to the difference between subcutaneous fat and visceral fat is another mistake that is too often made when we talk about training or how we approach food; this is a serious mistake because different types of fat respond different to stimuli.

Another very important thing to keep in mind is that the initial fat that is burnt by training and dieting is the one between the muscle tissue, and not the subcutaneous or visceral fat, as many erroneously claim.

When we talk about subcutaneous fat, we refer to white adipose tissue (WAT) located under the skin, which is distributed mainly in the lower areas of the body (gluteal-femoral area) and in the superficial abdominal area; on the other hand, when we refer to visceral fat, we mean the WAT located between the internal organs.

This helps us understand that, with the right approach, we can focus specifically on the type of fat we want to lose. Many studies have shown that in order to eliminate subcutaneous fat, the ideal exercise is aerobic activity at medium-low intensity, maintaining an FCmax of 60-65% with a training duration of 30-40 minutes; to eliminate visceral fat, on the other hand, it has been shown that it is more appropriate to do aerobic exercise following HIIT (High-Intensity Interval Training) protocols.

There are basically two schools of thought: the first claims that to burn fat you need to train at low intensity for a long time, otherwise, if you train at high intensity, you burn sugars. Some studies by Dr. George Brooks of the University of California have shown that the body uses fat more as an energy substrate during low-intensity workouts. It has also been observed that, by performing exercises below 65% of one's maximum capacity, the body implements a real "change of direction", exploiting fat as "fuel" rather than carbohydrates, while the opposite happens if you go beyond this percentage.

In essence, the rate of fat burning as a percentage of fat cells decreases as exercise intensity increases. Put like this, the best way to lose weight seems to be a real piece of cake: just train at low intensity and the body will use fat as an energy source. But is this really the case?

The second school of thought states that while it is true that during low intensity and high duration training more fat is oxidized for energy purposes, it must also be noted that high intensity training causes a stimulation of hormones, such as GH and catecholamines, which cannot be stimulated by low-intensity training.

Fat oxidation following exercise is closely related to exercise intensity which, in turn, is related to peak GH and catecholamine secretion. The GH peak has been proven to be the greatest predictor of fat utilization after an exercise (Pritzlaff et al., 2000). Although low-intensity aerobic training promotes increased fat burning for energy during exercise, excess post-exercise oxygen consumption (EPOC) does not lead to increased fat burning, unlike aerobic exercises at high intensity, like interval training, which alternates aerobic periods with anaerobic periods.

Although blood flow to adipose tissue is lower during high-intensity training (vasoconstrictor effect of catecholamines), fat oxidation after exercise is increased. But, in the end, what does it matter if less fat is burned for energy during physical exercise, and then if more is burned during recovery, given the metabolic stimulus coming from lipolytic hormones?

Returning to the debate between the two schools of thought, they both agree on one thing: compared to low-intensity training, training at high intensity for the same amount of time burns more fat overall, even if in percentage terms you burn less fat. Low-intensity training burns about 60% of fat for energy purposes, while high-intensity training burns only 30%.

However, if, for example, we burn 200 kcal in a one-hour low-intensity workout, and in a high-intensity workout we burn 600 kcal, we must consider that 60% of 200 kcal corresponds to 120 kcal burnt and 30% of 600 kcal is 180 kcal. In other words, we will still have used more fat for energy purposes. Recent studies carried out by Laval University in Canada have shown that subjects who trained more intensely had more muscle mass and less fat tissue compared to those who trained more moderately. This is because the former had a higher calorie consumption.

In conclusion, it is important to reiterate that, while there may be more or less efficient training methods in terms of calories and fat burnt, **to achieve weight loss nutrition plays a key role**. Those who go to the gym or do physical activity cannot neglect this aspect. The balance between these two components promotes optimal weight loss.

However, since we should not compare apples to oranges, we must evaluate the amount of fat burnt not by considering the time compared to the calories, but by considering the fat burnt for the same number of calories. According to this logic, the amount of fat that is burnt for the same number of calories is higher during low-impact aerobic activity. In a study published in the *International Journal of Sports Medicine* (Cho et al., 2011), Korean researchers studied three groups of obese, sedentary, middle-aged women: one group maintained a sedentary lifestyle; the second group walked three times a week at a VO_2 max of about 40-50%, consuming 400 calories per session starting from the fifth week; the third group ran three times a week at a VO_2 max of 70-75%, consuming 400 calories starting from the fifth week.

After 12 weeks, various blood tests and body measurements were taken to see which group had the greatest improvements in cardiovascular benefit, body composition and lipid profile (cholesterol and triglycerides). Unsurprisingly, the running group had the best cardiorespiratory benefits, as the 70-75% VO_2 range is particularly beneficial for improving cardiorespiratory parameters.

However, in terms of body composition, even though both the running and walking groups lost weight, the walking group lost more subcutaneous and visceral fat. This was in contrast to the total weight loss, which was greater in the running group, implying a greater loss of muscle mass. Both groups had an improvement in their lipid profile (higher HDL) and a decrease in insulin resistance, especially the walking group, although not significantly.

Other studies have shown that, for the same caloric expenditure, low-intensity exercise is equivalent to high-intensity exercise in promoting weight loss, visceral fat loss and fat loss throughout the body. Furthermore, some studies (Houmardja et al., 2004) seem to show that the duration of exercise, rather than the intensity, is the most important factor for improving insulin sensitivity. The reason why individuals subjected to more intense physical activity did not burn more fat due to increased post-exercise oxidation and higher hormonal stimulation is related to the fact that they did not follow a specific diet. It's well documented that high-intensity workouts often lead to higher calorie intake for the rest of the day. Moreover, fatigue leads to a subsequent decrease in motor activity. Training at a lower intensity favors lipolysis at the level of the subcutaneous and visceral tissue, by avoiding the hormonal vasoconstrictor effect and by stimulating circulation. HIIT is undoubtedly a cardiovascular workout that, based on the alternation between high and low-intensity workouts with short but intense training sessions, has positive metabolic effects with relatively little time requirements. However, it doesn't seem ideal for fat loss. A Canadian study found improvements of up to 17% in maximal oxygen uptake after just 20 minutes of exercise over 2 weeks. This is not enough time for high-calorie expenditure and

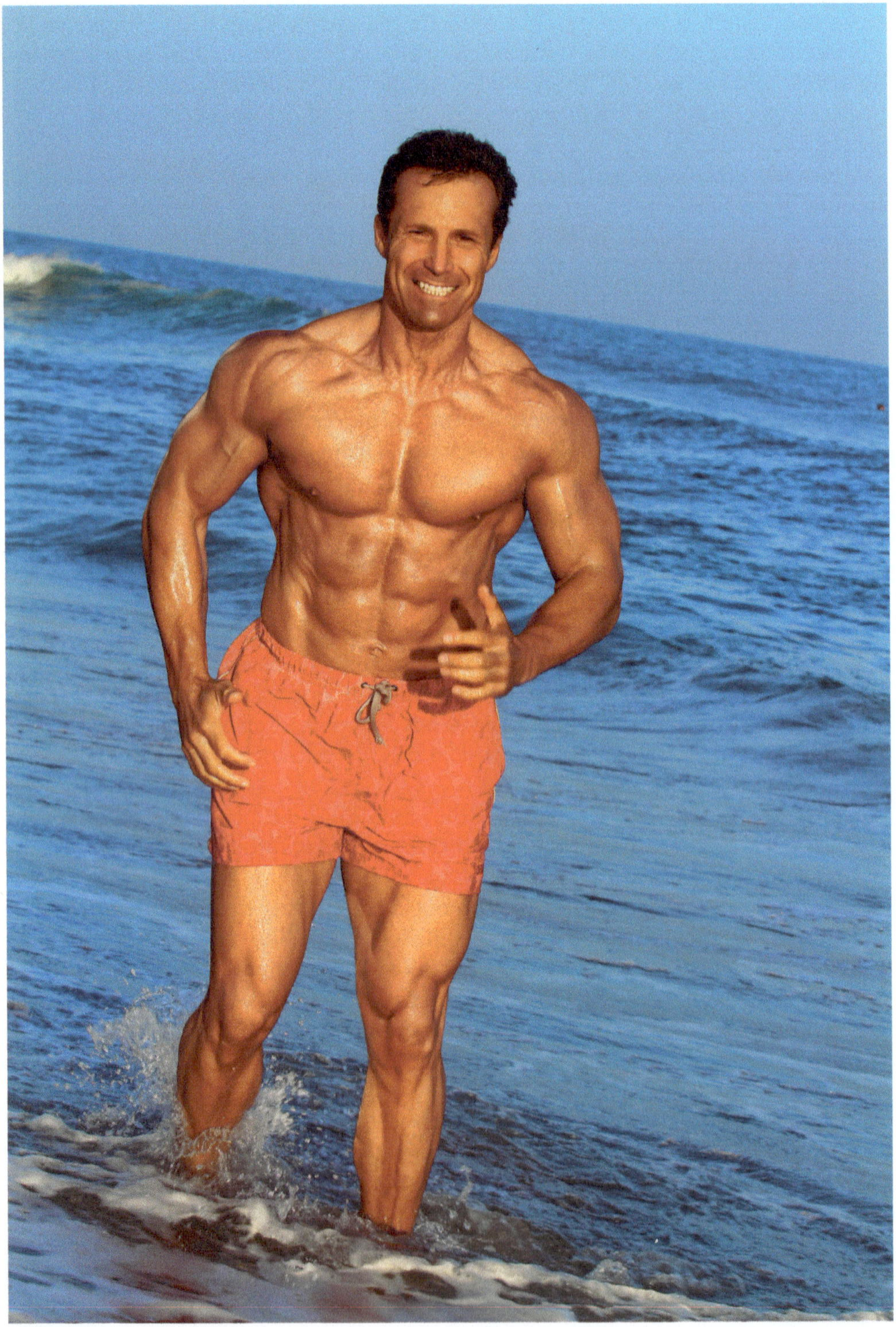

accelerated fat loss. An Australian study conducted by Shelley Keating found that in sedentary and overweight adults, training with continuous exercises for 12 weeks led to more significant fat loss compared to HIIT workouts. The increases in exercise capacity were the same (22-24%), but continued exercise reduced abdominal fat by 3.1% versus no change with HIIT training.

HIIT training is a great way to get metabolically fit but produces poor results for altering body composition when performed in short sessions (*Journal of Obesity*, 2014). Therefore, even high-intensity training (HIIT) should be structured for a sufficiently long period, say at least 30 minutes, alternating high-intensity phases (from 4 to 6) of about 30-60 seconds (sprint) with moderate intensity phases of about 4 minutes.

In a recent meta-analysis reviewing 6000 publications, 31 were included in the study comparing Moderate Intensity Continuous Training (MICT) with High-Intensity Protocols (HIIT), showing a greater overall reduction of body fat with MICT training. One reason why continuous training seems to ultimately produce better results in terms of weight loss may also be due to the correlation between GH production and training duration. The National Weight Control Registry is a database that identifies people who have lost a minimum of 15 kg and have kept the weight off for at least 1 year. Most of these "successful weight loss subjects" exercise for at least 60 minutes a day. Growth hormone is an amazing fat mobilizer, and this may be an important reason why people lose weight during prolonged exercise. Researchers at the University of North Carolina at Greensboro have found that the increase in growth hormone levels during aerobic exercises is directly proportional to the duration of the workout. Growth hormone levels progressively increase with 30, 60 and 120 minutes of exercise. If it lasts more than 120 minutes, the effect is counterproductive. However, it is equally true that HIIT training has a minor negative effect on muscle mass. A study published in the *Journal of Obesity* reported that men who practiced 20 minutes of HIIT pedaling (8 seconds of sprinting with 12 seconds of recovery) three times a week lost 2 kg of fat in 12 weeks and gained 500 g of muscle, obtaining a better result compared to pedaling for 40 minutes three times a week with the equivalent energy expenditure. Obviously, as with all studies, the results need to be contextualized and interpreted. The muscle response in a sedentary obese person in which even just 20 minutes of HIIT can induce an adaptive response, is different from a bodybuilder, who is used to very different stimuli. Furthermore, 40 minutes of exercise at low intensity probably does not represent the necessary time threshold to best activate fat burning and GH production.

As we have seen previously, doing cardio after training has a negative effect on the increase in muscle mass, but doing it before (excessively), can compromise the performance of weight training. However, if the goal is weight loss, it is better to do cardio after weight training, precisely to activate the AMPK pathway which also has a catabolic effect on fat. This was confirmed in a study by sports scientists at the University of Tsukuba and it was published in *Medicine and Science in Sports and Exercise*.

The researchers conducted a trial that included 10 male students with an average age of 23. On one occasion, the students pedaled for 60 minutes (group E) at an intensity of 50% of VO_2 max, which is equivalent to a slightly more intense effort than pedaling calmly, but it still allows you to talk without the slightest breathing difficulty. On another occasion, subjects performed weight training before cycling. The workout consisted of four sets of shoulder presses, flyes, bicep curls, squats, bench presses and lat pulldowns, all performed with weights that barely allowed the subjects to complete 10 repetitions. After they rested for 20 minutes (group RE20), they did aerobic training; then, on another occasion, they rested for 120 minutes (RE120 group) after weight training and then performed aerobic training. The final result was that subjects in the RE20 group lost more fat than the E and RE120 groups (Fig. 28.1).

Researchers believe that this is due to the release of adrenaline and norepinephrine during weight training, which promotes lipolysis at the cellular level by releasing circulating fatty acids. Another advantage is that doing cardio after weight training results in better stimulation of GH, which is a powerful lipolytic hormone, while some studies have verified that GH production in athletes who performed cardio before weight training fell short of expectations. The researchers concluded that their study demonstrates that fat utilization for energy purposes is increased when submaximal cardio is performed after weight training. However, this effect is only achieved if submaximal cardio is performed after weight training with a short rest.

So, how can we include aerobic training in our daily lives? A study that was recently published in the *Performance Training Journal* reported that post-exercise metabolism increases most when you do cardio first and weightlifting second, which

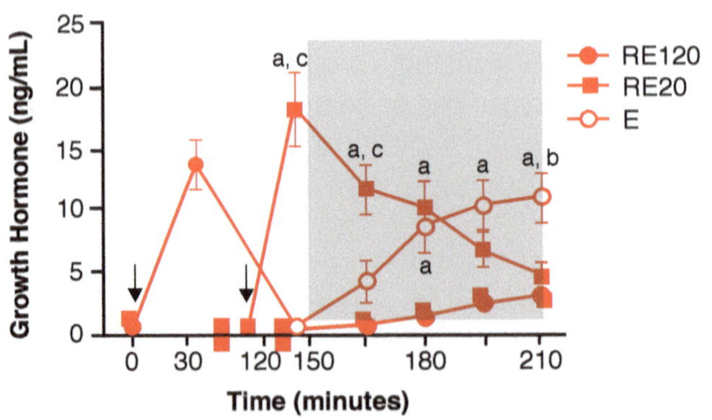

Figure 28.1 Serum growth hormone concentrations during three types of exercise regimens. The arrows in the graph indicate the time points of resistance exercise in the RE120 and RE20 trials. Submaximal exercise is indicated as a shaded area. (Modified by: Goto K et al. Effects of Resistance Exercise on Lipolysis during Subsequent Submaximal Exercise. *Med Sci Sports Exec.* 2007 Feb;39(2): 308-15)

could have an impact on the total daily fat oxidation. This is interesting news, however, we must consider that doing aerobic exercise first could compromise the quality of weight training because it consumes energy and causes muscle fatigue. It is also true that doing it afterwards activates the AMPK pathway, which has a catabolic effect.

These considerations make us aware that if we want to both increase muscle mass with weight training and do aerobic exercise to maintain lower levels of subcutaneous fat, it would be advisable to distance the two types of training. Considering that the stimulation of mTOR following weight training lasts for at least 5 hours, it would be appropriate to distance any aerobic activity that activates AMPK, which in turn inhibits mTOR.

The general rule is that if you do aerobic training before weight training, you will be using up glycogen during cardio, whereas if you train with weights, you will be depleting the glycogen reserves in this first part of the training, and then when you move on to aerobics, you will burn more fat at the subcutaneous level. The fact that, while subcutaneous fat decreases more with the stimuli given by aerobic training combined with weight training, visceral fat responds better to the stimuli provided by diet (primarily a decrease in carbohydrate intake) should not be underestimated.

Almost always, attention is mistakenly directed mainly towards the subcutaneous fat, but it is of fundamental importance to get rid of visceral fat as soon as possible, which is very dangerous as it increases the risk of cancer (colorectal, breast), type 2 diabetes, insulin resistance, high blood pressure, sleep apnea and cardiovascular disease, and it is often related to metabolic syndrome.

The factors that favor the formation of visceral fat most are stress, poor quality of sleep and foods with a high glycemic load. It has also been established that people with persistently high blood glucose levels have large amounts of visceral fat.

Visceral fat, fortunately, is a fat that is generally lost quickly if you follow an appropriate diet and if you train and pursue a healthy lifestyle.

In addition to visceral fat and subcutaneous fat, it is good to pay attention to perivascular fat, which is the fat found inside the arteries. Yudkin's research shows that perivascular fat produces signal molecules that interfere with insulin and alter blood flow in arterioles in response to insulin, another confirmation of the correlation between blood flow and localized fat.

Now let's move on to the last aspect concerning cardio, fasted cardio. Slimming protocols often recommend training in the morning on an empty stomach. This suggestion is appropriate, but it is not always motivational or, to say it better, it depends on the circumstances. The timing of physical exercise is closely linked to the nutritional state in which the body is found, therefore it is clear that if you train in the morning, after fasting overnight, the body will tend to use fat for energy. In this condition, in terms of substrates, we find a very low availability of sugars, which forces the body to use fats. Researchers at the University of Bath, including Dylan Thompson and Yung-Chich Chen, have found that fasting for 12 hours before a 1-hour brisk walk leads to greater fat mobilization and increases gene activity in adipocytes compared to consuming a meal 2 hours before training.

Eating before exercising inhibits long-term adaptation to fat use in endurance exercises. Therefore, this is an ideal moment for aerobic training, but since cortisol levels tend to be higher in the morning, it is also a bad moment for physical activities that use weights that are particularly intense and, if performed in this part of the day, could lead to a catabolic condition instead of having an anabolic benefit.

In conclusion, given the organic hormonal conditions and their timing, **it is more productive to do aerobic exercise in the morning** to ensure that fat is burnt more efficiently, and **physical activity with weights in the late afternoon or, in any case, towards the evening**, where we find a hormonal condition more favorable to anabolism, always carefully evaluating the morphological and psychophysical characteristics of the subject.

Regarding the calculation of the maximum heart rate and exercise prescription, the internationally validated formulas are given below:

1. HRmax = 220 – age in years (for men)
2. HRmax = 226 – age in years (for women), or:
3. HRmax = 227 – age in years (for women)
4. To evaluate the maximum heart rate, other researchers propose a different formula for adults: FCmax = (210 – 0.5) × age in years
5. Another formula according to Liesen et al.: HR training = (180 beats/min – age in years) + 5 beats for each decade of age starting from the third decade of life
6. HRR (Heart Rate Reserve) or Karvonen formula = [(220 – age – RHR) × % of chosen intensity] + RHR (Rest Heart Rate)
7. Ball State University formulas, very popular in the USA:
   - HRmax = (214 – 0.8) × age in years (for men)
   - HRmax = (209 – 0.7) × age in years (for women)
8. "Pulse rate" formula according to Martin et. to the. (1989): training heart rate = HRmax – (0.45 × HR at rest)
9. Tanaka's formula: HRmax = 208 – (0.7 × age in years)
10. Mellerowicz (1985) formula:
    - HRmax = (170 bpm – age in years) for adults
    - HRmax = (180 b/min – age in years) for young individuals
11. Cerretelli formula, for both sexes: HRmax = 216 – (1.1 × age in years)
12. Formula for determining the optimal and subjective HR training: HR training = HRrest + 0.6 × (HRmax – HRrest)
13. The formula for calculating training HR in swimming: [(% prescribed HRmax) × (HRmax –13*)]; * where 13 is a fixed correction factor
14. The Conconi test, a test with increasing loads, correlates the presumed FCmax detected in the so-called deflection point to the presumed anaerobic threshold; however, this has no correlation with the HRmax estimated in tests for individuals with sedentary lifestyles. Therefore, this cannot be taken as a model for FT (Fitness Test), but only for athletes

CHAPTER 29

Targeting fat loss

Massimo Spattini and Riccardo Gaspari

When we talk about *spot reduction* or targeted fat loss, it is very important to clarify that it is not a matter of losing weight only in specific regions, but rather of increasing lipolysis even in the areas where fat is more stubborn. The cornerstone of concept is to promote local vasodilation at the level of the capillary circle of the adipose tissue overlying the activated muscle, which favors an imbalance at the level of fatty acid esterification, thus limiting their accumulation in the target areas.

The two biggest mistakes that are still being made today are: thinking that targeted fat loss does not exist and that it is a topic exclusive to females. We will now look at some of the most important scientific research that has amply demonstrated the validity of targeted fat loss to understand to what extent its indications are also applicable to bodybuilding.

Before delving into the world of targeted fat loss, let's discuss the importance of **angiotensin II**, a topic that we will discuss in depth later. A study published in the *Journal of Physiology* proved the existence of a hormone, angiotensin II, produced by adipose tissue that is capable of reducing blood flow, thus causing the inhibition of fat burning in adipose tissue and skeletal muscle. Therefore, when blood flow is low, there is an increase in the production of angiotensin II.

This hormone stimulates an increase in fat not only by reducing blood flow, but also by stimulating α_2 receptors and is therefore decisive in increasing the activity of some enzymes responsible for the accumulation of fat and for the increase of insulin resistance. A good method to reduce the α_2 antilipolytic receptors, ensuring a decrease in stubborn fat levels, consists in following a low-carb diet for 4 days which does not contain more than 20% of total carbohydrates and is richer in fat compared to normal diets: this will allow us to deactivate the α_2-agonist receptors, i.e., the antilipolytic ones.

Negative factors that increase angiotensin II levels are smoking, high-fat diets, high estrogen levels and stress. In terms of dietary approaches, the best nutritional approach in the search for targeted fat loss is undoubtedly the **COM Diet**, an acronym for the Italian "CronOrMorfodieta", which is based on personalization, focusing on hereditary characteristics, metabolic and hormonal influences, dietary habits and environmental factors that affect everyone's life; this approach identifies a specific diet which can help each person achieve their best physical shape and health status, maintainable for life. The two pillars on which the ChronHorMorphodiet (from CHRONobiology, HORmones and MORPHOlogy) is based are a normocaloric diet in relation to the basal metabolic rate and physical activity. The innovation of the COM Diet lies in identifying how to achieve targeted fat loss, proposing diets that take into consideration the person's morphology and the rhythms that regulate hormones and metabolism. This leads to the extreme customization of the COM Diet which bases all its foundations on the characteristics of the individual. Starting from the morphology of the individual (pear, apple or pepper shape), the COM Diet has identified four main categories of subjects, the hyperlipogenetic, the hypolipolytic, the hypermixed and the hypomixed.

The accumulations of fat in different areas of the body are determined by the hormonal structure and the individual's eating habits, therefore hormones and food choices condition each other, resulting in accumulations of fat in specific parts of the body. Another crucial fact, which should not be underestimated, is that hormone secretion varies throughout the day, so even the intake of certain foods at different times of day has different effects on the accumulation of fat. This points to the extreme importance of the timing of food intake.

Given the link between nutrition and the hormonal system, food timing is crucial for achieving success in a dietary program designed for fat loss. There are countless studies that show that the decrease in body fat depends on the time of food intake, rather than the number of calories; therefore, the aspects of a diet (food composition and their distribution during the day) have a direct influence on body fat, which is independent of the quantity and, consequently, of the number of calories.

Given that the vast majority of hormones are not secreted on a regular basis during the day, but follow a well-defined circadian rhythm and vary during the day, thus conditioning and determining the distribution of fat, we can say with certainty that **by acting on all these variations, it is possible to manipulate, and therefore change, the distribution of fat in the human body**.

But let's go back to where we were: in addition to our publications (*The Com Diet and Spot reduction*, and dozens of other articles), further research and studies have confirmed the validity of training methods based on targeted fat loss. I would like to begin by mentioning a piece of research carried out by Dr. Marco Neri and by Prof. Antonio Paoli of the Nutrition & Exercise Physiology Laboratory at the Department of Biomedical Sciences, University of Padua and by that by Dr. Bente Stallknecht of the Panum Institute in Copenhagen: their studies have shown that exercising with a higher number of repetitions and heavier weights reduce localized fat deposits.

A research study from 1994, carried out by the team of Italian researchers Dussini, Neri, Paoli and Velussi, which illustrated a particular method of aerobic circuit training for the localized reduction of fat, was published in the *European Journal of Physiology*. It demonstrated how the selective stimulation of certain body areas, given by a circuit training consisting of weights and aerobics, performed continuously without any breaks, reduced skin folds in the targeted regions more than traditional aerobic training. To corroborate this research, in addition to the fact that moderate aerobic intensity (65-70% HRmax) allows for an increase in lipid expenditure, we can also mention that in periods of active recovery (the aerobic phase) there is a predominant passage towards the aerobic system, i.e. an energy system that allows for significant acute oxidation of fat deposited in adipose tissue, without forgetting that weight training recruits the muscle groups distributed in the areas in which it is intended to reduce localized fat. The alternation between aerobic activity and weights stimulates the circulatory system which leads to a greater outflow of liquids from the areas in which these are excess.

In a study carried out by Dussini et al., a total of 48 moderately trained male and female subjects aged 17 to 30 years were tested. They were divided into two groups, one experimental group (16 males, 14 females) and one control group (15 males, 13 females). The study involved three training sessions per week, similar in terms of exercises, but with a different training setting. The experimental group, i.e., individuals in which the spot reduction method was tested, performed Aerobic Circuit Training (ACT) consisting of trisets which targeted the parts that were intended to reduce localized fat (triceps, abs, obliques), interspersed with cardio machines (bike or stepper). The aerobic portion of this program was 28 minutes long. At the end of the circuit, the upper body muscles, which had not been directly exercised previously, were stimulated with traditional weight training (3 sets per exercise and 1 minute of rest between sets).

The control group, on the other hand, performed a workout consisting of weightlifting and cardio performed consecutively. Cardio training was performed in the form of circuit steady state training, with various aerobic stations (stepper, bike, treadmill), which also lasted 28 minutes. The other half of the control group's program was set on regular weight training for the upper body only. All subjects continued to follow their lifestyle, with no nutritional changes, to ensure that the research results could be clearly attributable solely and exclusively to the training program and not to the addition of pre-set external factors, such as the diet. At the end of the 6-week study, both groups experienced significant fat loss.

The proof of the effectiveness of the experimental protocol in terms of targeted fat loss was the greater reduction of skin folds in the muscle areas of the subjects in the spot reduction group (triceps, abdomen, obliques). Furthermore, a significant decrease in thigh folds was found in female subjects of the same study group.

Thanks to the positive findings obtained by Dussini et al. in this study, the name "spot reduction" was attributed to this type of Aerobic Circuit Training (also known as Cardio Fit Training), which has fat loss localized to specific areas of the body as its primary objective. Furthermore, it has been widely observed that the execution of a traditional steady state aerobic program is not optimal for achieving targeted fat loss in the areas stimulated by exercise.

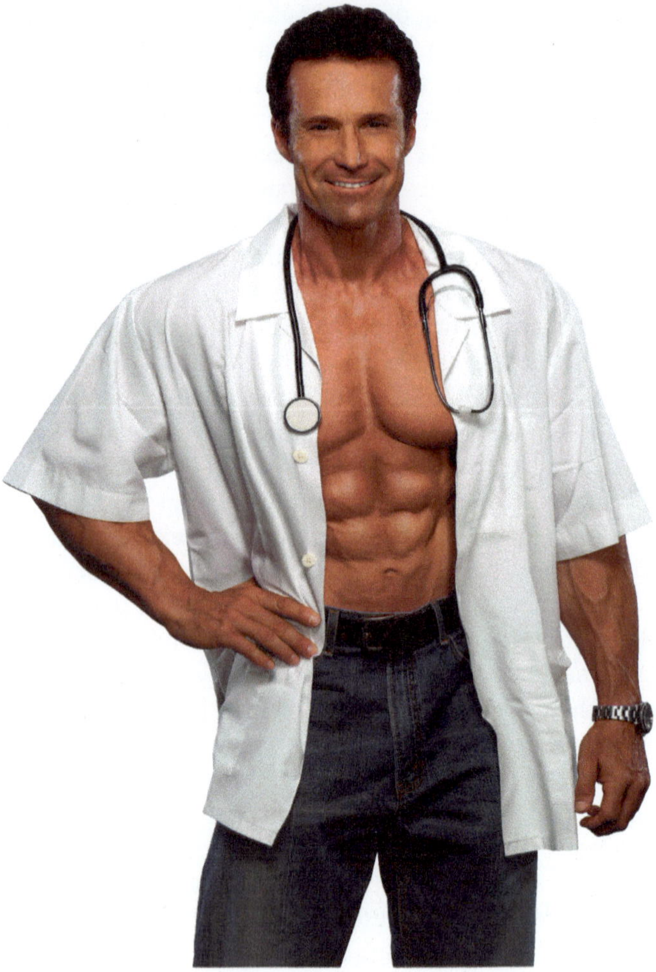

Given the fact that classic aerobic and anaerobic workouts lead to a generalized weight loss with a predetermined fat reduction, the spot reduction methodology aimed to combine aerobic training with typically anaerobic weight training, giving rise to the aerobic circuit training method (ACT) specialized in the reduction of localized fat.

The following table shows the different training protocols performed by the two study groups mentioned above.

Study by Dussini et al. (1994) *	
Study group	**Control group**
Mixed part (spot reduction) • Stationary bike for 8 minutes • Crunch 20 reps • Seated stick twist 100 reps • Push down 20 reps • Stepper 5 minutes • Reverse crunch 20 reps • French press 20 reps • Treadmill 5 minutes • Jackknives 20 reps • Seated stick twist 100 reps • Push down 90° bent torso 20 reps • Stationary bike for 5 minutes	**Aerobic part (steady state training)** • Stationary bike for 8 minutes • Stepper 3 minutes • Treadmill 3 minutes • Stationary bike for 3 minutes • Stepper 3 minutes • Treadmill 3 minutes • Stationary bike for 5 minutes
Anaerobic part (resistance training) • Dumbbell incline bench press 3 × 10 reps, 60 seconds of rest • Front lat pull-up 3 × 10 reps, 60 seconds of rest • Dumbbell lateral raise 3 × 10 reps, 60 seconds of rest • Seated alternating biceps curl 3 × 10 reps, 60 seconds of rest • Stationary bike for 5 minutes	**Anaerobic part (resistance training)** • Dumbbell incline bench press 3 × 10 reps, 60 seconds of rest • Front lat pull-up 3 × 10 reps, 60 seconds of rest • Dumbbell lateral raise 3 × 10 reps, 60 seconds of rest • Seated alternating biceps curl 3 × 10 reps, 60 seconds of rest • French press 3 × 20 reps, 50 seconds of rest • Crunch 3 × 20 reps, 50 seconds of rest • Seated stick twist 1 × 100 reps, 1 second of rest

*Dussini N, Martino R, Neri M, Paoli A, Velussi C. Multifactorial analysis of circuit-training induced regional fat reduction. *Eur J Physiol* 1994;424:R159-R188.

Another study, published in the *American Journal of Physiology*, highlighted some interesting results that seem to indicate that targeted fat loss is actually possible, although it is not clear to what extent.

In a study conducted by the University of Copenhagen (Denmark), researchers had one leg extension exercise performed with a light weight for 30 minutes consecutively, then measured the amount of blood flow in the subjects' subcutaneous fat in both the trained leg and the other leg that was left at rest. They also measured the amount of lipolysis (release of fat) of the fat cells in the subcutaneous tissue. The researchers found that subcutaneous tissue cells of the trained leg experienced a significantly higher increase in blood flow and lipolysis compared to the untrained leg. During the exercise, the fat cells around the trained muscle area released more fatty acids into the blood, meaning that more lipolysis was stimulated in the target area to supply fat for energy. This study suggests that, when training a certain muscle group, you burn fat preferably in the area you are training, especially if you use a high number of repetitions at high intensity with reduced breaks. After the publication of this study, more results appeared on the web under the heading "spot reduction" expressing a positive opinion; however, despite this, the majority of results are still negative.

Another study is often cited by the detractors of the concept of targeted fat loss: 13 men performed targeted abs training for 27 days. They started with 140 repetitions in the first week and reached 336 repetitions at the end of the last week, for a total of 5000 repetitions of sit-ups during the course of the research. The size of the abdominal fat cells in the subscapularis region and the glutes were then measured (by biopsy). This showed that fat had decreased equally at all three sites. But we know, and it is unanimously recognized, that the last areas to lose weight are those in which an individual tends to accumulate fat. In most men, and in some women, the abdominal region is the most resistant, while the glutes, thighs and hips are a problem mostly for women and for some men. Therefore, if we approach this study from this point of view, the fact that the fat loss occurred to the same extent in the abdominals compared to the other regions is already a success, because, in men, the abdominal region has more stubborn subcutaneous fat. In order to draw a definitive conclusion, the researchers should have used a control group with morphological characteristics similar to those of the study group, or they should have used the same group in a subsequent phase and subjected them only to a low-calorie diet without training.

Well, we are convinced – and our decennial experience confirms it – that in this case, the percentage of fat loss would have penalized the abdominal region since it is precisely the most resistant region in most men. On the other hand, if the accumulation of differentiated fat in specific areas is a fact, why can't the same be said for fat loss in specific areas? Recent research on obesity has shown that blood flow is highly dependent on localized fat accumulation. Excess local fat tissue increases the so-called "perivascular fat," which is the fat inside the arterioles. Excessive perivascular fat produces signaling molecules that interfere with insulin and alter blood flow in arterioles in response to insulin (Yudkin, 2005). This means two things:

1. If you gain fat in a certain area of the body, the excess carbohydrates will more likely be stored as fat in that region
2. This implies a close correlation between vasodilation and localized fat accumulation

Put simply, research suggests that there is a relationship between excess localized fat, which impairs the vasodilation of arterioles, and the promotion of localized fat. For this reason, if you are trying to lose weight, the areas where there is more fat are disadvantaged. Anyone who has followed weight loss diets will have noticed that it is easier to lose fat in certain parts of the body than in others. New research on vasodilation and fat accumulation suggests that areas of the body where more fat has accumulated have impaired vasodilation which makes it more difficult to get rid of fat there. The reduced blood flow to adipose tissue is known to be a major cause of the non-mobilization of fat. Fat mobilization requires a rich blood supply blocking blood flow in the adipose tissue is equivalent to having a knot in hose while watering the lawn: the flow is reduced. As mentioned above, the study published in the *Journal of Physiology* proved the existence of a hormone produced by adipose tissue that can reduce blood flow to adipose tissue, cause impairment of nutrient blood flow, and inhibit the burning of fat in visceral adipose tissue and skeletal muscle. In the past, adipose tissue was considered only a deposit of fat; however, it has been clearly shown to produce a variety of hormones that exert multiple effects. It is currently known that more than one hundred substances are secreted by adipose tissue, which are part of a wide range of protein families, as well as fatty acids and prostaglandins. Adipose tissue is highly vascular and contains many blood vessels, meaning it has a rich blood supply.

It has been recognized that the blood flow to adipose tissue is not constant and that it increases during periods of stress (diet or exercise), when the need for lipid mobilization increases. Compared to other tissues in the body, white adipose tissue can dramatically change cell size over time, depending on caloric intake. The creation of new fat cells is always accompanied by an increase in the number of blood vessels. A new fat cell is like a newborn baby, it needs nutrients to grow, and that means it needs new blood vessels to carry nutrients to its hungry mouth. Conversely, the hypertrophy of old fat cells produces no change in blood vessel formation. Both the storage and mobilization of fat are tightly controlled by blood flow. In order to burn body fat, adipose tissue must be able to release stored triglycerides into the blood. The fact that there is a reduction in the blood supply to adipose tissue in obese people compared to leaner people which could be the result of an increase in the production of angiotensin II produced in adipose tissue, has attracted a lot of interest. Being overweight is associated with many metabolic disorders, but a common problem with obesity is high blood pressure. When weight and fat gain occur, the body tries to restore the correct weight by increasing the production of catecholamines or adrenaline to burn fat. It is known that adrenaline and catecholamines not only increase fat mobilization, but they also increase blood pressure through the increased activation of the nervous system. Long-term activation of the sympathetic nervous system is thought to be one of the keys to the underlying mechanisms of hypertension and associated obesity.

Angiotensin II is a powerful hormone that increases blood pressure by causing vasoconstriction (when blood vessels narrow, the blood supply is restricted or slowed down). Many people with high blood pressure are treated with drugs called ACE inhibitors, which slow down the activity of enzymes that decrease the production of angiotensin II. As a result, blood vessels dilate or enlarge, and blood pressure is reduced. It has recently been documented that angiotensin II is present in both white and brown adipose tissue cells. In a recent study, injections of angiotensin II into subcutaneous adipose tissue led to an inhibition of fat mobilization in healthy volunteers. When you want to increase fat burning, having a rich blood supply facilitates the mobilization of fat from adipose tissue. It has been shown that when angiotensin II is infused into the forearm during exercise, it reduces the blood supply to it. This effect of reduced fat burning could be, at least partially, dependent on the vasoconstriction capacity of angiotensin II in the subcutaneous adipose tissues. Angiotensin II reduces blood flow to the adipose tissue in a dose-dependent manner (the more angiotensin II is produced by adipose tissue, the lower the blood flow to adipose tissue will be). Interestingly, blood flow to adipose tissue is lower in obese subjects and weight reduction is followed by an increase in the adipose tissue blood flow. In addition, approximately 5% weight loss led to a 20% reduction in angiotensin II in the adipose tissue. Reducing angiotensin II via the pharmacological blockade with ACE inhibitors in obese people will not only lower their blood pressure, but it will also increase the blood flow to the adipose tissue, resulting in weight loss.

Angiotensin II not only reduces the blood supply to adipose tissue, thereby inhibiting fat burning, but it can also stimulate fat mass gain through the following mechanisms:

- angiotensin II stimulates α_2 adrenoceptors, which inhibit the mobilization of fats; an increase in α_2 receptors translates into an increase in fat storage
- angiotensin II also increases the storage activity of enzymes which accumulate fats (glycerol-3-phosphate dehydrogenase and fatty acid synthetase)
- angiotensin II causes insulin resistance in large fat cells and an increase in lipid storage. Administration of ACE inhibitors (angiotensin II production blockers) has been shown to improve insulin sensitivity and also to reduce fat mass
- angiotensin II levels are increased by plasma cortisol, smoking, a high-fat diet and estrogens

A team of researchers from the University Medical Center Hamburg-Eppendorf led by Prof. Bamberger, director of the Medical Prevention Center Hamburg, verified the effectiveness of the Hypoxi Method, which is based on the combination of treatments that exploit the alternation of positive and negative pressure ("vacuum effect"), promoting peripheral circulation, and slimming exercises on a sample of 20 overweight women and 16 men, aged between 30 and 50, dividing them into two groups. The first group had to complete a 4-week cycle of exercises on a conventional cycle ergometer or treadmill, while the second group had to do the same exercises with the vacuum effect of the Hypoxi Method.

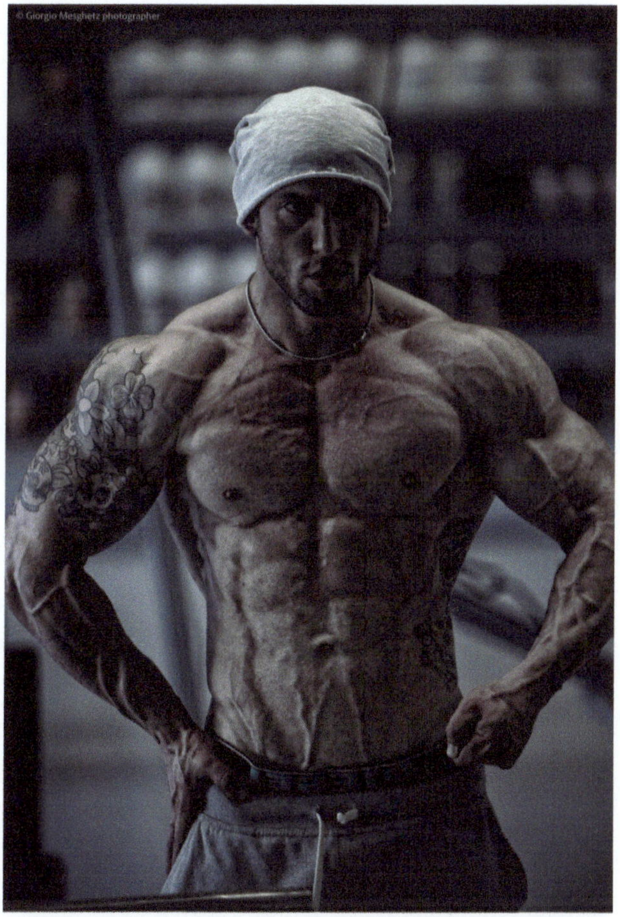

The checks conducted after 4 weeks showed that the subjects of the Hypoxi group, both women and men, obtained significantly better results on the localized reduction of circumference: women that were part of the Hypoxi group lost an average of 13.1 cm around the hips, glutes and thighs, while those who did traditional exercises showed a reduction of the same areas by 4.8 cm. For men, however, the critical areas that were treated and analyzed were the abdomen and hips: in this case, the Hypoxi group recorded 9.4 cm reduction in circumference compared to a 2.9 cm reduction in the first group. All of this indicates that localized exercise that stimulates blood flow to the area where fat is stored can have the effect of relieving local vasoconstriction caused by excess fat. Furthermore, it suggests the possibility of improving the ability to burn fat in a specific area simply by increasing blood flow by any method. Thus, any system (exercise first) that can increase blood flow to a certain area has a positive effect on insulin sensitivity and, as a result, allows for burning fat in "problematic" areas at a faster rate, which can be equal to that of "non-problematic" areas.

Another noteworthy study demonstrating the real effectiveness of targeted fat loss, was the one carried out by Italian researchers Alessandro Scotto di Palumbo, Enrico Guerra, Carmine Orlandi, Ilenia Bazzucchi and Massimo Sacchetti, published in *The Journal of Sports Medicine and Physical Fitness* (2017).

Scotto di Palumbo and his collaborators verified the possibility of reducing a localized fat mass through training programs focused on specific body regions.

Sixteen inactive women (age: 31 ± 4, BMI: 27.5 ± 2.1), i.e., doing less than 1 hour of physical activity per week, were recruited and randomly assigned to two different groups. The first group was labeled Upper and performed upper-body weight training followed by aerobic training, featuring circuit exercises for the lower body.

The second group was named Lower and performed weight training for the lower body and, subsequently, aerobic training with exercises for the upper body, always repeated in circuits. After their respective weight training sessions (which consisted of 5 exercises, each of 3 sets, for 10 repetitions performed explosively, i.e. emphasizing the speed of the movement, with 30 seconds of rest between sets), both groups had to perform a 30-minute aerobic workout with 50% VO_2 max. The study lasted 12 weeks and training was repeated three times a week. The authors hypothesized that the combination of exercises involving different body regions could induce different effects on localized body composition, which they were able to prove. At the end of the study it was found that the Upper group had a greater reduction in fat mass in the upper limbs than in the lower limbs. In contrast, in the Lower group, the fat loss was more significant in the lower body. The measurement was obtained both by DEXA and by the evaluation of the triceps fold and the quadriceps fold of the thigh. The significant difference found in this study than in previous investigations was the combined use of weight-bearing exercises and aerobic exercise. Therefore, it is necessary to explain how this could make a difference mechanically.

The focus of this entire discussion is blood circulation. It has been hypothesized that fat mobilization is hindered, to some extent, when there is poor blood circulation to a specific area of the body. Likewise, muscle exercise has been shown to increase blood flow to adipose tissue in nearby areas. Therefore, it is plausible that specific muscular work favors the mobilization of local adipose tissue reserves to a greater extent compared to adipose tissue reserves in other areas of the body (you will certainly have noticed how even really overweight people still have a low amount of subcutaneous fat in their forearms and calves. Generally, these are the leanest areas of the body and they are also the ones where muscles are most often contracted, thus favoring blood flow).

The result is always the same: **the greater the blood flow, the less fat is accumulated and vice versa.**

In April 2020, a very interesting article was published in the *International Journal of Medicine and Health Development*, which was the result of a study conducted at the University of Nigeria.

The researchers, in particular, wanted to study the effect on muscle mass and localized fat of two specific exercises for the glutes: squats and donkey kicks. The controlled-randomized study involved 111 women aged between 18 and 30, who were divided into three different experimental groups who followed a predetermined training program for 6 weeks:

- 1st group: squat (SG)
- 2nd group: donkey kick (DKG)
- 3rd group: control (CG) (no intervention)

The Squat group performed a workout structured as follows three times a week:

- 5 minutes warm-up
- 5 sets of 20 reps of squat with a 5 kg barbell, with a 2-minute break between sets (for a total of 100 reps)
- 5 minutes of stretching and a final cool-down

The Donkey kick group performed a training structured as follows three times a week:

- 5 minutes warm-up
- 5 sets of 20 reps per leg of donkey kicks using 2.5 kg ankle straps, with a 2-minute break between sets (100 reps per side, for a total of 200 reps)
- 5 minutes of stretching and a final cool-down

It is interesting to note how, in the sample of subjects used for the study, the researchers followed the principle of *progressive overload*: in phase 1 (weeks 1-3) they used a load equal to 5 kg for the squats and 2.5 kg for the donkey kick; in phase 2 (weeks 4-6) they used a weight equal to 10 kg for the squat and 5 kg for the donkey kick.

At the beginning, in the middle (third week) and at the end (sixth week) of the program, the following parameters were measured:

- strength of the gluteal muscles (GMS)
- muscle mass of the glutes (GMB)
- adiposity located in the glutes (GA)

The comparison between these groups revealed **a statistically significant difference in the glutes for parameters related to glutes fat, glutes strength and glutes muscle mass.**

In particular, it was noticed that the group of women who performed **the squat had a greater increase in the strength and growth of the glutes**, while the group of women who performed **the donkey kick obtained significant results in terms of localized adiposity**.

In conclusion, the researchers stated that a training program including squats and donkey kicks can be used to increase glute strength and toning and to decrease surrounding fat tissue in young women.

The study carried out by Paoli et al. (2021) further demonstrates the validity and feasibility of targeted fat loss theories. The researchers, starting from the assumption that performing physical activity regularly has a strong influence on body composition, reducing fat mass and improving the individual's state of health, selected 14 subjects and divided them into two groups; both groups trained with a frequency of three training sessions per week following a protocol with the same types of exercises, duration and volume, but with different execution and recovery times between one exercise and another.

The targeted fat loss (SR, Spot Reduction) group underwent a circuit training consisting of abs, triceps and aerobics training, and targeted the remaining muscle groups with traditional overload training (the mobilization of localized subcutaneous fat was stimulated by target exercises and fat oxidation was ensured by aerobics); the control group (RT, Resistance Training), on the other hand, first performed all the aerobic exercises, and then moved on to resistance training.

Spot Reduction Group (SR)		
Exercises	**Sets × Reps/Time**	**Recovery**
Treadmill	5 minutes	–
Crunch	20 reps	–
Dumbbell overhead extension	15 reps	–
Bike	5 minutes	–
Crunch	20 reps	–
Dumbbell overhead extension	15 reps	–
Step	5 minutes	–
Crunch	20 reps	–
Dumbbell overhead extension	15 reps	–
Treadmill	5 minutes	–
Crunch	20 reps	–
Dumbbell overhead extension	15 reps	–
Bike	5 minutes	–
Dumbbell flat bench press	3 × 10	60 seconds
Lat pulldown	3 × 10	60 seconds
Shoulder press	3 × 10	60 seconds
Curl	3 × 12	45 seconds
Leg press	3 × 10	60 seconds
Leg extension	3 × 12	45 seconds

Continues

Continued

Control group (RT)		
Exercises	**Sets × Reps/Time**	**Recovery**
Treadmill	5 minutes	–
Bike	5 minutes	–
Step	5 minutes	–
Treadmill	5 minutes	–
Bike	5 minutes	–
Dumbbell flat bench press	3 × 10	60 seconds
Lat pulldown	3 × 10	60 seconds
Shoulder press	3 × 10	60 seconds
Curl	3 × 12	45 seconds
Dumbbell overhead extension	4 × 15	45 seconds
Leg press	3 × 10	90 seconds
Leg extension	3 × 12	60 seconds
Crunch	4 × 20	45 seconds

The premise of the study was to verify spot reduction in the abdomen and triceps areas, which corresponded to the target exercises in the SR circuit. At the end of the study there was a notable decrease in body mass in the SR group, but not in the specific RT group, and the body fat percentage of the individuals showed a notable decrease only in the SR group; skinfold measurements reported by the RT group revealed no difference, while significant reductions in the suprailiac and subscapularis landmarks were reported in the SR group, but no direct effect was observed on triceps measurements.

The authors hypothesize that it is possible that, due to their beginner level, the participants engaged the stabilizer muscles of the shoulder and scapula more than the triceps when performing the dumbbell overhead extension exercise, thus reducing its effect on the specific site.

The study, however, confirms what has already been argued for some time, specifically that lipolytic activity is associated with an increase in blood flow in the adipose tissue and, therefore, with the oxygenation of the adipocyte.

Another very important factor that emerged from the study is that in order to reduce the body mass, the intensity of training is more important as a variable compared to the type of exercise. Training intensity can be changed in several ways: by increasing the loads or the level of oxygen consumption, but also by reducing the rest intervals or by altering the speed of movement. In the initial part of the mixed circuit of the SR protocol, the subjects did not rest between the exercises, which increased the overall metabolic demand of the workout.

We also know how body fat distribution divides overweight gynoid and overweight android morphotypes. As the name indicates, the android morphotype is generally more common in male individuals and it usually refers to men who accumulate subcutaneous fat particularly on the abdomen and in the lumbar region. It is easier to lose weight in the upper part of the body than in the lower part (yes, men are luckier in this case!), and this happens because the subcutaneous fat of the upper part is more sensitive to lipolytic processes than the subcutaneous fat of the lower part; precisely for this reason, the subcutaneous fat of the abdominal region responds better to caloric restriction and training which, in this case, can be a sufficient solution. Undoubtedly, hormones are the basis of this different distribution of fat, above all testosterone and cortisol which are at the basis of the android morphotype; according to the various circumstances, these hormones can favor or limit the accumulation of fat in certain regions of the body.

Adipose tissue is highly vascularized and blood flow increases with exercise as the need for fat mobilization increases. In order to use body fat for energy purposes, the adipose tissue must be able to release the fatty acids that come from lipolysis into the bloodstream.

The lipolytic effect caused by diet and training is mainly mediated by catecholamines, which are mainly responsible for lipolysis, while the others, such as GH, sex hormones, cortisol and thyroid hormones, are mostly synergistic. Catecholamines, i.e. adrenaline and noradrenaline, exert their lipolytic effect by binding to receptors distributed in the adipose tissue. The most important receptors for the lipolytic processes are β_2 and α_2; a lipolytic effect is obtained by stimulating the former, while by stimulating the latter, lipolysis is inhibited. Hence the distribution of these receptors in the adipose tissue is very important, since, if β receptors prevail in a specific area of the body, there will be a good level of lipolysis; vice versa, if the α prevail, this will not exist (it is important to remember that the sex hormone testosterone increases β receptors in the abdomen).

Let's be frank: the goal of every "fitness addicted" or "fitness oriented" individual is to get particularly fit to achieve a low percentage of body fat to highlight muscle definition but, above all, the so-called "six-pack", i.e. sculpted abs. It is clear that this can be achieved through an intensification of training, both aerobic and anaerobic, training localized at the abdominal level, a diet with both qualitative and quantitative restrictions, and also the use of supplements that promote lipolysis.

Unfortunately, the common idea is that it is enough to make changes to diet and supplementation to solve the problem of abdominal fat, but the truth is that, on the contrary, what is extremely useful is to find training strategies that can promote blood circulation critical areas (in our case, the abdomen).

In light of the above, we can confidently say that a localized physical exercise that stimulates blood flow in the area with excess fat can have the effect of relieving the local vasoconstriction caused by this excess.

We will see shortly how to deal with a workout that increases blood flow in our "resistant" area (the abdomen), increasing its ability to burn fat at a rate equal to that of the "more responsive" areas and simultaneously maintaining an important hypertrophic stimulus on other areas of the body to avoid finding ourselves with a defined abdomen, but without muscles in the rest of the body. In this phase, even more than in the others, it is of great help to rely on the indications of the COM Diet which, based on constitutional biotypes, will allow us to maximize our workouts.

Following a low-calorie food plan is absolutely necessary to achieve our goal of having a defined six-pack for the following reasons: a person who "goes on a diet" will lose weight faster in the areas that are already thinner; fat contained in the adipocytes is not stable but in continuous renewal (it is completely renewed every 3 weeks); with a normocaloric diet, a lot of fat is released and a lot of it is re-synthesized (a lot of fat leaves the adipose cell and a lot goes back there, and this renewal mechanism also occurs when there is a calorie deficit, but in this case, the input is lower than the output).

A man who diets to sculpt a great set of abs will certainly decrease his waistline, but the "love handles" and that fat that hides between his abs will not go away that easily. This is due to the fact that a large amount of fat loss occurs at the expense of visceral intra-abdominal fat and not subcutaneous fat, which "covers" the abs. If all the fat came from the subcutaneous region, our abs would be evident in a few weeks, and this result could be achieved by increasing the workout intensity of target areas and by maximizing blood circulation, thus limiting the esterification of fatty acids, which are necessary for depositing fat. Let's put this targeted work into practice.

Example 1 of Men's Spot Reduction Workout

Trained muscles: chest, deltoids, triceps

- **Circuit 1** (repeat 5 times without rest): chest press (4-6 reps) + crunch (maximum possible reps) + reverse crunch (maximum possible reps) + cardio 75-80% (1 minute)
- **Circuit 2** (repeat 4 times without rest): incline bench press (8-10 reps) + crunch (maximum possible reps) + reverse crunch (maximum possible reps) + cardio 75-80% (1 minute)
- **Circuit 3** (repeat 3 times without rest): pectoral machine (10-12 reps) + crunch (maximum reps possible) + reverse crunch (maximum reps possible) + cardio 75-80% (1 minute)
- **Circuit 4** (repeat 5 times without rest): slow forward (6-8 reps) + cross crunch (maximum possible reps) + V-sit crunch (maximum possible reps) + cardio 75-80% (1 minute)
- **Circuit 5** (repeat 4 times without rest): lateral raise (10-12 reps) + cross crunch (maximum possible reps) + V-sit crunch (maximum possible reps) + cardio 75-80% (1 minute)
- **Circuit 6** (repeat 3 times without pause): close grip bench press (6-8 reps) + jackknife (maximum possible reps) + leg pull up on the bar (maximum possible reps) + cardio 75-80% (1 minute)

Continues

Continued

- **Circuit 7** (repeat 3 times without rest): push down with rope (10-12 reps) + jacknife (maximum possible reps) + leg pull up on the bar (maximum possible reps) + cardio 75-80% (1 minute)

Example 2 of Men's Spot Reduction Workout

Trained muscles: back, posterior deltoids, biceps

- **Circuit 1** (repeat 5 times without rest): deadlift (4-6 reps) + sit-up (maximum possible reps) + Russian twist (maximum possible reps) + cardio 75-80% (1 minute)
- **Circuit 2** (repeat 4 times without rest): rowing (8-10 reps) + sit-up (maximum possible reps) + Russian twist (maximum possible reps) + cardio 75-80% (1 minute)
- **Circuit 3** (repeat 3 times without rest): pull-up (10-12 reps) + sit-up (maximum possible reps) + Russian twist (maximum possible reps) + cardio 75-80% (1 minute)
- **Circuit 4** (repeat 5 times without rest): 90° flyes (6-8 reps) + mountain climber (maximum possible reps) + oblique crunch (maximum possible reps) + 75-80% cardio (1 minute)
- **Circuit 5** (repeat 4 times without rest): chest pulls (10-12 reps) + mountain climber (maximum reps possible) + oblique crunch (maximum reps possible) + cardio 75-80% (1 minute)
- **Circuit 6** (repeat 3 times without rest): barbell curl (6-8 reps) + leg Bar raise (maximum reps possible) + crunch (maximum reps possible) + cardio 75-80% (1 minute)
- **Circuit 7** (repeat 3 times without rest): concentrated curl (10-12 reps) + leg bar raise (maximum reps possible) + crunch (maximum reps possible) + cardio 75-80% (1 minute)

Example 3 of Women's Spot Reduction Workout

Total body training on 5 circuits with a predominance of quadriceps, hamstrings, glutes, abs

- **Circuit 1** (repeat 5 times without rest): squat (3-5 reps) + hip thrust (15-20 reps) + sit-up (maximum possible reps) + reverse grip lat machine (12-15 reps) + steady state cardio (3 minutes)
- **Circuit 2** (repeat 5 times without rest): deadlift (3-5 reps) + adductor
- machine (20-25 reps) + crunch (maximum possible reps) + lateral raises (12-15 reps) + steady state cardio (3 minutes)
- **Circuit 3** (repeat 5 times without rest): 45° leg press (3-5 reps) + squat jumps (15-20 reps) + reverse crunch (maximum possible reps) + pulley
- **Circuit 4** (repeat 5 times without rest): squat (3-5 reps) + hip thrust (15-20 reps) + sit-up (maximum reps possible) + kick back (15 reps) + dumbbell curls (15 reps) + steady state cardio (3 minutes)
- **Circuit 5** (repeat 8 times without rest): walking lunges (30 total steps) + bridge for glutes (30 reps) + sit-up (maximum possible reps) + steady state cardio (2 minutes)

CHAPTER 30

Training timing: Is "when" you train as important as "how" you train?

Massimo Spattini

It's common knowledge that people have preferred times when they can train at their best. It is not easy to generalize and in my clinical practice as a sports doctor and coach I have met people who find it best to train early in the morning, others around noon, and most towards the afternoon/evening. The reasons for these different performances can vary. Individual biorhythms, especially hormonal ones, are different for different people (we know that there are so-called "morning birds" and "night owls") and they depend on contextual situations: for example, a person who has to face a long tiring workday will probably have less psycho-physical energy at the end of the day; a person with a fast metabolism will probably have already consumed the energy from the previous evening's meal in the morning and will need at least a couple of meals to recharge and have a better workout. However, if we want to generalize, I can say that athletic performance capacity is better in the afternoon. This is supported above all by laboratory tests which have highlighted that:

- the **reaction time to visual or auditory stimuli** peaks in the late afternoon, in correspondence with maximum body temperature values. One explanation can be found in the fact that for every degree Celsius (°C) increase in temperature, nerve conduction velocity increases by 2.4 m/s
- **explosive strength** and **maximal strength** are at their highest levels between 4 and 6 pm; the same is true for joint mobility
- **both aerobic** and **anaerobic metabolisms** are higher in the late afternoon when the maximum values of oxygen consumption, pulmonary ventilation, stroke volume and cardiac output are present. In this part of the day, an athlete's resistance to high-intensity exercise and the ability to produce lactate are higher.

A recent study by the University of Birmingham (UK) which included 20 female hockey players and was published in the journal *Current Biology*, shows that athletic performance can vary by 26% throughout the day and that the best time to do sports is late afternoon. Another reason why it may not be a good idea to train as soon as you get up in the morning, especially when the goal is to increase muscle mass, is that

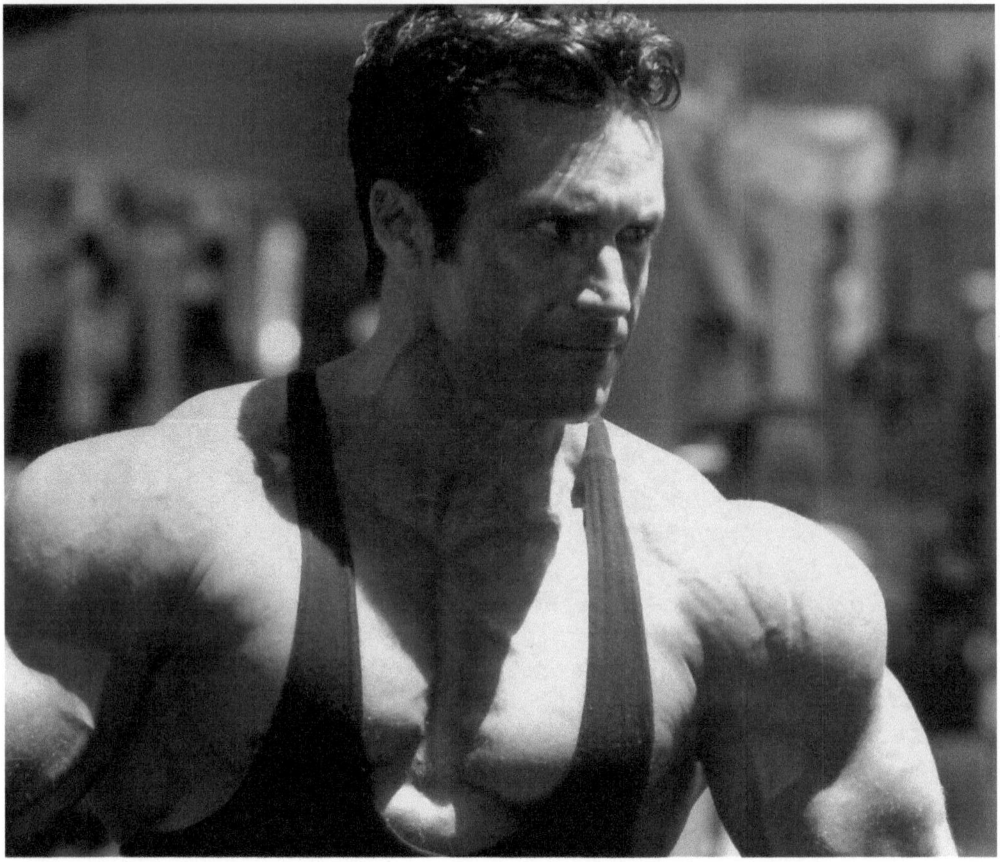

cortisol levels are higher in the morning, especially in certain individuals, and as a result, the catabolic effect of training may dominate.

If, on the other hand, the goal is to increase strength or lose weight, then there is a system used unconsciously by most of us, which alters our biological clock and can drastically increase athletic performance: **caffeine**! To test caffeine's promising ability to improve athletic performance in the morning, Rodriguez et al. tested 12 fit men performing squats and flat bench presses at 75% of maximum weight, at different times of the day, with and without caffeine, in a double-blind placebo experiment. The result was that the group that trained in the afternoon without caffeine was significantly stronger than the group that trained in the morning, which was given the placebo, confirming the negative impact of training in the morning. When both groups received caffeine, there were no significant differences in both squats and bench presses, indicating that caffeine manages to bridge the performance gap between the morning and the afternoon. Caffeine can trigger the AMPK enzyme, an energy regulator at the cellular level, which in turn activates SIRT 1, which is an enzyme that is normally activated by low energy levels (for example, a low-calorie diet), which accelerates the production of energy from fats and glucose. In conclusion, caffeine's ability to stimulate SIRT 1 promotes a better biological clock for a morning workout.

Furthermore, a study carried out by researchers at the University of Toledo (Spain) found that caffeine improves bench press and squat performance when it is administered in the morning more than in the afternoon. Most athletes believe that they perform best in the late afternoon or early evening, but it is difficult to attribute this result to an internal biological clock or to various influencing factors, such as sleep status, nutrition, external environmental factors, etc.

Laboratory conditions are much more stable than the real world, and the variables studied in the laboratory are intentionally dissociated from other variables. Thus, a given percentage of performance variation found in the laboratory may be insignificant in the world of competitive sports. However, if we take into consideration the competitive sector, i.e. the evaluation of performance in a competition, it is important to know that competitive performance is conditioned not only by circadian variations of strength and endurance, but also by innate and acquired skills, by the level of training, motivation, and concentration; as a result, the time of the day when you compete is a secondary factor.

The time of day does not seem to influence overall performance in non-competing athletes either. In one study, 25 subjects who were frequent visitors at a fitness club were examined and they were asked to train at different times of the day. The maximum number of repetitions performed for certain exercises was then evaluated and only a small, non-significant increase in strength was found in the afternoon. Moral of the story: the time of day in which you train is one of many variables that characterize overall performance, but it is not the deciding factor. Consistence, motivation, concentration, rest, nutrition and supplementation can make the circadian rhythm negligible.

Take home message: if you don't have time to train in the evening, "no excuses": get up early, have your coffee and train!

CHAPTER 31

Strength training in bodybuilding

Antonio Squillante

Bodybuilding is a sport that enhances the physical development of an athlete to the extent that muscle mass, highlighted by optimal body composition that tends to minimize subcutaneous fat levels, defines a symmetrical and aesthetically well-proportioned body. The search for robust muscle hypertrophy becomes, without a shadow of a doubt, a necessity for a bodybuilding athlete, while strength training plays a secondary role, which is often overlooked. Over the years, different schools of thought have developed regarding the world of bodybuilding, ranging from supporters of high-volume training, such as Arnold Schwarzenegger and Serge Nubret, to athletes like Mike Mentzer and Dorian Yates who have made high-intensity training a dogma. However, recent studies seem to demonstrate that the intensity of the training stimulus – expressed as a percentage of the maximum (1RM), according to a more rigorous and scientific approach, or as a measure of the muscular effort, according to a pragmatic approach – represents the only confirmed factor to ensure a superior hypertrophic response. As explained by Dr. Carl-Etienne Juneau (2019), a researcher and lecturer at the University of Montreal, muscle growth confirmed depends on co-factors such as training volume and frequency, but these seem to have a degree of variability such as preventing the identification of optimal guidelines; **the only factor that can truly support muscle growth is the intensity of the training stimulus**.

Proper strength training – the method of maximal effort, basic exercises with barbells and loads between 80 and 90% of the maximum, 2-4 sets of 2-5 repetitions per exercise, and complete recovery times lasting an average of 3-5 minutes – aims to improve intramuscular and intermuscular coordination without necessarily producing a significant hypertrophic response. It is also true that a properly structured period of strength training is capable of maximizing an athlete's potential for muscle growth. Training intensity, expressed in terms of absolute (tonnage) or relative (%1RM) training load, seems to play a fundamental role in the regulation of myostatin or Growth Differentiation Factor 8 (GDF-8), a protein produced at the level of muscle cells, which tends to inhibit the processes of protein synthesis, limiting the hypertrophic response to overload training or resistance training.

A lower production of myostatin induced by the application of the overload principle facilitates muscle growth through the inclusion of new genetic material at the level of the muscle fiber itself, often described as *satellite cell-mediated myonuclear addition* (Petrella et al., 2008). Satellite cells are dormant cells normally present and located close to the muscle fiber. The cellular damage induced by particularly vigorous muscle contractions – a prerogative of training for muscle hypertrophy – can stimulate the proliferation of satellite cells, creating the necessary conditions for transferring a part of the genetic material contained in them to the adjacent muscle fibers, whose protein synthesis capacity, controlled by messenger RNA transcription and translation phenomena, can increase (Kadi et al., 2004; MacKenzie et al., 2013). Although it is possible to define an ideal intensity range to stimulate an optimal hypertrophic response (the canonical 8-12 repetitions at 70-80% of the maximum), in the absence of progressively increasing the training stimuli over time (progressive resistance training), the ability to promote appreciable gains in muscle mass decreases significantly. An increase in muscle strength, therefore, can translate over time into significant gains in lean mass where, by virtue of a periodized training program that alternates periods of strength training with periods of training for muscle hypertrophy, an increase in progressive training loads in compliance with adequate recovery times is guaranteed (Rhea et al., 2002). Defining a periodization model that is particularly suited to a bodybuilder's needs is difficult. To date it is not possible to establish a periodization model that is capable of guaranteeing better gains in terms of muscle mass with scientific rigor (Mansor et al., 2014; Rhea and Alderman, 2004). Numerous meta-analyses have concluded that periodized training, i.e. training organized over time in a way that manages the central and peripheral fatigue processes, thus facilitating the supercompensation processes necessary to improve physical performance, produces better results compared to training that lacks adequate organizational rigor (Baker et al., 1994; Kraemer et al., 1996; Stone et al., 1999). However, it is not possible to establish with certainty which, among the numerous periodization models (linear periodization, non-linear periodization, daily undulating periodization, weekly undulating periodization, block periodization or self-regulation) is actually capable of ensuring superior results in terms of physical development.

Regardless of the periodization model adopted, strength training in bodybuilding must respect the following characteristics (Bosco, 1997):

- **Use training loads (intensity) heavier than 80% of the maximum**, increasing the executive speed as much as possible during the concentric phase of the movement. This training method is also known as Compensatory Acceleration Training (CAT) and was made famous in the early 80s by Dr. Frederick C. Hatfield (1942-2017), author of the book *Bodybuilding: A Scientific Approach* (1984). Some studies show that, regardless of the speed of movement, the ability to give the balance wheel maximum voluntary or intentional acceleration, even if the balance wheel moves in a relatively slow and controlled manner, as often happens when using loads heavier than the 80% of the maximum – is able to maximize the number of motor units recruited, producing significantly greater strength gains compared to traditional training (Jones et al., 1999). This technique is often defined as *maximal intended velocity training* (González-Badillo et al., 2014).

- **Adopt a bi-weekly training frequency**, with two sessions at high intensity that include barbell exercises for both the lower and upper limbs (Graham, 2002; Kraemer & Fleck, 2007). If the weekly frequency increases, introduce an active recovery session (60-70% of 1RM) in the 24-48 hours immediately following a session of high-intensity training. You can increase your weekly training frequency by adopting a push-pull split or by simply adopting an approach known as *heavy, medium* and *light*, which involves high-intensity sessions followed by maintenance-load sessions. This approach uses intensities of no more than 90% of the training load and is preceded by sessions with a light load. It can also involve active recovery sessions, for which a training intensity equal to about 80% of the training load is envisaged (Squillante, 2020). Studies conducted in the early 80s on Soviet weightlifters demonstrated how a similar approach to the management of training loads allows for significantly lower blood levels of urea, a marker used in the laboratory to measure muscle damage (catabolism) (Verkhoshansky and Verkhoshansky, 2011).
- **Maintain relatively long recovery times**, 2-3 minutes long, where the goal is to increase the absolute maximum strength, or even a longer rest, of about 4-5 minutes, where the goal is to increase relative maximum strength. Active recovery strategies can be adopted by alternating low-intensity exercises for parts of the body not directly involved in the session. Strength training, even in bodybuilding, can never lead to *muscle failure*. If you need to increase the training volume, you can use *cluster sets*. The term cluster set is used to describe an interrupted set mode whose goal is to manage the progressive build-up of fatigue to maximize force and power levels and/or vertical barbell speed (average/peak). It is a training method that has been used successfully by Eastern European weightlifters for over 30 years, but was only recently made famous in the world of athletic training through the work of Dr. Guy Haff (2016). Cluster sets – also known as interrupted sets – utilize short 15-20 second rest periods between sets of 2-3 reps, up to a total of 18-20 reps per set, with training loads at or above 80% of the maximum (Haff et al., 2008; Morales-Artacho et al., 2018). In this way, relatively stable intracellular levels of creatine phosphate are maintained, while muscular acidosis due to the accumulation of hydrogen ions is avoided.

Regardless of what the ultimate goal is, whether it is aimed at improving physical performance or increasing muscle mass, **it is necessary to specify that hypertrophy and muscle strength are not necessarily synonymous.** While muscle strength is directly proportional to the cross-section of a muscle – which, in physiology, is called Muscle Physiological Cross-Sectional Area (PCSA), i.e. the cross-section of the muscle perpendicular to the orientation of the fibers, which considers the pennation angle and the number of sarcomeres in parallel per unit area – a hypertrophied muscle is not necessarily capable of developing higher levels of strength.

Similarly, we cannot say that a muscle capable of expressing particularly important levels of force is a markedly hypertrophic muscle. The maximum isometric force, i.e., the maximum capacity of a muscle to express force in static contractions, normally measured in the laboratory through the use of dynamometers, depends on a series of unique structural and functional characteristics of the neuromuscular system.

- **Myogenic characteristics**: this term defines a series of structural characteristics concerning the skeletal muscle tissue, strongly conditioned by the genetic makeup of an athlete (genotype). Expressing high levels of muscle strength depends on the unique properties that define muscle composition and architecture. These include the cross-sectional area of the muscle, the pennation angle of the muscle and its tendon insertion, muscle fiber composition and the relative percentage of white or fast-twitch fibers, and finally, the composition of the skeletal muscle tissue itself. The relationship between PCSA and isometric/dynamic muscle strength depends on the percentage of dry muscle tissue, which represents, on average, 20% of lean body mass, and should be taken into consideration. The contractile component of the sarcomere is represented by the protein filaments of actin and myosin and, to a lesser extent, the elements that form the cytoskeleton of the muscle fiber (titin, nebulin, etc.), which make up most of the dry weight of a muscle. Increasing the protein component – i.e., increasing muscle density or the ratio between the contractile component (actin and myosin) and sarcoplasmic volume, a phenomenon known as myofibrillar hypertrophy or functional hypertrophy – corresponds to a more relevant increase in strength. An increase in intracellular water retention is associated with an increase in intramuscular glycogen stores (sarcoplasmic hypertrophy or non-functional hypertrophy), whose impact on physical performance is completely negligible.
- **Neurogenic characteristics**: this term defines a series of functional characteristics that concern the neuromuscular system, which are less influenced by the genetic makeup of a subject and, for this reason, they are easily conditioned with training. The central nervous system is able to modulate the amount of force expressed during static and/or dynamic muscle contractions by altering the number of motor units recruited during near-maximal efforts, intervening at the level of intramuscular and intermuscular coordination. We can identify different types of *intramuscular coordination*, divided into spatial recruitment (i.e. the recruitment of a higher number of motor units), temporal recruitment (i.e. the recruitment of a higher number of motor units in the unit of time), and *intermuscular coordination* (i.e. coordination mechanisms that regulate the synergistic activity of agonist muscle groups and the corresponding relaxation of antagonist muscle groups). Furthermore, levels of muscle force produced can increase when the central nervous system is able to generate action potentials (the nerve stimulus that reaches

the pool of recruited motor units from the primary motor cortex) at a higher frequency. This is traditionally known as "firing rate".

A muscle's ability to express adequate levels of force depends predominantly on the number of actin and myosin filaments that are present at the level of a single muscle fiber and the muscle belly in its entirety. Each cross-bridge – the link between the myosin head and the active site at the level of the actin chain, i.e. the functional complex that regulates muscle contraction according to the sliding filament model described by Andrew Huxley and Hugh Huxley in 1954 (sliding filament theory) – is able to generate from 3 to 6 pN (picoNewton) of force. Consequently, a hypertrophic muscle, i.e. a muscle that has an increased number of actin and myosin filaments in response to an increase in protein synthesis, is a muscle potentially capable of expressing higher levels of strength. In this case, we are talking about structural adaptations, to which it is possible to attribute an important, albeit secondary, role in strength training. Strength training by itself results in an almost negligible hypertrophic response, as demonstrated by Fry et al. (1994) in a longitudinal study of a group of Olympic weightlifters. Data collected over 12 months of strength training in a group of young weightlifters have shown that changes in muscle mass levels are negligible, even completely irrelevant when compared to gains in muscle strength. In 9 male subjects aged between 16 and 18, subjected to a battery of laboratory tests completed 1 year apart, a net increase in body weight of 1.8 kg (2.5%) was recorded against a very modest increase in lean body mass and a modest decrease in body fat levels. In contrast, muscle strength levels demonstrated very substantial increases, equal to 7 kg (12%) in the snatch and 11 kg (10%) in the swing turn (Fry et al., 1994).

Table 31.1 shows the increases in the parameters of maximum relative strength recorded after 12 months and 24 months respectively.

Table 31.1 Strength training in bodybuilding: relative maximal strength

Parameters	12 months	24 months
Body weight (kg)	63.9 ± 3.6	65.7 ± 3.9
Fat-Free Mass (kg)	60.7 ± 3.4	62.5 ± 3.6
Body Fat (%)	5.0 ± 0.3	4.7 ± 0.5
Snatch (1RM)	91.9 ± 7.3	98.9 ± 6.7
Clean & Jerk (1RM)	116.7 ± 8.3	127.8 ± 7.7

Modified from: Fry AC, Kraemer WJ, Gordon SE et al. Endocrine responses to overreaching before and after 1 year of weightlifting. *Canadian Journal of Applied Physiology* 1994;19(4):400-410.

Functional adaptations, on the contrary, play a fundamental role both in athletic training and bodybuilding. Greater intramuscular and intermuscular coordination makes it possible to increase the workload or, with the same training load, this coordination can increase the number of reps, thus increasing the level of intensity during training sessions for muscle hypertrophy. Many authors, including Prof. Emilio They (1939-2000) and Dr. Fred Hatfield (1942-2017), have tried to define the concept of intensity applied to the world of bodybuilding using a pragmatic approach. Their effort has helped outline the importance of what is now defined in the literature as *Resistance Training (RT)-induced skeletal muscle hypertrophy*, or muscle damage induced by resistance training, i.e. by training with overloads. This concept can be quantified scientifically through the measurement of specific inflammatory markers and the histological study of muscle tissue in vivo through needle biopsies. As Dr. Brad Schoenfeld explains in an article published in the scientific journal *The Journal of Strength and Conditioning Research* in 2010, muscle hypertrophy is the product of three physiological conditions required to stimulate an increase in protein synthesis, as listed below.

- **Muscle damage**: tissue-level muscle damage is normally associated with an inflammatory response and is mainly due to this includes a series of microtraumas caused to the contractile and non-contractile structures of the muscle cell. In addition to actin and myosin, this includes a series of supporting structures of the cytoskeleton, often described as "disarray" or the loss of the structural integrity at the level of the sarcomere, which compromises the correct alignment of the myofibrils inside it. This is directly proportional to the degree of tension generated from the muscle during contraction (Mobley et al., 2018). Consequently, the greater the degree of external resistance (%1RM), i.e. the greater the training load and, consequently, the tension that the muscle generates, the greater the degree of muscle damage that is created. Muscle damage increases in a particularly important way where the eccentric component of the movement is emphasized. Numerous studies have demonstrated a significant increase in the concentration of proinflammatory cytokines following training programs with a strong submaximal eccentric component.
- **Mechanical tension**: The degree of mechanical tension represents an independent stimulus for muscle growth. Recent studies have demonstrated how mechanical transduction or mechanotransduction (Hornberger, 2011) represents a powerful anabolic stimulus capable of increasing the levels of protein synthesis by acting at the level of the mTOR complex. Mechanical transduction depends on the time of tension produced during the eccentric phase of the movement, normally indicated as Time Under Tension (TUT), a metric that also includes the times of isometric contraction and possibly the duration times of the concentric phase of the movement. It is possible to correctly quantify the time under tension during submaximal eccentric contractions (60-80% of 1RM), as the training load that can allow for the execution of the concentric phase of the movement.

Erroneously, supramaximal eccentric contractions (100-140% of 1RM) are associated with an increase in protein synthesis processes and, consequently, with an increase in muscle mass. Actually, supramaximal eccentric contractions have a much shorter duration than submaximal eccentric contractions, which are much more suitable for workout programs for muscle hypertrophy. Recent studies have shown that global TUTs of 60-70 seconds per set are optimal for increasing the protein synthesis processes.

- **Metabolic stress**: this term refers to a temporary or transient hypoxic condition, i.e., a condition of insufficient oxygen supply to the muscle tissue, normally associated with anaerobic-lactacid efforts. The more or less complete occlusion of the blood vessels at the level of the muscle belly – a consequence of isotonic-type exercises performed with loads equal to or greater than 30% of the maximum and with a marked isometric component, a prerogative of weight lifting – and/or the use of extremely short recovery times between successive training sets, often lasting an average of 30-60 seconds, favors the establishment of a cellular environment with a reduced pH, stimulating a marked increase in protein synthesis levels (Feriche et al., 2017). Hypoxia generated by normal high-volume training methods is defined as transient because, when the training stimulus disappears, blood flow is restored without compensating the oxygen debt (EPOC). The accumulation of waste metabolites, such as hydrogen or phosphate ions, and cell swelling particularly accentuated by reperfusion (also known as the "pump" associated with high repetition sets performed with incomplete recovery times) create a metabolic environment at the cellular level which is especially suited to supporting an increase in the rate of protein synthesis.

If it is true that the use of training loads greater than 80% of the maximum – a prerogative of strength training, but not necessarily a common approach in the world of bodybuilding – would maximize the mechanical damage at the level of the muscle cell, it is equally true that a reduced number of repetitions per sets, relatively short tension times and complete recoveries would reduce the degree of metabolic stress, making it difficult to obtain appreciable gains in muscle mass. Lighter loads, between 60 and 80% of the maximum, allow for a significant increase in the time under tension, exploiting sets of 6-12 repetitions with an emphasis on the eccentric phase of the movement, for a total of 4-6 seconds per repetition, facilitating the use of incomplete recovery times (60-120 seconds) and therefore supporting a markedly superior hypertrophic response. This approach, known as the Repeated Effort method, is nothing more than a variant of the original DeLorme method proposed in 1951, modified over the years to adapt to the needs of modern bodybuilding, by introducing intensive techniques and high-volume workout protocols such as German Volume Training (GVT). Table 31.2 shows the traditional work parameters for the Repeated Effort method:

Table 31.2 Strength training in bodybuilding: hypertrophy

Parameters	Myofibrillar hypertrophy	Sarcoplasmic hypertrophy
Number of exercises	2-4	3-6
Exercise sets	3-4	4-8
Reps per set	5-8	10-15
Load (%1RM)	70-80	60-70
Rest (seconds)	90-150	45-90
Time Under Tension per set (seconds)	30-50	60-70

Modified from: Squillante A. *Allenamento della forza*. Giacomo Catalani Editore, Arezzo, 2020.

Short periods of strength training with basic exercises, loads equal to or greater than 80% of the maximum, and short sets of 2 to 5 repetitions with complete rests, also have their own role in the world of bodybuilding. Even a relatively short period of strength training, lasting 6-8 weeks, can improve muscle strength levels by 10-15%. Strength training creates the necessary conditions to increase the intensity of the training stimulus. It is possible to distinguish two variants of the maximal efforts method, both applicable in the context of strength training for bodybuilding: an intensive-type variant, more suitable for supporting functional-type adaptations affecting the central nervous system with a relatively low impact in terms of muscle growth, and an extensive variant, which offers an ideal compromise between gains in muscle strength and increases in lean mass. Table 31.3 shows the main reference parameters.

In strength training, the importance of managing central fatigue processes, which can compromise the ability to express adequate levels of muscle tension, is important to consider. Therefore, unlike the Repeated Effort method, in which it is possible, but not necessary, to bring a set to muscular failure, in the Maximal Effort method using a more conservative approach which, allows you to maintain the same training

Table 31.3 Strength training in bodybuilding: muscle strength

Parameters	Relative strength	Absolute strength
Number of exercises	2-4	3-5
Exercise sets	3-4	4-6
Reps per set	1-3	3-5
Load (%1RM)	90-100	80-90
Recovery (minutes)	3-6	2-4

Modified from: Squillante A. *Allenamento della forza*. Giacomo Catalani Editore, Arezzo, 2020.

Table 31.4 Strength training in bodybuilding: programming

Maximum reps	Maximum load	Target load	Target reps
1 RM	100%	92-95%	1-2
2 RM	95%	88-90%	2-3
3 RM	90%	82-85%	3-4
5 RM	85%	78-80%	4-5
8 RM	80%	73-75%	5-6
10 RM	75%	66-70%	6-8
15 RM	70%	62-65%	10-12

Modified from: Squillante A. *Allenamento della forza*. Giacomo Catalani Editore, Arezzo, 2020.

load over several successive sets with the help of complete recovery times is more preferable.

This approach is called "set across" and makes use of a strategy known as "buffering". The number of repetitions prescribed per set (working set) is reduced by 10-20% compared to the maximum number of repetitions foreseen for a given load range (RM). Such an approach not only preserves adequate training volumes but also, above all, supports an explosive execution by maximizing the recruitment of type II or fast-twitch muscle fibers. The same principle of buffering can be applied to the workload, reducing it by 5-7% of the maximum. Table 31.4 shows the load parameters.

The bottom line is that **short bouts of strength training can be extremely beneficial to bodybuilders**. Programs lasting 4-6 weeks with a frequency of two or three times in the space of a year (macro-cycle) make it possible to maintain a positive trend of adaptations at a neuromuscular level which, year after year, guarantees improved physical performance. On the one hand, basic traditional weightlifting exercises performed with a barbell according to the Maximal Effort method (extensive) make it possible to avoid detraining that often occurs during particularly long periods of training for muscle hypertrophy, the so-called "muscle-gaining phase" in bodybuilding, or "bulking". On the other hand, basic traditional weightlifting exercises performed with a barbell according to the Maximal Effort method (intensive) have proven to be able to exert a protective action against lean body mass during periods of low-calorie diets, the so-called "getting-shredded phase" in bodybuilding, or "cutting". Strength training has been shown to have a distinctly anabolic, but also anti-catabolic, effect, significantly increasing the rate of protein synthesis up to 24 hours post-workout and thus contributing to maintaining a positive nitrogen balance even during periods of calorie restriction (Atherton and Smith, 2012).

CHAPTER 32

Posture in bodybuilding

Ciro di Cristino

"What does posture have to do with bodybuilding?" This is the question that the students of the first NABBA bodybuilding instructor course asked themselves in 1990 in Parma.

To explore this topic, I have to first describe to my background and my special "training partner".

Despite having practiced various sports in L'Aquila during the ISEF 1976-1979, thanks to Prof. Giuseppe Valentini, the study of corrective gymnastics fascinated me. When I got to Parma, I was lucky enough to meet Prof. Giuseppe Gussoni, who was like a father to me from a professional point of view and made me even more passionate about the complexity of the mechanisms that regulate our posture and our motor skills. Being a member of the UNC (Unione Nazionale Chinesiologi) and the SIGM (Società Italiana Ginnastica Medica), in addition to continuously attending courses and conferences as both a student and a speaker allowed me to deepen my knowledge of the study of posture more and more, eventually becoming a professor of academic and university courses.

In 1983, I realized my dream of opening my first gym, Palestra Life (150 m^2). I taught traditional bodyweight gymnastics and with equipment such as wall bars, medicine balls, hoops, ropes, iron sticks, wooden sticks blocks and supports, but bodybuilding was a continuous evolution. A young man, Alfredo Delporto, who enrolled in my gym did not follow my lessons but used the bench, dumbbells and barbells to perform his exercises in a fairly rational way. He really wanted to participate in a bodybuilding competition, an environment he was familiar with. I proposed that we train together, albeit with different objectives: he would participate in the competition and I would improve these exercises from a kinesiological point of view. All this gave me the opportunity to analyze, correct and verify the quality of the workouts, so Alfredo made his dream of participating and winning his bodybuilding competition a reality, taking home the FIACF-IFBB Regional Champion title. Meanwhile, my experience was enriched.

In 1989 I opened the new Palestra Life (500 m^2) and on the day of the inauguration, I was honored by the presence of many participants, including Dr. Massimo Spattini (Italian Heavyweight Champion and a physician specialized in Sports Medicine and Food Science), with whom, given his skills, it was not difficult to establish an interesting dialogue on my choice of bodybuilding equipment, after having tried and selected them from three different manufacturers, but also on the presence of squared mirrors and equipment for corrective gymnastics and rehabilitation. At the end of our chat, he invited me to his studio the following day to further explore how to use my experiences in the practice of bodybuilding.

After this second meeting, he decided to train with me in my gym, which proved to be very interesting experience. Spattini has always been an idol in this environment because of his skills and the results obtained by himself and his students: every year he would go to Gold's Gym in California, and in addition to having shared workouts with the best bodybuilders in the world, his training partner was the great Samir Bannout! It was easy for us to merge skills, collaborate for the development of our students, and, given our mutual respect, we were able to establish a friendship.

From the first training session with Massimo, I noticed a big difference in posture. Despite being considerably more muscular than me, he had started off with a relatively light weight; I noticed the difference in how he used weights, not seeking out heavy loads but training the single muscle, as hard as possible, during each set and repetition. Despite having lifted fewer kilos than my usual workouts, I felt the famous feeling of fullness that all bodybuilders seek. Therefore, we paid close attention to the most correct execution for each exercise, respecting kinesiology, biomechanics and physiology.

The most important goal for this discipline is to recruit fibers, isolate, stimulate and innervate the muscle through a correct and efficient posture, to avoid traumas and micro-traumas, and exploit biomechanics to ensure optimal planes, amplitudes and angles until you feel the burning, the pain, the fatigue of the contraction and the pumping of the single muscle, avoiding associated movements, synergies, oscillations, leaps, automatisms and even controlling the "adrenaline rush".

During exertion, an involuntary mechanism, the "Valsalva maneuver" is triggered, which consists in closing the glottis and all the orifices of the diaphragm, closing the abdominothoracic cavity. This way, the pressure increases considerably and transforms this cavity into an expandable structure located anterior to the spine, capable of transmitting effort to the pelvic girdle and perineum, contributing to the decrease of D12-L1 disc compression by 50% and L5-S1 by 30%, as well as reducing tension in the spinal muscles by 55%. However, although this mechanism is very useful for reducing effort by the spine, it can only act for workouts with short periods of exertion and long periods of rest (as in weightlifting). So, to reduce this major increase in pressure, the main rule to follow is that, during effort, which usually corresponds to the "concentric" phase, you must exhale, just as you inhale in the "eccentric" phase. In "isotension" training, the matter is not so simple, but in any case, the diaphragmatic block must be avoided (and therefore the Valsalva maneuver) in order not to put yourself at risk due to the pressure increase in the intracranial venous system, the decrease in venous return to the heart and in the amount of alveolar blood, and the increase in small circulation resistance, cerebrospinal fluid pressure and blood pressure.

In addition to the obvious risks to life itself, this condition, protracted over time, leads to a dysfunction of the diaphragm, which causes a pathological circumstance characterized by hypertonicity, pain and shortening. The diaphragm also has another strategic function, as it is connected to both the anterior and posterior postural chains through the phrenic center. For this reason, it plays a primary role in the body's balance: its dysfunction, therefore, determines a series of compensations that lead to assuming altered postural habits.

How do postural studies intersect with the discipline of bodybuilding?

Posture is **personalized adaptation of the individual to the physical, mental, and emotional environment**.

Posture represents one's own experience. Everything that happens to us leaves an imprint, which generates a deformation of posture, a memory in our limbic system (related to the fundamental functions for the conservation of the species).

Let's take into consideration the management of our posture, which can be defined as the ability to perceive one's body both when stationary and in its mobility in space. It is characterized by the need to overcome the force of the Earth's gravity. There are several components capable of altering the mechanisms that serve to get the better of this fight, such as mechanical, kinesiological, neurophysiological and psychomotor components; the last ones are due to an inexact collection and integration of data, i.e. a kinesthetic misinterpretation.

Humans are the most evolved of all animals; our upright posture represents the final moment of a very long process of adaptation, or transformation and evolution, understood as the gradual acquisition of a set of privileges that have given us control over the environment.

The upright position obeys the sole necessity of the projection of the center of gravity within the polygon circumscribed by the footprint; the same need will reappear when this balance is disturbed.

Some kinetic reactions ensure the return to the initial equilibrium:

- *static reactions*, which maintain the fundamental status
- *rebalancing reactions*, which maintain equilibrium in the presence of unbalancing forces
- *adjusting reactions*, which free the voluntary motor activity from the task
- to recover the lost balance, through the use of anti-gravity muscles, which are largely made up of tonic fibers (red), which respond to the stimulation of a prolonged contraction and which, under normal working conditions, are "tireless"

These reactions, if directed by the cerebral cortex, would have an energy expenditure that would not be logical, so everything will have to be analyzed through postural education aimed at making this game more efficient, without recourse to the will or the control of the conscience.

Neurophysiological considerations

Kinesiology is the study of movement, more specifically of rational movement.

A **movement** is a complex act, the result of the action of the pyramidal motor system and the extrapyramidal motor system. These two systems are not separate, as the movement itself is controlled by the pyramidal system, which intervenes in voluntary movements, but the series of adjustments represented by the maintenance of correct posture, balance and relationships between the antagonistic muscles are controlled by the extrapyramidal system, which intervenes in muscle tone and automatic movements.

The pyramidal pathway is very fast; the extrapyramidal pathway is formed by chains of neurons and is slower. Both converge in motor neurons, which are found in the anterior horns of the spinal cord but travel through different areas.

The **pyramidal system** consists of motor fibers that originate from the posterior part of the frontal lobes of the motor cortex (area 4 of Brodmann, pre-Rolandic) and is defined as such because these fibers gather in a bundle that passes in correspondence with the "pyramids", which are two protrusions of the ventral surface of the bulb ending in the nerve centers of the pons, in the medulla oblongata and in the anterior horns of the spinal cord.

The main function of the pyramidal system is to control voluntary motor activity of our body; in particular, it initiates previously planned fine and precise voluntary movements in the cerebral cortex.

Damage to the pyramidal system can impair voluntary movements, while injuries to the pyramidal system can cause serious and irreversible motor deficits (paralysis).

The **extrapyramidal system** is a set of pathways and nerve centers that act directly or indirectly on correct motor action, controlling instinctive reactions and adapting them to the voluntary movement (coordinated by the pyramidal system). The extrapyramidal tracts are found primarily in the reticular formation of the pons and medulla and target motor neurons in the spinal cord, which are involved in reflexes, locomotion, complex movements and postural control. The thalamus and hypothalamus participate extensively in the motor integration performed by the extrapyramidal system.

The extrapyramidal system is responsible for the control of automatic activities, however, it also influences voluntary movements, where it determines the tonic accompaniment and the syncinetic activity.

Damage to the extrapyramidal system generally preserves voluntary movements but causes hypertonicity, hypokinesia, the appearance of involuntary movements (such as tremors and tics) and spasms: classic examples of extrapyramidal system disorders are represented by Parkinson's disease and Huntington's disease.

The **muscle** has three simplified functions:

- sensory (sends and receives information through the central and peripheral nervous system)
- phasic (dynamic, movement)
- tonic (static, supportive)

These three functions are present in all muscles, but in some, one prevails over the others, regardless of strength, mass, speed, etc., on which they do not depend, but they can still favor an improvement.

The pyramidal system acts selectively and is mostly used in the phasic function. The extrapyramidal system, after having stored experiences, controls and coordinates global movements and kinetic chains, and it is mainly used in the tonic function.

The muscle, as a motor organ, is functional if it is elastic. For it to remain elastic, there is a need for a tonic balance between the agonist muscles which carry out the movement, and the antagonist muscles, which control it by limiting it in time and space (while one shortens, the other lengthens and vice versa). If this does not happen harmoniously, it means that there is a hypertonicity problem.

Hypertonicity, caused by overworking or even organic-visceral or neuropsychic reasons, leads to loss of the "wakefulness" function (brain control). Hypertonicity tends to shorten the connective tissue that surrounds the sarcomeres (the contractile unit of the muscle) and no longer spontaneously returns the previous length, except through special techniques.

When these "retractions" occur, there are inevitable alterations in posture, joint compressions, non-physiological axial rotations of the joint heads and bad muscle synergies, therefore joint inflammation, tendonitis, bursitis, arthrosis, etc.

Hypertonic muscles, therefore, have limited functions and are less willing to expand (mass), which is one of the main goals of the bodybuilder.

First of all, when facing this type of situation, a medical opinion and certification with the relevant indications are recommended, followed by information from the student regarding their condition and their objectives, which will then be followed by a functional evaluation and a postural observation. After having investigated the origin of this hypertonicity, proceeding with myotensive practices to return to the eutonic condition will be possible.

Typical bodybuilding exercises are divided into:

- *fundamentals*: squats, deadlifts, rows, bench presses and pull-ups; the tools used are barbells, dumbbells and bars; the muscles involved act synergistically, favoring the extrapyramidal function
- *complementary*: chest, pulley, leg extension, delts, etc.; these exercises use the so-called isotonic machines; the muscles are stimulated through the pyramidal function in an isolated form

When **planning a workout**, it is necessary to calculate the type of stress that the student will be subjected to based on the volume, intensity and density of the workout.

I will not dwell excessively on this topic, since it has already been covered by other authors, but I will mention it because it concerns the topics that are discussed in this chapter.

With regard to a **single exercise**, set and repetition, **and not training as a whole**, I usually distinguish three types of loads:

- *external load*: the real weight of the barbells or machines that I am using and the number of repetitions performed
- *internal load*: how much stimulus I am sending pyramidally to the target muscle, and with what intensity and in which phase (concentric or eccentric, or in both) regardless of the weight used
- *support load*: the muscular effort that I have to produce to maintain a correct posture

Generally, the goal in sports is the pursuit of maximum performance with minimum effort; therefore, after having mastered a very expensive movement – through the pyramidal system – one tries to repeat the same movement until it becomes automatic and, therefore, cheaper, by activating the extra-pyramidal system, the storage of the automatisms, coordinated by the cerebellum.

In summary, the athlete activates the pyramidal system to acquire a motor skill, then repeats it many times until it becomes automatic, so there is no longer any need for the intervention of the brain, which will be busy with other functions.

Below are two examples:

- in weightlifting, whoever lifts the heaviest weight (external load) wins. In order to perfectly learn the snatch and sprint technique (pyramidal system), the athlete must use a relatively low external load, in order not to incur traumas or technical errors. When they manage to automate, making the movement efficient, acquiring greater mastery in the management of the correct posture, and therefore using a low support load (extrapyramidal system), they will consequently be able to lift the heavier external load
- in bodybuilding, during the mesocycle dedicated to the development of strength and *myofibrillar hypertrophy* (increase in the cross-section of the muscle fibers thanks to the increase in the contractile proteins actin and myosin), the effort made is comparable to that of a weightlifter; on the other hand, for training aimed at seeking the stimulation of the satellite cells, capable of increasing the number of nuclei in the muscle fibers, the basic posture will have to be optimized to make it more efficient and less risky during exertion, therefore the support load will have to be closer to zero (extrapyramidal system). The internal load, in this phase (pyramidal system), will be as heavy as possible, trying to get to the exhaustion of ATP as soon as possible, so that the processes stimulating the growth factors can take place. The external load, on the other hand, may vary and will be related to the choice of training technique, the type of exercise and the experience of the bodybuilder who is training

Bodybuilding competitions vary according to the regulations of the organizing federation. The evaluation criteria also change according to the categories. In any case, it is a competition based on the sensations that the athlete manages to convey to the judges, as there are no measures or times. Usually, a bodybuilding competition takes place in two rounds:

- in the first round, the athletes, divided into categories, go up on stage and, directed by the head judge, in an upright position, perform the obligatory poses, first semi-relaxed and then in contraction, in frontal, sideways and back positions. For this round the evaluation criteria are:
  - *line and general appearance*: static-dynamic posture, musculoskeletal fitness condition
  - *symmetry and proportion*: evaluated according to planes and axes, which make it possible to show a human body in a static form, front and back, right and left, top and bottom
  - *muscularization*: "mass", i.e. muscle volume; "definition", fat elimination, to highlight the muscles; "vascularization", which highlights the veins; "separation", which highlights the muscular bellies
  - *the ability to perform the mandatory poses*, through which the athletes can highlight their qualities
- in the second round the athletes appear on stage individually and show the best of themselves through a performance routine, interpreting a series of poses and movements, in tune with the music of their choice, suitably prepared for the occasion. The judging criteria for this round are:
  - *presentation*: posture and body hold (poise) during the static phases and performance dynamics
  - *interpretation*: understood as the choice of music suited to the competition and the character being played, sense of rhythm, expressed through poses performed in time and in harmony with the musical piece; originality and ability to impress the audience
  - for some categories, even *functional abilities*: demonstrations of strength, resistance, elasticity, balance and coordination

Motor activity in the field of education, training, rehabilitation or performance must start from a postural examination of the subject. The data collected from the postural investigation can reveal the true conditions from the psychophysical and neurophysiological point of view of the subject in question and, from these, it is possible to deduce the short-, medium- and long-term objectives to decide the most appropriate means that should be included in the program; rationally, it is a technique that adapts to the subject and not vice versa. The subject must remain at the center of the study.

The search for physical harmony is sometimes affected by accumulations of localized fat and muscle deficiencies.

Through the detection of body composition and postural control, the related problems are highlighted, for which we try to make the most appropriate adjustments. The following must be established:

- *where it is located and what the extent of the accumulation or deficit is. The gynoid or android prevalence (shape: apple, pear, pepper)*: to recognize this, it is essential to carry out a correct assessment of the body composition, through plicometry, impedancemetry, etc. In order to be able to draw up the ChronhOrMorphodiet, a subject should evaluate the supplements and the most appropriate training
- *whether the subject is training too much or too little and with what density and/or intensity; whether the diet is adequate for the type of expenditure*. Individuals are divided according to their morphology, in ectomorphic, mesomorphic and endomorphic, as well as other mixed forms. These morphologies must be taken into consideration when planning training and nutrition, because hormonal influence, metabolism and reaction to the type of training are different
- *if there are deficiencies in the stabilizing muscles (rotator cuffs, pelvic floor, core, etc.)*: it is difficult to follow training schedules that indicate sets of exercises for the muscles that stabilize the joints and allow the body to maintain balance and stability during the execution of the movements. Their function is mainly tonic, so they have a high degree of resistance. They are classified according to the joint involved (for example, stabilizers of the shoulder, knee, trunk, etc.)
- *if myofascial dysfunctions are present due to an accident*: when dealing with physical trauma, three aspects can be considered in determining the consequences on the connective tissue: the force of the impact, the anatomical site involved and the experienced emotion. Stretching is often referred to as a form of treatment for myofascial dysfunction. Stretching with positions held for a short time and non-specific breathing (perhaps even with small rebounds) is contraindicated in myofascial syndrome

Actually, they should be considered aggravating factors. Only once the myofascial problem has been solved does the picture stabilize through a reconditioning program that involves both stretching and strengthening the imbalances in the treated areas. A suitable rebalancing protocol aimed at obtaining the best muscle extensibility, joint flexibility and strengthening of the hypostenic districts is essential to resume of normal activity and for stabilization of the case:

- *identify the functional characteristics of the muscle in question; if the muscle under examination is hypertonic or hypotonic*: if it is a muscle with a mainly tonic function (support), tending to be hypertonic or phasic (dynamic), consequently, the direction and quality of the proposed stimulus must be different; exercises with weights do not always cause an increased tonus, it depends on the type: concentric, eccentric, isotonic, isometric, etc. Therefore, it is important to adapt the stimulus according to the functional characteristics of the muscle to be recovered

- *if the antagonist muscle (opposite to the one involved) shows hypertonicity that could prevent the correct use of the muscle in question*: you have to proceed by releasing the hypertonic muscle through exercises and/or treatments suitable for this purpose in order to then be able to recover the desired muscle
- *if the intervertebral foramen, through which the vessels and nerves pass to the muscle, has an obstruction due to the disc compression of the same vertebrae; if there is therefore a vascular problem, with consequent lack of venous return and/or lack of muscle nutrition, or if it is a question of a nerve stimulation defect, with consequent lack of sensitivity and fiber recruitment*: the vertebral column is subjected to unbalanced forces which can lead to a decrease in the intervertebral spaces mono- or bilaterally, with the consequent crushing of the intervertebral discs. Incorrect resistance workouts can strain the spinal muscles. This can lead to a worsening of the physiological situation, with the consequences already described; in this case, analytical stretching would be insufficient, so more advanced myotensive techniques and decompensated global stretching will be used
- *if the subject is unable to send a complete stimulus to the desired muscle via the pyramidal route, via the pyramidal route, or if they use another muscle in synergy to contract a deficient muscle*: generally, this problem is due to a lack of muscle sense (the ability to feel the body and its parts, in time and space) and surely the subject will not have been properly initiated into the discipline; insisting on increasing the external load (as usually happens) is not convenient. On the contrary, it will be necessary to decrease the weight and improve the ability to be in tune with the muscle, through proprioceptive and exteroceptive stimulations, thus reaching the goal
- *if the entire kinetic chain of the postural muscles presents an incorrect situation, whereby the assumed habits and positions do not respect favorable conditions from a biomechanical point of view and, therefore, determine a useless expenditure of energy derived from reasons of imperfect integration at the kinesthetic level*: in this case, it is clear that postural education will be fundamental. You should never put muscle strengthening or toning before postural work. If you strengthen a structure that has some defect or problem, you will upgrade the defect or problem as well. In this case, it would be even more difficult to correct an altered posture. First, it will be necessary to re-stretch the contracted muscles and rebalance the posture, and then, possibly, strengthen the structure that has the correct parameters with exercises suitable for the case. If tensions are eliminated, blood circulation will improve and the muscle will get more vascularized. Consequently, we will have a more nourished muscle, with a relative increase in the volume of the elements that compose it (hypertrophy process). Constant practice will allow for better acquisition of the complete perception of the muscle, thus achieving a better isolation capacity (in the phases of concentric and eccentric contraction): in this way, both greater recruitment of latent fibers and an increase in the number of cells will be obtained. After applying the right remedies, you can proceed to the more specific training techniques of bodybuilding

Recovery

After cooling down at the end of each workout, it is good practice to make students aware of effective postural recovery through analytical and global stretching for the superficial and deep muscles. During this phase, it is essential to perform correct deep diaphragmatic breathing, trying to prolong the expiratory phase to stimulate the vagus and the parasympathetic nervous system. Decreasing breathing stimulates the pituitary gland, which regulates all others to ensure the right hormonal balance. Nasal breathing, in the paranasal sinuses, produces nitric oxide (nitrogen monoxide), which is a vasodilator (it also acts on erectile dysfunction), lowers blood pressure, is antithrombotic, and relaxes smooth muscles. During breathing, being in tune with the heart produces a slower heart rate and general relaxation.

This practice is of fundamental importance so that the direct and reflected stresses, due to the overload, are completely recovered, with the extra advantage of avoiding injuries, optimizing the supercompensation phase in the best possible way and avoiding the predisposition to asymmetrical and disproportionate development. It must be kept in mind that training is a stress and that benefits are obtained during recovery. Optimizing recovery also helps improve the performance.

CHAPTER 33

Motor evaluation in bodybuilding

Davide Antoniella and Ivan Martellato

Both amateur and competitive bodybuilding are disciplines which can put a strain on the joint integrity of the whole body if performed with little attention to our morphological individuality.

A good percentage of alterations affecting the musculoskeletal system derive from muscular imbalances that have never been resolved and, therefore, have persisted over time. Muscles that are too weak or too strong, muscle retractions and asymmetries between the two sides of the body, and continuous joint stress generate a condition of limited joint stabilization capacity. Chronic joint stress, if not solved at the root of the problem, is the main cause of inflammation and loss of function in the injured tissue, which will reach the point of no longer being able to compensate for progressive cartilage damage. Furthermore, it must be kept in mind that the chronically contracted muscles of many bodybuilders are also responsible for joint pain. Neglecting the myofascial treatment of areas subject to retraction (trapezius, pectoralis minor, subscapularis, hamstrings, iliopsoas, piriformis, but also wrist and finger flexors) induces our system to create a compensatory motor pattern that inevitably leads to joint inflammation and pain.

As mentioned above, bodybuilders are chronically subjected to overload in all joint compartments and, although this behavior can partly be good for bone calcification, joint lubrication, and for the stimulation of chondrocytes (cells that synthesize cartilage), it becomes bad when in macro-cycle joint mobility exercises, volume deload intended as total tonnage and exercises aimed at promoting greater joint lubrication are not implemented.

If it is therefore established that a macro-cycle must necessarily include prevention exercises, with the aim of allowing the athlete to train longer and with greater intensity without incurring more or less serious injuries, it is also true that these exercises should be evaluated based on the athlete's anthropometric, morphological and performance characteristics.

To ensure optimal performance, combined with injury prevention, we must necessarily use tests to measure various parameters.

- **Strength tests**: they assess maximal, sub-maximal, isometric and explosive strength. Their limiting factor is that they do not discriminate the difference in strength between the two sides of the body; in this case, a dynamometer (displacement, speed, power, force) is essential.
- **Metabolic performance tests**: they measure cardiovascular capacity. Although these tests do not represent the bodybuilder's metabolic demands, the cardiovascular function needs monitoring given the potential myocardial restructuring which occurs in people doing resistance training. Tests that measure the maximum amount of oxygen that can be used to produce power (VO_2 max), heart rate variability and its recovery, blood pressure, and blood lactate, when performed every six months, can provide important information on mitochondrial health and, therefore, on the cardiovascular state of the athlete.
- **Postural evaluation tests**: they evaluate the position of body segments in the different planes (frontal, sagittal and transverse). They allow us to quickly detect any asymmetries or postural imbalances deriving from retractions or pre-existing muscle weaknesses.
- **Mobility tests**: they evaluate the range of motion of a given joint. They assess active mobility (the degree of movement that a subject can achieve with their muscles) and passive mobility (mobility is measured by an operator without the intervention of muscle strength). There are also free and compensated tests and non-compensated guided tests.

Strength tests

Strength tests are extremely important to evaluate the level of an athlete regarding the recruitment and synchronization of the motor units of the tested muscle. Unlike powerlifters, bodybuilders wish to lift an increasingly greater tonnage, exclusively for the action that the mechanical load has on the stimulation of the biochemical pathways linked to protein synthesis.

Verifying the behavior of the various organic-functional qualities (in this case strength) of different muscles of the body before, during and at the end of a bodybuilder's mesocycle is of fundamental importance to outline the changes that should be implemented in the subsequent training program. In summary, strength tests, when they take into consideration not only personal and anthropometric data but also the athlete's current training program, are a great way to understand:

- the trend of strength gain
- the difference in strength between the various body regions
- the difference in strength between two limbs, often assessed with the aid of a digital dynamometer

In this way, they offer a point of reference for future feasible programming.

Strength tests include **maximal strength** tests, including dynamic and static or isometric tests, **explosive strength** tests and resistant and reactive strength tests.

This discussion will be limited to describing some explosive, dynamic and static strength tests.

Maximal strength

Maximal strength means the maximum tension that the neuromuscular system can express with an isometric contraction against an immobile (static) or moving (dynamic) load. Static strength measurement is one of the most reliable methods for measuring the strength of a particular body region. Unlike dynamic maximal strength, when measuring static or isometric maximal strength, there is no need to research the ideal weight to use for 1RM (Repetition Maximal). If we take the same exercise into consideration, the force generated during a maximal strength test in isometric conditions is 20% greater than that generated by a concentric push. Compared to a dynamic strength test, the isometric strength test exclusively measures the force produced by the generation of action potentials of the motor units of the target muscle and, contrary to what happens in dynamic strength tests, it depends on the mobility and joint stability of the subject.

To implement a static isometric maximal strength test, the exercise you decide to perform must be accompanied by dynamometric cells connected to a data logger.

The dynamometer measures the strength of a muscle group during an isometric action that reproduces the postures of the technical movement (i.e., flat bench and leg extension).

Static isometric strength tests

These tests measure the maximum tension that the neuromuscular system can express with an isometric contraction in the absence of changes in the distance between the origin and insertion of the evaluated muscle:

- leg extension or leg press to assess the strength of the leg extensors on the thigh
- pushes on the multipower with stops positioned so as to lock the balance wheel with the arm parallel to the ground and the forearm perpendicular to the arm, to evaluate the strength of the pectorals and triceps
- rotator cuff: lock the elbow adjacent to the torso and do an initial internal rotation, which is maintained isometrically, then turn around and do an external rotation; this test is used to identify any discrepancies and problems in the rotator cuff muscles

Dynamic strength tests

They measure the maximum tension that the neuromuscular system can express with a contraction characterized by a shortening and lengthening of the muscle.

The method used is that of incremental repetitions with a barbell or an isotonic machine.

- If the force to be evaluated is the maximal one, the 1RM is performed with a load that is assumed to be the maximum possible based on the athlete's history or calculated with approximate formulas, such as the Brzycki formula. Brzycki formula

is often used by bodybuilders **to get a rough idea of the weight that they can potentially lift through 1RM**. It takes the mechanical load used to bring a muscle to exhaustion (number of repetitions equal to or less than 12) as a reference. **The fewer repetitions completed with the target weight, the greater the reliability of the test** (the weight with which the 1RM is evaluated will be more accurate if the starting point is the tonnage lifted for a total of 4 repetitions instead of 12); as a matter of fact, **the more the repetitions, the greater the contribution of the resisting force**. In order to avoid misleading calculations, it is also necessary to evaluate the presence of compensation during the execution of the repetitions: the reliability of the formula drastically decreases if the lifts are compensated by the contribution of other muscles not involved in the movement. Brzycki formula has gained more and more ground due to its less dangerous execution compared to the 1RM test.
- **If the strenght to be evaluated is submaximal, 3 to 6 repetitions are performed; these tests are optimal to indirectly measure the 1RM with good reliability**.

As previously stated, dynamic maximal strength tests also take joint mobility into consideration, and, especially when evaluating the 6 repetitions, can help outline when the athlete begins to "cheat" by compensating with other muscle groups.

It is important to identify the MRU (maximum useful repetition) or the MRT (maximum technical repetition). These are concepts of precision and maximum muscle stimulation.

The dynamometer

The muscle dynamometer is a portable device used in rehabilitation medicine and sports for measuring strength and musculoskeletal resistance. The dynamometer is an instrument whose usefulness is not limited to the reliable and precise measurement of the strength differences between muscle groups, as it can also be used to calculate how long it takes an athlete to recover after performing a given movement (be it injury or intense training); moreover, if positioned in the right angle, it allows you to understand which angle of the movement is better in order to improve the movement.

The dynamometer helps measure the strength of single muscles, evaluated approximately through the exclusive perception of the operator, which is far more reliable.

The device has electronic force translators that provide acoustic and optical biofeedback and is equipped with a large contact surface that improves its precision during measurement.

In summary, the dynamometer can measure:
- maximal strength
- strength endurance
- peak of maximum force
- time necessary to express maximum force
- speed needed to reach peak strength

Explosive strength

Even though at first glance one might think that in bodybuilding the explosive component has a marginal importance in the performance, the muscle fibers capable of contracting faster are also the most hypertrophiable. These fibers, which are responsible for the explosive performance and represent only a small percentage of the muscle fiberpool, are type IIx fibers.

In humans these fibers represent the type of fibers with the highest power and speed of contraction, thus fulfilling the role of the IIb fibers of rodents. In the rodents that are used as experimental models, histotype IIx has intermediate biomechanical (speed of contraction) and metabolic characteristics (between IIa and IIb).

An insight into the classification of muscle fiber histotypes was accomplished with the identification of all myosin contractile protein intermediates: 1 ↔ 1/IIa ↔ IIa ↔ IIa/IIx ↔ IIx. These fibers with intermediate characteristics are always present in the skeletal muscle and can be seen as transitional forms between pure-type fibers. Returning to the explosive force, we can confirm that, in humans, type IIx and IIa/IIx fibers are both the strongest and most hypertrophiable, and the best way to stimulate them is through an explosive contraction, using 40% of the load for a maximal contraction or using submaximal loads.

Explosive strength tests

For the lower part, the most used tests are the Squat Jump (SJ) and the Counter Movement Jump (CMJ) of the Bosco Tests.

These tests are performed with instruments capable of measuring the **time of the movement**, the **fast force** of the extensor chain of the lower limb, and, in the case of the CMJ, the ability of the limb to accumulate and recover its elastic energy.

Performing the Bosco Test: Squat Jump (SJ)

- Starting position with hands on the hips, knees bent at 90° and heels resting on the ground.
- The trunk must be as vertical as possible in relation to the ground.
- Execution of a vertical jump at maximum speed, limiting any countermovement with the lower or upper limbs as much as possible.
- Cushioned landing to avoid injuries.

When performed with meticulous attention to the position of the body, this test is an excellent way to evaluate the explosive strength of the lower limbs (gluteus, psoasand quadriceps).

To analyze the speed of movement and to calculate the **speed of the take-off** and the **acceleration of the body upward**, markers must be applied to the joints involved in the movement.

In the absence of markers, the calculation of the reached height can also be used to evaluate the explosive force.

It should be noted that the Squat Jump is never perfect, precisely because the countermovement, even if minimal, is always present. The evaluation will therefore have to take into account **the lack of precision derived from this error**.

A test that is very similar to the Squat Jump, which also includes the countermovement in the evaluation, is the Counter Movement Jump (CMJ). Unlike the Squat Jump, this exercise also measures the elastic strength of the extensor muscles of the lower limbs.

Performing the Bosco test: Counter Movement Jump (CMJ)

- Starting position with hands on the hips, upright position and heels resting on the ground.
- The trunk must be as vertical as possible in relation to the ground.
- Execution of a vertical jump at maximum speed, preceded by a rapid bending of the knees to 90° with the heels staying on the ground.
- Landing with straight legs, toes first, with subsequent cushioning to avoid trauma.

As for the upper part, the flat bench or the multipower is used. Since the power (P) is equal to the force (F) multiplied by the speed of execution (V), and the greater the load the lower the speed, the load used must allow the subject to perform the lift at a sufficient rate to generate the desired power. Explosive strength is evaluated by setting a load equal to 40% of your 1RM and by placing a marker in the balance wheel to measure its acceleration.

Ballistic test

A baropodometric platform can also be used to evaluate foot support. The ballistic test is used to analyze the various phases of a ballistic movement, such as a jump in its various components:

- the eccentric descent and, therefore, the stretching phase
- the phase of change of elastic reusage
- the concentric ascent phase
- the take-off phase from the ground
- the relapse and stabilization phase

Knee stability, ankle strength and calf squeeze phases are then taken into consideration. It can be performed with one or both feet. The use of the baropodometric platform during the execution of this test gives us very useful information on foot support, especially for women, because it often involves problems that can later easily translate into poor circulation and cellulite.

Metabolic tests

For a successful increase in muscle mass, the bodybuilder must adhere to precise training schemes aimed at the hypertrophy of the desired muscle group.

When it comes to the type of training in bodybuilding, it must be kept in mind that each scheme is strongly dependent on the sensations of the athlete. However, although it is impossible to find two athletes who train with the same exercises, the same repetitions and the same recovery, we can say that when it comes to increasing muscle mass, the repetitions range from 6 to 15, the time under tension from 15 to 60 seconds, and recovery times from 60 seconds to 3 minutes.

Since the intensity used during the repetitions performed is always above 50% of 1RM, the vasoconstriction of the arterioles involved in muscle oxygenation is such as not to allow efficient oxidative metabolism. It follows that, for the first 3-7 seconds of exercise, energy is drawn from the immediately available ATP and is resynthesized by phosphocreatine, while for the following 40 seconds, energy comes from anaerobic glycolysis. The end of each set occurs when the desired muscle failure is achieved, both from the increase in the levels of lactic acid produced by the anaerobic metabolism and from the inability of the motor neurons to re-establish the potassium gradient inside the cell. The increase in acidity derived from the catabolism of lactic acid produced during training is responsible for the increased amplitude of somatotropin (GH) secretion by the pituitary gland. It has not yet been confirmed whether the lipolytic and/or anabolic effect is achieved from the GH secretory increase or from the intensity and density at which training is performed. This is due to the multifactorial nature of the stimuli (training, energy expenditure), behaviors (nutrition, supplements, sleep), and lifestyle (stress, sedentary lifestyle). However, since GH is a pulsatile hormone, with a frequency of secretory peaks ranging from 4 to 8 and whose amplitude is strongly dependent on lifestyle (sleep, carbohydrate intake, protein intake, cortisol levels, leptin levels, training type and use of some specific amino acids), workouts with short recovery time and a time under tension of 40 to 60 seconds, which lead to a huge increase in blood levels of lactate and hydrogen, can be further stimuli for the increase in GH. The anabolism triggered by lactic acid is not limited to the increase in GH but it also depends on its direct role in the lysosomal activation of mTOR, one of the most important protein kinases when it comes to hypertrophy.

Although lactic acid is rightly sought after by the bodybuilder, it is also directly responsible for the fatigue and loss of strength that precede muscle failure. These unpleasant events derive from the ability of lactic acid to counteract the action of the processes involved in muscle contraction:

1. Lactic acid inhibits the cytosolic enzyme creatine kinase, responsible for the resynthesis of ATP.
2. Lactic acid, when it reaches a certain threshold, blocks the interaction between the Ca^{2+} ion and troponin C, the protein that, together with tropomyosin and another troponin, allows for the interaction of myosin with actin.
3. Lactic acid derives from pyruvic acid and its production underlies the inability of the mitochondrion to respond to energy requests. The mitochondrion needs

pyruvate in order to synthesize acetyl-CoA and, therefore, to produce energy with oxidative phosphorylation; however, if lactic acid is produced, mitochondrial energy production is also impaired.

At this point, it is clear that lactic acid is negative and positive at the same time. The role of the bodybuilder will therefore be to exercise, in order to tolerate ever higher levels of lactate, both to exploit its anabolic effect (GH and mTOR) and to increase the volume of work through a longer time under tension.

To do this, metabolic tests of VO_2 max and lactic threshold are essential, remembering that, although bodybuilding involves very little cardio, the resynthesis of energy during recovery passes through a good aerobic metabolism.

Speeding up the resynthesis of ATP in those 60-120 seconds is crucial to improve the performance in the following sets. VO_2 max, in this case, measures not only the maximum intensity at which you can efficiently use oxygen to produce strength but it also monitors the progress of your cardiac physiology at each month-cycle. When you improve your VO_2 max, you become more athletic than before, because the heart and mitochondria have improved their efficiency and, consequently, your general well-being. A low VO_2 max is most likely representative of cardiac restructuring towards concentric hypertrophy, very present in those who practice weightlifting and correlated to the early onset of cardiovascular disease.

Metabolic Tests: Maximal Oxygen Uptake (VO_2 max)

Maximal oxygen uptake is a measure of maximal aerobic metabolic power and, therefore, of the maximal intensity of exercise that an individual can tolerate for long periods of time.

More precisely, VO_2 max is the amount of oxygen that the body can take from the air through breathing, transport to the lungs and heart, and consume in the mitochondria of the muscles under effort within a given unit of time.

The greater the efficiency of the organs involved in each stage of the process (lungs, heart, red blood cells and mitochondria), the higher the VO_2 max will be.

If the energy demand exceeds the capacity of the maximum aerobic power, there will be an involvement of anaerobic glycolysis, with increasing production and, consequently, accumulation of lactic acid.

VO_2 max can be expressed as an absolute value (L/min) or it can be normalized for body weight (mL/kg/min), and it can be measured through direct tests or indirect tests.

Direct tests for VO_2 max

These are laboratory tests. They are more specific, more reproducible and more valid compared to indirect tests. These tests use gas analysis to measure the cellular respiratory quotient.

- **Exercise tests with integrated analysis of exhaled gases** (O_2 and CO_2)
- **Breath by breath**: enables instant measurement of the concentrations of O_2 and CO_2 in the volume of exhaled air

- **Mixing chamber**: the exhaled flow is collected in a chamber where the gases are mixed every 30 seconds

Exhaled gas analysis is the method used to evaluate both the amount of oxygen used during effort and the fuel used by our cells in cases of increased energy demand.

The respiratory quotient (RQ) is the ratio of the CO_2 emitted to the O_2 utilized by respiration. It should be noted that, through the respiratory quotient, it is possible to estimate cellular consumption. A QR close to 1 indicates the prevalent use of carbohydrates, while a QR close to 0.7 indicates that the metabolism mainly consumes lipids. Intermediate values, on the other hand, correspond to the use of both nutrients and this is what happens under physiological conditions.

A QR of 0.8 is representative of a predominantly lipid metabolism, excellent metabolic flexibility and high mitochondrial efficiency, while a QR >0.9 describes a predominantly glucosidic metabolism. The QR derived from the use of lipids is lower than the one derived from the use of carbohydrates, simply because the oxidation of fatty acids produces less CO_2 than the oxidation of glucose. However, when particularly high intensities and large concentrations of lactic acid are reached, CO_2 production begins to be independent of oxidative processes. This event is called external respiratory quotient; under these conditions, the QR can reach values of up to 1.10, a value that we will see later as a marker of the achievement of VO_2 max.

Test instrumentation

- **Bicycle ergometer**: equipped with an electromagnetic braking system and an analog-digital interface with an ergospirometric system
- **Treadmill**: manual and automatic elevation speed, immediate stopping capabilities, with an analog-digital interface

Test type

- **Ramp protocols**: small increments in short times (Balke test)
- **Scale protocols**: long increments in long times (Naughton test)

Since bodybuilding does not necessarily involve the use of cardiovascular equipment, in order to choose which machine to use during the test, it is necessary to know the type of machine preferred by the athlete. If the athlete does not use a cycle ergometer or treadmill, the treadmill is preferable due its user-friendliness.

Criteria for determining VO_2 max

- Reach the point in the test where oxygen consumption no longer increases
- Reach peak VO_2
- Achieve a lactate concentration of 8-10 mmol
- Reach the maximum heart rate for your age
- External respiratory quotient >1.10 (large production of lactic acid)

Indirect tests for VO_2 max

These are field tests that measure a parameter correlated with maximum oxygen consumption. Although they are less valid, not reproducible and less specific than direct tests, they offer useful indications both on the athlete's state of fitness and aerobic metabolism. Indirect tests can be **maximal** or **submaximal**; the latter represent the anaerobic threshold, i.e., the intensity at which a change from aerobic to anaerobic metabolism occurs.

Maximal indirect tests

They include continuous or escalating intensity trials with a pre-set distance or duration. They start from the assumption that the maximum intensity that a subject can withstand through aerobic metabolism represents their VO_2 max, and that the greater the aerobic power generated, the greater the VO_2 max.

Test types

- **Cooper test and Blake test:**
  - *they measure the maximum distance covered in 12 minutes (Cooper's test) and 15 minutes (Blake's test)*
  - *the distances obtained correspond to approximate values of VO_2 max*
  - *motivation and environmental conditions are limiting factors for the test result, as well as the ability to choose the right running pace*
  - *estimate VO_2 max through reference tables*
  - *a final sprint is not advisable, as it would derive from the anaerobic lactacid metabolism*
- **Shuttle run bleep test:**
  - *a test with increasing intensity*
  - *running 20 m or 50 m from signal to signal*
  - *can be performed by running in one direction or back and forth*
  - *speed of 7.5 km/h in the first minute and 8 km/h in the second minute, with 0.5 km/h increments every 2 minutes up to a maximum of 18 km/h*
  - *the test ends when the subject fails to keep up with the bleeps*
  - *estimates VO_2 max through reference tables*

Submaximal indirect tests

Submaximal tests are performed at constant intensity for a duration of about 5 minutes and aim to measure the relationship between heart rate and work intensity. They have a bigger margin of error compared to maximal tests, which take as reference the linearity existing between VO_2 max and the heart rate recorded during submaximal workouts. It should be kept in mind that heart rate normally reaches its maximum value at an exercise intensity representative of VO_2 max. For the bodybuilder, it is important to monitor the modification of these parameters from time A (beginning of the mesocycle) to time B (end of the mesocycle). In this case, the goal is to have in time B, with the same intensity, a decrease in heart rate and VO_2 max compared to time A.

Limitations

- VO_2 max is overestimated in athletes and underestimated in sedentary people, with a 10-15% margin of error
- The relationship between VO_2 max and heart rate is not perfectly linear
- The 220 – age formula is not always reliable

Submaximal tests (anaerobic threshold)

They are the most important tests for bodybuilders since they determine the intensity beyond which there is an increase in lactate levels to a value associated with energy production not only through oxygen but also thanks to anaerobic metabolism. Improving these parameters is equivalent to improving the time under tension, the resynthesized energy with the same recovery, the quality of the contraction and the extracellular buffer systems (bicarbonate, phosphate, albumin).

These tests are useful for monitoring an athlete's progress over time.

- Intensity is evaluated with incremental tests
- May be affected by parameters such as age, gender and altitude
- Test duration: 15 minutes
- Typical increments of 2.5 km/h when running and 12-18 W when cycling, with a pedaling frequency of 60 to 80 rpm
- The length of the steps must allow the subject to reach the steady state

Submaximal test types:

- **V-slope method**: evaluates the variation of ventilation. The relationship is linear until ventilation increases more than VO_2 max
- **Mader Anaerobic Threshold Test**: evaluates blood lactate concentration by doing a fingertip test. A blood lactate level of 4 mmol/l is used as a general estimation point of the aerobic threshold. Once this value is reached, greater intensities can be obtained with the progressive increase in lactate

Postural assessment and mobility tests

Postural evaluation

The standard anatomical position for postural evaluation is erect, facing forward, with the arms along the sides and the palms of the hands facing forward, with all the fingers extended. It is a reference location for all definitions and descriptions of body planes and axes.

Considering the standing position, the posture must always be analyzed on two different planes, i.e., the frontal plane (anterior and posterior analysis) and the sagittal plane (lateral analysis).

Anatomical planes are imaginary lines drawn across the body. These lines allow you to objectively describe the movements and positions of the body.

- **Sagittal plane**: it is vertical and is thus defined by the name of the sagittal suture of the skull. It is also called the anteroposterior plane. The midsagittal plane divides the body into left and right halves
- **Frontal or coronal plane**: it is vertical and extends from side to side. It is defined after the direction of the coronal suture of the skull. It divides the body into anterior and posterior portions

The frontal plane postural assessment

On this level, postural imbalances of the flexor-extensors are analyzed. To analyze them correctly you need to imagine a plumb line dividing the body into two equal parts (left and right). The analysis must be performed both anteriorly and posteriorly.

In the cranial to caudal direction, the physiological alignment should be as follows:

- head and neck must remain in the axis (no rotation, no lateral inclination)
- equal distance between the ears and the head
- straight spine, without lateral curvature
- equal size of the paraspinal muscle: nose, chin, suprasternal notch, sternum and navel are cut into two equal halves
- equal shoulder height (dominant shoulder may be lower)
- medial edge of the scapulae equidistant from the vertebral column
- lower angle of the shoulder blades must be equally distanced
- symmetrical rib cage
- elbows with equal resting angles
- iliac crests of equal heights
- ASIS and PSIS at equal heights
- greater trochanters of equal height
- gluteal folds at equal height
- equal size of the hamstrings
- equal distance between the knee joints
- kneecaps facing forward and at equal height
- popliteal fossae of equal height
- equal size of calf muscles
- Achilles tendon and heel in neutral alignment
- equal distance between the ankle joints and the medial malleoli
- longitudinal arch of the foot not excessively high or flat
- fingers in natural alignment
- feet apart from 5° to 18°

In both the anterior and posterior view, the ears, shoulders, iliac crests, peroneal headsand lateral malleoli should be in the same plane. In athletes who have played a throwing sport in the past (volleyball, tennis, baseball) or in people who have a dominant arm, it is common for the dominant shoulder to be lower than the other.

The arms must be equidistant from the trunk, with an equal angle (5°-15°). Your palms should be facing your body, with your thumbs pointing forward. The posterior view should show the scapulae being equidistant from the spine and level with each other in a superior-inferior direction. Normally, the scapulae, at rest, are located 5-8 cm from the vertebral column, between the T2 and T7 thoracic vertebrae. The spinous processes along the spine should be in a vertical line, with no noticeable curvature in the frontal plane (scoliosis). The iliac crests should be at the same level. The rib cage and trunk should be symmetrical on each side, with no lateral displacement or trunk deviation appearing in the frontal plane.

Posteriorly, the gluteal crease should be vertical and the gluteal masses should be symmetrical. The knees should be in a slight valgus position with the kneecaps pointing directly forward. Posteriorly, the popliteal fossae should be at the same level and horizontal. The feet should be slightly abducted (5°-18°), remaining symmetrical. Posteriorly, the Achilles tendons should be relatively vertical and symmetrical to each other.

Postural assessment in the sagittal plane

Postural assessment in the lateral view should be performed from both sides. As with the anterior and posterior view assessments, the assessment should begin cranially (above) to caudally (below). As a result, when viewed from the side, the plumb line should ideally line up:

- through the external auditory meatus
- through the odontoid process
- through the bodies of the cervical vertebrae
- through the acromioclavicular joint of the shoulder
- slightly anterior to the thoracic kyphosis
- slightly posterior to the lumbar lordosis
- through the greater trochanter of the femur
- slightly posterior to the center of the hip joint
- slightly anterior to the center of the knee joint and posterior to the patella
- slightly anterior to the lateral malleolus, across the calcaneocuboid joint of the ankle

A conformation often found among people with poor postural hygiene is the lower and upper cross syndrome. This syndrome is characterized by neuromuscular imbalances in which gluteal and abdominal weaknesses are compensated for by excessive iliopsoas and thoracolumbar extensor tone (lower cruciate syndrome) or forward head posture due to excessive extension of the occiput and rhomboid hypotonicity, with suboccipital muscle stiffness and deep neck flexor weakness (superior cross syndrome).

In this syndrome, certain muscle groups tend to be tight (tonic muscles) or weak (phasic muscles). Muscles prone to tension are usually readily activated with any movement, creating abnormal movement patterns.

Individuals with this postural dysfunction are prone to posture-related headaches and cervicogenic headaches. A common postural dysfunction, which is also present in individuals with a forward head posture, includes bilaterally rounded and internally rotated shoulders.

Tight muscles in these individuals probably include the latissimus dorsi and pectoral muscles. Tight pectoral muscles also commonly contribute to increased thoracic kyphosis, which is correctable (if functional dysfunction) with verbal and tactile cues. As we will see later, retracted hip flexors commonly contribute to the postural dysfunction of increased lumbar lordosis and limited hip flexion. Weak hip abductors can contribute to static and dynamic postural dysfunction (walking, running and jumping) and increased knee valgus. Weak external hip rotators may contribute to an increased internal rotation of the femur, a common component that has been described as lower extremity medial collapse (increased hip adduction and medial rotation beyond normal limits, with dynamic tasks). *Pes planus* (flatfoot posture) is a common postural dysfunction that may be static due to structural abnormalities or dynamic due to lack of muscle control, either proximal to the hip locally in the foot (e.g., the performance of the tibialis posterior and peroneus muscles). The presentation of kypholordotic posture is characterized by excessive kyphosis in the thoracic spine and corresponding excessive lordosis in the lumbar spine. A flat back posture is one in which the lumbar spine has less than normal lordosis or is flattened.

All of these postural dysfunctions (Fig. 33.1) can result from **structural** or **functional defects**. Structural defects result from congenital or developmental abnormalities, disease or trauma. Structural defects include excessive thoracic kyphosis due to Scheuermann disease, scoliosis or congenital leg length discrepancy. Structural defects often require bracing, specific exercise prescriptions and occasionally surgical corrections (if needed). Functional defects are those that typically result from poor posture habits. Upper and lower cross syndromes are common examples of functional defects.

Mobility tests

Similar to other sports, bodybuilding involves physical overloads deriving from the chronic repetition of a certain movement.

At first, the continuous contractile stresses to which the muscles are subjected have a protective role towards the joints. Precisely, it must be remembered that the mechanical pressure applied to the bones through weightlifting directly increases their mineralization and joint lubrication. The somatic perception derived from this discipline allows for an approach to the outside world such as placing front-line muscle contraction during all daily activities (moving weights, walking, running, sitting, etc.), thus preventing the joints from overloading, something which, without sufficient muscle mass, would be inevitable.

However, if on the one hand bodybuilding can be protective for the joints, exercises performed incorrectly, body asymmetries, poor rest and contractile stimulations

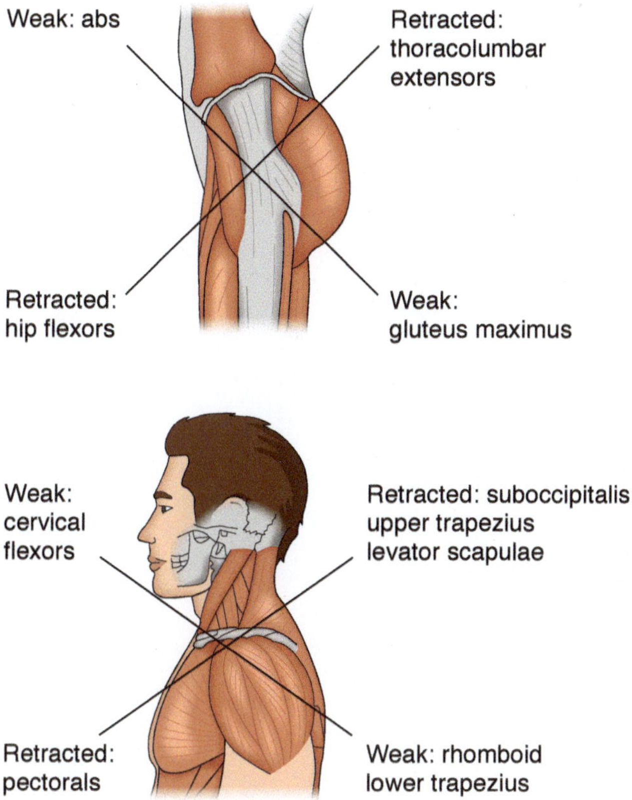

Figure 33.1 Inferior and superior cross syndrome: a consequence of weak and retracted muscles.

not accompanied by appropriate stretching sessions can be responsible for muscle contractions that, if ignored or otherwise not treated, can alter what should be the normal motor pattern used during an exercise.

This contractile shift is not only responsible for an incessant loss of strength, but it is also the main cause of joint pain that, sooner or later, affects all athletes.

Although the average bodybuilder begins to be interested in the hygiene of their joint mobility only after the onset of pain, mobility tests should have a mainly preventive role, not a curative one.

Since we have already dealt extensively with postural imbalances in the previous paragraph, here we will limit ourselves to describing the most useful mobility tests that can be administered to a bodybuilder.

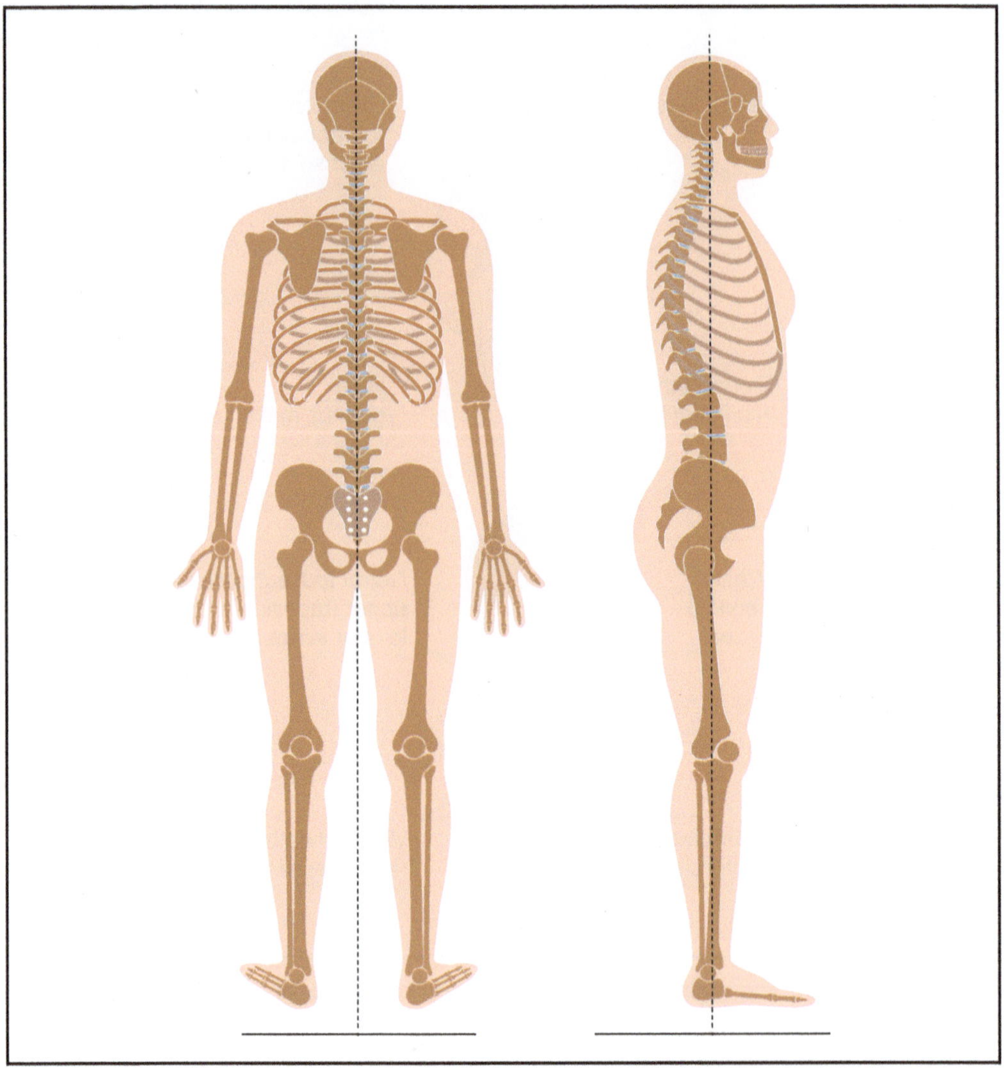

Figure 33.2 Posterior view (frontal plane) and lateral view (sagittal plane) of the skeleton.

Premise

To evaluate the active or passive mobility of a joint, it is always necessary to generate the movement opposite to that physiologically expected by the muscles of the tested joint. The greater the resistance generated by the muscle during the test, the more limited the mobility of the joint will be.

Mobility tests are a great way to detect which muscles are responsible for impaired joint motor efficiency and give us the opportunity to find out which muscles need to be stretched and/or strengthened.

Mobility tests are often combined with strength tests. However, it must be kept in mind that a contracted muscle is also a weak muscle; maximal myofibrillar recruitment can occur only after an optimal pre-stretch.

Shoulder mobility test

Rotator cuff

The assessment of shoulder mobility mainly passes through the analysis of the rotator cuff in order to evaluate the capacity for extra- and internal rotation. The rotator cuff muscles are particularly active with 0° to 90° flexion and abduction.

The rotator cuff is the most active muscle-tendon complex of the joint; its function is to force the humeral head into the glenoid "cavity", ensuring joint co-action.

However, it must always be kept in mind that, to analyze the correct scapulohumeral rhythm, muscles such as the trapezius, serratus and deltoid must also be evaluated in order to have a more complete picture of the athlete's muscular balance.

The rotator cuff includes the following muscles.

1. Supraspinatus: extrarotator and abductor
2. Infraspinatus: external rotator and adductor
3. Teres minor: external rotator and adductor
4. Subscapularis: intrarotator and adductor

Trapezius and serratus major

Scapular rotation from 90° to 150° is evaluated through the analysis of the sternocostalclavicular and scapulothoracic joints.

The trapezius and the serratus major work in synergy to allow for the physiological scapulothoracic pattern, coordinated with the movement of the glenohumeral joint.

Latissimus dorsi and thoracic mobility

The range of motion of the latissimus dorsi and pectoralis major muscles and of the spinal column muscles is evaluated from 150° to 180°. The latissimus dorsi, like the pectoralis, are humeral intrarotarors: the more they are retracted, the sooner the anteversion of the pelvis (lordotization) will be observed following the flexion of the limbs.

Assessment of active mobility

It is the degree of articular movement that a person can reach with their muscles. The movements that are evaluated are always the internal and external rotators.

Apley's Scratch Test (Fig. 33.3)

The abduction/external rotation/flexion are evaluated with the hand above the head; the subject should arrive at the spine of the opposite scapula.

The adduction/internal rotation/extension are evaluated with the hand behind the back; the subject should touch the inferior corner of the opposite scapula.

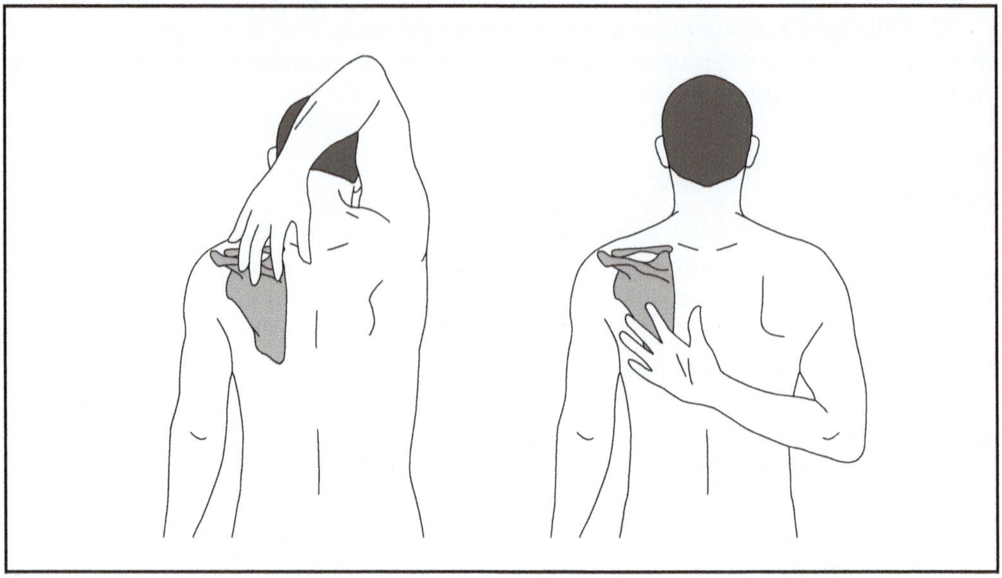

Figure 33.3 Apley's Scratch Test.

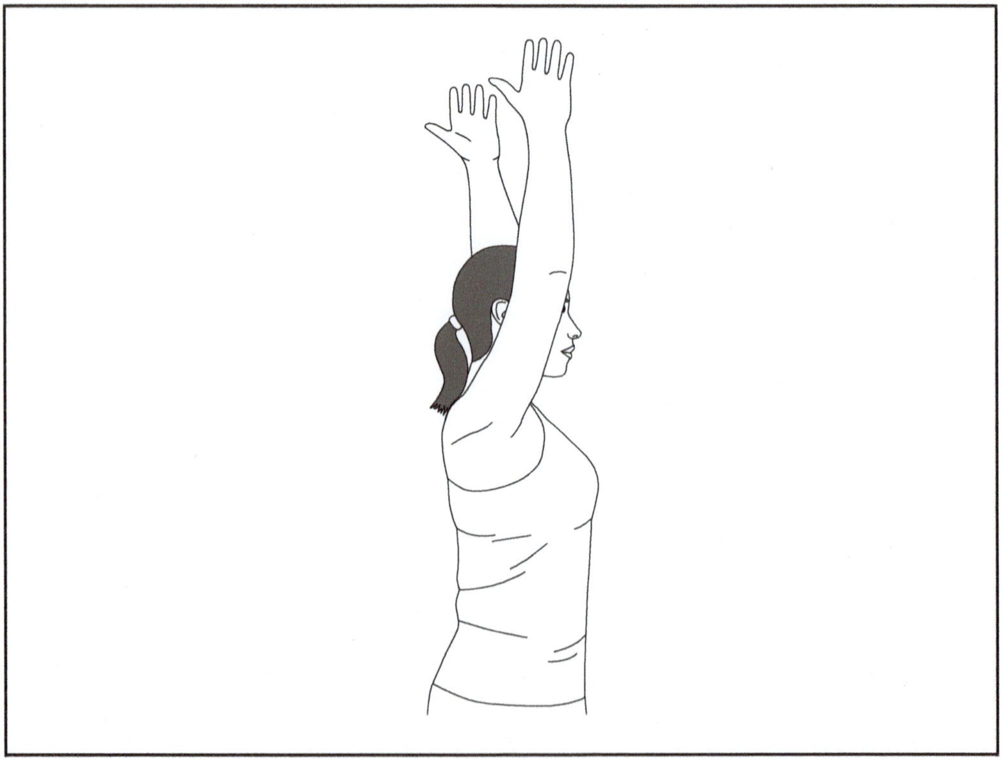

Figure 33.4 Global abduction and flexion test.

Global Abduction and Flexion Test (Fig. 33.4)

The subject is asked to perform an abduction in the frontal plane with straight arms and a flexion in the sagittal plane. On three sides, we observe:

- the fluidity and the range of motion
- symmetry
- scapulohumeral rhythm
- compensation and postural deviations during or at the end of the movement
- onset of pain

Assessment of passive mobility

Passive mobility tests examine internal rotation and external rotation thanks to the intervention of an operator. The athlete must remain in the supine position without applying any resistance.

The test shown in Figure 33.5 evaluates the etiology of joint stiffness, which can depend on a too-stiff musculature (mild stiffness), on a capsule-ligament block (significant stiffness) or on a bone block if the resulting resistance is insurmountable.

Along with mobility exercises, some exercises must be avoided in order not to further overload the blocked joint.

Although it is not uncommon for an athlete to have retracted external rotators (excessive training volume of the posterior shoulder lodge, resulting in low plasticity and muscle stiffness), the retracted intra-rotator muscles are responsible for alterations in the shoulder, including the glenohumeral joint.

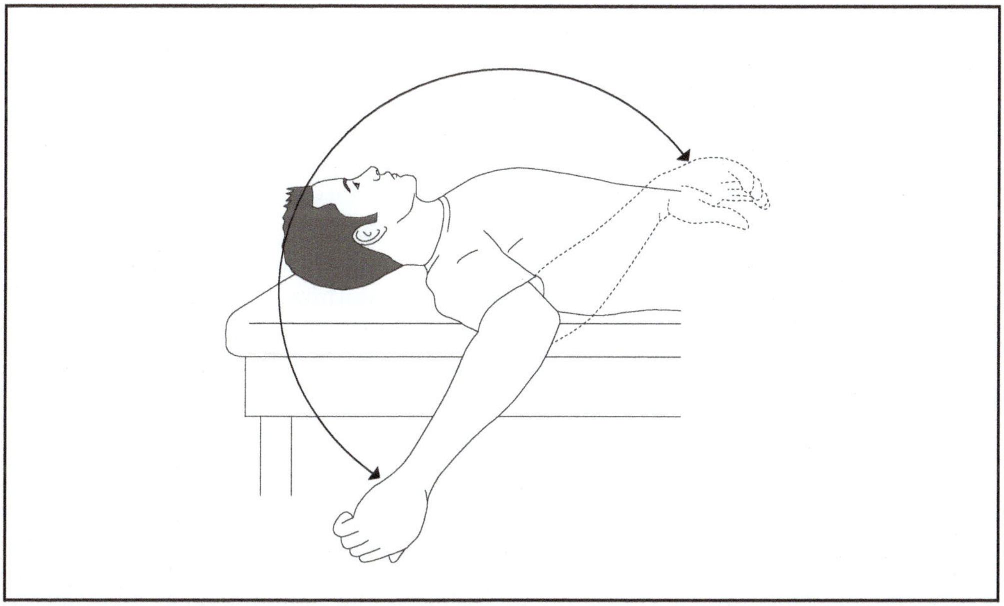

Figure 33.5 Passive mobility assessment test.

Since internal rotation is not generated exclusively by the subscapularis (the only intra-rotator of the rotator cuff), but also by the pectoralis major and latissimus dorsi muscles, which are decidedly larger and stronger than the extra-rotators, it is important to focus simultaneously on their stretching and on strengthening the external rotation muscles (posterior deltoid, rhomboid, infraspinatus).

Due to the poor external rotation derived from the rigidity of the internal rotators, the exercises to avoid will be those that force the joint to bear an overload in the externally rotated position. The overhead press with the barbell, the seated or standing French press, and the back squat are the first to avoid; vice versa, single-arm open kinetic chain exercises, with handlebars, can be preparatory for improving the perception of movement and adjusting the trajectory freely, without the rigidity imposed by a barbell.

As for squats, they should be replaced with front squats, Bulgarian split squats or hack squats.

As far as exercises involving the pectoralis major and latissimus dorsi are concerned, the execution must be carried out in maximum lengthening and minimum shortening. This will induce a positive muscle restructuring, with an increase in the contractile component to the detriment of the tendon component.

Test for posterior capsular retraction (scapulothoracic mobility)

With the subject in a prone position, with the arms rotated internally behind the back and the hands at the height of the sacrum (position of the lift-off from the lying position), the arm is released to evaluate the scapular excursion. If the scapula does not descend, a blockage of the posterior compartment is assumed and the following treatment should be focused on the mobility of the serratus and external rotators, and on the strength of the subscapularis.

Together with mobility exercises, the exercises to be used to improve the scapular pattern and, therefore, to regain mobility of the scapulothoracic joint are:

- pullover, lying down with the dumbbell or standing on the cable, always using one arm at a time and controlling the eccentric phase (about 4 seconds)
- tractions or lat machine exercises with scapular movement; summing up, at the end of each eccentric or ascent phase, an elevation with subsequent depression of the scapula is applied. Besides increasing scapulothoracic mobility, this movement allows for a significant anabolism of the latissimus dorsi muscle. It is also preferable to perform this exercise with one arm at a time

Tests to evaluate subacromial impingement or impingement syndrome

It is a pathology of the shoulder involving the rotator cuff, determined by the dysfunctional passage of the supraspinatus tendon through the coraco-acromial tunnel.

- **Neer test**: flexion against resistance with the arm internally rotated and with a locked scapula
- **The Yocum Test**: hand of the affected shoulder is placed on the opposite shoulder, and then the examiner elevates the elbow

- **Jobe test**: test for the rotator cuff integrity and for the supraspinatus strength; with the limbs internally rotated in the scapular plane, a push against resistance is required
- **External rotation test**: with arms adducted and elbow flexed, the patient actively rotates the arm externally against the resistance of the examiner's hand

The hip mobility tests

The evaluation, with the consequent correction, of the mobility of the muscles that fit into the hip joint, represents one of the main anamnestic targets both for the improvement of the performance in multi-joint exercises, such as squats and leg presses, and, given their anatomical proximity, for the efficiency of the respiratory, reproductive and excretory systems.

Tests for assessing hip mobility include tests which evaluate several muscles:

- hip flexor length test (Thomas Test)
- hip rotator muscles tests (Freiberg Test, FAIR Test, Heel Contra-Lateral Knee [HCLK] Test)
- tests to measure the flexibility of hip extensors, whose tightness results in a forward tilt of the pelvis (Seat and Reach Test, Lasègue Test, Hamstring Test, Squat Test)

Hip flexor mobility test

The iliopsoas is the main hip flexor, along with the quadriceps. A hypertonic state of these two flexors can lead to an excessive lumbar lordosis, with consequent overloading of the intervertebral discs and deactivation of the gluteus maximus, due to a constant pre-stretching of the latter.

Thomas Test

On a firm table without padding, the subject lies on their back with their thighs half outstretched, one lower limb extended and the other flexed, bringing the knee to the chest. This exercise evaluates whether the contraction of the iliopsoas affects the other limb by raising the thigh.

The Thomas Test is one of the gold standard tests for assessing the iliopsoas length and can present several scenarios:

- **typical length of hip flexors**: this is the physiological position of a non-retracted iliopsoas (Fig. 33.6); the thigh stays on the table and the angle between the leg and thigh is 90°
- **typical length of one-joint hip flexors (iliopsoas) and shortness of two-joint hip flexors (quadriceps)**: the thigh stays on the table, but the angle between the leg and thigh is >90°. In this case, the quadriceps is retracted. Stretching and foam roller exercises for the rectus femoris are recommended
- **shortness of both one-joint and two-joint hip flexors**: the thigh lifts off the table and the angle between the leg and thigh is >90°. In this case, both the quadriceps and the psoas are retracted. Stretching exercises are recommended for both the iliopsoas and the rectus femoris

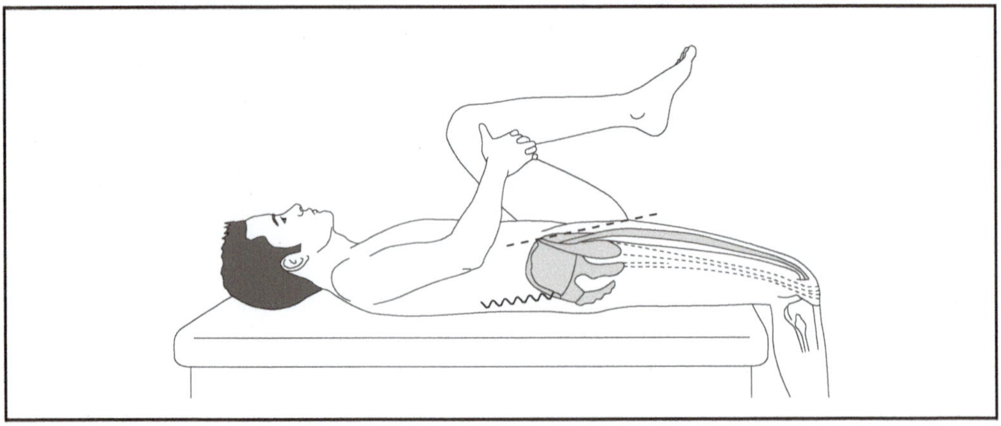

Figure 33.6 Thomas Test: The physiological position of a non-retracted iliopsoas.

- **typical length of two-joint hip flexors and shortness of one-joint hip flexors**: the thigh lifts off the table but the angle between the leg and thigh remains stable at 90°. In this case, only the psoas is retracted. Stretching exercises for the iliopsoas are recommended

The other flexors potentially involved in hip and knee problems are the tensor fascia latae and the adductors (the latter also act as extensors). Foam rollers are used for the former (including the iliotibial band) and stretching is used for the latter.

Mobility tests for the deep external rotator muscles of the hip

The deep external rotator muscles of the hip are mainly responsible for the external rotation, adduction (obturators, gemelli, quadratus femoris) and abduction (piriformis) of the hip. A retracted pelvis is often associated with weak gluteus medius and gluteus maximus muscles. Postural imbalance associated with a weak glute and retracted piriformis may be one cause of tension felt near the ischial tuberosity, subgluteal region and posterior thigh near the gluteus maximus.

- **Freiberg Test**: with the patient in the supine position, the examiner forcefully brings the hip into internal rotation and adduction, keeping the knee extended.
- **FAIR Test**: the patient's hip is passively flexed to 90°, adducted and internally rotated, with the knee flexed to 90°. The test can be performed with the patient in the supine position or lying on their unaffected side.
- **Heel Contra-Lateral Knee (HCLK) Test**: lying in the supine position, the patient places the heel of the foot of the affected limb on the contralateral knee, thus bringing the hip into external rotation and flexion beyond 90°.

The muscles tested are external rotators of the hip: excess resistance to internal rotation of the leg of the affected part of the hip is indicative of retraction of the piriformis.

However, the opposite should also be taken into consideration: excess internal rotation represents a weakness of the external rotator muscles of the hip and requires strengthening through specific exercises.

Mobility test for the hip extensors

Hamstrings are the main extensors of the hip and act synergistically on the glute. A hypertonic state of these two extensors can lead to hypolordosis, with consequent overload for the vertebral facet joints. Tight and weak hamstrings are the leading cause of anterior cruciate ligament rupture in soccer players. If hamstrings are extremely tight, the athlete experiences muscle weakness with symptoms made worse by repeated eccentric contractions, trunk flexion and hip flexion in activities such as running or maintaining a sitting position.

- **Bent-Knee Stretch Test**: with the athlete in the supine position, bring the thigh into the position of maximum flexion, with the leg perpendicular to the thigh; at this point, extend the leg as much as possible. The test is positive when the subject perceives pain at the level of the ischial tuberosity. It is very important to distinguish between pain derived from muscle stretching and neuropathic pain.
- **Squat Test Position 2**: originally created as a NASM test protocol (National Academy of Sports Medicine, USA) and of the Fizkultura i Sport, University of Moscow, Russia, the Squat Test includes five tests which, together, evaluate the global and functional active mobility of all the joints of the body. Position 2 is specific for the hamstring range of motion.

Squat Test Position: Hands at sides with fingers forward and elbows back. The hands resting on the iliac crests force the trunk to be supported by the quadratus lumborum, allowing for greater joint mobility of the lumbar spine. Position 2 is the position where the operator focuses on the pelvis and lower back.

Errors that can be detected: the following errors are representative of poor mobility of the muscles of the posterior chain (lower back and hamstrings):

- excess bending of the torso forward
- loss of lumbar lordosis
- torso rotation

The alterations of the muscles associated with the pelvic girdle cause various limitations in the quantity and quality of the exercises that an athlete should be able to perform.

Very tight anterior musculature (femoral quadriceps and iliopsoas) leads to postural hyperlordosis, which will only get worse if the muscles involved in the posterior pelvic tilt are weak.

In these conditions, it is necessary to strengthen the abdominal, gluteal and hamstring muscles to adjust the morphological compensation.

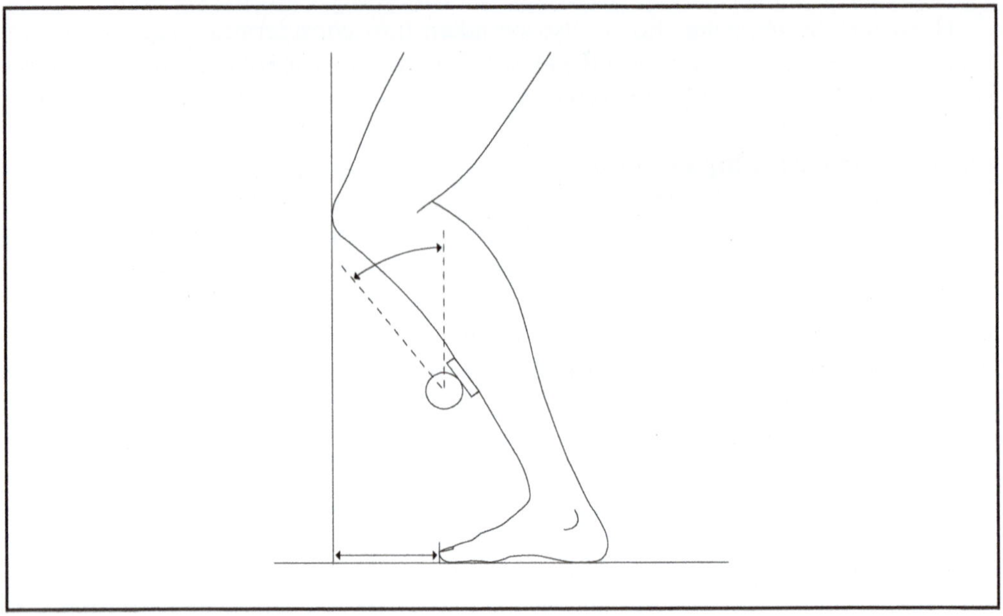

Figure 33.7 5 Fingers Wall Test.

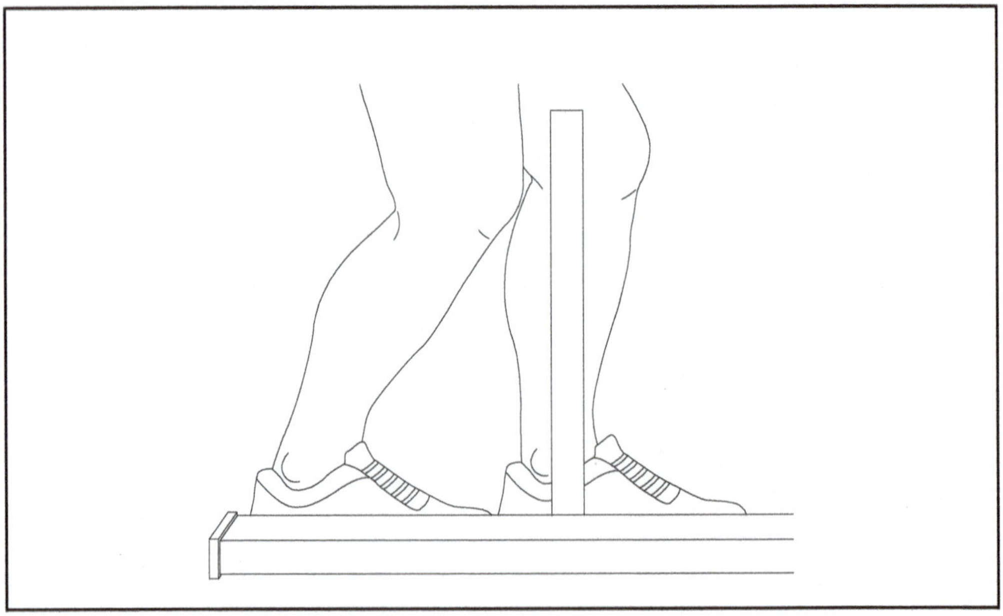

Figure 33.8 Ankle Clearing.

Starting the leg session with leg curls, including exercises such as deep squats and hip thrusts, and training the abs at least three times a week, together with daily stretching, can be sufficient to improve postural balance.

Conversely, severely tight posterior musculature (hamstrings) may cause hypolordosis, weak deep vertebral muscles and hamstring strains/tears.

In these conditions, in addition to the daily stretching of the posterior chain, the hamstrings should continue to be trained, emphasizing the eccentric phase as much as possible and limiting the movement in the concentric one. You must continue to do exercises such as squats, possibly with an angle of 140° between one leg and the other in order to limit the resistance that the shortened hamstring would apply in the descent phase, or with a one-inch thick plate placed under the heel to deduct the contribution of the triceps surae from the descent phase.

Ankle mobility test

The evaluation, with the consequent correction, of the mobility of the ankle represents one of the main anamnestic targets for the improvement of the performance in multi-joint exercises such as squats and leg presses. Ankle mobility tests evaluate the range of motion of the triceps surae (gastrocnemius) and soleus.

Wall Test

It is the simplest and most effective test for analyzing ankle dorsiflexion:

- lay measuring tape on the ground with the zero marking at the wall
- position yourself with your toes pointing toward the wall
- find and mark the maximum distance that allows your knee to touch the wall (keeping the heel on the ground)
- do the same with the other ankle
- longer distance achieved equals better ankle dorsiflexion

Five-inch Wall Test

It is the same as the previous one, the only difference being that, in this test, your big toe is five inches from the wall (Fig. 33.7).

If your knee can touch the wall, you have good dorsiflexion; vice versa, you need to work on ankle mobility with active mobility exercises or foam rolling for your calves.

Ankle Clearing Test (Fig. 33.8)

- Position your feet so that the toes of the rear foot touch the heel of the front foot.
- The ankle of the rear foot is evaluated by sending the knee as far forward as possible.
- Take the tip of the knee of the rear leg as a reference, with the malleolus of the front foot.

Poor ankle mobility, in addition to limiting the performance in multi-joint exercises such as presses and squats, predisposes the knee joint to more rapid wear.

Poor mobility of the ankle joint is the main cause of poor performance during exercises such as squats, hack squats and lunges.

Stretching and/or myofascial treatment of the gastrocnemius and soleus should be performed daily to achieve significant improvements; however, other precautions can also be applied to avoid an excessive overload of the patello-femoral joint directly connected to tibio-tarsal inefficiency:

- 1-inch thick plate under the heel during the squats
- prefer split squats to lunges, so you can place the plate under the heel
- prefer the front squat to the back squat
- train the calves and emphasize the eccentric phase as much as possible. Limit the movement of the concentric phase. Intraset stretching can act as a passive stretch for the soleus and the gemelli

CHAPTER 34

Back pain and abdominal muscle training

Steven Giuffrida

Unfortunately, in bodybuilding athletes, vertebral pain problems are often encountered, especially in the lumbar region, which is stressed with heavy loads that alter the functional biomechanics of the lumbar lordosis. If we consider the vertebral column as a complex network of anatomical structures subjected to precise physical and biomechanical laws, it is easy to understand that simple alterations significantly modify its physiology and function. Due to the proximity of vital anatomical elements, cranial nerves, spinal cord, brain stem, arteries and other blood vessels, any change in the biomechanics of the spine will have negative effects on these structures, significantly affecting the athlete's training ability.

Upper and lower abs

Although, from an anatomical point of view, we speak of rectus abdominis and, therefore, not of a horizontal separation into upper and lower abdominal bundles, some studies (Willett et al., 2001) in which four abs exercises were examined (abdominal crunch, reverse crunch, twist crunch, V-sit) showed that in the reverse crunch, there is greater activation of the sub-umbilical part of the abdomen, and the activation of the external oblique is strong in the V-sit. The upper part works in a similar way in almost all the exercises, both in dynamics and in isometric contraction (Figs. 34.1-34.3).

While examining the possible exercises in case of back pain we should pay the deserved attention to an exercise called "Janda sit-up", conceived by Dr. Vladimir Janda. The exercise looks like a normal sit-up, with the difference that it is performed through the contraction of the extensor muscles of the leg, thigh and buttocks, together with the trunk coming close to the pelvis; this contraction can be facilitated by using a support on which the heels can carry out an isometric contraction against resistance. The ratio exploits the law of "reciprocal innervation" (Sherrington's principle), according to which "the contraction of an antagonist muscle can induce relaxation of the agonist muscle"; this way, the action of the hip flexors should be reduced, making the exercise doable also by subjects suffering from lower back pain.

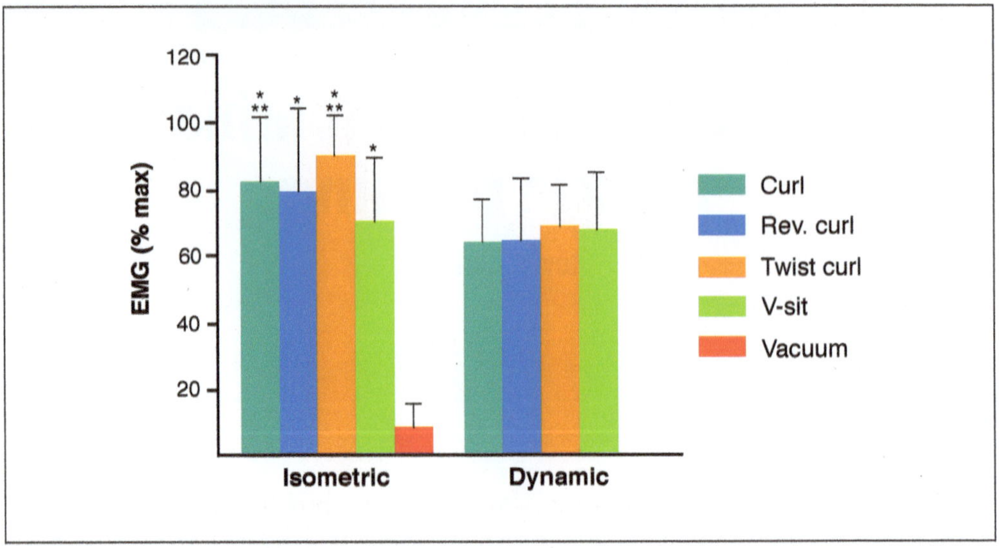

Figure 34.1 The graph shows the activation percentage of the upper portion of the rectus abdominis during the execution of the exercises, both in dynamics and in isometrics, compared to both the vacuum exercise and the V-sit. (Edited by: Willett GM et al. Relative activity of abdominal muscles during commonly prescribed strengthening exercises. *J Strength Cond Res* 2001 Nov;15(4):480-485)

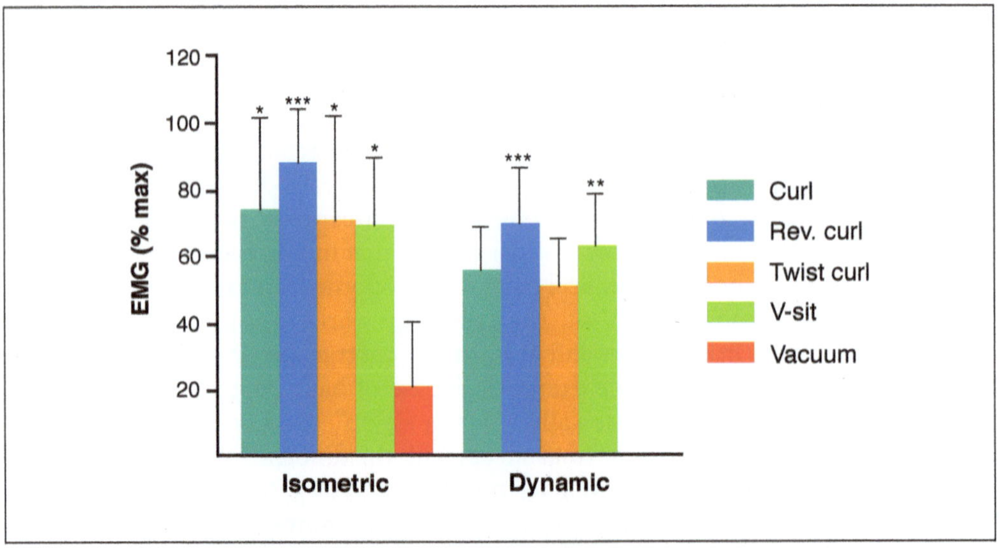

Figure 34.2 The graph shows the activation percentage of the lower portion of the rectus abdominis during the execution of the exercises both in dynamics and in isometrics, compared to the vacuum and to all the lifting exercises of the trunk, also with torsion. (Edited by: Willett GM et al. Relative activity of abdominal muscles during commonly prescribed strengthening exercises. *J Strength Cond Res* 2001 Nov;15(4):480-485)

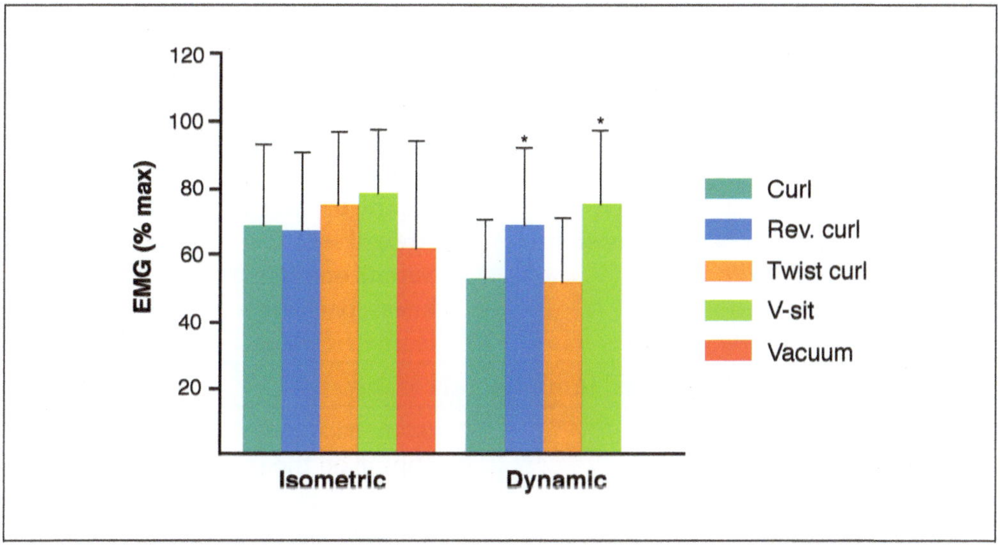

Figure 34.3 The graph shows the activation percentage of the lower portion of the external oblique during the execution of the exercises both in dynamics and in isometrics, compared to all the lifting exercises of the trunk, also with torsion. (Edited by: Willett GM et al. Relative activity of abdominal muscles during commonly prescribed strengthening exercises. *J Strength Cond Res* 2001 Nov;15(4):480-485)

This exercise finds scientific confirmation in Workman et al. (2008), where the following muscle groups are also examined by electromyography:

- URA (Upper Rectus Abdominis)
- LRA (Lower Rectus Abdominis)
- EO (External Obliques)
- LAS (Lower Abdominal Stabilizers)
- rectus femoris and hamstrings

The results of this study indicate that hamstring activation during the Janda sit-up not only reduces the rectus femoris activation, but also induces high levels of muscle activation in the LRA and URA.

Another study (Axler and McGill, 1997) examining the relationship between abdominal activation and spinal compression demonstrates that the exercises considered "safe" in case of spinal pain are not those that ensure better activation of the abdomen.

This study was performed using an EGM (electromyograph) and examined a series of common exercises and, among them, the relationship between compression of the lumbar spine and greater or lesser muscle activation.

The best relationship between URA and spinal compression	
1. Anchored foot crunch 2. Straight leg raise with legs in suspension 3. 90° ¼ leg sit-up 4. Anchored foot twisting crunch 5. Leg raise, bent knees in suspension 6. Free foot crunch	7. Straight leg sit-up 8. Sit-up, bent knees, anchored feet 9. Supine on the mat, leg raise, bent knees 10. Supine on the mat, leg raise, straight legs 11. Supine on the mat, leg raise bent knees, back arched (lordosis) 12. Isometric plank
Increased lumbosacral compression	
1. Straight leg sit-ups 2. Supine on the mat, leg raise with bent knees 3. Sit-up, bent knees, anchored feet 4. Leg raise, bent knees in suspension 5. Anchored foot twisting crunch 6. Leg raise, straight legs in suspension	7. Isometric plank 8. Supine on the mat, leg raise, straight legs 9. 90° ¼ leg sit-up 10. Anchored foot crunch 11. Free foot crunch 12. Supine on the mat, leg raises bent knees, back arched (lordosis)
Best URA activity	
1. Straight leg sit-up 2. Leg raise straight legs in suspension 3. Sit-up, knees bent, feet anchored 4. Leg raise, bent knees in suspension 5. Anchored foot twisting crunch 6. 90° ¼ leg sit-up	7. Lying on the mat, leg raises with bent knees 8. Anchored foot crunch 9. Free foot crunches 10. Supine on the mat, leg raise with straight legs 11. Isometric plank 12. Supine on the mat, leg raise bent knees, back arched (lordosis)
Best EO activity	
1. Leg raise with straight legs in suspension 2. Sit-up, knees bent, feet anchored 3. Supine on the mat, leg raise with bent knees 4. Anchored foot twisting crunch 5. Straight leg sit-up 6. Leg raise with bent knees in suspension	7. Isometric plank 8. Anchored foot crunch 9. 90° ¼ leg sit-up 10. Supine on the mat, leg raise with straight legs 11. Free foot crunch 12. Supine on the mat, leg raise bent knees, back arched (lordosis)

Continues

Continued

Conclusions	
1. ¼ sit-ups	Better stimulation of the rectus abdominis
2. Isometric plank	Better stimulation of the oblique
3. Supine on the mat, leg raise with straight legs	Not recommended in relation to the URA/compression ratio
4. Supine on the mat, leg raise bent knees, back curved (lordosis)	Not recommended in relation to the URA/compression ratio
5. Lying on the mat, leg raise with bent knees	Not recommended in relation to the URA/compression ratio
6. Leg raise with bent knees in suspension	Not recommended in relation to the URA/compression ratio

From the examination of the exercises, the plank in its infinite variations, both on stable and unstable planes, proves to be particularly important due to its effectiveness and reduced impairment in a spine that is already affected by pathologies, capable of further stimulating the proprioceptive system and the consequent response of the neurological system.

The role of the proprioceptive system

Balance is a complex function, integrated and correlated the posture. Both are the result of the elaboration of vestibular, visual, auditory and proprioceptive afferents at the brainstem level, under the constant modulation of the postural tonic system. Any alteration of the postural tonic system, linked to the receptor activity or to a bad integration of the relative information by the central nervous system, involves a loss of the harmonic relationships in the three dimensions of space, between the various skeletal elements, resulting in an asymmetrical deconstruction of joint mechanics and muscle synergistic chains.

In recent years, physical preparation experts have increasingly recommended exercises for the muscles of the central part of the body, known as "core" in sports training and rehabilitation programs.

Janda and Va'Vrova (1996) state with certainty that the use of the Swiss ball has the advantage of minimizing joint stress, but above all, it contributes to a significant increase in proprioception and balance.

The results of various studies, in the long term, seem to indicate that exercises aimed at improving core stability can reduce the intensity of pain in the spine as well as prevent any recurrence (Rasmussen-Barr et al., 2003; Stuge et al., 2004).

In this regard, Marshall and Murphy (2005) have minimized the importance of isolated activities of the rectus abdominis muscle in report with the overall muscle action, in stabilizing the pelvic girdle and lumbar region. Therefore, the notion of the overall receptor balance of the central part of the body is privileged and it must fit into a neurophysiological concept of posture, not just a biomechanical one.

We must also consider the fact that exercises on unstable surfaces cause an increase in the electromyographic activation of the muscles through the simultaneous contraction of the muscles of the abdominal wall. As a reflex, there is also an important and diversified receptor activity, which is expressed in an improved neuromuscular control, with stabilizing effects that are demonstrated both during complex sports movements and common daily activities.

According to Lehman et al. (2005), the prone bridge (or plank) performed on the Swiss ball gives rise to an increase in the electromyographic activity referred to the rectus abdominis and the external oblique muscles. During a supine bridge, however, the Swiss ball exercise does not affect the rectus abdominis or external oblique muscles. On the other hand, the side bridge, if performed on a Swiss ball, produces a higher electromyographic activity both in the internal oblique and in the spinal erector muscles.

In conclusion, current scientific guidelines show that exercises designed to improve strength, if performed on a Swiss ball (Bosu ball), i.e. on an unstable surface, lead to a greater increase in electromyographic activity and a higher involvement of core stability, with significant advantages for the static-dynamic balance of the athlete.

CHAPTER 35

Training with back pain: our experience

Riccardo Gaspari, Massimo Spattini and Federico Focherini

Training with back pain

Riccardo Gaspari

August 2, 2019, was one of the most traumatic awakenings of my life: my right leg was barely responding to my commands. After a few moments of panic, I did what seemed right to me (in those moments, and for a few more hours, I was hoping it was a tear). And the statement "I was hoping for a tear" should already give you an idea of the pain and the psychological situation I was in, even if, in hindsight, I probably already knew the cause but denied it to myself). I called Massimo (the co-author of this book and constant lifeline to my problems), who immediately sent me to get an MRI.

I went to one of the most avant-garde centers in Northern Italy where they performed an examination with Swiss precision and after a few minutes (which seemed like hours) they gave me the report. I still don't know whether to consider it a medical report, a court verdict or a life sentence: L5-S1 expelled hernia (with the physician's assistant specifying the significant dimensions of the extrusion).

I think I sat in my car in the facility's parking lot staring into space for at least an hour.

I had already abandoned my competitive career and all that follows for personal and professional reasons. I trained to feel good, to be healthy and fit, and to indulge in a photo shoot every now and then, but this report made me realize that I would be limited in my everyday life, both in private and at work. I panicked and called Massimo.

Upon hearing the news, Massimo bent over backwards to offer a range solutions for me. This is where the true (fortunately successful) journey begins, which has strengthened my ties to my job even more, making me pay attention to details and research, study continuously, and above all, introducing me to the pleasure of helping people get better (I consider my job a privilege).

After a cycle of ozone discolysis (supervised by Dr. G. Sarcletti) and a few rehabilitation sessions with Dr. R. Carniel, I began to feel brand new and at this point I called Massimo again...

This is where Davide Antoniella, professor, trainer, osteopath and professional athletic trainer, as well as collaborator of the Spattini Medical Office came into the picture.

Davide and I already knew each other, and I knew about his professional and personal value, but he proved to be really important in my journey, as he became a constant support with a continuous exchange of opinions and impressions, until he developed the pre- and post-workout postural program that I still follow today at the beginning and end of my workout.

The exercises given below serve to warm up and stretch all the muscle chains that are in some way connected with L5-S1, preparing them adequately for the training session. They help lengthen and loosen the overloaded muscle chains during training, always “linked” to L5-S1. Believe me, these exercises are of vital importance in terms of safeguarding and prevention and will guarantee you considerable athletic longevity.

In preparatory terms, performing the pre-workout schedule, even on rest days, when I woke up proved to be very useful. Before describing the exercises, it is essential to highlight the importance of correct breathing – something that is always taken for granted but is often lacking – using lung capacity to the maximum and putting into practice the correct mechanics of breathing, which consists of two phases, inhalation and exhalation, and which involves the diaphragm and the intercostal muscles, thanks to which we can expand the rib cage by increasing its volume in the inhalation phase and decreasing its volume in the exhalation phase.

Over time, this mechanism that is automatic in children and changes in adults, can be partially conditioned by predominantly psychosomatic causes.

Breathing is a very powerful tool because **it allows you to regulate the balance between the sympathetic nervous system**, which is activated in stressful situations, prepares for the fight-or-flight response, and generates rapid and superficial thoracic breathing (chemical mediators: norepinephrine, adrenaline and cortisol), and the parasympathetic nervous system, which is activated in calm, recovery and immune defense situations, favored by slow and deep diaphragmatic breathing (release of acetylcholine).

Diaphragmatic breathing stimulates the vagus nerve, a long bundle of motor and sensory fibers that connects the brain and brain stem to the heart, lungs and the digestive system: the **vagus nerve**, among other things, stimulates the parasympathetic nervous system, manages inflammation, controls cardiac variability (HRV, functioning index of the interaction between the cardiovascular, nervous and respiratory systems) and regulates emotions, generating positive ones, as well as helping for a better management of the negative ones.

On the other hand, when the activation of the sympathetic system prevails, we find ourselves in situations of generalized hypertonicity which also negatively affects the anti-gravity kinetic chain muscles and the diaphragm itself, which would cause further traction on the lumbar tract of the spine and would limit the natural respiratory function, forcing the use of accessory muscles.

Using deep diaphragmatic breathing (in normal conditions, the diaphragm lowers during inspiration and, meeting the viscera, causes the belly to swell), **emphasizing the expiration phase activates and stimulates the vagus nerve**. Maintaining the right respiratory condition allows you to improve the situation, thanks to the exercises described below.

Pre-workout table by Prof. Davide Antoniella

Stretching of the adductors, lying frog-leg posture

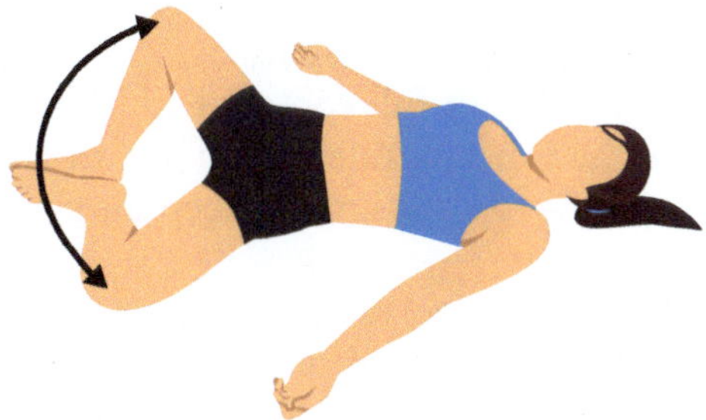

A simple but effective exercise to stretch the entire group of adductor muscles.

- Lie on your back with your knees bent and externally rotated at the hips. The soles of your feet are facing each other and your back is flat on the ground, while your arms rest on the ground along your sides with the palms of your hands facing upwards. Bring your chin towards your chest; to facilitate the movement, you can put a riser under your neck.
- From this position gently push your knees downwards to tense the adductors without taking your back off the ground and hold for about 20-30 seconds, breathing deeply.
- Changing the distance between your feet and pelvis or bringing your knees lower or higher allows you to manage and adapt the tension during the stretching phase.
- To accentuate the stretching of the adductors it is possible to press your hands against your knees, but the pressure must not be exaggerated. A feeling of slight discomfort is natural, but not pain. Finally, avoid sudden, jerky or bouncy movements, which can injure or tear the muscles.

Hip rotation in a supine position

This exercise is suitable for stretching your lower back and it also increases the flexibility and mobility of the hip extensors (glutes and hamstrings) and the oblique abdominals.

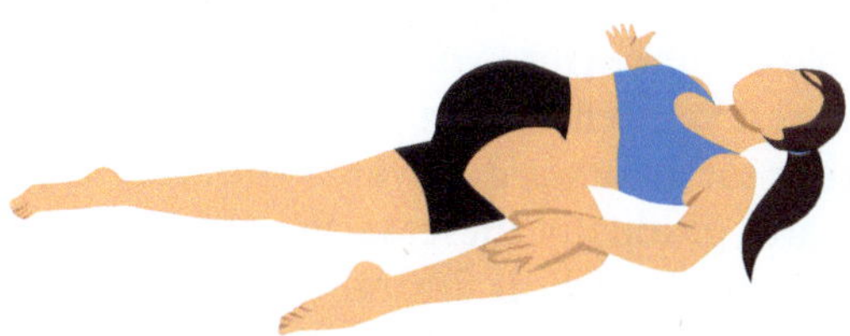

Continues

Continued

- Lie on your back (supine position in lateral decubitus) with your arms stretched out at your sides. From this position, lift the leg you want to work on with your knee slightly bent and bring it over the opposite leg, letting your foot fall to the floor.
- Keeping your shoulder on the ground, grasp the outside of the flexed knee with your opposite hand and rotate your lower body, pulling your knee down. The rest of your body must remain as still as possible.
- The nonworking limb remains in full contact with the ground and, if flexibility allows, the shoulder on the working side should not lift off the ground. Your head can be turned away from the turning limb to keep the clavicle still and to increase torque.
- Push your knee down until you feel tension in your buttock and lumbar area (in subjects with good flexibility, the knee can touch the ground). When you reach the maximum stretch, hold the position for at least 30 seconds then repeat the exercise for the other side. Breathing is slow and regular.

For a better focus on the hip muscles, the knee of the rotating limb should be flexed. In the extended limb and knee variant, there will be a greater involvement of the hamstrings.

Seated hip abduction with the heels together – Posterior chain and crossed stretching

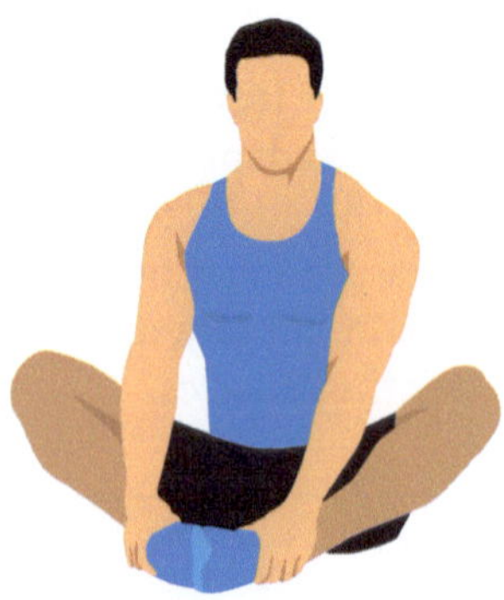

This is an exercise that stretches the adductor muscles, upper back and shoulders.

- To start the movement, sit on the floor with your legs opened in abduction, your knees bent and the soles of your feet together in a butterfly (or breaststroke) position at a comfortable distance from your pelvis.
- From this position, rest your elbows on your knees, pressing them gently towards the ground. Flex your torso forward, towards your feet, trying to keep the lumbar curve unchanged, and gradually increase the tension in the adductor muscles, until reaching maximum stretch. If flexibility allows, place your forearms on the floor in front of your feet and bring your hands together.

Continues

Continued

- Relax your legs and spine to allow gravity to work with your body weight. Hold the position for 45-90 seconds and breathe deeply.
- Your heels must remain close to the pelvis for the entire duration of the movement, about 30 cm away from it. During the stretching phase, do not force the inclination of your torso, but flex to the point where your flexibility allows it, usually until you feel a consistent but not painful tension on your inner thigh muscles.
- To come out of the pose, push your hands into the floor and unroll the spine in a controlled manner. Bring your knees together with the help of your hands. Next, place your arms behind your body and bend your trunk back to straighten your hips and legs.

Cross-legged supine buttock stretch

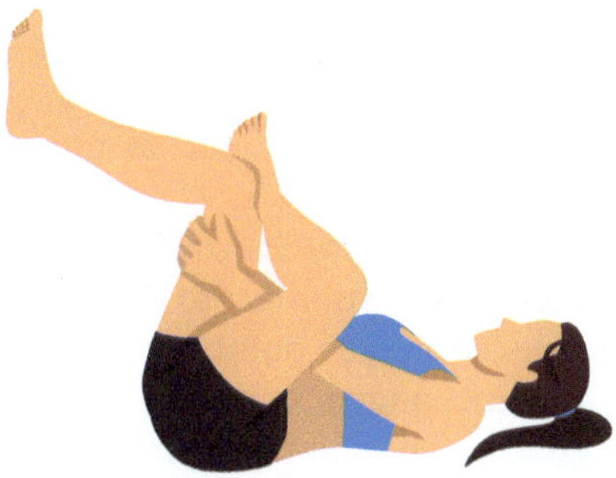

This exercise increases the flexibility and range of motion in your hamstrings and hip flexors (iliopsoas), with a particular focus on the gluteus maximus. The lying position facilitates the execution in subjects with little flexibility.

- Start the exercise in the supine position. Place the soles of your feet on the ground and flex your knees, then cross the limb you want to work on, placing your ankle over the opposite knee. Grasp the back of the supporting thigh with both hands and gently pull it towards the chest to activate the glute stretch. Your back must remain close to the ground for the entire duration of the exercise.
- Having reached the point of maximum tension on the buttock, hold the pose for about 30 seconds then repeat the movement on the opposite side.

Continues

Continued

Quadrupedal hip abduction – Frog split

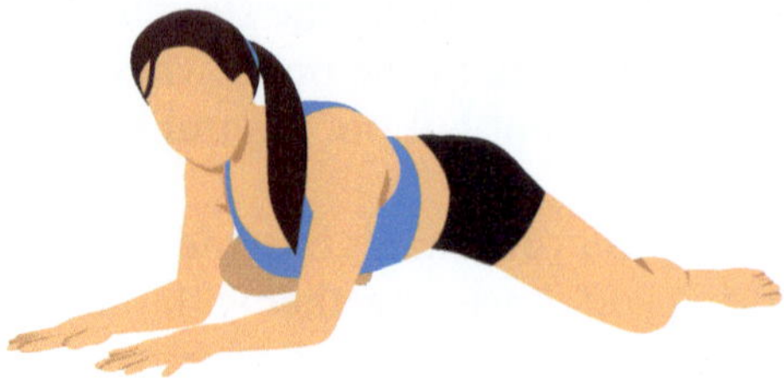

This exercise is suitable for increasing the mobility of the hips and the elasticity of the adductor muscles.

- To start the movement, position yourself in a quadrupedal position, resting on your hands, with your knees at 90°. Hands and knees are shoulder-width apart, your back is in a neutral position and your gaze is directed downwards. Abduct the hips, therefore spreading your knees apart as much, maintaining a comfortable position.
- Make sure that there is a 90° angle between your leg and thigh and that your knees are aligned with each other. Rotate your feet to allow the inner side of the ankle to touch the ground. Your toes should be pointing up.
- Keeping the lumbar curve unchanged, push on your hands and lower your pelvis vertically, towards the ground, and not backwards as if you wanted to sit on your heels (in this case the stretch of the adductors will decrease). Relax your muscles and lean back to help lower the pelvis and push your hips outwards to emphasize the stretch in your hips and inner thighs.
- Palms remain on the floor to support the stretch, flat on the floor or joined together for added support.

To emphasize the stretch and to have a more comfortable posture, with the lumbar spine always in a neutral position, it is possible to rest your forearms and elbows on the ground.

> *You have to stretch coming into the poses and then work with your breathing; remember that inhalation should last half as long as the exhalation, approach it as an exercise in concentration.*
>
> David

Post-workout table by Prof. Davide Antoniella

Kneeling psoas stretch

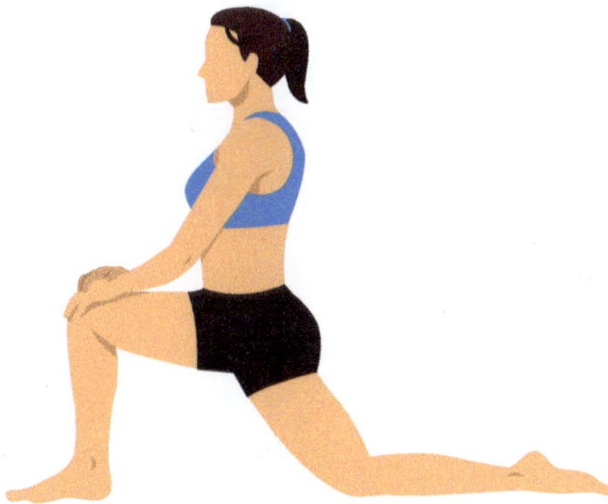

This is an exercise that combines knee flexion and hip extension. It is particularly suitable for stretching the hip flexors, the muscle group that includes the iliopsoas.

- Start from the standing position and bring your body forward with a big step, without lifting your back foot off the ground. From this position, bend your rear knee, ensuring that most of your body weight is supported by your front leg. Your front knee is at a right angle and should not go past your toe. Your rear knee rests on the floor and is semi-extended, while the tibia and back of the foot are fully supported.
- Keeping your back straight, push your pelvis forward and squeeze your glutes until you feel the front hip muscles stretch. To maintain balance, place your hands on your front leg or on a lateral support, as balance is essential for the correct execution of this exercise. For a more marked stretch, smoothly turn your body to the side of your front leg.
- Maintain the position for 20-30 seconds, breathing deeply, then switch legs and repeat on the opposite side.

Continues

Continued

Piriformis stretch on a bench

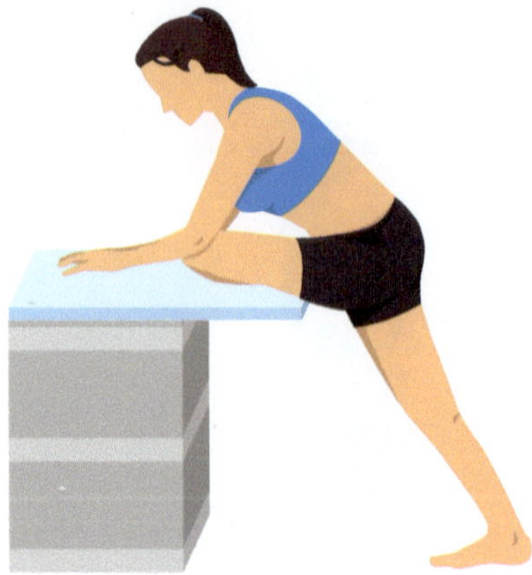

This movement is suitable for stretching the external rotator and hip extensor muscles (for example, glutes and piriformis), and it also helps to improve hip joint mobility, reduce lower back pain and improve performance in exercises such as squats and deadlifts.

- The starting position is standing. Lift one leg and place your foot on a table or stable support at hip height, keeping your leg and thigh at a 90° angle and your knee in line with your hip. If mobility permits, your knee may remain in contact with the supporting surface. The supporting leg is placed on the ground with the knee slightly bent. Place your hands on the support, either side of your leg or in front of it, to emphasize the stretch and maintain a neutral curvature of the spine, especially in the lumbar spine. Your chest and hips are both leaning forward.
- From this position, while maintaining the correct alignment of the spine, bend your torso forward until you feel the tension on the muscles of the gluteal region. If your flexibility allows it, rest your forearms on the table to emphasize the stretch. Hold the position for about 90-120 seconds before repeating on the other side.
- The height of the stand depends on the degree of flexibility of the subject. If you have severe muscle weakness, choose a lower platform. Finally, if you do not feel the stretch, make sure that your chest and hips are extended forward. To help the stretch, try leaning more or bringing your support leg closer to the center of your body.

You may feel tension in the front side of your thigh during the movement. If tension prevails in this position, reduce the step, bringing your rear leg as close as possible to the table/bench. Be careful if there are problems with your knee ligaments, as the latter twists slightly during the exercise. In such cases, this movement is not recommended. Finally, in subjects with good flexibility, lowering the neck during the stretch phase allows for good stretching and relaxation of the neck muscles.

Continues

Continued

Bridge – Lengthening of the column

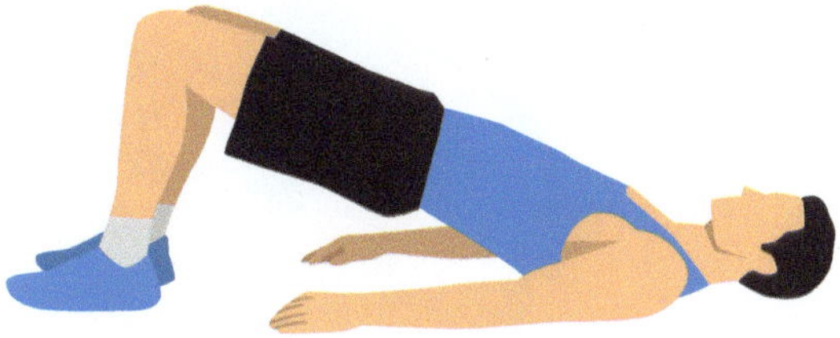

This exercise is suitable for everyone and has countless benefits. The bridge is a back extension movement that involves the whole body and helps to lengthen the column, with particular emphasis on the lower back.

- To start the movement, lie on the floor on your back, with your stomach facing up and your arms at your sides, in contact with the floor. Legs are spread hip-width apart. Flex your legs, keeping your feet firmly on the ground, and bring your heels backwards, towards your pelvis, up to about 20-30 cm from the buttocks.
- From this position, without taking your arms off the ground, press your feet on the floor and lift your buttocks, hips and back from the ground, until you create a straight line from your knees to your shoulders. Contract the buttocks and pull the abdominal wall inwards, towards the column, keeping the abdomen contracted for the entire duration of the movement.
- In the position of maximum stretch, only your feet, shoulders, neck and arms remain in contact with the ground. Pay attention not to shift the support of the body only on the neck; instead, the weight should be supported by your shoulder blades and upper back.
- Having reached maximum stretch, breathe deeply, trying not to contract muscles not involved in this movement.

The exercise can be done both in a static way, holding the pose for 20 to 60 seconds, or in an active way, bringing the hips up and down without touching the floor, for the recommended number of times.

Back extension, a movement at the base of the bridge, has always been considered dangerous because in subjects with hernias or protrusions it could push the nucleus pulposus (a pad that supports the compression forces on the column) posteriorly and worsen the clinical picture.

In healthy people, extending the back improves vertebral health, as arching the spine helps return the nucleus pulposus to its natural location.

This exercise is not recommended for people with neck injuries, abdominal hernia and excessive lumbar lordosis, as well as pregnant women, due to the pressure placed on the lower abdomen and internal organs.

Continues

Continued

Child Pose

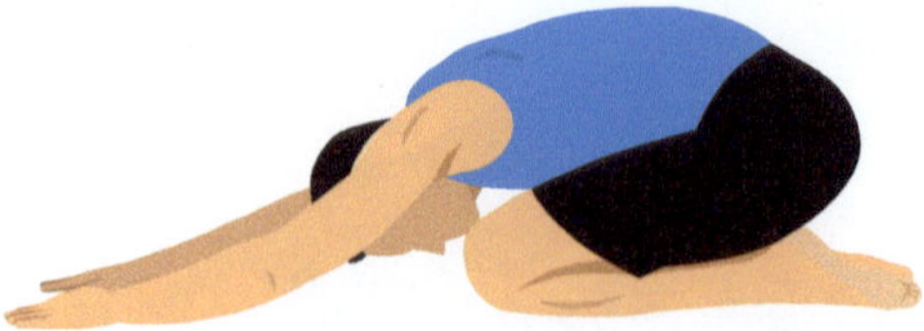

This exercise is suitable for stretching the latissimus dorsi, but based on the posture, it can also be very useful for stretching the pectoralis major. In addition to the benefits for these muscle groups, this movement also stretches the spine, lower back, hips and glutes.

- To begin the movement, kneel on the floor with knees at a shoulder-width distance and big toes touching. Inhale deeply and as you exhale, lower your hips back, trying to sit fully on your heels.
- From this position, bend your torso forward and extend your arms on the ground, forward, beyond your head. Keeping your arms straight with your elbows straight and your hands planted on the floor, press your torso down, trying to stretch your neck and spine.
- In the stretch position your chest rests over your thighs and your shoulders press into the floor. Consciously try to move your ribs away from your tailbone and the top of your head away from your shoulders. Maintain the pose for the time needed to achieve maximum muscle relaxation.
- Your hands remain in line with your shoulders for the entire duration of the movement; if they spread more, beyond shoulder width, there will be greater involvement of the pectoral muscles. Finally, a variant of the exercise involves placing your arms next to your legs, with your palms facing upwards.

In subjects with limited mobility, it is possible to perform the exercise in a similar way by placing the hands on a support.

Focus on breathing deeply with your belly, allowing your ribs to expand as you inhale and gently settle as you exhale and relax. Maintain the position for at least 20-30 seconds.

You need to stretch by getting into the positions and then work on your breathing; remember that inhalation lasts about half as long as exhalation, approach it as an exercise in concentration.

Davide

Don't wait for a protrusion or a herniated disc: adopt these two training programs and implement them on the days you train if you can't do them daily; after the first few days, you will feel a clear lightening of the lumbar area and a better contraction of the muscles of the lower body during your workouts.

When put into practice, the two tables above will really help many people. Almost 1 year after my injury, I felt almost completely recovered but not yet 100%, which I then achieved by incorporating proprioceptive exercises and bodyweight micromovement workouts. Proprioception helps to ensure balance, stability, coordination and the correct execution of the movements, while micro-movement training ensures excellent motor recovery of deep muscles and stabilizing muscles, ensuring strengthening and decompression at the joint level.

I performed the proprioceptive exercises at the beginning and at the end of my workout, while micro-movement training had to be done daily. I did it in the morning as soon as I woke up and in the evening before going to sleep, and I won't deny that I still have the habit of dedicating 15 minutes to it every night before going to bed.

This last step guaranteed me a full and total recovery from the injury. As far as training is concerned, I compared myself to Massimo; the injury literally blocked me for 6 months, so I found myself having to start from scratch. We decided to use a big TUT, 5 seconds in the concentric phase and 5 seconds in the eccentric phase on each rep, 15 reps per muscle group, all done with non-stop continuous tension; this allowed me to deeply stimulate the muscle while using a low workload. I started with three training sessions a week and the split routine was divided as follows:

Workout A	Workout B	Workout C
• Chest: 6 sets • Deltoids: 4 sets • Triceps: 3 sets	• Back: 6 sets • Trapeze: 3 sets • Rear delts: 3 sets • Biceps: 3 sets	• Quadriceps: 6 sets • Hamstrings: 4 sets • Calves: 3 sets

I maintained this pattern for 3 weeks, at the end of which I began to increase the frequency of my workouts every two weeks until I got to training all my muscles twice a week; I maintained the six workouts a week for 4 weeks and then, starting again with the same pattern described above, I started training four times a week, increasing the volume every two weeks. I found myself doing my training pattern (reported in this book) in no time, with even heavier weights than what I used before my injury.

An important aspect is the care with which you start, and never stop, training your abdomen and lumbar spine. I perform 15 sets of abs every other day using crunch movements and avoiding any type of twisting. I perform each set in a slow and controlled manner until I reach positive exhaustion. On the days when I don't train my abdomen, I perform 15 sets of 15 repetitions of exercises for the lumbar spine, usually deadlifts with semi-flexed legs with dumbbells and hyperextensions, without ever reaching exhaustion and maniacally attending to the execution method (I kept the TUT described above and maintained the same tension without reaching exhaustion).

Training with back pain
Federico Focherini

The first neurosurgeon to get his hands on the three expelled hernias in my lumbar spine in 1993 stated that my spine was very thin and that I should stop weight training. Not a pleasant diagnosis for a 26-year-old athlete who would do anything to build muscle and compete.

Unfortunately, my foramina, where spinal nerves roots pass, are narrow by nature and the use of heavy weights in squats, deadlifts and rows, and "cheat" movements performed with poor technique (major mistakes, which may be why I became a maniac of perfect execution of weightlifting exercises) have contributed to increasing their narrowing in the position below the facet joints, causing a stenosis. My hernias at the lumbo-sacral level (L-4/L-5 and L-5/S-1), and later at the cervical level, caused various disabling muscular atrophies over the years from both a functional and aesthetic point of view.

After three surgeries, dozens and dozens of treatments and, in the last 15 years, even resorting to rhizotomy every 2 years in South Africa (where I used to live), I never stopped training. I have not undergone this type of mini-surgery for several years, but I can say that, with some training, stretching and a minimum of anti-inflammatory support as needed, I have always managed to work out to the maximum of my abilities every day, even taking part in bodybuilding competitions, without ever finding myself semi-paralyzed in bed with my back blocked.

What has my training looked like? What precautions did I have to take in 32 consecutive years of competitions and at least 35 years of heavy daily workouts, to ensure that my paravertebral, abdominal and lumbar muscles always carried the load of my body, taking it off the spine?

The spine is not made to withstand the constant loads lifted for a lifetime by a bodybuilder. It can be considered the mast of a ship, and the tie rods and cables of this mast are our abdominal and lumbar muscles: the core muscles. The ship's mainmast would break if it weren't for the steel cable structure that supports it.

To all those who have a problem similar to mine, i.e. having had hernias or even just lumbar and cervical disc protrusions and bulging with consequent muscle spasms and very strong pain, I advise you to train your abdominal and lumbar muscles every day for your whole life. With the abdominal movements, you will be able to create a good elasticity of the spine which, over the years, tends to stiffen, forming osteophytes as a result of numerous processes of degeneration of the vertebral discs. Therefore, a lot of elasticity is needed to have a back that can last a long time.

What daily exercises should you do?

In addition to simple stretching exercises of the often stiffened lower back, glutes and hamstrings, you must perform **exercises that aim to bring the rib cage closer to the pelvis and the pelvis closer to the rib cage**.

- **Pelvis lifts at the bar**: 4 × 20 reps. Raise the pelvis, even slightly, rotating it upwards and consequently shortening the rectus abdominis muscle without using the iliopsoas muscle. Therefore, you don't need to lift your legs, but only to tilt the pelvis.
- **Kneeling cable crunches**: 4 × 20 reps. Kneeling, with a 90° angle between the tibia and femur and between the femur and vertebral column, with the rope over your head, roll up and try to bring your head between your knees, forming a "cat's hump". It can also be done at home, on the floor, on all fours, pushing your belly towards the floor, and then hunching over while contracting your abdomen. It is exceptional for spine mobility.
- **Horizontal hyperextensions**: 4 × 20 reps. Start with a back extension with a locked pelvis, then continue as a hip extension, descending with the pelvis until exhaustion, to finish with locking the trunk parallel to the ground in isometry for as long as you can resist. It's great for all back, hamstrings, glute and lumbar muscles. This exercise offers great back stability, improves the upright posture and tends to give a greater lumbar curvature. It is also very important for all women who are unable to activate their glutes when performing squats and lunges, and for those who seek greater anteversion of the pelvis.

It is therefore necessary to create a very strong kinetic chain of posterior muscles (hamstrings, glutes, lumbar and spine erectors) and an equally strong abdominal wall in order to shift the load away from the spine, which is no longer as strong as before. This work must be performed **daily**, never overshadowing it or even omitting it from your training plan! So, **always do it at the beginning** of the training session. **I advise not doing any movement that causes torsion, rotation or asymmetrical contraction**. The safest thing is to always train a muscle according to the way it is supposed to be used. Don't do any kind of work other than that for which it was meant to do.

For everything else in your weekly weight training, I highly recommend doing a classic **deadlift**. Once a week, 4-5 sets of no more than 10 repetitions, without getting exhausted to avoid making mistakes in the form of execution.

Using a symmetrical or asymmetrical grip (whichever you think is better), position yourself with the barbell on the ground as at the start of the Olympic snatch exercise, with a flat back, head up, butt down and heels on the ground: start pushing with your feet, then with your legs, squeeze your glutes, bring your shoulders back by slightly adducing your shoulder blades as you rise to a vertical position, never arching your back. Therefore, I advise you to mentally follow these steps (which the older weightlifters would shout in my ears when I was a kid), developing them in a chain order: **"make two holes in the ground with your feet, legs, glutes, shoulders, freeze it, hold it squeeze it, then go down"!**

I find deadlift exercises to be safer for the lower back than barbell rows.

As for free-weight exercises for the thighs, I don't recommend heavy squats but I really like free front squats with a 1cm wooden board placed under your heels. Descend deeply on your heels keeping your back straight and the lumbar arch neutral (never flex the lumbar area, stop just before this happens) and push with your heels without ever fully extending your legs. I repeat this sequence: head up, barbell tucked under your Adam's apple, go down in an upright position, then go back up by pushing with your heels, legs and glutes, and just before fully extending your thighs, go down again. In this exercise, your glutes must always be squeezed to support the back.

When Tom Platz, "the Lord of the Squat", came to my gym in 1995 for a seminar, he explained how to squat correctly for at least an hour. He used to say that the perfect squat was that of a 1-year-old, who sits and stands up inside the box where he plays and does it without hesitation, without mistakes. The secret, if we want to talk about a secret, of Tom Platz has always been this: contracting the muscles of the glutes throughout the movement, both going down (not easy, as the glute muscles tend to lengthen on the way down) and going up, in which the glute acts as a "setter" as in the game of volleyball, in which the ball is pushed up with a clear touch, just like the gluteus maximus, always contracting, pushing the weight of the body and the load of the barbell up. This is precious help that takes the weight and effort off the weak link of this kinetic chain, i.e. the quadratus lumborum and spinal erectors. Therefore, to avoid spinal damage, you should concentrate on the buttocks throughout the range of motion and **"let go" of the thighs in the negative/eccentric phase**. Your legs are already doing their best on their own, so don't worry.

We have already addressed this topic in Chapter 17, where I explain how to perform repetitions correctly, i.e. how to slow down the descent with the antagonist muscles in order to sensitize other muscles, to use heavy loads, and above all to avoid injuries to the weak links of these exercises. In barbell curls, you descend with the triceps; in overhead presses, the shoulders descend with the rhomboids, infraspinatus and teres muscles; in chest dips, one descends with the trapezius and so on. When descending with squats, front squats, hack squats and presses of all types, the muscles that we cannot see and which, for this reason, are even more difficult to activate, must be activated in order to be able to slow down the descent by removing stress from the joints, which would otherwise be overstretched.

As for cervical disc protrusions and bulging, with consequent stiffening of the neck and traps, I recommend stimulating blood flow into the area with lateral and rear shrugs, and also upright rows with two 5-10 kg plates that allow you to rotate once you reach your chin. Just as if you were taking off a sweater, cross your arms, raise them until the plates reach under your chin, then rotate outwards. It's an excellent exercise to free yourself from the continuous muscle discomfort that prevents you from moving your neck toward your shoulder. *After training chest and shoulders, I always perform 10-12 minutes of neck traction with a cervical traction device under my jaw and wrapped around my face, under the occipital area of the skull, sitting at the lat machine with my shoulders towards the weight stack.* I recommend never exceeding a 6 kg counterweight, to avoid dizziness and a sense of nausea. This practice, performed after training, offers wonderful sensations: sometimes you relax to the point that you can fall asleep. I think it's the simplest thing to do.

This is a static mechanical stretching exercise for the cervical spine. If you have a weight that weighs on the vertebral discs crushing the nerve roots, with consequent rectification of the cervical spine, just lift that weight, creating a minimum of extra space, to obtain a guaranteed benefit. Everyone claims to have understood this concept, but I have not yet seen a single person who practices this technique with consistency. Everyone has neck pain, but no one has the patience to do this exercise, which is much more effective than anti-inflammatory drugs and doesn't have the same side effects.

Blood, in my opinion, is the most important factor of all and is the common denominator of all the joint, muscular and nervous pathologies affecting athletes.

If you want to help your lower back, you have to keep it active and well-supplied with blood. Never let it cool down. The more blood we can bring to the site, the greater the benefit and, consequently, the muscle relief. After training, I don't recommend stretching exercises, which athletes will hardly go through, partly due to lack of time or laziness, so I recommend simply lying down on the ground with your legs together and the soles of your feet on the floor, with the heels close to the buttocks, to relax and do nothing. This way your erectors and lumbar muscles will slowly relax, gliding smoothly to the floor. When you have a stiffening in the lumbar area, the first thing to do is lie down on the floor in a supine position. Always on a hard surface.

Training with back pain

Massimo Spattini

In Chapter 25, I described the injury I sustained while squatting in a powerlifting contest. This lesion in the lumbar muscle, not adequately treated because I was preparing for a bodybuilding competition, evolved into fibrosis with calcification, which lead to muscle retraction, creating a torsion of the spine and causing me a dislocation of the facet joints at the L4 and L5 levels. However, I kept training and, when I consulted an orthopedist for possible sciatica, disc protrusion or hernia, normally treated with ozone therapy, he looked at my x-rays and my magnetic resonance and invariably told me that I had a "wheelchair" back but that, thanks to my highly developed paravertebral muscles, I was able to keep everything more or less under control and therefore, basically, I had to continue doing what I was doing.

And I trained heavily and frequently, only limiting heavy squats above 300 lbs. Obviously, over the decades, my lumbar muscles have also shrunk and my back pain has increased, while remaining within the limits of tolerability. The turning point came when I had a motorcycle accident 4 years ago, in which I fractured my talus (an ankle bone) and had to use crutches for 2 months. This dealt the final blow to my lumbars, which lost strength and mass; consequently, the vertebral instability due to the dislocation of the facet joints generated chronic inflammation that favored an arthritic process. Unfortunately, according to the explanation given to me by the neurosurgeon, if I hadn't had well-preserved intervertebral spaces, the generated arthrosic would have practically "welded" the L4, L5 and S1 vertebrae, increasing my stiffness but also my vertebral stability and thus solving the pain caused by the continuous inflammation as a result of the dislocation of the facets.

Instead, the arthrosis had wedged itself into the vertebral canal, narrowing it and causing a stenosis, and also causing me neuropathic symptoms. According to the surgeon, the only possible solution was arthrodesis surgery (insertion of a plate with screws that fix the vertebrae) with surgical enlargement of the canal. What I didn't understand was why, if the problem had been amplified by the loss of the lumbar muscles, by restoring the latter I would not have been able to solve the situation. According to the surgeon, once this compensation was lost, it was not possible to recover it; he had already seen many football players who, forced by an injury to inactivity, were no longer able to recover. But "I am not a football player, I am a bodybuilder!" I set aside the idea of the operation and devoted myself religiously to rehabilitation under the guidance of my friend and collaborator, Davide Antoniella.

My workout

At this point, however, it is appropriate to describe my training. Without a doubt, I gave more space to training aimed at muscle relaxation, especially of the anti-gravity muscles, while simultaneously strengthening the "core" muscles with daily workouts, which I perform early in the morning after my 20 minutes of meditation, in which I visualize my spine realigning itself properly. In the morning, I perform alternating days with aerobic activity, which I do on a stationary bike, a few sets of free standing bodyweight squats on the balance board to improve the proprioception and stability of the injured ankle, and subsequently, every day, a whole set of exercises for stretching and core strength (including meditation, my morning routine lasts about 90 minutes).

In the evening, I do my bodybuilding session, during which I have no problems performing the various exercises for the shoulders and arms, which I do best in a sitting position. Obviously, no problem for the pectorals and lats; when I'm at home I use the reverse rower.

Reverse rower

- Set the multipower bar at approximately pubis height. The higher the bar, the easier the movement.
- Position yourself under the bar, lying face up. Lie on the floor under the bar (which should be positioned just above where you can reach it from the ground).
- Grab the bar with an overhand grip, slightly wider than shoulder-width.
- Contract your abs and glutes and keep your body in a completely straight line.
- Bring your shoulder blades down and back towards each other as you move towards the bar. Don't shrug. Imagine trying to hold a table tennis ball between your shoulder blades to keep it from falling.
- Pull yourself up to the bar until your chest is almost touching the bar.
- Lower yourself back down with proper form all the way down until your arms are fully extended and then pull yourself back up.

If I train in the gym, I perform the **row with bench support** so as not to burden the lumbar area. Another exercise I perform is the dumbbell row with my torso at 90°, resting my forehead on the support of the Larry Scott bench, which reduces the effort at the lumbar level.

I have eliminated squats because of both the direct load on the vertebral level and because I naturally have poor joint mobility in my ankles, further worsened by the fracture, so I tend to overly flex my torso forward. I prefer to use the **45° leg press** where I don't go beyond the 90° angle between the thigh and leg to avoid losing the normal physiological curve at the lumbar level, and the single-leg horizontal leg press, where I can go down more and involve the buttocks more by performing it both in a frontal and lateral position, i.e. lying on one side to engage the gluteus medius more.

I later realised that by doing leg presses, I could also go down, using light weights, with my knees up to my chest, which was beneficial because this opened up the spinal canal more, and the neurological problem related to stenosis decreased.

Lumbar training

I train my lumbar spine at least twice a week: I've verified that always maintaining excellent muscle tone at that level has a stabilizing effect. I start with the **good morning exercise** by performing three sets of 15 repetitions, then I move on to deadlifts with a light weight and a slow and controlled movement, three sets of 15 repetitions, both in the ascent and descent phases; I start with the barbell positioned on risers to avoid the first part of the movement, which is the most demanding for the lumbar spine, and after a few sets, I start with the barbell off the ground, paying attention to perfect execution without losing my lumbar lordosis, for three sets of 10 repetitions.

Finally, I do three sets of 6 reps for strength with the bar positioned on padded mats, using a relatively heavy load and dropping the bar onto the mats after completing the concentric phase, thus completely avoiding the harder-to-control eccentric phase, which puts me at a higher at risk of injury. I do this **lower back workout** after three warm-up sets of **banded core extensions**. Sometimes, I use the reduced version in my morning routine and the full version in my evening workout.

Hip thrusts

While it is certainly true that strengthening core muscles is highly recommended for those suffering from back pain, it is equally true and essential to have an optimal glute tonus. We know that deep squats and back lunges are among the best exercises for the glutes, but the problem is that, given the direct load on the spine, squats may not be a good solution; moreover, also single-leg squats and lunges, even if performed with lower loads, can stress the piriformis area and trigger a neuropathic-type pain (false sciatica) in those who already have back problems.

An excellent exercise used in functional recovery of the lower back is the hip thrust, which requires fundamental prerequisites and a correct form of execution. Basically, you must avoid accentuated lordosis or a straightening of the lumbar spine, otherwise the stress will fall on the lumbo-sacral tract or the dorso-lumbar tract, and less on the buttocks. Furthermore, you must not have "blocked" sacroiliac joints, which limit glute engagement.

Correct execution involves positioning your feet so that, when your hips are fully raised, your shins are perpendicular to the floor. Avoid arching your lower back too much without bringing your hips higher than your shoulders and knees in a slow, controlled motion, just as you shouldn't bring your head back by hyper-extending your neck. The exercise must be performed by stabilizing the core in advance in order to stiffen your trunk, like a plank. Pelvic floor control is also fundamental as, through the activation of the core, it contracts and stabilizes the lumbo-sacral complex, avoiding the intervention of accessory muscles such as the piriformis.

Your knees must remain centered on your shins and must not go inward. For this you can use a light resistance band around your thighs, just above your knees, to oppose resistance. In this way, your glutes are activated by reflex and your femurs are kept centered. I prefer doing hip thrusts to increase glute activation and functional back re-education, almost daily, with lighter loads and higher repetitions.

At the end of my workout, I usually hang on the **reverse bench** for a few minutes, since I have a small spondylolisthesis, a sliding of one vertebra on the other, which can occur anteriorly with respect to the underlying vertebra (anterolisthesis) or posteriorly (retrolisthesis).

I often hear a small "pop" which probably corresponds to the realignment of the vertebrae and I feel an immediate benefit. Some osteopaths and physiatrists I had consulted told me that if I wanted to improve my problem, I would have to completely abandon weight training to avoid the muscle tension that it generates. Maybe, but it's a possibility I haven't even contemplated for a second, and I've managed to improve my problem by training even more.

CHAPTER 36

The heart and training in the gym

Luca Silvestrini

Basics of anatomy

The heart is a hollow muscular organ found in most animals. In humans, it lies in the middle of the thoracic cavity, more precisely in the mediastinum, between the two lungs, behind the sternum and the costal cartilages that protects it like a shield, in front of the vertebral column, from which it is separated by the esophagus and the aorta, and it rests on the diaphragm, which separates it from the underlying viscera.

It is made up almost exclusively of striated muscle tissue and is surrounded by a fibrous sac called pericardium.

The organ is divided into two unequal sections, the left which contains oxygenated blood, and the right which contains deoxygenated blood that "returns" from the systemic circulation; each of these sections includes an upper cavity, the atrium, with thin walls, and a lower cavity, the ventricle, with thicker walls.

Atria and ventricles communicate with each other through valves: the mitral valve, on the left side; the tricuspid valve, on the right. The left and right sections of the heart do not communicate directly with each other, but, as a system in series, through the systemic and pulmonary circulations.

The heart acts like an alternating pump, capable of filling and emptying rhythmically (systole-diastole alternation), guaranteeing, also thanks to the elastic component of the arterial vessels, a continuous blood flow to the organs it has to supply. The efficiency of the heart as a pump is based, on the one hand, on almost simultaneous contraction of all the ventricular muscle fibers (cells), and on the other hand on the rhythmic, organized and coordinated contraction of the cardiac muscles, made possible by a conduction system, which prevents the heart muscle from contracting randomly.

The atria act as a reservoir for blood returning from the veins, which can thus be rapidly forced into the ventricles; the latter, with their contraction, act like a pump that is capable of producing sufficient pressure for blood circulation.

The two main arteries arise from the upper portion of the anterior side of the heart, the aorta on the left and the pulmonary artery on the right, which spreads into a left and a right branch. The bases of these arteries are surrounded by the atrial appendages or *auriculae* (which take their name by their wedge-shaped conformation which resembles a dog's pendulous ears).

Posteriorly, there are two blood vessels that flow into the right atrium, the venae cavae, divided into the superior vena cava and the inferior vena cava.

The pulmonary veins, which flow into the left atrium, lie between these four vessels, two on the right side and two on the left side.

On the surface of the heart, we can see the right and left coronary arteries originating from the ascending aorta; the coronaries branch out, covering the whole heart up to the apex.

The left coronary is generally the main artery of the heart and includes the anterior descending artery – also known as the anterior intraventricular artery, the circumflex artery, and the smaller, inconstant, intermediate artery; from the origin of the right coronary artery rises the sinus node artery, and the atrial arterioles, while the main branch is the posterior interventricular artery plus some more smaller vessels. The arterioles that supply the ventricles enter the myocardium where they terminate in small tufts. The collateral channels allow communication between the main arteries and their branches, or between the two coronaries through the vasa vasorum; if a pressure gradient is determined through a stenosis of the large epicardial branches, the collateral canal can dilate over time and provide blood flow beyond the obstruction.

We could summarize it as follows: the left coronary supplies two-thirds of the heart, as it reaches almost the entire left ventricle, the anterior part of the interventricular septum and a small part of the right ventricle; the right coronary supplies most of the right ventricle, the posterior part of the septum and most of the posterior wall of the left ventricle. The papillary muscles are reached by both arteries, while the conduction system of the heart is predominantly, if not entirely, supplied by the right coronary artery.

The right coronary and the two branches of the left coronary (anterior descending and circumflex) are considered the three main vessels for blood supply to the heart and, if affected by atherosclerosis, they play a fundamental role in the pathogenesis of ischemic heart disease.

The vessels that bring blood back to the heart are the cardiac veins: they run parallel to the branches of the coronary arteries and flow into a venous trunk which can be found in the diaphragmatic surface of the heart, in the coronary sulcus, in the coronary sinus, to then flow into the right atrium.

The heart contains several lymphatic vessels, which are divided into a subendocardial network and a myocardial network; both networks reach a third network, the epicardial one, from which large collecting vessels are formed. These reach and flow into the tracheobronchial lymph glands and the tracheal bifurcation.

The coronary and venous vessels run on the outer surface of the myocardium, immersed in adipose tissue which prevents the vessels from being constricted during the myocardial contraction, which allows blood flow to be constant both in the systolic and diastolic phase. This facilitates blood circulation especially during the systole, i.e. the moment in which the demand for energy and oxygen is maximal.

Assessment criteria for cardiac function

There are many criteria that provide information about the functioning of the cardiac muscle, some of which are better known than others.

Two of the most commonly used, even among non-experts, are **heart rate** (HR) and **blood pressure** (BP).

HR refers to the number of systoles in a well-defined time and correlates with the subject's characteristics, such as age and training status. It is common knowledge that the heart of an athlete thanks to structural adaptation which allows it to function "extraordinarily" both in the filling (diastole) and emptying (systole) phases, tends to have lower resting heart rates compared to the general population.

BP is the force with which blood is pushed by the heart pump into the vessels; it takes the name of arterial pressure if it concerns arteries or venous pressure if it concerns veins. The higher the pressure, the greater the work (and the "effort") that the heart has to do. It is influenced by factors such as the cardiac contractile capacity (inotropism), the tone of the arterial vessels (which goes hand in hand with their elasticity), and the peripheral resistances, which are generally proportional to the overall surface of the vessels and the type of tissue to be perfused.

Another assessment criteria for cardiac function which is rather widespread is **ejection fraction** (EF), which represents the difference in percentage terms between the heart volume at the end of filling (end-diastolic volume) and at the end of emptying (end-systolic volume). A value ≥50% is considered as normal. It is fundamentally influenced by parameters such as the amount of healthy myocardial tissue available for simultaneous contraction and by the pressure regimes existing within the cardiac chambers and immediately below.

Other parameters, such as cardiac output (and derived indices such as cardiac index), isovolumetric relaxation time, strain and strain rate, represent further assessment criteria for cardiac function, useful in assessing uncertain clinical cases or in those requiring more accurate diagnostic tools.

This is only to provide the non-expert reader with an idea of how the cardiovascular system represents a very fascinating sector of medical knowledge. It may be difficult to understand for those who do not have a specialist's knowledge, despite the fact that we often have to deal with positions that persist in the use of only the cardiac hypertrophy parameter as a divider between healthy and sick individuals...

Why a chapter on cardiology in a book dedicated to overload training?

The medical literature has begun to be interested in cardiac models in non-sedentary subjects since the first uses of diagnostic imaging, such as teleradiography and echocardiography.

The work of Morganroth in 1975 was a real milestone. Based on the data coming from compared anatomy with the animal world, a concentric type of cardiac remodeling (hypertrophic cardiac walls and normal-sized ventricular cavities) was postulated in people doing weightlifting assiduously (therefore, basically subjected to pressure work), compared with a pattern of eccentric hypertrophy (hypertrophic heart walls and symmetrically enlarged ventricular cavities) among those who practiced endurance training (thus, subjected to volume work).

All this is confirmed by the data provided by hemodynamics, which show an increase in peripheral resistance and a decrease in venous return during isometric/isotonic movements, in spite of a general reduction in peripheral resistance and an increase in central venous return during long-duration, low-intensity exercises.

This led to the observation of clinical data as well as post-mortem data, which confirmed that a heart with hypertrophic walls was a potentially and chronically hypoperfused heart in its endocardial – or innermost – portions. These areas are anatomically more distant from the large coronary vessels and it is no coincidence that they are defined as epicardial due to their location on the external surface of the heart. Their position comes from the need to prevent vessels which are essential for the oxygenation of the heart muscle from undergoing external pressures capable of rhythmically occluding the lumen, thus potentially causing frequent ischemic strokes.

The year 1975 marked the start of a twenty-year period in which this anatomical-functional model was never questioned (probably also due to poor scientifical and epidemiological interest), hence an attitude of substantial skepticism from medical professionals toward the utilisation of overload physical activity for both recreational and therapeutic purposes.

Such certainties began to crumble in the last decade of the last century, a time when publications about the absence of cardiac adaptations in subjects resistance training were published.

However, the concept of concentric cardiac hypertrophy as a dangerous adaptative pattern is never questioned. What is called into question is rather the presence of adaptations of such kind in those who practice weightlifting. Such stances ought to be reexamined by medical professionals, especially given the strength of epidemiological data over pathologies that impact most on healthcare costs, such as diabetes, ischemic heart disease and osteoporosis, which would benefit significantly from a better muscle and metabolic efficiency in general.

My personal experience as a sports cardiologist with almost twenty years of professional activity

Always passionate about weight training and doing resistance exercise myself, I began to be interested in studying the cardiac response to weight-bearing activities, starting from myself as the "object" of observation over time. To date, I have accumulated so much data that I can understand how my body is dealing with certain types of stress (and I don't mean just the one imposed by training) based on the changes in the electrocardiogram at rest, just to name one.

Inevitably, my innate curiosity led me to observe what was happening in other hearts, perhaps those of more experienced athletes (in terms of number of years of practice) and extraordinary sportspeople.

I do not hide my enthusiasm in seeing the data from the literature of the 90s partially confirmed, with a personal addition of absolutely non-univocal data about the heart model detectable in athletes doing resistance training. The lack of parameters that are distributed in a statistically "ordinary" way (as happens in athletes such as runners, cyclists or football players, grouped in with those having the same role, etc.) must be searched in the only factor that is capable of inducing the same morpho-functional changes: training.

The type of training program carried out (number of sets, repetitions, percentage of load with respect to the theoretical maximum, frequency of training of the same muscle group, etc.) makes resistance exercise one of the most flexible and adaptable types of training based on the needs and goals that the athletes set for themselves. You can train in an attempt to set a record in a lift or as physical therapy after a trauma... between these two extremes, there is a very wide range of possibilities.

Hence, once again, just imagine my disappointment in seeing the medical professionals of the new century turn a deaf ear to the possibility of combining the well-known therapeutic protocols, based on the administration of one or more drugs, with a weapon at practically zero cost, but with indisputable effectiveness.

Bodybuilding and the heart: a dangerous relationship?

From what has been said so far, the answer would be a resounding "no", since there are no large-scale prospective studies that unequivocally demonstrate how the constant practice of resistance training can pose a risk to the health of a healthy heart.

And here comes the sore subject: a healthy heart requires periodical checkups, as in any other sport. A lack of clear rules, together with the creeping certainty of "I'm fine anyway, why do I have to do a checkup?" means that very often, people with more or less serious cardiovascular problems, practice weightlifting while being unaware of a potential condition which can manifest itself sooner or later, even dramatically. Obviously, and fortunately, we are talking about small numbers compared to the enormous number of those who lift weights, but they are still subjects who encounter serious health problems that are not always possible to remedy.

Returning to the title of the chapter, I can confidently say that a healthy heart, checked periodically, can do this sport with absolute tranquility and with the certainty that, over time, this can bring undoubted advantages in terms of quality of life.

Why then are medical professionals so skeptical about prescribing weight training to patients, while they keep recommending the very well-known, yet little practiced "20/30-minute-a-day walk"?

Certainly, what hospital doctors often meet are bodybuilders that can be defined as anything but athletes: their BP values are out of range, their HR at rest recalls that of an advanced cardiopathic patient, rather than an athlete's bradycardia, their heart is more or less markedly hypertrophic and their functional data are utterly pathological (ejection fraction, diastolic filling phase, isovolumetric relaxation time, presence of late enhancement on magnetic resonance, etc.).

This whole situation is even more alarming if we consider that more and more young people show these signs, confirming an absolutely wrong path taken by the sports world. If we add the fact that many people, due to their progress both at an aesthetic and a well-being level, keep on training hard even at an age when they shouldn't anymore, the picture is quite clear.

Prescribability of resistance training and major cardiovascular and metabolic diseases

How to reconcile an enormous number of people (not all in perfect health conditions) who exercise with dumbbells and barbells, or equipment which has nothing to do with the latter, but which puts the cardiovascular system under the same stress, with the need to ensure that sport itself does not become a source of additional risk?

How to prescribe resistance training following the principles of good clinical practice and medico-legal ethics in the presence of hypertensive heart disease?

Let me go back to what I said before: training programmes which are flexible in the choice of loads, repetitions and %1RM allow everyone to get the benefits of a better use of energy substrates coming mainly from carbohydrates and, to a lesser extent, from fat.

In the case of hypertension, for example, a fundamental premise is a good pharmacological control of basal BP. The second step is the assessment of potential co-morbidities through the use of the so-called second-level investigations (but without using methods which could pose risks to the patient's health), such as the color-Doppler echocardiography, the carotid Doppler ultrasound, exercise testing, circadian monitoring of ECG and BP monitoring.

Cardiac exercise testing makes it possible to evaluate up to what HR (and, therefore, muscular effort) the pressure stays within the limits of safety. This is the core of the prescription: the use of that HR cut-off must be taken into account as the maximum cardiocirulatory effort possible, regardless of the equipment used or, more generally, of the exercise performed.

A certainly more complex picture is that of ischemic heart disease, where time must necessarily be considered. A subject with a history of acute coronary syndrome (ACS) must spend at least 3 months avoiding exertion of any kind, except for common daily activities; at that point, residual functional capacity assessment plays a fundamental role in the possibility of prescribing resistance exercise.

The discussion, at this point, would become extremely technical, but it suffices to say that, if there are no significant arrhythmias, there is no risk for them to be induced by an increase in HR, there is no remodeling of the ventricle characterized by areas of marked thinning of the wall and there is a residual EF still within the limits, then resistance training with an HR cut-off in an absolutely safe range improves the metabolic profile which brought the patient, perhaps in the presence of other risk factors, to develop an acute coronary syndrome or ischemic heart disease.

Therefore, a wide array of diagnostic tools easily usable by all cardiologists/sports doctors/physiatrists would allow any minimally experienced medical professional to support theoretical principles of physiology with indications tailored on the patient in question. This would determine how far they can push themselves with resistance exercise, while minimizing the risks and maximizing the benefits.

At this point, the only missing link in the virtuous circle of an attentive doctor's ability to do the right prescription, would be a qualified instructor who knows how to interpret and put indications and programming into practice and who has maybe also read this book...

CHAPTER 37

Psychology and bodybuilding

Marco Tullio Cau

According to the general understanding of sports psychology, it deals with discovering, experimenting and implementing techniques aimed at improving sports performance, in diverse disciplines.

Today, this branch of psychology is held in considerable regard in Italy (while in other countries this has long been the case). When I was a member of a team that dealt with motorcycle riders, which also included an athletic trainer and a sports doctor, a chief mechanic said to a young motorcyclist "But what's the point of having a psychologist: just hop on your bike, start it and go...".

It was one of the reasons that prompted me to attend a two-year master's degree in sexology, a topic, as I said on the first day of attendance, that certainly "aroused" me the most!

In reality, the definition of the national Order of Psychologists is decidedly more complex, and therefore, it is necessary to quote it in its entirety, because it better frames its areas: "Sport psychology studies the cognitive, emotional and behavioral processes associated with the performance of athletes and teams in the sporting context, in physical exercises, and when participating in sporting activities". A distinction to keep in mind concerns the objectives of the research and intervention of a sport psychologist.

This means that some psychologists characterize their work by the fact that they are in contact with high-level athletes or teams, with the aim of developing and applying techniques that maximize the athlete and/or the team's chances of achieving their competitive goal. The main areas of research focus on areas like:

- the relationships between perceptions, representations and motor behaviors
- intrapersonal, interpersonal, motivational and situational factors that influence individual and group performance
- the most effective techniques for mental preparation for the competition
- the characteristics of optimal sports performance
- processes for improving personal and collective efficacy beliefs
- the definition of objectives (goal setting)

- psychophysiological and cognitive self-regulation techniques
- the study of attentional processes in relation to the different demands of different sports disciplines
- general tolerance and pain tolerance in competitive activities
- learning and applying psychomotor and psychosocial skills in different types of physical and sporting activities
- group dynamics and leadership in team sports
- the relationship between psychophysical and motor activity, and personal development and psychological well-being
- individual differences in sports activities
- the role and functions of sports coaching etc.

Furthermore, especially in recent years, sports psychologists have drawn on numerous contributions deriving from the psychology of organizations, framing the performance of the high-level athlete in a broader context. On a professional level, in addition to psychological support for achieving optimal performance of the athletes and increasing their psychophysical well-being, sport psychology turns its attention to aspects related to sporting practices that are not directly aimed at achieving an objective, but rather at the relationship between sports practice and improvement of the quality of life in the different stages of development, from infancy to adolescence, youth, adulthood and old age.

From this perspective, the contributions of different disciplines and study methods are taken on: from those typical of general psychology to those connected to developmental psychology, clinical psychology or social and applied psychology. The covered topics range from the effects of physical activity on physical health and psychological well-being, on sleep and on cognitive processes (for example, mental efficiency and reaction times) to psychophysiological reactions to stress; from the perception of effort to the concept of the physical Self, from psychogenic eating disorders to excessive exercise and doping".

Sport psychology involves interdisciplinary approaches both from other branches of psychology (cognitive psychology, psychophysiology, neuropsychology, clinical psychology, developmental psychology, social psychology, applied and organizational psychology, etc.) and from sport and movement sciences such as physiology, sports medicine and educational sciences. In their professional work, sports psychologists collaborate with coaches, technical staff, managers of sports clubs, students and teachers of primary and secondary schools, parents, students, and operators of university sports organizations.

Here we will deal in particular with bodybuilding techniques, both in terms of training and in the practice of posing routines, and we will continue with a few of the obvious, as well as hidden reasons that lead to lifting weights.

However, I think it is best to comprehensively address the topic, so, here's some advice: "Psychological strategies included by strength and conditioning coaches in applied strength and conditioning" (Radcliffe et al., 2015) is certainly a book to consult, as well as "Sport psychology: technologies ahead", by Jeunet et al. (2020), which deals with new options such as virtual reality associated with MT (Mental Training), which still hasn't been fully investigated but is a very promising procedure. Another interesting work is "A Systematic Review of Self-Directed Cognitive Strategies Effects on Strength Performance" (Tod et al., 2022), which, as the title suggests, provides a summary of what has been written on the subject, including a discussion on the validity of the various techniques, although there is (as expected) no unanimity in general, including on what exactly determines these results at a physiological level.

Among the "classic" techniques, the ones related to relaxation take the lion's share: there are many, and here we will limit ourselves to progressive relaxation and autogenic training (AT), mindfulness and yoga; these methods are useful before a workout because they can free the mind from other disturbing thoughts, so as to be able to fully concentrate energy on the upcoming session, to decrease excessive levels of arousal (excessive or absent motivation are both negatives!) but also to promote recovery, which if used before bedtime, becomes a particularly important factor for "natural" or senior athletes.

If all roads lead to Rome, the practices just mentioned lead to the same physiological effect and the same type of brain waves and breathing in one phase of the procedure or in another.

Even the very recent bi-Olympic champion Marcell Jacobs said that he attaches great importance to breathing in general, in order to unlock some emotions and to better expel toxins, especially before competitions, to become more "centered".

Progressive relaxation was proposed by Jacobson in 1938 and consists of a sequence of contractions and decontractions of specific muscle groups (particularly suitable for bodybuilders, who have above average muscle control), while **autogenic training** was popularized a few years earlier (1932) by Schulz, who had been perfecting it since the 1920s, exploiting personal experiences and psychophysiological studies of other scientists who had preceded him; broadly speaking, it provides self-suggested instructions of heaviness and heat in various parts of the body.

Many studies have shown that, despite the methodological differences at the psychophysiological level, the outcomes are similar, including the practical results. Some of these include Nicassio et al., in 1974 and more recently Singh et al., in 2018, whose work is actually more inherent to the topics covered here since concentration was the most influenced parameter. Furthermore, Schulz himself believed that relaxation was only one of the effects of AT, which instead was aimed at reactivating an individual's bionomic resources. The term "bionomic" refers to the set of "laws of life" that regulate the functions of an organism in its biological-psychological-spiritual totality.

These "laws of life", which Schultz describes in his work "Bionomic Psychotherapy – An Essential Experiment" in 1951, are innate, binding, and finalized, and lead the organism, through various passages, towards a state of dynamic equilibrium where its potentials are fulfilled. Failure to observe the laws of life or improper adherence to them is at the origin of the pathological developments of the organism. So, **the main purpose is to restore energy and health** that allow the individual to live an active life, to their fullest potential... just what we need for our workouts!

A brief mention of a **yoga** technique (a very ancient discipline that needs no introduction): Savasana, or... corpse pose! Once again, conscious relaxation is sought, trying to lighten the various parts of the body and using breathing. As for the other methodologies, there is not enough space here to accurately describe the different ways of using this important tool to our advantage, which is normally taken for granted as involuntary. Diaphragmatic or thoracic breathing, depth of breath and frequency are all parameters that can greatly influence our bodily and mental parameters. Deep, slow breathing is naturally associated with a state of calmness, while shallow, "short," jerky breathing correlates with a state of anxiety or excessive activation.

There are many books to draw from to learn all the techniques listed above, even if a good instructor can certainly facilitate learning.

In any case, AT entails a more important role for the subject, even if the term "autogenic" refers (mainly) to the fact that the change is generated without the will of the subject, thanks to suggestions induced by the "commands" expected and their psychophysiological effect.

Clearly not everyone will be successful on their first try. Others, on the other hand, will too much... success, ending up falling asleep, which is only good if it happens right before bedtime!

I'd like to dedicate a few lines to **mindfulness**, or the human ability to be fully present and aware of where we are and what we are doing rather than being overly reactive or overwhelmed by what is happening around us. Kabat-Zinn, the creator of a scientifically researched Mindfulness-Based Stress Reduction program, explains how mindfulness "turns on" parts of our brains that aren't normally activated when we behave mindlessly, on autopilot. In an interesting study (Hope et al., 2020) the authors explain: "To be clear, 'mindful' strength training is not about feeling calm or peaceful, but about being deliberate and aware of every action and thought regarding the task that you are about to perform".

By regularly practicing mindfulness, an athlete can set up their workout with greater awareness and attention, which can increase the efficiency and effectiveness of the workout, and ultimately can improve the execution of the athletic movements, making them more powerful and decisive. The authors go on to state that mindfulness practices include conscious breathing (participants focus their attention on their breathing), body sensations, the flow of thoughts and emotions, and body scanning (in which attention must be focused on the parts of the body in a sequential and non-critical way). Finally, one must cultivate conscious movements, i.e. implement a "mindful" awareness of the body while it is in movement. The researchers then focus on the research on attentional focus (internal/external) and also provide a series of practical advice.

This case also has some basic procedures to follow, but they will not be explained here for reasons of space: this practice, however, is one of the various tactics that can be used in order to reach a level of concentration that brings results, in the gym and outside of it... we just need to find the one that best suits our personality.

Turning to **arousal**, the previously mentioned study by Tod et al. obtained excellent results (even if the same researchers in "Psyching-up and muscular force production" delve into the subject and, while confirming the validity of the various approaches, leave some questions open).

The study by Perkins et al. ("The effects of elevated arousal and mood on maximal strength performance in athletes" from 2001) also reports highly positive effects, with high arousal levels *in very simple tasks* measuring hand strength, a movement that does not require a lot of coordination or fine motor skills. We know that each sport (and each person) has its own optimal level of activation, including on the basis of expected technical difficulties, conventionally evaluated with an inverted U-shaped curve (Yerkes-Dodson law), in which the level in the center is more than the correct one (with the caveats previously mentioned), while at the beginning and at the end of the continuum the levels are too low or too high: remember that minimal activation is correlated with slowed movements, generalized state of distraction, lack of concern for performance, anticipation or enthusiasm, a sense of heaviness and minimal elasticity. On the other hand, an excess is connected with awkward, jerky, uncoordinated movements, excessive muscle tension, negative thoughts and high respiratory/heart rate.

The most recommended techniques are "imagine yourself energetic, increase your heart rate, use positive phrases and statements, listen to your favorite music, visualize energizing images or a successful training session".

A bodybuilder who has an hour or more of training ahead of him will not be able to start lifting like a powerlifter at the last set, just as an Olympic lifter will not be able to start the third clean & jerk attempt like the aforementioned bodybuilder at the first set!

Scientific data aside, I believe that experience has its importance: I remember that exactly 40 years ago, at the age of 18, I wanted to try to lift 180 kg for the first time on a bench press: I had no idea how much weight I could lift because I used to do flat bench dumbbell flyes first, since doing the presses first put too much emphasis on my anterior deltoid. I "charged" myself up for 5 minutes, both mentally and with suitable music (for me), at full volume. I was very determined, but I was equally amazed when I managed to perform three repetitions, in perfect style, without bouncing or arching! A success? Not completely, because everything else in the session was pitiful... I had exhausted all my nervous energy and in each subsequent exercise, I lifted much less weight than usual: a lesson I have not forgotten!

Without examining it with further research, I believe that it is necessary to experiment with both the type and the optimal activation/relaxation level, because never as in this case a personalized approach is the only way, also depending on the moment of the training periodization that one is facing in a given contingency.

Regarding the importance of **music**, there is one particularly interesting, but also long study: Karagheorgis and collaborators carried out an extensive series of studies, which are all very interesting, among which I recommend "The psychological, psychophysical and ergogenic effects of music in sports: A review and synthesis" (Routledge Online Studies on the Olympic and Paralympic Games, 2012) because, as the title suggests, it is a synthesis of their work and also contains numerous bibliographic references.

There are many topics ranging from the differences between asynchronous synchronous and *oudeterous* (that is to say neutral) music, to the number of bpm or decibels. I also want to add "Music and strength training. The influence of sound stimulation on strength performance" (by Gollin et al., 2014), in which a volume of 75 dB and a number of bpm between 120 and 145 guaranteed substantial improvements in squats and overhead presses, and also "Using auditory stimulation to enhance athletes' strength: An experimental study in weightlifting" (Murgia et al., 2012), because he obtained good results in the bench press by using an auditory stimuli formed by a sound of 60 dB and one of 95 dB, respectively in the eccentric and concentric phases.

Another factor to consider is freeing our mind from the unconscious chatter that occupies it uselessly and that we are not fully aware of: after exercises like the ones described above (or even meditation, for those interested in Eastern disciplines), our brain is ready to attack the weights, but a latent, negative inner dialogue could choose that moment to present itself: our **critical inner voice** is not an auditory hallucination, it is experienced as "thoughts in your head" and this flow of destructive thinking forms a negative narrative that discourages individuals from acting in their own best interests.

In this regard, it is useful to replace both the "background buzz" that distracts us and any negative dialogues that bring us down: as mentioned, these thoughts are often not fully apparent in our conscious brain because they are deeply rooted in some previous experience (childhood, sports, work or love) and are "introjected" without realizing it.

A not so recent study (Lodge et al., 1998) demonstrates how negative dialogues play a role in generating or maintaining anxiety levels. Newberg and Waldman (2012), on the other hand, state that positive words can alter the expression of genes, strengthening areas in our frontal lobes and promoting the cognitive functions of the brain, prompting the motivational centers of the brain to take action and maximize resilience. In their book, the two scholars state: "formulating positive and optimistic words in your mind stimulates activity in the frontal lobe. This area includes specific language centers that connect directly to the motor cortex responsible for taking action. And, as our research has shown, the more you focus on positive words, the more they begin to affect other areas of the brain as well. Functions in the parietal lobe begin to change, which changes your perception of yourself." Conversely, hostile language can turn off specific genes that play a key role in the production of neurochemicals that protect us from stress. Humans are hardwired to worry – part of our early brain protects us from threats to our survival – so our thoughts instinctively go in that direction. A single negative word can increase the activity in our amygdala, massively implicated in reactions of excitement, fear, alertness and aggression, and this releases hormones and neurotransmitters that produce stress, which in turn hinders the functioning of our brain (especially in regard to logic, reason, and language). The scholars add, "angry words send alarm messages throughout the brain, and in part deactivate the centers of logic and reasoning located in the frontal lobes".

And, as Sonja Lyubomirsky, one of the leading researchers in Positive Psychology and the pursuit of happiness, confirms, if you want to maintain a fulfilling life throughout your existence, "you need to engage in positive thinking about yourself and do this by sharing your happiest events with others – through language. If you use your words – your self-talk and your conversations with others – to engage in optimism and positivity, you will find yourself moving in a more invigorating direction."

These internal dialogues must therefore be replaced with mantra-like affirmations (in the Western sense) and must be: repeated continuously, short (fundamental!), realistic (*I will probably squat 500 kg* is beyond the possibilities of most of us...), incisive and, generally, positive (better to say "today I will do 10 sets of squats" than "today I will not stop at the seventh set of squats"). In fairness, it should be noted that a quite recent study (Papeo et al., 2016) *partially* contradicted the "two-step model of cognition" cognitive model, which claims that positive meaning is first fully activated and then modified to reflect the negation and, to a certain extent, the statements reported in the previous lines are based in relation to preferably formulating positive concepts; but, as always – and fortunately – there are never univocal opinions.

However, mantras must be "felt" by those who develop them, therefore they must arise from one's needs/requirements, verbalized with the words chosen by the subject; in any case, they can and must evolve into new ones, once their needs require it. Frank Zane is the champion who has perhaps made the most of the diverse psychological techniques: "The Chemist" declared that he had made extensive use of various mantras, starting from the year of his first victory at Mr. Olympia in 1977 when he declared to everyone from the rooftops (as well as himself, several times a day) that this was "the year of Zane"; in 1978, however, he chose "you've already won" and used it for quite a while!

Frank also uses meditation a lot and currently sells equipment designed to facilitate the achievement of the desired state of activation or relaxation.

Let's move on to **associative visualization**, a technique that has been widely used for a long time: remaining in "our" field, who does not remember Arnold, who visualized his formidable biceps increasingly massive during every training session, until they filled up the whole room? Schwarzenegger himself, who from a young age imagined himself as the winner on the top step of the podium in a bodybuilding competition, has always attached great importance to mental abilities and setting goals: "What makes you be at the top? It's the mind that actually creates the body, it's the mind that really makes you work out for four or five hours a day, it's the mind that visualizes what the body should look like as an end product."

In Italy, Massimo Spattini told me about similar experiences: at the beginning of his training he had a very vivid dream in which he imagined the physical form he wanted to have, and he always kept a strong memory trace of it, using it as a spur during the years that led him to victory at the IFBB Italian heavyweight championships: well, his physical condition revealed on that occasion was precisely the one that "appeared" to him many years before in his sleep... he had finally reached his goal!

Dr. Spattini has always said that he has used his medical knowledge to perfect his approach to training and diet, but what many do not know is that he has also used autogenic training and other techniques, availing himself of a psychiatrist expert: from the sensations of heat, gradually more and more localized, of which we have previously written, to the use of visualization, ending with the use of a mantra, very similar to the one used by Zane in 1978.

In a 2014 interview, Arnold argued that "you have to be inside the muscle, that's the difference"... yet how many times have I seen, purely by way of example, someone doing set after set of alternating dumbbell curls, following an almost "aerobic class" rhythm, without any concentration on the work itself. Of course, in half-pronation lifting the elbows up to the ceiling and religiously flexing the wrists!

However, very recently, I was surprised (watching a so far unpublished video interview of Steve Reeves) to discover that even the great American champion, god of Physical Culture, was already using visualization in his time, and in a similar way to Arnold, envisioning the muscles he was training with the proportions and dimensions he wanted to achieve!

The quintessential cinematic Hercules used internal focus (which we will discuss later), focusing on the contraction of the muscle he was training; a technique that proves to be successful for maximum hypertrophy.

Steve adds that the mind is also essential in drawing on the last supply of energy needed to overcome one's limits in the gym (and beyond): "mind over matter", textual words!

Frank Zane, on the other hand, used the following technique: "I sit in a quiet place, preferably in a dark room; I close my eyes and focus my attention on my forehead. I imagine a big movie or TV screen in front of me, then I see an image of what I look like, then I gradually transform into what I want to look like." In a 2011 interview, Frank stated: "When you do a set of exercises in the weight room, there is nothing else. One must learn to get in touch with the sensation of performing the exercise. Don't focus on anything but the sensation, not even the breath." He concludes by stating that breathing will come by itself, once you feel like you are one with the aforementioned set... true, maybe after a little practice, though!

And what about Tom Platz: the "Golden Eagle" attaches great importance to the mental aspect, which he calls "Mind Doctrine". On his site, he dwells on visualization, goal setting (annually, monthly, weekly), "commitment" (attitude to sacrifice), positivity and the ability to face fear... Tom used mantras that he expressed loudly ("Tom Platz, Mr. Michigan!") or visually, sticking phrases similar to those that he verbalized on the bathroom mirror. There would be much more to write about the ideas of "Mr. Legs", who is also known for his incredible concentration that allowed him to have a superhuman intensity in his workouts.

Even the long-lived Bill Pearl (who enjoyed 20 years of success in competitions and died recently at over 91 years of age from bacterial infection contracted in the hospital after an accident), the multi-time winner of Mr. Universe and author of many books, including *Keys to the INNER universe* (in which he included the chapter entitled "You are what you think"), argued that one must exercise for a purpose, to train a muscle and not to impress onlookers or to simply lift the maximum weight; Bill also suggests discovering the exercises that make us better perceive the contraction of the muscle of interest and performing them for a greater number of sets, always thinking about the muscle and not about the performance; and this didn't stop him from training with weights, which were decidedly impressive at the time!

Speaking of heavy loads, Reg Park (many times winner of Mr. Universe and Schwarzenegger's idol) made it clear that *the mind is the limiting factor*: during one of their meetings in South Africa, Arnold saw the old champion use 360 kg on the calf raise while he was only using 135. After hearing Reg's words, before long Arnold was training with... 450 kg!

In this field, stories relating to Franco Columbu also abound: Arnold talks about how the Sardinian champion, during a workout, for once, was less performing than him: the Austrian did 6 repetitions of squats with 225 kg, while Franco only did 4! At that moment, however, a group of girls that the two had already met on the beach entered Gold's, and Schwarzenegger, after greeting them, said to his training partner: "Look, they told me they don't believe you can lift 225 kg in the squat", relying on his mental strength and the desire to make a good impression in front of the pretty exponents of the fairer sex. Indeed, Franco put the barbell on his shoulders again and performed 10 repetitions without apparent effort! His willpower had transformed him in minutes!

Another time at Gold's, Arnold and Dave Draper had done a set of T-bar rows with over 130 kg and they challenged Franco to do better: some Italians had just entered and the future two-time Mr. Olympia, not wanting to make a bad impression in front of fellow countrymen, concentrated for a moment and doubled the number of repetitions performed by the two giants!

Let's move on to **Mental Training** (MT): it is now a widely used practice in the sports field and ideomotor training, which is part of it, and it has obtained numerous results. One that stands out is the discovery of mirror neurons (initially in non-human primates and then in humans) by our Rizzolatti in the 1990s, who provided a (further) explanation of the importance of MT: these are neurons that are present in motor and premotor areas of the brain that are activated both when an action is performed and when an action is seen performed.

For humans, we speak of a "mirror system", because it is not possible to record the activity of a single neuron during the execution, observation, or even the imagination of an action, while it is feasible to detect the presence of brain activity with instrumental assessments. Brain activation is mainly recorded in the posterior parietal cortex, secondary motor cortex and Broca's area.

This type of neuron allows the motor gesture to be acquired through its visualization (already present in children and very important for their learning); it will settle for a second time, so to speak, and it will be possible to reuse it at will, which is very useful (also) for sportsmen. It can also be used in rehabilitation, as show in "Mirror neurons and cognitive and motor functions" (Fugassi, 2008).

A similar potential can also be exploited by bodybuilders: many go to Venice to take advantage of being able to train alongside so many champions, which, in addition to having a high motivational value, allows them to learn better execution of the exercises or perhaps to make it their own, maximizing the aspects best suited to their structure, according to the Latin concept of *aemulatio* compared to that of *imitatio*.

I went to California in 1983 to see the "mecca" of bodybuilding up close and to "experience" the invigorating atmosphere which, especially at that time, reigned at Gold's and at the World's Gym. It was right there where I met Massimo Spattini, a regular since the early 80s: for decades, Spattini spent his holidays (mainly) in the States, even after retiring from competitions, in order to keep his motivation – which is not easy after several decades of practice – and to stay updated on all the news that arises year after year. This also applies at an academic level, given the fact that in the USA, topics are addressed or in any case treated in a more exhaustive way, which might be considered inconvenient elsewhere.

In 1825, Johann Friedrich Herbart tackled the subject by asserting that "the image of perceptual effects can favor the relative movements" and, in 1854, William Benjamin Carpenter stated that **simply imagining a movement can determine a stimulation** of the muscles involved in the imaginative activity itself (as also confirmed by recent research which has scientifically proven these assertions, even if in a lower percentage compared to the real action). The resulting neuromuscular feedback promotes learning of the displayed motor skills ("Carpenter effect"). Furthermore, in 1890, William James (a well-known American psychologist, doctor and philosopher) wrote that "every representation of a movement awakens the real movement to some extent ".

Much more recently, Pascual-Leone and collaborators (1995) found that after a session of MT, the changes in the map of the sensorimotor cortex are similar to those obtained with physical exercise, thanks to the modulation of the neural circuits involved in the early stages learning motor skills. Not only does this modulation result in a marked improvement in performance, but it also appears to put subjects in an advantageous position for learning other motor skills with minimal physical practice. Furthermore, thanks to these physiological effects, MT can help not only with learning new motor patterns, but also with maintaining what has already been learned in subjects who are temporarily unable to do so because of injuries.

In a much-cited study, Kosslyn et al. (2001) wrote that, until recently, MT was part of the realm of philosophy and cognitive psychology, which were able to raise important questions, but made no progress in answering them, due to a lack of objective procedures. Through brain imaging research, new constantly evolving technologies are finally revealing the ways in which imagination acts on the mechanisms used in other activities, such as perception and motor control. Therefore, they have proposed the existance of a kind of functional equivalence (not to be confused with similar definitions in psychology and ecology) emphasizing how ideomotor training recruits structures and/or neural processes that are analogous to the real activity of visual perception and motor activity.

Here, it is not possible to further explore the physiological processes of the improvements obtainable with MT (also because there are still no certainties), but I recommend reading: "Neural mechanisms of strength increase after one-week motor imagery training" and "Spinal plasticity with motor imagery practice" by Grosprêtre et al. (not cited), in which the volunteers who underwent MT obtained significant results; the study by Ladda et al. and "Mécanismes neurophysiologiques de l'imagerie motorice: effet d'une stimulation somatosensorielle associée" by Elodie Traverse (not cited), is decidedly exhaustive, considering the length of almost 180 pages!

An attempt to give order to this matter can be seen in a study by Martin et al. (1999), which proposes a model that conceptualizes sports, the type of imagery used and the ability to use imagery as factors influencing the way images can condition an athlete. Three broad categories of image effects were examined: (a) skill and strategy learning and performance; (b) cognitive modification; (c) regulation of arousal and anxiety.

Another interesting work is that of Pakulanon (2016), who examined the effective use of mental imagery in athletes, based on the models of Paivio and Hall, which divide MT into five types (motivational specific: MS; motivational general-mastery: MG-M; motivational general-arousal: MG-A; cognitive specific: CS; cognitive general: CG). According to the results, MG-M and CS images appeared to be the most effective and most used by athletes and, CS in particular improved skill learning, while MG-M allowed for greater sport-specific confidence.

Mental training, while obviously not being able to replace real training, has an effectiveness that is now out of the question, as demonstrated by numerous studies. I myself, after injuring a hamstring during a 30m sprint on the track, used ideomotor training to avoid losing my discus throwing technique, during the forced stop: I still remember the incredulity and skepticism when I returned to the ring, and threw even better than before, so much so that one of those who were present said in untraslatable slang: "Marco Tullio, have you finally learned to throw?" moreover, he was the only one who, apart from the joke, gave the right value to the unexpected improvement and, not by chance, he was the only one of those present to have a past as a champion (called up for the national team in two totally different disciplines).

The result, therefore, is a strengthening of the mnestic trace of the performed movement, which, session after session, facilitates the learning of the real movement, with which it mutually consolidates or maintains its level in those who cannot train. This also applies to the bodybuilder's posing routine: in my day, I practiced it religiously, several times a week (I also obtained different versions of the chosen classic song, to find the one that had the rhythm that best suited my style, since every conductor has a way of making the score in front of them come alive), to synchronize myself with the beats of the music, acquire fluency and execute each position at its best (*not to mention the improvement in muscle separation and mind-muscle connection*).

Visualizing the sequence mentally, in addition to the actual exercises, is of great help and, in my opinion, remains an overlooked factor: I have seen some Mr. Olympia competitions live, including in California, and I have always been amazed at how champions performed the poses badly even at that level, being totally out of sync and, last but not least, choosing poses that were not very suitable for their physique... a real mess!

Obviously, a good poser with a 35 cm arm won't go far, but I wonder how this important aspect can be ignored, given that it allows us to best show the result of the sacrifices that we know are behind those two or three minutes of poses which are performed on the day of the competition and which are only the final moments of a long process.

In this case, "friends" of the competitor do not help, as, due to inexperience or not to disappoint him (a collusion in the psychological sense), they are not critical enough: constructive criticism is actually fundamental, since it helps to improve the weak points and also to avoid many disappointments.

A little personal anecdote: at the evening show of a national competition, I was called to pose, but my tape (old times...) was nowhere to be found and I had to perform without music, after all my detailed work! I was beside myself. When I was declared the winner, miraculously the tape "reappeared" and I was very insistent that I could perform my routine again, this time with my longed-for music!

In addition to what has been said above, ideomotor training makes the displayed sporting movement "familiar", so that it is no longer anxiety-producing (if it were in the first place): let us remember the negative internal dialogues, that chatter mentioned above, often unconscious, which frequently sabotages us...

As mentioned previously, there are now numerous studies relating to the effects of MT on sports, while there are few relating to the world of resistance training (as we can see in the sarcastic "Mind–muscle connection revisited: do 100 studies about beanbag tossing, stick balancing, and dart throwing have any relevance for strength training?" by Andersen and Calatayda) and in any case, they are slowly accumulating.

Another very important aspect to take into consideration is whether to set up the movement from an internal point of view (in which the subject imagines himself performing an action and experiences the sensations as if they were performing it in reality) or external (seeing ourselves from outside, in the third person): I think it is necessary to experiment with both methods and find the one that best suits one's aptitudes; eventually they can be alternated if necessary, since, as we will see, the two methods seem to be more or less valid depending on the planned goal.

One certainty is that of the benefits of this approach for untrained subjects, as can be read in a study by Chaiwanichsiri et al. (2006), who reports that "eight weeks of mental weight training resulted in a 40% and 30% ($p<0.000$!) gain in arm muscle strength in sedentary adults. It is easy to perform and practice frequently, and it does not cause any serious side effects." Incredibly, the exercise that subjects had to "do mentally" was a bicep curl (external focus), but 30% of the previously reported increase (that of $p<0.000$) was earned by the extensor, the triceps!

The researchers also carried out EMG measurements of the arm muscles with both "imaginary" and real (4 kg) weights: in the first case, simultaneous contractions of agonists and antagonists were recorded, while in the second, only contractions of biceps and brachioradialis were recorded. Very interesting! Some studies, however, such as the one from Lebon et al. (2010), obtained less striking results, but sufficient to allow the authors to recommend MT "because it optimizes the execution of the exercises [in the present case, those for the lower limbs] and increases intrinsic motivation".

Three uncited works (Wakefield and Smith, 2011 a/b; Smith et al., 2018) used the PETTLEP model to evaluate any improvements (once again) on the bicep curl (in external "mode"), reporting noticeable improvements in the lifted load, in some cases around 15%! In one of the studies, the results were comparable to those of subjects performing two sets of curls... *Of course, in all cases, the subjects were not people that regularly exercised with weights.*

PETTLEP is an acronym that represents a checklist of seven points to follow when conceiving an imagery intervention (physical, environment, task, timing, learning, emotion and perspective). It is based on solid neuroscientific foundations ("The PETTLEP approach to motor imagery: a functional equivalence model for sports psychologists", Holmes et al., 2007) and supports the thesis that states the brain stores memories in the form of an accessible central representation from the execution of a physical movement and, more importantly, from motor images associated with this execution.

A large body of evidence supporting shared core frameworks suggests that sports psychologists should more closely consider all aspects of their athletes' subjective responses when providing imagery interventions, and not rely only on clinically oriented "traditional" methods.

Perhaps the most marked difference between the PETTLEP approach and more traditional image methods is that images have often been thought of as something entirely separate from the actual physical practice. This method, however, conceptualizes physical practice and imagery as being on a continuum, and posits that the closer imagery interventions are toward the physical side of the continuum, the more effective they are likely to be.

One study worthy of mentioning is that of Alexander et al. (2019) because it provides theoretical foundations and practical advice in relation to powerlifting, but it is interesting for anyone because we are talking about exercises that are widely used in all sports and because it deals with strength, motivation and self-confidence, anxiety and arousal control, and post-injury rehabilitation.

Speaking of injuries, a 2019 study (Paravlic, not cited) on recovery after total knee arthroplasty found significantly better results compared to the control group that only performed routine physical therapy, leading the authors to determine that it is certainly advantageous to add MT to normal therapies.

A substantial review in 2016 (Slimani et al.) also showed how the combination of MT and "real" exercises is more effective than the latter alone: this is true for both the "injured" and "healthy" control groups; unlike what has been seen in other works, in this case, it was the "internal" group that had the best results, and the authors gave some reasons for this (one, the higher number of "internal" studies they examined), and they formulated numerous hypotheses at various levels on the scientific motivations underlying these results, too many to mention, but not too many to read!

Paravlic et al. (2018), again, found good results both without "real" exercises and in association with them, writing that "the practice of Mental Training can be considered a substitute or additional training tool to preserve muscle function when athletes are not exposed to maximum training intensities".

In this regard, and given the moment in which I am writing these lines (September 2021, after several lockdowns due to the Covid-19 pandemic), the study by Dello Iacono et al. (2021), in which 30 professional basketball players were randomly assigned to three counterbalanced groups is very interesting: two MT training groups, who completed ideomotor training by mentally rehearsing muscle-loaded upper and lower limb RT exercises 85% of a repetition maximum (85% 1RM) or optimal power loads (OPL, the value of the maximum power output, evaluated by special machines), or to a control group.

Well, physical performance improved significantly following both MT protocols (range ~2% to ~9%) but was reduced in the control group, compared to preintervention (P 0.016). There were some differences between the two modalities, but the researchers still concluded that "during periods of forced reduction, mental imagery appears to be a valid tool for maintaining and increasing physical performance capacity among professional athletes."

A very recent study by Bouguetouch et al. (August 2021) in which we can appreciate the crossover effect on an untrained limb, is equally interesting: what happens with actual training also partially happens with MT! Think of the importance of these findings for recovering after an injury!

In this regard, a study by Neige et al. (2020) shows us how pain caused by an injury inhibits not only muscle contraction but also the neurocortical excitability normally elicited by MT, which is a factor to be taken into consideration.

Neige herself also proposed other interesting research, with Célia Ruffino as the main author. They are worth a read.

Another notable work is that of Buck et al. (2016), in which the maximum performance of some volunteers on three repetitions of the front squat was initially evaluated, together with their Self-Efficay (SE) with respect to their 3RM (SE, according to Bandura [1977] is the belief in one's own ability to organize and execute the courses of action necessary to produce certain results).

Subsequently, subjects in the experimental group followed a structured imaging protocol that incorporated video recordings of both their 3RM performance and a reference lifter with excellent technique; all this, twice a day for 3 days. Control group subjects spent the same amount of time watching a placebo video. After 3 days without physical training, the front squat 3RM and self-efficacy measurements were repeated. The subjects of the experimental group tangibly increased in self-efficacy after the intervention and showed a marked improvement in the 3RM compared to those of the control group (almost 10 kg vs 2.5). It was evaluated that self-efficacy was a fundamental cornerstone for the purposes of the results that were described above.

Not bad indeed!

A study by Gilson et al. ("An examination of athletes' self-efficacy and strength training effort during an entire off-season", 2012) has demonstrated the validity of SE in terms of improving results in strength training. Also, a work by Khan et al. ("Effects of imagery and video modeling on self-efficacy during resistance exercise", 2019) demonstrated the importance of MT, combined this time with video images of the movement to be performed (lunges), in achieving superior performance compared to the control group; the authors also add two sobering concepts because, citing two previous papers (Debarnot et al., 2014 and Weinberg et al., 2008, not cited), they point out how watching ad hoc videos helps beginners in particular, whereas the first-mentioned study proved the different activation of neural circuits activated by imagery between novices and advanced athletes, obviously in favor of the latter (as in less activation due to expertise levels), while Weinberg et al. have remarked how video and imagery help subjects with poor imaginative skills, thanks to the combination of the two techniques: an invitation to experiment and not to throw in the towel at the first sign of failure!

So, self-efficacy aside, one of the most successful modalities seems to be AOMI (action observation and motor imagery), thanks to the combination of observing a movement demonstration, usually via video, while imagining the feelings and sensations involved in the execution of the observed action: the recent publication "Recommendations for combining action observation and motor imagery interventions in sport" (Wright et al., September 2021) addresses all the nuances and offers numerous bibliographic ideas, as well as several practical tips.

Previously Di Rienzo et al. ("Effects of action observation and action observation combined with motor imagery on maximal isometric strength", 2019), had obtained (again on the arm flexors) worthy results, given the statistical value ($p < 0.001$) being much higher than the control group. These results were also achieved in a previous study of the same working group ("Short-term effects of integrated motor imagery practice on muscle activation and force performance"). Another composite procedure can be evaluated in "Does performance-related information augment the maximal isometric force in the elbow flexors?" (Miller et al., 2021), in which visual and verbal input were compared individually or in pairs with the goal of improving performance in the "usual" bicep curl: all were superior to the control group, but the visual one obtained the best results compared to the verbal one, or to a combination of both at the same time.

Richter et al. (2012) proposed an imagery model to maximize the execution of an exercise (in this case the deadlift, but it is obviously valid for all the others), dividing it into pre-workout, pre-lift, during and after the lift, and recommended its implementation, while suggesting customization for the best results.

In other research papers, such as that of Chan et al., again related to the deadlift (2019, not cited), there were no significant improvements in performance, but there was progress in posture and in the regularity of the various repetitions, evaluated from an external point of view, thanks to greater automation of the movement. The same can also be seen in Kal et al. (2013, "External attentional focus enhances movement automatization: a comprehensive test of the constrained action hypothesis"), a factor that in the long run can protect against injuries, as well as allow gains in strength, thanks to the better exploitation of key positions.

Several studies have reported how the results of MT performed by holding the tool(s) that are used in a sport are decidedly superior; a more recent study ("Motor experience with a sport-specific implement affects motor imagery", Zhang et al., 2018) deals with the topic, also including the bibliographic data of previous works, and is an interesting procedure in the RT field while using an empty barbell or dumbbells!

However, regarding the increase in strength, from what we have seen, the external focus seems to prevail over the internal one: in "The effect of attentional focus on gluteus medius recruitment and force production" (Grace Golden, 2020), the external focus allowed an improvement in strength, similar to interesting research by Marchant et al., where it allowed an increase (what else!) in a bicep curl that obtained a statistical significance of <0.05, *while the internal one increased the activation of the muscle being examined.*

In recent work by Ghorani et al. (2021), researchers found (through EMG) only a greater activation of the "visualized" muscles without a corresponding increase in strength or change in lumbar posture (another investigated variable).

A study by Schoenfeld et al. (2018) gives us further scientific proof of what has just been reported: the purpose of this paper was to study the effects of the use of an internal rather than an external attentional focus on muscle adaptations during an RT session. Thirty untrained college students were randomly assigned to an *internal* focus group (Internal) that focused on target muscle contraction during training ($n = 15$) or an *external* focus group (External) that focused on attention to the outcome of the lift ($n = 15$). For both groups, the training consisted of three weekly sessions, on non-consecutive days, for 8 weeks. Subjects performed four sets of 8-12 repetitions per exercise. Strength changes were assessed with 6RM in bicep curls and isometric strength changes with maximal voluntary contraction in knee extension and elbow flexion. Muscle thickness changes for the brachial flexors and quadriceps were evaluated by ultrasound. The results showed a significant increase in brachial flexor thickness in the Internal group compared to the External group (12.4 vs. 6.9%, respectively), while there were no statistically significant results for the quadriceps. Isometric resistance in flexion was greater for the Internal group, while isometric knee extension was greater for the External one, although no conclusive statistical significance was reached in either case. The results seem to confirm the importance of the mind-muscle connection for the purpose of muscle hypertrophy in the Internal mode. The authors also explain that the difference measured in the results of the lower limbs could be due to the lower control of the thigh muscles exhibited by untrained participants, and also because they are used to using the biceps for "fine" movements. Trained athletes would probably have achieved better results due to their superior control of all muscles, including those of the lower body, as described in "Importance of mind-muscle connection during progressive resistance training" by Calatayud et al. (2016). The same thing was described in "Mind-muscle connection training principle: influence of muscle strength and training experience during a pushing movement", by the same authors (2017).

Similar results emerged from a study by Collum et al. (2020, not cit.), this time on pectoralis contraction as measured by electromyography. The "internal" attention prevailed in this study (incidentally, the conditions were more complex in this case).

Also, let's consider that focusing on the dichotomy internal/external could be the wrong way to look at the "problem" and a good starting point could be found in work by Peh et al. (2011, not cited) where the authors state that "Investigations into the relative effectiveness of either focusing on movement form (internal focus) or movement effects (external focus) have tended to dominate research on instructional constraints. However, rather than adopting a comparative approach to determine which focus of attention is more effective, analysis of the relative efficacy of each specific instruction focus during motor learning could be more relevant for both researchers and practitioners. Theoretical advances in the motor learning literature from a nonlinear dynamics perspective might explain the processes that underlie the effect of different attentional focus instructions".

Another line of research related to the potential of the internal focus was developed by a group of researchers from some Brazilian universities, led by Fujita, who have carried out a series of studies on training without equipment consisting in contracting agonist and antagonist muscles and determined that a different verbal instruction allows a subject to focus more on the triceps or biceps (as can be read in "Influência de diferentes instruções verbais sobre a atividade mioelétrica dos músculos flexores e extensores de cotovelo during a co-contração muscular co- muscular contraction"); however, they give more explanations about this method (which they themselves define as unorthodox) in other papers, such as "Co-contraction training: myoelectric activity and recruitment strategies in an unorthodox resistance training", this time by Dos Santos Silva, in which they also provide several bibliographic sources (for example, Mackenzie et al., "Neuromuscular adaptations following antagonist resisted training", 2010).

A study by Snyder et al. (2009, not cited) showed how inexperienced subjects executing a lat pull-down exercise were able to shift the focus to the back after adequate instructions, while the "standard" execution had mainly involved the arm flexors: proof of what has been seen in the gym, in my case for decades... The right advice allows the beginner to perform the exercise more profitably: the expert eye can understand when the target muscle is not being addressed.

This brings to mind an experience I once had: I was called to award the medium class at the 1985 regional bodybuilding championships, and I noticed how the winner had exceptional forearms and arms and front deltoid nearly as good, while pectorals and back were less and less developed the more you approached the center of the chest... By chance, I met him after 2 weeks in a Roman gym and, after seeing his poor execution on the lat machine and lat pulley (he put more strain on the upper limbs – especially the brachioradialis and forearm flexors – than the back), as well as in bench presses, with the elbows too close to the body (thus putting more stress on the deltoids and triceps), I was able to understand his unusual development, attributable both to his genetics and to the wrong focus and biomechanics!

Another study that proves the effectiveness of internal focus is that of Catalayud et al. (2016/17, not cited), in which the authors demonstrate through EMG how it is possible to shift the focus to the triceps or pectorals, at least up to 60% RM, while at 80%, the subjects failed to achieve significant results. Personally, I believe that an advanced athlete can do better, provided that he trains "with his head": the subjects in question were "experts" (8 years of training on average), but with a ratio of 1 RM max of 1.25 kg per kg bodyweight on the bench press, hardly elite. A brief aside: we have seen how "feeling" a muscle, knowing how to contract it, and having a "feeling" with "it" is important, as Arnold already stated and as we have scientifically "discovered". I saw myself assigned an extra point in the Clinical Psychophysiology exam after having appropriately piloted the discussion on the skills that a good bodybuilder should have in this regard and after having argued about it at length!

This should be the case, in theory, because as we can see in "A study of body-part(s) training consciousness using a picture of a single-joint exercise" (Oshita et al., 2018), 90% of those who had viewed a photograph of a leg extension exercise responded that the exercise trains numerous other muscles in the trunk, the back of the leg, the upper limbs, in addition to the "front thigh muscles"... and if these subjects did not train, 80% of the experienced ones gave broadly similar answers, as did 60% of those who had practiced under professional supervision: if you don't know which muscle to activate, you won't be able to contract it with maximum efficiency!

A study, once again by Schoenfeld (et al., 2016), a very prolific author in the field of RT, puts a definitive point on the matter: a long theory of research indicates that results-oriented tasks are optimized through the adoption of an external attentional focus. A recent literature review including over 50 publications on the topic (Wulf, 2013) is cited, showing that more than 90% of these studies have shown superior improvements in motor learning and strength when using an external focus compared to the internal one (in 1998 Wulf et al., had already demonstrated that adopting an external focus of attention enhances accuracy, balance, jumping performance and other sport-specific exercise outcomes). The same is stated in a paper by Halperyn and Vigostsky ("The mind–muscle connection in resistance training: friend or foe?"), which found that a strength performance can be affected by the "internalization" of attention, due to the co-contraction of agonists and antagonists.

But, Schoenfeld continues, if the external focus is more profitable when the goal is to improve performance, with regards to resistance training, its superiority has been attributed to a greater force production but by virtue of an increased economy of movement associated with reduced muscle activity (as seen in Marchant et al.). However, while a more efficient movement pattern facilitates the acquisition of better motor skills and greater strength, it may not be optimal for muscle development: when the goal is to maximize hypertrophy, indirect evidence suggests that an internal focus may be the best approach. As we have seen, bodybuilders have long preached the importance of developing a "mind-muscle" connection during the training session.

Inner focus involves visualizing the target muscle and consciously directing neural input to the muscle during an exercise. Theoretically, this approach should increase the activation of the target muscle, while decreasing the contribution of the secondary muscles. Research seems to support this thesis. The attentional focus should correspond to a specific goal: athletes such as powerlifters, weightlifters or strongmen, who aim to maximize force/power production, should use an external focus. The same principle applies to basketball players or those who practice athletics and want to increase their jumping height or distance; it also applies to runners or rowers that are looking to improve the efficiency of their movements and also dart throwers, golfers and pool players who are chasing pinpoint accuracy. Instead, when attempting to increase muscle activation, an internal focus of attention would appear to be a better choice. This could also be attributed, as Grgic et al. wrote recently (2021, not cited) to the constrained action hypothesis. The authors rightly add that "while our findings suggest a benefit of using an external focus of attention for muscular strength, such recommendations should not be generalized to other resistance training adaptations such as muscular hypertrophy". By the way, the above hypothesis came to the light thanks to McNevin, Shea, & Wulf (2000; see also Wulf et al., 2001) that proposed a "constrained action hypothesis", according to which trying to consciously control one's movements constrains the motor system by interfering with automatic motor control processes that would "normally" regulate the movement. Focusing on the movement effect, on the other hand, might allow the motor system to more naturally self-organize, unconstrained by the interference caused by conscious control attempts, resulting in more effective performance and learning. Moreover, quite recently Saway et al. (2022, not cited) summarized the effects of internal focus and external focus on brain activity, performance and motor learning, focusing on various types of rehabilitation: "the use of attention focus has the potential to improve patient performance during rehabilitation without the need for special equipment". They wisely conclude "that based on conflicting findings, both internal focus and external focus should be implemented during rehabilitation, and the most optimal attention focus for individual patients should be considered". Maybe they're not taking a strong stance on the matter, but one cannot blame their emphasis on individuality, as there is no single recipe that is good for everyone!

So, most likely, bodybuilders and others seeking maximum hypertrophy will find it advantageous to focus on the target muscle during an exercise rather than the result or environment. Of course, one could argue about the importance of increasing strength for subsequent greater hypertrophy, but we don't have enough space for such a complex debate here! However, it is likely that the molecular signal for all three primary mechanisms of hypertrophy, namely mechanical strain, metabolic stress and muscle damage, are increased when athletes focus their attention inward, which could lead to greater muscle development compared to a specific load in a given exercise, especially for sessions with loads that are *commonly* called "light", technically definable with 50/60% 1RM. In my opinion, this precise control of the muscles is very useful, but the fact remains that more and more people practice RT: when the number was much smaller, being an almost niche activity, the number of enthusiasts was greater, in percentage terms; moreover, there were fewer machines and it is known that the use of free weights requires greater control (even if they're not always "fine" movements...) than that required by the many weight-machines that are present in gyms, preferred by trainers because less time is wasted explaining how it works and by the owners for the lower risks that they pose for beginners: for this purpose, equipment that gives feedback on the execution of individual exercises is being studied for both ways of lifting ("W8-Scope: Fine-grained, practical monitoring of weight stack-based exercises", Radhakrishnan et al., 2020; "ERICA: enabling real-time mistake detection and corrective feedback for free-weights exercises", Radhakrishnan et al., 2020).

These are welcome innovations because when I train in commercial gyms I see tremendously wrong executions. However, the human factor must not be neglected, given that a machine cannot replace our sensations... I believe that a mixture of the two factors is the best solution: you don't necessarily have to remain anchored to the good old days, you have to make the most of what technology offers us, without being overwhelmed by it.

In this regard, we can see how the aforementioned contribution of other disciplines can be helpful for sport psychology: in the last century, using some principles of psychophysiology, authors such as Rothemberg, proposed "touch-training" (an interesting review of their book appeared in *Physiotherapy*, April 1997, vol. 83, n. 4, edited by Phillips), which, as one can imagine, uses a certain type of dexterity to help "feel" a muscle and which is used in osteopathy in a different way.

If a clever practitioner can perceive the contraction of individual muscles, a novice, or even those who train *haphazardly*, will face difficulties, so a touch can help them to better perceive the target muscle through a series of physiological mechanisms: once the subject is able to master this ability, they will be able to train "normally".

The last study demonstrating that the use of mental training is not limited only to increasing strength is that of Silbernagel et al. (2007), in which the authors found that "the results showed that physical images (i.e. visions related to achieving a better body) were the most used and considered to be the most effective, followed by representations techniques (i.e. those related to the correct execution of the techniques and exercises) and energizing images (those relating to feeling "charged" or sensations of high energy)"; moreover, those who practiced MT appeared to have more self-confidence in the gym and more motivation.

Instead, for the purposes of the possibility of performing MT at different times, recent research (Dias Kanthak et al., "Revisiting the acute effects of resistance exercise on motor imagery ability", 2021), against the foreseen hypotheses, found that RT training and resulting fatigue improved MT-related performance; a factor to keep in mind.

It should be noted that the promotion of the effectiveness of MT must certainly be increased, because many coaches or athletes are still unaware of it or underestimate it, as highlighted by Xavier Wallace et al. (2019) in a study showing how, after watching a short explanatory film, the interest and appreciation of these techniques significantly increased in both groups.

The same group of researchers led by the aforementioned Radcliffe, in "Barriers to the Prescription of Psychological Strategies by Strength and Conditioning Specialists" (2019), analyzes the reasons that limit the use of MT and concludes that "it is clear that not incorporating psychological strategies in strength training or muscle building can be attributed to internal, personally self-determined beliefs, or to external situations governed by the environment".

Internal sources consist of insufficient knowledge regarding both the effectiveness of psychological strategies and the methods of implementation of these techniques; moreover, the realization of psychological techniques may be outside a trainer's mission or there is difficulty in demonstrating the validity of the interventions, while the external ones are due to lack of time, insufficient control of the contents of the training sessions and negative perceptions of the athletes themselves.

Let's broaden the discussion for a moment. In psychology, the Locus Of Control (LOC) is a term that refers to the fact that human behavior is not necessarily determined by objective descriptions of events, but rather by subjective meanings attributed to them. The LOC is one of the dimensions of personality that sits on the continuum between internal and external control. Individuals with internal LOC are identified by their belief that they are able to influence their own destinies. This facilitates the feeling of satisfaction with life and allows you to cope better with stress. Instead, individuals with external LOC make their lives more dependent on the influence of independent factors, such as other people, luck or coincidence. The LOC is acquired on the basis of personal and social experiences. It arises from an individual's subjective interpretation of the relationship between a behavior and its consequences, for example, successes versus failures. According to social learning theory, beliefs formed through various (even specific) social situations generalize over time, as well as personal ones.

Getting in touch with your body, identifying yourself with a muscle and with the sensation of its contraction is certainly easier for subjects with internal LOC. The LOC can also be exploited in relation to the fact that we cannot control what is happening around us: there will always be the person who "blasts" rap at full volume (it happened to me this morning, and in French...), the one who bangs weights or occupies a piece of equipment for an excessive amount of time by chatting or – easier these days – looking at their smartphone, perhaps using it for an endless series of selfies. We can't help it, but we can decide how to react, letting ourselves be distracted or getting extremely angry, or keeping our concentration on the next sets... or at least, after the first moments of anger, we can quickly fall back in line, perhaps using a mantra that we hold dear.

Another almost unexplored field is MT in relation to the fascia, which was considered an inert envelope for a long time but instead, it is being identified by contemporary scientific research as a system that plays an important role in human movement. A recent definition suggests that fascia is "a sheath, sheet or any number of other aggregations of connective tissue that forms under the skin to attach, enclose and separate muscles and other internal organs." Furthermore, we speak of the "fascial system", a term that refers to a "network of interdependent, interrelated and interactive tissues that form a complex whole". Fascia assists the human structure and function, including force transmission, some sensory functions, and wound regulation through its "collagen-fibrous tissues that are part of a larger system of tensional force transmission to the entire body".

The fascia comprises several cells with dissimilar characteristics: fibrocytes (i.e., fibroblasts and several types of myofibroblasts), adipocytes, migratory white blood cells, telocytes and fasciacytes. Furthermore, the fascia includes ground substance (an acellular component of the connective tissue, mainly made up of proteoglycans, which associate with long chains of hyaluronic acid) and collagen, which contribute to the formation of the extracellular matrix; there are also other physical and neural components (very important for the purposes of this discourse), but their precise examination goes beyond the discussion here; however, the fascia is considered to be among the richest sensory organs in the human body, as the vast majority of sensory nerve endings in musculoskeletal tissues (such as in the perimysium and endomysium) originate from it.

The extent of its nerve connections, both in an afferent and efferent sense, has not yet been fully understood, but the discoveries that are envisaged will certainly open many paths, as we can read in "Integrating mental imagery and fascial tissue: a conceptualization for research into movement and cognition" (Abraham et al., 2020), which offers a comprehensive review in which we conceptualize the ways in which MT could reciprocally interact with the fascial tissue to support performance, recovery from injuries and cognitive functions.

Among the listed conditions, we can include the positive effect on proprioception, on body pattern and the alleviation of pain. Drawing on the cellular, physiological and functional similarities and associations between muscle and fascial tissue, it can be argued that MT has the potential to influence the fascial tissue, but the latter may also exert feedback. The authors expose a number of biomechanical, psychological and neurosensory mechanisms that could be involved. It is truly interesting work, which cannot be further explored here, but merits opening a debate that can lead us far...

Another technique worth mentioning is dissociative imagery, which involves moving away from the situation one is experiencing in the here and now: in a moment of great effort, one can fantasize about being elsewhere, in a pleasant condition, but I see it more practicable for aerobic activity (possibly on equipment where there is no risk of tripping/falling!) than during weight training, which requires a certain amount of attention, especially with the use of free weights.

A further element to take into consideration is "self-control", which in our case can be defined as the ability to voluntarily control behavioral tendencies or even to resist immediate temptations in order to achieve long-term goals. Athletes are regularly confronted with a variety of demands for self-control: they must control their emotions during competitions and concentrate in high-tension contexts, but also, and above all, they need to achieve goals that are not immediate and they must resist immediate temptations to achieve goals in the long term: after a stressful day, finding the will to go to the gym, find a parking spot, do a heavy session, perhaps in a crowded room, is not a breeze. In this context (according to a self-control "model"), all acts of self-control are based on a single pool of metaphorical energy (the force of self-control): obviously, every person, even in this field, has different skills and abilities.

Some are able to recruit and maintain this energy better, but in addition to this characteristic, individuals also differ in the amount of self-control they can access in a given situation, as it can be depleted ("ego-depletion") for a prolonged period of time after being confronted with a primary self-control question (for example, emotion regulation during a sports competition or constantly working on an unpleasant task); at this point, athletes are less persevering during intense exercise, are less likely to stick to their training programs and tend to perform athletic feats under pressure less effectively. A vast line of research has arisen on this subject, and it is advisable to read the entire mass of works by Englert and his collaborators, who have expertly examined the various aspects of it.

A technique that has proved to be very useful (not only in the gym) is goal setting which, combined with a periodization of training, is essential in any sporting activity: having a focus is essential for reaching a goal, much like having a route or an itinerary if you want to reach a place.

An acronym is used to indicate the right implementation, SMART: S for specific, M for measurable, A for attainable, R for realistic and T for time-based; lately, some have added ER (SMARTER), i.e. exciting and recorded.

This brings us once again to Zane, the American athlete who planned all his preparation, from workouts to diet, to photos to see progress, to poses. He had to do it because until 1977 he was a full-time professor and had to maximize the available time: teaching mathematics, he could only use rational methodologies!

Zane used a training diary (the final R of the acronym) both to evaluate progress and responses to a specific type of program and to overcome the sticking points that can occur in some muscle groups (in many years of training – now more than 60 – surely it had already happened to him, like for everyone that trains hard) and he even published a summary, which includes everything he did up to about fifteen years ago!

Zane isn't my favorite bodybuilder, but I talk about him extensively because he's the one who got the best out of his physique with certainly inferior potential compared to the other Mr. Olympias, in part thanks to his intellectual curiosity, which also includes a long series of university studies in psychology.

Moreover, another, more "recent", Mr. Olympia, Dorian Yates, has used goal setting a lot and has maximized the use of training diaries: the English champion often reiterates the importance of putting pen to paper (in the actual sense of the word, no computers!) about everything you do in the gym to be able to evaluate the pros and cons of the various routines.

In a broader context, goal setting can be framed in the concept of "behavioral change for the purpose of a high-level performance", which provides for the identification of an intention, or a goal, to be translated into actions aimed at achieving it (which can be facilitated or hindered according to the personal characteristics of the subject or the surrounding environment), which must be repeated until they become habitual, with a process similar to that described by Schwarzer and Luszczynska in "Health action process approach" (2008), which is worth exploring further.

Now let's talk about **motivation**, which is essential for being able to train over time.

The simplest way to look at motivation is to divide it into extrinsic and intrinsic: the former comes from external sources (for example, while watching a bodybuilding competition, reading a fitness magazine or receiving a compliment about the shape we are in). As useful as this typology is, its duration is limited if it is not connected with something more personal and intimate.

Then we come to the motivation that arises from our inner goals, desires and needs, which, even without being flashy, are the ones that keep us focused, consistent, committed, and in a word, motivated!

Intrinsic motivation, however, is like wood that can be added to the fire of inner motivations, which we must analyze carefully, introspectively, because we can make the most out of it only if we are aware of it.

Thus, also in relation to extrinsic motivations and our goals: to renew the former and to keep the fire burning, and honestly evaluate the attainability of the latter. A positive mental attitude is one of the concepts to keep in mind because always seeing the glass half empty won't get us far... A sort of self-fulfilling prophecy (a sociopsychological construct coined by Thomas and perfected by Merton: an assumption, or prophecy, which, by the mere fact of having been pronounced, makes the foretold event materialize also through unconscious behaviors, thus confirming its own reliability); I repeat, it can also be something that is not consciously explicit, but that still influences us.

This is true in a general sense, regarding the common attitude or specific situations.

An example that comes to mind, because it happens all the time, is not being able to follow a pre-set schedule because the gym is overcrowded or because there is someone doing very long circuits, perhaps while chatting. You can get angry and maybe you can argue with that person, or you can try some new combinations or an exercise that you haven't done for a long time and possibly derive an unexpected benefit from it... It's up to us to choose!

Another cornerstone is to surround yourself with positive people, since the negativity around us can sabotage every aspect of what we do, just as positivity brings benefits on many levels.

There are other ways of examining the motivation that prompts us to practice resistance training: I like to quote (briefly, even if it deserves much more space) the one used by an American colleague, Edward Smith, who many years ago wrote a book that revolved around the world of weights (bodybuilding, powerlifting and weight lifting, as well as what people in the USA call "odd lifts", such as bicep curls with a barbell). Edward (who also competed in the last two disciplines mentioned above), who I occasionally exchange opinions with, divides motivation into four categories: "I have to do it", "I must do it as a means for a specific end", "I want to do it for the experience in itself" and, last but not least, "I want to do it for personal growth", which is the most interesting category for those who are truly passionate about "iron".

If the first typology refers to some sort of external pressure (from the doctor, the family, peers, etc.) and almost contains a moral obligation (the subject lives a standard imposed by others), the second is conditioned by an imperative ("I must lift to achieve something"), but it is anyway aimed at a goal, such as post-accident rehabilitation, athletic training for a different sport or even winning some Mr. Something contest; in any case, the activity is not carried out for the mere pleasure of doing it, unlike what happens in the third type of motivation, which makes it intrinsic.

This feeling can only be understood by those who, even in another field or in another sport, have made enormous efforts and sustained great sacrifices, always loving what they did. The fourth, on the other hand, leads to personal growth, which, while encompassing it, goes beyond physical growth: it unites them in a whole that includes areas that would otherwise be distinct, such as the physical, mental, emotional and spiritual ones. In a few words, a holistic development, using weights to explore yourself, getting to know yourself more intimately and on multiple levels, confronting conflicts, personal fears and unresolved psychological issues, and being able to overcome them.

The idea that training with weights can increase one's self-awareness fits into a line of previously explored studies: George Leonard (Ultimate Athlete), in the 70s, wrote that "sport and physical education, reformed and renewed, could give us the best possible path for self-knowledge, also for the purpose of a social transformation".

The four motivations that we described are to be considered in an incremental form – from the simplest to the most complex – and often partially coexist and can evolve; indeed, this is often the case.

For example, the great Oliver Sacks, the neurologist who wrote a series of very interesting books on the clinical cases he treated (including *Awakenings*, from which the homonymous film nominated for numerous awards was made, including three Oscars, played by Robin Williams and Robert de Niro), was also an excellent powerlifter: in the late 1950s he began training at Muscle Beach with, among others, Dave Draper; in one impromptu challenge, he managed to lift 260 kg in the front squat, without knee wraps or other equipment and without doping (shortly after he set the California open record for squats, no weight limit). He wrote that he started out not because he was skinny, but because he was an introvert, and he continued because he gained greater self-confidence in every aspect of life, as well as a better physique and a passion that accompanied him for the rest of his life. However, due to poorly executed stiff-legged deadlifts and with too much weight and two disastrous accidents at sea and in the mountains, he had to fall back mainly on swimming, where he could fully unleash his deep passion for physical exercise.

Since this is a book on weight training, I can report, out of curiosity and for a comparison with what is done today, that the hotshot doctor performed 5 sets of squats of 5 repetitions with 555 pounds (about 250 kg), every 5 days... Rather than focusing on the possible numerological value, I would give more thought to the potential and simplicity of "old-time" equipment and schedules!

Moreover, in line with what has been reported above, Sacks assigned an important role to music as a modulator of human feelings and moods, thanks to a privileged relationship with the brain, so much so that he dedicated a book to this subject and also included numerous mentions in another book, in which he spoke of his neuro-muscular re-education after one of his accidents that we mentioned.

I would like to conclude with an insight into the "path", quoting my friend Smith, who resorts to Castaneda, who makes "his" Don Juan say "There are many paths, each one is a candidate among millions, the idea is to sift through many and, after careful examination, choose one: if, after having traveled on a path for a while you realize that it is not the right one, abandon it and try another one. This must only happen after a disciplined experience with it. You will have to ask yourself: does this path have a heart? If it does, it's the right one; if it does not have it, it is useless... both paths lead nowhere, but one has a heart, and the other doesn't. One will give you a blissful journey and as long as you follow it, you are at one with it. The other will make you curse your life. One makes you strong, the other makes you weak." And sometimes, I add, it's the journey that counts more than the destination.

In short, a path that you follow with your heart will strengthen you, externally as much as internally, and will help you overcome an impasse during a set of a training session, a period of poor results or of life itself.

Everyone must find the path that makes them happy. You may not win Mr. Olympia, you won't squat 400 kg or do a 250 kg clean and jerk, but you will become a different person.

Unfortunately, what I see on social media nowadays makes me realize how iron disciplines have taken a wrong turn... but I think it's a sign of the times.

CHAPTER 38

Bodybuilding and hormones

Andrea Militello and Massimo Spattini

The muscle: an endocrine organ

Bodybuilding and hormones: an inattentive and mischievous reader could interpret the title incorrectly.

In this chapter we will analyze how weight training, i.e. the noble art of bodybuilding, can influence and modify the hormonal balance of our body.

Therefore, we won't discuss the use of hormones to become a strong and muscular athlete but, on the contrary, will explain how exercise with weights together with our genetics will allow us to achieve a body to die for and restore a hormonal balance that is essential for our psychophysical well-being.

First, let's consider the latest developments in scientific research regarding the muscle itself: not only is the muscle cell capable of exerting mechanical contractile activity, but it can also have a personal endocrine profile which, stimulated by repeated physical exercise, allows for the activation of enzymatic stages otherwise quiescent, which are responsible for endocrine-metabolic modifications (Pedersen et al., 2020).

Skeletal muscle has recently been identified as an organ that produces and releases cytokines, called "myokines," and given that it is the largest organ in the human body, discovering that it can secrete protein sets a new paradigm: skeletal muscle is an important endocrine organ that can affect metabolism in other tissues and organs.

After discovering that exercise causes an increase in a number of cytokines, a possible link between **skeletal muscle contractile activity and immune alterations was also established** (Hoffmann et al., 2017). Based on the current state of knowledge, the main physiological function of myokines is to protect the functionality and enhance the exercise capacity of the skeletal muscle itself. Myokines control adaptive processes in skeletal muscle by acting as paracrine regulators of oxidation, hypertrophy, angiogenesis, inflammatory processes and the extracellular matrix.

We infer that the endocrine functions attributed to myokines are involved in body weight regulation, low-grade inflammation, insulin sensitivity, tumor growth suppression and improvement of cognitive function, and indeed, the study of metabolites of muscle-derived regulators, as well as the design of modified myokines, are promising new paths in the treatment of chronic diseases.

The importance of regular physical activity to prevent and treat chronic and degenerative diseases is widely recognized. This does not only include metabolic diseases, such as type 2 diabetes and morbid obesity, but most – if not even all – the widespread and common diseases of an aging society (Schnyder et al., 2015).

There is growing evidence among exercise enthusiasts as well as medical professionals that regular exercise is a powerful treatment for the progression of cardiovascular disease, cancer, neurodegenerative diseases, psychiatric disorders and chronic lung disease.

To prevent these non-communicable diseases, the World Health Organization (WHO) developed "Global Recommendations on Physical Activity for Health" (WHO, 2010).

If we go back in time, we can see how, for decades, researchers have focused on elucidating the mechanisms by which the energy-demanding mechanical work of skeletal muscle can impact the entire body to promote significant health benefits. It was not possible to understand what the link or the decoder was between physical exercise and well-being.

In 1961, Goldstein conducted cross-transfusion experiments between resting dogs and dogs in which muscle contraction was induced by electrical stimulation (Goldstein et al., 1961). This brilliant researcher had already postulated the existence of humoral components induced by muscle work that improve the utilization of glucose in resting dogs; please, take note of this, as we will return to this important concept towards the end of the chapter.

But here is a first game changer: the detection of increased expression of the cytokine interleukin 6 (IL-6) in human muscle biopsies obtained after exercise (Ostrowski et al., 1998) and the concurrent release of this IL-6 derivative from muscles into the blood flow (Steensberg et al., 2000) was the starting point for a new branch of research. Since then, the list of myokines has been steadily growing, and the classification has been interpreted more broadly to include any secreted protein produced in skeletal muscle that acts in an autocrine, paracrine or endocrine manner.

Discovering that the muscle secretome consists of several hundred produced and secreted peptides provides an entirely new conceptual basis and paradigm to understand how muscles "communicate" with other organs such as adipose tissue, liver, pancreas, bones and the brain. Therefore, we are beginning to look at our "muscle tissue" with much more respect and attention.

Based on current knowledge, the main physiological function of myokines is to protect the function of skeletal muscle and to enhance its exercise capacity. Myokines control the adaptive processes in the skeletal muscle by operating as paracrine regulators of oxidation, hypertrophy, angiogenesis, inflammatory processes and in the regulation of the extracellular matrix. The endocrine function of myokines has to do with the regulation of body weight, low-grade inflammation, insulin sensitivity, tumor growth suppression and the improvement of cognitive function. Among the most there is Irisin, which may serve as a potential pro-myogenic factor in human pathological conditions and Interleukin-6 (IL-6), which is the most extensively studied myokine detected in 2000 and is secreted by skeletal muscle cells into the bloodstream in response to muscle contractions through which skeletal muscles communicate with central and peripheral organs. IL-6 increases insulin-stimulated glucose disposal in humans, as well as glucose uptake and fatty acid oxidation in vitro through AMP-activated protein kinase and PI3K-Akt signaling pathways. Another myokine which also affects metabolism is myonectin which is released into the bloodstream through muscle contraction and, similarly to insulin, promotes fatty acid uptake into cells by increasing the expression of fatty acid transport genes. As regards cancer research, SPARC (Secreted Protein, Acidic and Rich in Cysteine) was studied. Training- stimulated SPARC secretion has been shown to inhibit colon tumorigenesis by enhancing apoptosis in colon cancer cells. Brain-derived neurotrophic factor (BDNF) is the second member of the neurotrophin family of growth factors which regulates neuron survival, plasticity, growth and death trough tropomyosin-related kinase B (TrkB) receptor. High systemic levels of BDNF are frequently reported following hard workouts. If only did I have the time and space we would have dozens and dozens of these to describe and comment on.

All of this above could give rise to the following right observation: if many proteins produced by skeletal muscle depend on its contraction and its use with adequate training, then physical inactivity probably leads to an altered response to the production of myokines, which could provide a potential mechanism to understand the association between **sedentary behavior and the onset of many chronic diseases** (Pedersen et al., 2012).

Let's now focus on the hormones with a systemic action which are released during a bodybuilder's muscle effort. We will, therefore, find out how to optimize physical exercise to obtain the best production of hormones.

GH: growth hormone

GH (Growth Hormone), also known as somatotropin or somatotroph hormone (STH), is a peptide produced by the pituitary gland.

During adolescence, plasma levels of GH increase considerably, stimulating growth, increasing nitrogen retention and favoring the oxidation of lipid storage.

All of these effects are mediated by IGF-1 (somatomedin or insulin-like growth factor), a powerful anabolic hormone produced by the liver in response to somatotropin. After this period of life, GH levels decrease, but the hormone continues to be produced.

Even in adulthood, somatotropin carries out an important regulatory action on metabolic processes.

In humans, plasma GH values range from 1 to 5 ng/mL, with peaks of up to 10 ng/mL under stress or after overtraining; the secretion is pulsatile, with more frequent and wider peaks in the first hours of nocturnal sleep.

A GH deficiency in children impairs body growth (pituitary dwarfism) and the development of genitals and somatic features; at the same time, fat deposits in the abdominal region also increase.

If growth hormone deficiency affects adults, there is instead a reduction in muscle mass and a simultaneous increase in fat mass, the onset of metabolic alterations, increased bone fragility and reduced exercise tolerance (Nicholls et al., 2016).

Growth hormone secretion is controlled by the interaction of hypothalamic GH-secreting hormone (GHRH) and somatostatin, which inhibits the effect of GHRH. Certain specific conditions, such as the heat, the deprivation of carbohydrates and calories, or the intake of protein or amino acids in free form, as well as also an adequate and restorative period of sleep favor the production of GH. Let us not forget – in this chapter we must highlight this concept – that physical exercise represents a powerful stimulus for the secretion of GH.

So, what are the training strategies to increase GH levels?

First of all, let us not forget that we could never isolate the "hormonal concert" that is activated in our body, as agonist and antagonist hormones will always be produced in search of a constant balance.

As a matter of fact, high-intensity training will always increase testosterone, GH and IGF-1 levels, but it will inevitably also promote cortisol peaks, which will try to go help our body which is experiencing a stressful situation.

Secondly, it should also be noted that the stimulus to release GH will be more easily increased in a less trained subject. For what reason?

The production and intervention of GH are closely linked to the presence of lactic acid, which is certainly produced to a greater extent in a less trained subject. In poorly trained subjects, workout intensity being equal, there will be a greater production of lactate, with a consequent decrease in blood pH. **The reduction in blood pH is an inducer of somatotropin release.** In the case of resistance exercises, such as weightlifting and bodybuilding, the greater GH response is observed especially in exercises that require a higher use of anaerobic glycolysis, therefore with greater production and concentration of lactic acid, such as squats (Werlang Coelho et al., 2002). Indeed, no one can deny that the first few months in the gym are the ones in which exciting aesthetic improvements are made.

So, what should an experienced athlete do to stimulate their GH during training? In order to obtain the maximum release of GH, specific training techniques must be considered, which we can summarize as follows: **intense and heavy workouts with little recovery, in order not to give the lactic acid time to be partially recovered**; therefore, from a general point of view, the workouts that induce higher GH production are **intense ones with maximum loads**. It will be useful, then, to focus on basic compound exercises (i.e. exercises that work multiple muscle groups at the same time) such as bench presses, squats and deadlifts, which are excellent for inducing the release of lactic acid and therefore of GH. What about recovery times? Would long rest periods be better to recover strength? Absolutely not: **recovery time must be incomplete between sets, between 60 and 90 seconds**, in order to keep ATP levels low, which leads to the production of polyribosomes (protein synthesis) and keeps lactic acid levels high.

Shot recovery times between sets, therefore, favor GH production (Kraemer et al., 1990). The exercise carried out as described above causes the depletion of muscle glycogen reserves, with the consequent production of lactic acid which induces a decrease in blood pH. Nowadays, this concept is very clear.

Now we know how to train. Will a couple of hours of training be enough? Not at all, and this would be a serious mistake that would ruin everything: the hormonal response of GH, which is activated within 10 minutes of training, reaches its maximum peak 30 minutes from the start of the session and then drops, reaching the minimum threshold after 60 minutes of training. Let's say that 45 minutes of a well-performed training session will have us in the shower with our body fully producing of GH.

So here's a recap: **volume that allows high intensity, short rests, workouts of about 45-70 minutes, basic exercises.**

It is not recommended, for those who want to optimize the release of GH and testosterone, to combine cardio and weight training, especially cardio after weights. Cortisol secretion suppresses all others and favors the AMPK pathway, which is catabolic, compared to the mTOR pathway, which is anabolic.

Let's now analyze another hormone that often works in harmony and synergy with GH and that we would certainly have already produced in the 45 minutes we have just mentioned; however, there are differences in the approach that can favor its secretion. Let's find out.

The king of hormones: testosterone

It was June 1, 1889 when a 72-year-old doctor, Dr. Charles Brown-Séquard, described miraculous improvements in his physical and mental stamina, and even in his urinary flow rate, since he regularly started injecting himself with a mixture of blood, semen and testicular fluid which he had extracted from the testicles of dogs and guinea pigs.

Brown-Séquard's "elixir of life" would be prescribed by over 12,000 doctors by the end of the same year. In 1935, the hormone responsible for these remarkable anti-aging, energy and performance-enhancing benefits was named after him: testosterone. In the same year, both Swiss researcher Lavoslav Ružička and German researcher Adolf Butenandt discovered how to synthesize it for commercialization and, in 1939, they jointly received the Nobel Prize in chemistry for this achievement (Morgentaler et al., 2020). Since then, the king of hormones has been one of the most controversial and sought-after substances in health, fitness and sports.

Both men and women produce testosterone in clearly different amounts, with the typical adult male producing around 5-10 mg per day and the typical adult female producing at least 10 times less. In men, almost 95% of testosterone is produced within a group of cells located in the testicles, the Leydig cells; women also produce up to 50% of their testosterone within their corresponding sex glands, the ovaries. The adrenal glands, located above the kidneys like a hood, are just a minor source of testosterone production in men but have a significant contribution in women.

Our body produces testosterone in other ways as well. The hormone is converted starting from dehydroepiandrosterone (DHEA) within the tissues, more commonly in women, but only a small fraction of the testosterone that our body produces locally affects its concentrations in the bloodstream. Regardless of the method of production in either sexes, the compound from which all these sex hormones are originally derived is the sworn enemy of every nutritionist: cholesterol. Testosterone uses two close "collaborators" to carry out its influence on tissues: DHT, a hormone that binds to specific intracellular receptors on target cells located in muscle, fat, liver, hair and brain tissue, and estradiol, a hormone derived from the aromatization of testosterone and often mistakenly considered a female-only hormone.

Before understanding how weight training can increase the production of our hormones, let's take a step back and review the endocrine axis responsible for its production.

The "orchestra conductor" is the hypothalamus, which releases GnRH, a hormone that stimulates the pituitary gland to secrete LH, the luteinizing hormone, and FSH, the follicle-stimulating hormone (gonadotropins).

LH binds to receptors on Leydig cells in the testis, thus stimulating the production of testosterone. At the apex of this hypothalamic-pituitary-testis regulatory axis are the nerve pathways that send information deriving from higher structures of the central nervous system and that modulate the secretion of GnRH.

GnRH secretion is conditioned by exogenous stimuli of a sexual, luminous, olfactory and emotional nature, and by endogenous hormone levels.

In summary, the regulation of GnRH secretion is therefore ensured by the interaction between the peripheral hormonal counter-regulatory systems, consisting of the pituitary gonadotropins (LH and FSH), the gonadal secretion products of the steroid type (testosterone, estradiol, progesterone) and substances with neurotransmitter activity (catecholamines and serotonin). In addition, other hormones, such as CRH (Corticotropin Relieving Factor), somatostatin, prolactin, and melatonin, interfere with its production.

GnRH stimulates LH, which in turn stimulates the production of testosterone in the testicles: it is the famous HPTA axis (Hypothalamic-Pituitary-Testicular Axis), often mentioned in the world of chemistry, the axis which is clumsily suppressed with the use of AAS (steroid hormones).

So, are we ready to go train and find out together how to increase testosterone production?

First, let's remember that testosterone secretion peaks in the early hours; our ancestors had to go hunting and high levels of testosterone and cortisol were essential to give them strength and energy.

Countless studies have now shown that regular **high-intensity** exercises help keep a man's testosterone at optimal levels.

Let's go from studies dating back to the late 1990s (Kraemer et al., 1999), in which the authors examined how intense weight training in both young people (23 to 35 years of age) and the elderly (58 to 65 years of age) affected their testosterone levels, to more recent studies confirming all these logical deductions (Stanton et al., 2012).

A famous study (Gunter Daxenbichler et al., 2009) showed that an intense and complete workout triggers three processes that are essential to promote muscle protein synthesis and this is how our hormones intervene:

1. Increased muscle tension
2. Increased testosterone
3. Increased androgen receptor activity

So what type of training and what rest periods are needed to optimize this production?

In general, **high-volume weight training performed at an intensity above the current threshold** stimulates testosterone production (Kraemer et al., 2008, Sokoloff et al., 2016). Free weights are best for building strength and size. Researchers at the University of Connecticut have shown that a total-body workout increases testosterone levels more than exercises working only the lower body (knee extensors).

And what about optimizing recovery times?

During weight training, an increase in testosterone production is observed during the recovery phase. While, as mentioned in the previous paragraph, short rest periods facilitate GH stimulation (Kramer et al., 1990), **longer pauses favor the recovery of fast fibers and testosterone secretion** (Bosco et al., 1995).

A significant increase in blood testosterone is promoted with a complete recovery of 3 minutes and repetitions performed with maximal as well as sub-maximal tensions at maximum power. High testosterone levels increase androgen receptor activity **during the recovery phase**, which presumably increases protein synthesis and muscle growth.

Thus, we have understood a concept: volume and intensity will certainly always be important (we don't hide it, they are what gives us the pleasure of training), but recovery can influence the different hormonal secretions of GH or testosterone. GH requires a lactic acid environment, an acidic pH; testosterone requires a full recovery phase in a non-lactacid environment.

As far as aerobic exercise and testosterone production are concerned, the news is not very comforting.

Aerobic exercise would not appear to be conducive to testosterone production. We know, in fact, that low-intensity aerobic exercise favors the release of serotonin, while high-intensity aerobic exercise induces the body to produce cortisol, a hormone which, in many situations, is seen as the bitter enemy of testosterone.

In some incremental-type tests carried out using a cycle ergometer, an increase in testosterone was observed 20 minutes after the test and a rapid decrease coincided with the beginning of an increase in cortisol. In some cases (running) testosterone levels decrease 30 minutes into the recovery phase.

Data in the literature are in agreement and indicate that weight training can lead to an increase in testosterone and that endurance sports (long-distance running), on the contrary, have a negative effect which is responsible for reducing testosterone levels. In the case of "chronic stress", a decrease in total and free plasma testosterone levels is induced. In these athletes, the lowering of testosterone levels could be due to an altered secretion of gonadotropins and a peripheral modification of the ability of Leydig cells to synthesize androgens.

Assuming that testosterone is one of the main anabolic stimuli and cortisol is one of the main catabolic stimuli, the ratio between the two quantities FT/CR (Free Testosterone/Cortisol Ratio) and its evolution over time are considered valid biochemical markers of the state of individual training, which is useful for monitoring the athlete.

FT/CR values lower than 0.35×103 or a decrease of 30% or more from the previous sample are considered indicators of overtraining, with free testosterone calculated in nanomoles per liter and cortisol in micromoles per liter. Many other studies have observed that prolonged low-intensity cardiovascular exercise can lead to the suppression of circulating testosterone levels for approximately 3 days. It has also been reported that low-intensity cardio not only reduces total testosterone levels, but also lowers the bioactive form of testosterone (free T). HIIT training improves insulin signaling and facilitates the uptake of glucose into muscle cells, providing them with more energy to improve muscle performance and therefore promote muscle protein synthesis.

Insulin and muscle training

We concluded the previous paragraph by mentioning insulin sensitivity and blood sugar control through training.

Bodybuilding training improves insulin sensitivity and glucose tolerance: it appears that people with type 2 diabetes (approximately 90% of diabetes cases) derive the greatest benefit from bodybuilding training, as insulin sensitivity is increased and, therefore, the problem causing this rise is addressed head-on. Individuals with type 1 diabetes also benefit from weight training, as most of them can confirm a reduction in the amount of insulin they need to take each day to manage their glucose levels.

Bodybuilding training increases the need to use glucose for energy: even moderate amounts of weight training (such as 30-40 minutes three times a week) increase muscle mass (Brinkman et al., 2017). Exercising with weights increases the expression of the GLUT-4 carrier on the membrane surface, a protein that allows glucose to be directly internalized within the cell (Spattini and Bevacqua, 2019). Having more muscle also means that more glucose is used throughout the day and during the exercise. In turn, this helps type 1 diabetes sufferers, as it may lead to a decrease in the insulin dosage (lower glucose levels mean a lower insulin dose).

We have understood the complex and articulated manner in which hormones respond to weight training. We are not able to catalog every single response, also because each hormone has a complexity related to different ways of action and interactions with binding proteins and receptor interactions.

Testosterone is the **primary anabolic hormone**, but its concentration changes during rest periods also depending on the up- or down-regulation of the androgen receptor in the muscle cell.

Growth hormone (GH) shows differential increases in recovery based on the type of GH dosed and the training used, but we have seen that the best route is that of high-intensity training with short rest periods.

IGF-1 shows variable increases in recovery and is strictly related to a number of binding proteins that are essential for its integrative actions and for mediating targeting effects. The muscle itself, during training, is able to release an isoform of IGF-1 called MGF (mechanical growth factor).

In contrast, the so-called "stress" hormones (cortisol, adrenaline, noradrenaline and glucagon) are able to supply the right amount of fuel to our body, until we exceed the tolerance threshold, beyond which we would enter a catabolic phase.

The stress caused by training correlates with the recruitment of muscle tissue through the glandular release of hormones that serve as signals to "tell" tissues to support homeostatic mechanisms for metabolism and tissue repair during the recovery process, the final stage of desired muscle growth. It is not yet clear how acute hormonal changes can have a real impact on the induction of muscle growth, but it is logical to assume it. A study that seems to support this theory is the one carried out on a group of athletes who underwent two differently structured workouts at different moments in time. In the first workout, the arms were trained alone, separately from leg training. In the second workout, the arms were trained together and immediately after leg training. The result was that, despite a drop in performance witnessed when doing arm training straight after leg training, due to the obvious fatigue that had taken over, there was a greater increase in muscle mass in the arms.

The authors hypothesized that this was due to the fact that arm training took place in a more favorable hormonal situation created by the previous leg training.

Cortisol is a hormone that is considered as the number 1 enemy. Let's debunk this myth.

Undoubtedly, a mantra that is repeated in gyms is "you mustn't produce cortisol".

Cortisol is a catabolic hormone that breaks down proteins and transforms them into glucose to provide the body with immediate energy: if this happens to the detriment of our muscles, it is not a positive thing. Hence it recommended not to exceed 40 minutes of training, because after that time there is excess cortisol production, and to use supplements such as phosphatidylserine, which is capable of reducing cortisol production during training. But is cortisol really that bad? Normally, if nature provides in a way, it means there is reason for that; let's see the reasons why cortisol is produced during intense training.

First of all, at the beginning of a workout with weights, catecholamines (i.e. adrenaline and noradrenaline) are secreted, and this facilitates the release of calcium ions from the sarcoplasmic reticulum, while triggering muscle contraction, increasing the production of heat by the muscle, and activating the beta receptors, favoring the vasodilation of the blood vessels of the worked muscles. Subsequently, other hormones come into play, especially the ones found in the adrenal cortex: glucocorticoids (cortisol and corticosterone), mineralocorticoids (aldosterone and deoxycorticosterone) and sex-anabolic hormones (DHEA, androsterone and androstenedione).

Cortisol production serves the purpose of enhancing the action of catecholamines to maintain blood pressure, which would collapse following the vasodilatory action of substances such as hydrogen ions and lactic acid, as well as enhancing their lipolytic effect in synergy with GH. It has a hyperglycaemic effect which stimulates gluconeogenesis, i.e., the production of glucose starting from non-glucide precursors, especially proteins, and at the same time favors the storage of glycogen in the muscles. It has an aldosterone-like effect by retaining sodium and therefore water, exerting a sort of "cushion" effect on the muscles and tendons, limiting the traumatizing effect of exercise. The anti-inflammatory effect of cortisol is also analgesic, so you feel less pain, both in the muscles and in the joints.

In this regard, in some subjects, the use of phosphatidylserine before a workout actually makes it more difficult to train precisely because of a greater tenderness in the tendon. Furthermore, DHEA is produced at the same time as cortisol, and it reduces any muscle catabolism induced by cortisol. In short, we could say that the production of cortisol during intense training is functional and we shouldn't worry too much about it; therefore, the myth that a workout should have a maximum duration of 40 minutes must be debunked, if it hasn't already been debunked by the practical demonstration given by the majority of high-level athletes in various sports, including strength and power sports, where they train longer than an hour a day.

What must be avoided is a chronically high cortisol level, which can occur in overreaching, i.e. when recovery is insufficient. This occurs more frequently in athletes who undergo frequent and exhausting workouts, such as bootcamp training, crossfit, training to failure, etc. As a matter of fact, adrenocortical hormone production meets the demands of the exercise, which can be done with less effort; the fitter an athlete is, the more this phase will have an early start and the longer it will last, while in untrained athletes it occurs later, leaving more space for the catecholamines (adrenaline and noradrenaline), and it can be maintained for a shorter time.

In addition to the relationship between the adrenocortical hormones DHEA and cortisol, which influences a series of metabolic activities, the cortisol/testosterone ratio is very important in athletes. A study examined the effects induced by both weight training and aerobic exercise on testosterone, DHEA-S and cortisol release in male subjects (the study included both sedentary people and expert athletes, either endurance athletes or weight lifters). Hormones were measured both before and after a 40-minute run or weight training session. Both exercise modes were structured in such a way that energy consumption was the same in order to obtain the same the level of effort.

The subjects that engaged in weight training had higher testosterone levels than those in the endurance group; moreover, the weight training group also had higher levels of DHEA-S and cortisol after the workout. The study authors suggest that having higher cortisol levels after weight training serves an important recovery function, promoting the breakdown of fats and proteins and, therefore, providing energy for recovery processes, which are of fundamental importance after a weight training session.

Australian researchers found that bodybuilding-type weight training (10 sets of 10 repetitions with controlled movements, using 75% of the max with 2 minutes of rest) increased testosterone and cortisol levels. Unanimous data in the literature show that weight training can increase testosterone levels and that endurance sports (prolonged running), on the contrary, have a negative effect on testosterone, obviously in relation to the type, intensity and duration of the workout performed.

Normally, weight training is considered the best for producing increases in strength and muscle mass. In one study, evaluating hormone secretions and comparing training with free weights and training with machines, training with free weights was found to produce a greater increase in testosterone, but also in cortisol, compared to training with machines. As we stated earlier, the problem is not cortisol in the acute phase, but cortisol secreted chronically under conditions of overtraining and chronic stress. In the case of "chronic stress", there is a reduction of both total and free testosterone.

In overtrained athletes, the reduction in testosterone could be due to an alteration in the secretion of gonadotropins (more typical of women) and a peripheral modification of the ability of the Leydig cells of the testis to synthesize androgens. Since testosterone is anabolic and cortisol is catabolic, what really matters is their ratio, which can be highlighted with the FT/CR value and its evolution over time, which can be a valid biochemical indicator of the training statue of the athlete and it can be used for programming. FT/CR values lower than 0.35×10^3 are considered indicators of overtraining, with free testosterone calculated in nanomols per liter and cortisol in micromols per liter. Even a 30% decrease in this value compared to a previous sample indicates a non-optimal recovery situation and should lead to a reduction in training.

Exercise with weights and the HPG (Hypothalamic-Pituitary-Gonadal) axis

The hypothalamic-pituitary-gonadal axis is, in both sexes, under the control of very complex neuroendocrine mechanisms, aimed both at reproduction and at modulating the production of sex steroid hormones.

The relationship between the HPG axis and physical exercise in women has always held a great appeal due to the high incidence of functional problems, such as amenorrhea, oligomenorrhea and delayed puberty in athletes dedicated to high-intensity training. However, other concurrent factors, such as modifications in body composition, alterations in eating behaviors, psychophysical stress, as well as genetic components should also be considered.

Unfortunately, there is no possibility of determining the complex pathophysiological situations regarding the relationship between the HPG axis and physical exercise. Alterations in gonadotropin secretion are most likely to be related to neuroendocrine changes affecting other hormonal axes involved in physical stress. For example, the hypothalamic-pituitary-adrenal (HPA) axis, with the production of ACTH and CRH; the hypothalamic-pituitary-thyroid (HPT) axis, with an alteration of thyroid hormones which, in turn, influence sex hormones; prolactin; opioid peptides, melatonin, arginine vasopressin, and neurotransmitters: dopamine, catecholamines, GABA. Even in men, there is a belief, but with less evidence, that physical exercise can influence the secretion of gonadotropins, again through complex hormonal regulation systems involved in the response to physical stress. Some studies have shown an early increase in LH following strenuous exercise, which could account for the increase in testosterone. Another cause could be a decrease in hepatic or extrahepatic degradation.

We are approaching the end of our chapter and, therefore, the end of a hypothetical training session. So, let's see what happened to our endocrine axis and what the positive repercussions could be if we persevere in doing our workouts. We have seen the wide array of hormones which are activated during training, even though, depending on the type of recovery and intensity, greater quantities of catecholamines, cortisol, testosterone and GH will be put into circulation (Hiroshi et al., 2016). As a matter of fact, heavy resistance training has been clearly shown to increase an athlete's ability to secrete greater amounts of adrenaline during maximum effort exercises.

Since adrenaline is involved in metabolic control, force production and other hormone response mechanisms (such as testosterone, GH and IGF), catecholamine stimulation is probably **one of the earliest endocrine mechanisms that occurs in response to exercise against resistance** (Haff et al., 2015). However, other hormones also enter the bloodstream with relatively predictable timing: DHEA (produced by the adrenocortical gland) intervenes to help us counteract the catabolic effect that cortisol has on proteins; androstenedione, another anabolic sex hormone, is released faster than testosterone.

The production of these sex hormones appears to be only partially linked to an increase in pituitary LH. In fact, the increase in testosterone during training appears not to be **LH-dependent, but rather to be strongly associated with the activation of the sympathetic system (catecholamines)**. Sex hormone binding globulin (SHBG) does not increase during exercise, which will consequently lead to an increase in the T/SHBG ratio.

Therefore, the highest and noblest part of the axis (hypothalamus and pituitary) seems to be only partially involved, while the sympathetic system and the adrenal gland (as well as the testicles, in humans) play a fundamental role.

Let's not forget the "core" benefits of training, too. As reported in an article which can be read on Dr. Spattini's website:

> *The muscle is now considered a true endocrine organ. It produces a whole range of elements, including neurotrophins. These, once secreted into the bloodstream by the muscle, pass the blood-brain barrier and influence the areas of the brain involved in neuroplasticity. This means that some areas of the brain involved in emotions and memory continuously produce new synapses as a function of stimuli from the external environment. Widespread inactivity is thought to have produced a decline in the rate of neuroplasticity in these areas. Resistance exercises would improve this situation, so much so that they could be included in the treatment of depressive syndromes and cognitive deficits.*

CHAPTER 39

Bodybuilding and strength training to protect your health

Fernando Finardi

When following a lifestyle plan aimed at improving and maintaining both mental and physical health, diet (understood as a well-structured personalized diet) and physical exercise, in which strength training should have an honorary place on your to-do list. By strength training we mean the use of one (total isolation is actually difficult to achieve) or more muscle groups to perform a specific exercise, such as lifting a weight (whether it is body weight, or, more commonly, an load). This type of exercise is aimed at increasing strength, muscle mass and endurance, all of which are essential for a successful aging process (Suchomel et al., 2018).

Having more muscle mass means being equipped with a true "health reserve" to draw on in case of need and to counter frailty due to hospitalization, illness, metabolic dysfunctions (overweight and sarcopenic obesity), osteoporosis or osteopenia, avoiding the risk of falling and counteracting cognitive declines and dementia, which are typical diseases of old age. Today, unfortunately, adults are advised (including at a health level) to have a few extra pounds of weight (fat) to avoid losing too much weight in case of hospitalization, instead of suggesting a safe and effective weight training program (which must be personalized and clear), aimed at increasing fat free mass, a true "treasure" for critical physical times. This is how bodybuilding rightfully plays a role in age management.

The scientific evidence that highlights the benefits of this type of training is now overwhelming and no longer questionable, to such an extent that even the WHO, in its latest guidelines issued in 2020, recommends introducing resistance training (or weight training or body building training) into your exercise routine to counter age-related or disease-induced sarcopenia and to improve your general health. **There are specific recommendations for resistance-based exercises** because it is clear that they have different and additional benefits to those of aerobic physical activity (Bull et al., 2020).

Strength is sustained by a combination of morphological and neural factors, including a muscle's cross-section area and structure, muscle-tendon stiffness, motor unit recruitment, speed coding, unit synchronization motor and neuromuscular inhibition. Bilateral training eccentric training, accentuated eccentric loading, and variable resistance training may produce the most comprehensive strength adaptations.

Programming a workout that combines heavy loads with light loads can improve endurance and enhance other strength-power characteristics. Multiple sets appear to produce greater training benefits than single sets; however, an athlete's training status and the dose-response relationship must be taken into consideration. Longer rest intervals between sets may produce the best strength-power benefits, while shorter intervals may be more effective for hypertrophy. Obviously, based on an athlete's training experience, the type of fibers he has, and their genetics (muscle fiber testing is an examination designed to determine what muscle fiber type is predominant in a given muscle group), it is possible to optimize training. To avoid potential injuries, beginner athletes should focus on developing strength before taking on power training.

We can, therefore, identify the following types of training, which are able to influence muscle strength, including the improvement of maximal force expression, and time-limited force expression. They include:

- **muscular hypertrophy**: it is an increase in the volume of muscle fibers, i.e. traditional bodybuilding; this type of training uses moderate to heavy loads to implement muscle growth
- **muscular endurance**: it is the ability of the muscles to support physical activity for a certain amount of time. Training usually involves high repetitions using body weight or light resistance
- **circuit training**: it is a form of total-body conditioning, useful for improving the ability to produce and tolerate lactic acid, where you go through a variety of exercises practically without interruption or with very short breaks, moving from one exercise to the next, and which generally works various muscle groups alternatively
- **maximum muscular strength**: it requires doing a low number of repetitions (usually between 2 and 6) with heavy weights to increase overall strength. It is a type of training recommended for experienced individuals who have learned the correct form of execution
- **explosive power**: it requires a mix of strength and speed (power = strength × speed) to improve power output. It is used by professional athletes, or at least experienced ones, to improve the ability to perform specific explosive movements preparatory to their sport

Bodybuilding and strength can obviously be trained either at home or in the gym, using one's own body weight that moves in space, and equipment such as dumbbells, barbells, kettlebells, elastic bands, ropes or straps, and specific machinery. There is no limit to imagination, and the important thing is that we can apply a resistance capable of causing muscular stress and taking us out of our performance comfort zone, allowing neuromuscular adaptations and consequent muscle growth over time.

Strength development offers many benefits to people of all ages and is of paramount importance for older adults. These benefits (simplified) are:

1. Increase in lean mass (improvement of body composition)
2. Increase in metabolic rate
3. Increase in bone density
4. Decreased risk of injury (improves balance and function)
5. Building back muscle tissue that is usually lost with aging (we will see below what this means in terms of overall health and improved quality of life)

Loss of skeletal muscle mass (sarcopenia) results in less available strength to perform basic necessary activities, such as standing up from a seated position, standing and preparing a meal, climbing the stairs and practice self-care. Skeletal muscle loss is also the main cause of decreased resting metabolic rate, which can lead to overweight or obesity. In short, **weight training has multisystemic benefits**, as specific mechanical resistance is converted into positive cellular responses (Thomas and Burns, 2016; Yand et al., 2019; Maestroni et al., 2020).

Furthermore, **weight training to build strength helps to improve an athlete's sports performance** where speed, strength and power are required, and it may also help to preserve lean body mass. Just as a more powerful engine usually corresponds to greater energy consumption, weight training, by increasing muscle mass, **helps to speed up metabolism**. This is not only because training already increases metabolism, but also because muscles are metabolically more efficient than fat and help burn more energy during rest (high energy requirement for the degradation and resynthesis of muscle fibers damaged by training, up to 3 days after) (McPherron et al., 2013; Gareth Burt et al., 2014; McMurray et al., 2014; Aristizabal et al., 2015; MacKenzie-Shalders et al., 2020).

Weight training reduces visceral fat which, although it is not as visible as abdominal subcutaneous fat, it is most dangerous when excess, as it is associated with an increased risk of chronic diseases, including cardiovascular disease, hepatic steatosis, Non-Alcoholic Fatty Liver Disease (NAFLD), type 2 diabetes and some cancers, as visceral fat cells produce high levels of a protein called fibroblast growth factor 2 (FGF2), which is associated with oncogenesis. In this regard, studies have shown that individuals who exercise regularly are less likely to develop cancer compared to those with a less active lifestyle (Moore et al., 2016; Chakraborty et al., 2017; de Mutsert et al., 2018; Xu et al., 2018; Nam et al., 2020; Silveira et al., 2020).

Resistance training can ultimately make you lose both visceral and subcutaneous fat, improving your shape and allowing you to appear leaner and more toned, since muscles are denser than fat and take up less space. This is observed more often by looking at yourself in the mirror (and by measuring the circumference of anatomical landmarks with a meter) than by stepping on the scale. Body mass can also be measured using impedancemetry, plicometry and other more complex methods. It is a fact that by gaining muscle mass and losing body fat muscles will be more evident (Mekary et al., 2015; Ihalainen et al., 2019; Vechetti et al., 2021; Yarizadeh et al., 2021).

In a randomized controlled clinical trial involving 141 obese older adults (who completed the study, out of a total of 160), the researchers evaluated the efficacy of different exercise modalities in reversing frailty and physical function and **in preventing reduction in muscle and bone mass induced by weight loss.** Participants were randomly assigned to a weight management program and to one of three scheduled exercise programs (aerobic training, weight training or combined aerobic and weight training) or to a control group (no weight management program or exercises). At the end of the 26-week study, those who did not exercise with weights lost fat, but also more muscle and bone mass than those in the groups who incorporated resistance training into their routine. Weight training proved to guarantee a conservative effect on muscles and bones during low-calorie regimes. A greater active lean mass corresponds to a lesser drop in metabolism levels even at rest, especially when on a diet. Incorporating weight training is a long-term guarantee that you will stay slim and structurally healthy (Villareal et al., 2017).

Strength training also has benefits on balance, coordination and posture; the latter also helps internal organs by facilitating the gastrointestinal system, acid reflux and evacuation, as well as allowing you to breathe deeply and correctly.

It has been established that **weight training**, by improving strength (especially when combined with proprioceptive training) **drastically reduces the risk of falls** (–34%), especially in the population over 60. As they strengthen the tissue around major joints such as ankles, knees, hips and wrists, they can support their bodies better and build up a sort of natural scaffolding, something like an armor, which provides additional protection against potential injuries. Should they occur, older adults who do resistance training will heal better with suitable and targeted physical activity. Naturally, this "armor" is also an enormous support for young professional or amateur athletes, as a tight core and strong hamstrings and glutes help prevent lower back injuries (–33%).

From the analysis of data collected in a study which involved thousands of athletes, resistance training was even found to **reduce the risk of injury in a dose-dependent way**, meaning that for every 10% increase in training volume there is a 4% reduced risk of injury (Gordon and Bloxham, 2016; Sözen et al., 2017; Benedetti et al., 2018; Lauersen et al., 2018; Walters et al., 2018; Calatayud et al ., 2019; Sadler et al., 2019; Sherrington et al., 2019; Edouard et al., 2020; Beato et al., 2021; Choi et al., 2021).

The heart also benefits from resistance training. Various studies have now established that regular weight training can reduce blood pressure, lower total and LDL cholesterol, increase HDL levels, improve blood circulation and oxygenation, strengthen the heart and blood vessels, maintain an ideal body shape, reduce visceral fat (visceral fat is linked to cardiovascular disease because it is associated with the release of specific inflammatory proteins and hormones that can damage blood vessels and increase blood pressure) and manage blood sugar levels, thus improving insulin sensitivity, reducing the risk of developing diabetes (up to –30%) and significantly lowering the risk factors for cardiovascular disease.

Muscle mass is inversely associated with insulin resistance, as muscle tissue helps manage blood sugar levels by using glucose for energy or by storing it as glycogen; otherwise, the sugars would be deposited around the organs, being stored as energy surplus (fat) thanks to the action of insulin, which "opens" the cells to let in the carbohydrate molecules. In other words, **skeletal muscle is the major site of glucose uptake after a meal**; as a matter of fact, the road to insulin resistance (a condition of multifactorial origin) opens just when you start to lose muscle mass significantly, i.e. around the age of 50. Maintaining toned and strong muscles, and actively opposing sarcopenia (which is physiological in older age), means maintaining a good insulin sensitivity.

Weight training reduces glycated hemoglobin values and blood pressure, given that **muscles capture between 70 and 85% of the available glucose, even without the intervention of insulin**: therefore, strong muscles serve as a defense line against the development of diabetes (strength is inversely related to metabolic syndrome) (Roberts et al., 1985; Srikanthan and Karlamangla, 2011; Colberg et al., 2016; MacDonald et al., 2016; Park et al., 2016 ; de Sousa et al., 2017; Lee et al., 2017; Shiroma et al., 2017; Costa et al., 2019; Liu et al., 2019; Mcleod et al., 2019).

While it's not exactly the type of training that would come to your mind when you want to develop flexibility, resistance training can actually **make you both more mobile and more flexible**. Flexibility is the ability of a muscle to stretch passively or without any particular effort. When you do static stretches (for example, in passive stretching) using your body weight, you are training the muscle's ability to relax and lengthen. Mobility, on the other hand, is the ability of joints to actively move through their full range of motion, such as lifting a limb to 90° and returning it to the starting position. Good flexibility is necessary for good mobility.

By good mobility, we mean being able to move in a wide articular range, maintaining stability while generating force. It goes without saying that weaker muscles will tend to have lower ROM (Range Of Motion) and flexibility (Leite et al., 2017).

A 2021 meta-analysis which compared resistance training to stretching to test their effectiveness in increasing ROM, found that both exercise protocols were equally effective (Alfonso et al., 2021).

Research from 2020 and 2021 tested the most effective range of motion for minimizing the risk of injury and maximizing resistance training adaptations. What was found was that a greater ROM (i.e. complete, and not partial) corresponds to better results in terms of maximizing muscle strength and the hypertrophy of the lower limbs. Similarly, functional performance appears to be enhanced by using full ROM exercises. In contrast, there are no major differences between full and partial ROM interventions in generating changes in muscle architecture (muscle architecture is the physical arrangement of muscle fibers at the macroscopic level, which determines the mechanical function of a muscle).

Of course, this means fully exploiting one's potential ROM while maintaining a perfect execution form (Pallarés et al., 2021). Conversely, research on the effects of ROM of the upper limbs is limited and conflicting, which prevents researchers from drawing strong practical inferences. To date, no research has investigated how ROM affects muscle growth in the trunk musculature. Finally, some evidence indicates that the response to ROM changes may be muscle-specific; however, this hypothesis deserves further investigation (Schoenfeld and Grgic, 2020).

Bodybuilding not only has a positive effect on muscles, mobility and flexibility, but it can also **prevent osteopenia** (i.e. the reduction of bone mineral density), effectively making the bones stronger. There are now many research studies that certify that those who constantly practice physical activity have better bone mineral density values than sedentary people, simply due to the fact that muscle contractions and tendon stresses on the bones positively stimulate bone remodeling. If this is particularly true for exercising with weights from a young age, the same cannot be said, for example, for swimming and cycling which, as much as they are excellent activities for the muscles, the cardiovascular system and the joints, are sports that are practiced in gravitational discharge, therefore, they don't cause overloading of the structures.

It goes without saying that having stronger muscles, tendons and bones greatly reduces the risk of falls, fractures and osteoporosis, which are particularly noticeable with advancing age. Also consider the recent training protocols of astronauts who, remaining for long periods in the absence of gravity ("accelerated aging" situation), counteract osteoporosis and sarcopenia both with exercise bike workouts (mostly to facilitate correct blood circulation and a positive action on the heart and lungs), barbell deadlifts (using elastic bands) and bodybuilding exercises.

The development of the law which describes bone remodeling due to stress belongs to German anatomist and surgeon Julius Wolff. Wolff's law states that a bone will adapt to the mechanical loads under which it is placed in such a way that an increase in loading will cause a strengthening of the internal and spongy bone architecture, followed by a strengthening of the cortical layer. Moreover, a decrease in stress applied to the bone will cause its layers to weaken. The duration, magnitude and rate of the forces applied to the bone dictate how the integrity of the bone is altered. As with any other choice in our life that affects our physique (and our mind), deciding how we age is a decision we make every day. Certainly, **weight training is the first therapeutic option in the fight against osteosarcopenia** (Mosti et al., 2014; Beck et al., 2017; Hong and Kim, 2018; Rowe et al., 2021).

Resistance training can also boost self-esteem and self-confidence, improving self-perception. "Feeling" a tailor-made armor made of stronger muscles, ligaments and joints also increases brain endorphins (endorphins are morphine-like chemicals produced by the brain, with analgesic and euphoria-generating properties). The results of some scientific studies indicate that **physical activity (especially strength training) is directly and indirectly associated with self-esteem**, and this is valid for all age categories, from adolescents to the elderly (Elavsky et al., 2005; Joseph et al., 2014; Ciccolo et al., 2016; Zamani Sani et al., 2016; Collins et al., 2019).

A review of several studies concluded that resistance training can significantly improve multiple dimensions of body image, including body satisfaction, aesthetic appreciation and social anxiety. Overall, weight training has the potential to improve body image in adults (as perceived by themselves and others), although more high-quality studies with rigorous, well-designed testing are needed (SantaBarbara et al. al., 2017).

The result of regular weight training extends to **a global improvement in mental health**, with consequent reduction of worry, anxiety and depression symptoms, better mood, self-esteem and feelings of safety, as well as the ability to carry out a task and an overall more positive outlook on life. Many studies support these data, which are valid both for healthy subjects and for those affected by full-blown pathologies: being physically active triggers the release of well-being hormones such as dopamine and serotonin, essential for modulating mood, intensifying one's motivation, and feeling more optimistic.

Furthermore, if it is true that any form of training improves mood because it increases endorphins, it is equally true that with strength training, due to the neurochemical and neuromuscular responses it offers, the positive effects on the brain are more powerful. Furthermore, there is evidence that moderate resistance training (in addition to stretching) can help you rest better, especially in the case of chronic insomnia, and we all know very well how a single sleepless night can negatively affect mood, energy and many other physiological parameters (Strickland and Smith, 2014; Jaggers et al., 2015; Gordon et al., 2017 and 2018; D'Aurea Carolina et al., 2019; Gordon et al., 2020).

We have certainly dispelled any doubts about the effectiveness of weight training to maintain (or regain) a healthy body, but... what does science say about brain health? This is quite an intriguing topic, especially for those who question the notion that weights and the brain have a connection. Let's take a look together at the scientific results.

Individuals who apply weight-training protocols may actually be in for better brain health and protection against senescence-related cognitive decline.

Cognitive frailty is defined as the presence of both physical frailty and cognitive impairment, in the absence of dementia. It is characterized by concomitant physical frailty and potentially reversible cognitive deterioration, and up to date, several studies on elderly subjects attest that **exercising with weights also generates significant improvements in cognitive function of those who do it as compared to those who don't**. It also appears that three workouts per week yield better results than two workouts per week (visible results with at least two workouts per week for at least 6 months) (Yoon et al., 2018; Li et al., 2018).

As we have already mentioned, aging is a degenerative process characterized by recognized functional, physiological and metabolic disorders, such as loss of strength and decreased cognitive ability. Therefore, the search for innovative strategies to prevent or delay such disorders is essential to ensure the independence and quality of life of a part of the population that is increasingly older.

Evidence suggests weight training is the physical strategy of choice for its neuroprotective effects, such as increasing tissue oxygenation as a result of improved blood flow (new capillaries are also formed), reducing systemic inflammation, and increasing the expression of brain-derived neurotrophic factor (BDNF), which is closely linked to memory and cognitive learning. These results are also valid for women, who are usually reluctant to try weight training.

In one study of 29 older women who underwent 12 weeks of resistance training, there were significant increases in average upper body strength (58%), lower body strength (68%) and cognitive ability (19%). This is due to the fact that **BDNF values increase in an effort-dependent manner (as the effort of the training session increases, plasma BDNF concentrations increase)**. Here's how weight training, started as a teenager and continued into old age, should be understood as body building (but also maintaining brain integrity and efficiency) in the finest and most ancestral sense of its meaning: *mens sana in corpore sano* (a healthy mind in a healthy body) (de Camargo Smolarek et al., 2016; Chupel et al., 2017; Mavros et al., 2017; Pereira et al., 2018; Wilke et al., 2019).

Europeans (Americans are of a different opinion), at the level of (induced) "common thought", tend to denigrate those who have more toned and developed muscles compared to their age group and the average population; however, it has now been understood that our muscles are much more than a mere aesthetic quirk, as they allow us to get up, walk, move in space, be independent and physically help others. This fundamental tissue, however, tends to decrease over time, so much so that, starting from the age of 30-40, muscle mass is lost at a rate that varies between 3 and 8% per decade, to then being lost at a much faster rate, which stays consistent after 60 years of age. Today we know that **the loss of muscle mass** goes hand in hand with the deterioration of the state of health, accelerating the onset of pathologies, and **it is even closely linked to premature death**. Studies report that muscle mass (muscle mass index, expressed as muscle mass divided by height squared) is a key indicator of survival in the elderly and one of the best predictors of total life span. In other words, **muscle mass is inversely associated with the mortality risk in the elderly regardless of their fat mass or cardiovascular and metabolic risk factors** (Srikanthan & Karlamangla, 2014).

The entire locomotor system (which includes muscles, tendons, ligaments and bones) is closely interconnected with the overall state of health: if a single link is weak, the whole organism will consequently become weak. The body is one and it is a complex machine, therefore stating that systems and organs are separate and have nothing to do with each other makes no sense from a scientific or psychological point of view. Traditional Eastern medicine has known this for millennia.

Take-home message: **weight training promotes a better health-related quality of life, especially as you get older**. Lean muscle mass is an anti-aging indicator and is the cheapest (and most dynamic) life insurance we can have, guaranteeing undeniable improvements and both physical and psychological benefits, regardless of our state of health. More strength and more stability mean greater energy and endurance, better control of inflammation and pain, improved mood and self-esteem, better body composition, proper management of stress and insulin sensitivity, improved bone mineral density, improved lipoprotein profile and markers of cardiovascular disease, better blood circulation, transport and metabolization of nutrients, reduction of oxidative stress and decreased risk of cancer: these are all fundamental factors for adding years to your life (Volpi et al., 2004; Canuto Wanderley et al., 2015; Kekäläinen et al., 2018; Hart and Buck, 2019; Sieczkowska et al., 2020).

Ultimately, even in the absence of chronic disease, aging is associated with a variety of biological changes that can contribute to decreased skeletal muscle mass, strength and function. Such losses reduce physiological resilience and increase vulnerability to catastrophic events. Therefore, strategies for both prevention and treatment are necessary for health and well-being in aging, regardless of gender (Fragala et al., 2019).

A "recently" discovered function is that **muscle tissue is an important endocrine organ** that expresses and releases myokines (cytokines with immunomodulatory activity), such as cytokine IL-6, which is involved in the oxidation of fats and in the metabolization of glucose. IL-6, moreover, inhibits the production of proinflammatory interleukin TNF-α (Tumor Necrosis Factor-α), which plays an important role in the pathogenesis of inflammation-associated insulin resistance (and we already know that the more body fat we have, the more "inflamed" we are).

We know that telomere length may be a potential indicator of real (biological) aging, as there is an inverse relationship between age and telomere length. Observational and experimental studies show a possible but still not completely clear **correlation between physical activity and telomere length**. Physical activity has been proven to reduce chronic inflammation and oxidative stress, especially in elderly and obese individuals, and may therefore reduce telomere shortening observed while aging (Mason C. et al., 2013) (Arsenis N.C. et al., 2017). Thus, exercise could have a protective effect on telomere length being particularly beneficial for high-risk individuals or suffering from chronic conditions with high level of oxidative and inflammatory stress.

A particularly intriguing study on muscle fibers (Jones RG 3rd, et al., 2022) carried out on mice and humans, has shown how working out affects gene expression. The Yamanaka factors are four protein transcription factors able to bring specialised and mature cells to a younger and more flexible state, specifically pluripotent stem cells Oct3/4, Klf4, Sox2 and Myc, also known by their acronym OKSM. Researchers compared the effects of OKSM factors on gene expression in the muscle fibers of mice that had or didn't have access to an exercise wheel. They also compared the effects of OKSM factors on muscles with the effects of a single transcription factor (Myc), finding that working out induces Myc expression to a greater extent than the other three factors. The mice belonging to the "physical exercise" group were free to run on a weightless wheel for the first week then, over the following 8 weeks, on a wheel made progressively heavier by magnetic resistances. In short, **working out makes the muscle fibers regress into a younger condition** through a greater gene expression, in particular Myc. Research carried out during the study has shown that alterations of gene expression through OKSM and the adaptation to exercise in mice's muscles are kept in human muscles after long-term training (muscle biopsy samples from women with at least 15 years of weight training).

It is understandable that, for many people, especially if they are older, obese or perhaps have pathologies, the label "weight training" can be intimidating for various reasons. However, we must realize that we are talking about improving one's ability to move safely, efficiently and effectively in their everyday life, i.e. being able to lift an object and put it away, walk and climb the stairs without feeling breathless, perhaps with shopping bags, bending the back, moving from a sitting position to an upright one, avoiding a fall or promptly getting up on their own after falling. Let's look at it this way: resistance exercise training is a primary countermeasure to age-related chronic disease (Mcleod et al., 2019).

Muscle growth and strength are possible up to a very advanced age, as many studies have now ascertained, and exercise with weights is essential to prevent the so-called "hypokinetic pathologies".

To conclude, I want to quote Jim Rohn's maxim, which gets straight to the point: "Take care of your body, it's the only place you have to live".

So, since muscle mass is a key biomarker for predicting survival as we age, do you want to live longer and better? Build and maintain your muscles by constantly training them like a real bodybuilder, under the supervision of an expert trainer.

CHAPTER 40

Warming up

Ciro di Cristino

Theoretical part

Warming up is essential for being able to face a workout, as the transition from a state of relative functional stillness to a state of particular commitment requires adequate gradualness.

You must **avoid** getting to your training session with tensions from the previous session, therefore this chapter will not take into consideration the methodologies implemented to treat these technopathies.

General warm-up has three objectives:

- mobilization
- raising awareness
- stabilization for safety

Dynamic stretching exercises (oscillations, twisting, circling) and static stretching (no more than 5 seconds per position) must be performed to **mobilize the joints** and their components in a progressive and dynamic way, freeing them and supplying them with synovial fluid.

As a result, the muscles begin to shorten and lengthen, without being forced.

It is necessary **to stimulate the deep stabilizing muscles** (core, rotator cuffs), which allow the body to maintain balance and stability during the exercise and to protect itself from injury or chronic injuries.

Activating control of breathing, diaphragm, pelvic floor and abdominal muscles is essential for constant and automated posture management.

Meanwhile, **the heart increases its rate and output**, providing more oxygen, heat and nourishment to the peripheral parts of the body.

Some exercises must be performed explosively, to increase coordination and intra/intermuscular recruitment as well as the perception and management of the various parts of the body in time and space.

Thinking about the warm-up as a sort of ritual, which also prepares you psychologically to face training adequately, is also very important.

After a day of working or other tasks, it is important to dedicate time to yourself. Therefore, living this moment to the fullest and however you want is only fair.

Precisely for this reason, I believe that, in addition to basic notions, warm-ups must mostly be performed in an individual and individualized way, both as regards form and duration, so that you can start with the right energy.

Practical part

General warm-ups

Not all individuals are inclined to perform this fundamental phase of training, as it is often underestimated, despite sometimes even sustaining injuries because of the lack of it.

The exercises indicated are only an example related to the purposes described in the theoretical part. I think this practice can be reduced even to 10 minutes, selecting only one or two exercises for the joint and muscle areas. By personalizing it, everyone will be able to develop the most appropriate warm-up, varying it in a rational way in order to avoid boredom and abandonment.

General warm-up exercises
Ankles • *No weight bearing* (standing: one foot in support): plantar-dorsal flexion, inside-out, inside- and outside-rotation, clockwise-counterclockwise circumduction • *In support* (on the tip of the foot): circling • *Weight bearing* (both feet in turn): lift the toes, heels, inner and outer foot
Knees • Semi-bent legs, hands on thighs, bring knees right-left, inside-out, clockwise, counterclockwise, inward, outward circles
Hip • With bent legs, circle, one leg at a time, in and out • With extended legs, swing, one leg at a time, forward-backward, inside-out
Pelvis • Anterior and posterior pelvic tilts, circumduction in both directions • Manage the movements of the pelvis using the superficial (abdominal-gluteal) and/or deep (pelvic floor) muscles

Continues

Continued

Trunk

- Inclined: hands on thighs, flexion-extension ("cat")
- Standing: forward-backward, lateral flexion, circumduction in both directions, twisting to the right and left (legs semi-bent)

Shoulders, elbows and arms

- Arms at the sides, lift-lower, front-back, and circle the shoulders
- Hands behind, arms thrust up-forward-out (simple, compound and combined exercises)
- Various swings and circles of extended arms
- From arms outstretched, adduct, abduct, intra- and extra-rotate, small and large-radius circumduction
- Flex, extend, twist and circle forearms on arms

Wrists and fingers

- Palmar-dorsal flexion, circles in both directions, even with fingers joined and/or crossed
- Open and close the palms of the hands, even with the use of balls
- Various mobilizations of the fingers

Neck

- Flexing the head back and forth, flexing right and left (looking forward), twisting right and left (looking left and right), swinging forward and circling in both directions
- Possibly carry out exercises with the head, even against resistance

Diaphragm

The choice of body position depends on the environment in which this activity is performed (recumbent, sitting or standing):

- inhale by inflating, in turn, only the chest and/or only the belly, to mobilize and sensitize the diaphragm, in order to manage it correctly during motor activities

Legs

- Jog on the spot, hops with feet together (2 × 3), stretching (5 seconds) right-left
- Jumps with feet together front-back, right-left, stretching (5 seconds) right-left
- Jumps on one leg (right-left), stretching (5 seconds) right-left
- Traditional jumping jack and front jumping jacks, stretching (5 seconds) right-left

Continues

Continued

Thighs

- Jog on the spot, rear kick (3 seconds), right-left flexor stretches (5 seconds)
- Jog in place, high skip (3 seconds), right-left quadriceps stretch (5 seconds)
- 3 forward lunges (on the third, iliopsoas stretching for 5 seconds)
- 3 back lunges (on the third, iliopsoas stretching for 5 seconds)
- 3 lateral lunges (on the third, stretching the adductors for 5 seconds, right-left)
- 3+3 jump lunges and torso twists (right-left)
- 3 squats: controlled descent, explosive ascent
- 3 box squats: parallel squat (stop 3 seconds), explosive ascent
- 3 squat jumps: parallel squat, ascent with leap (cushion the landing)
- 3 counter movement jumps: fast descent and countermovement jump (cushion the landing)
- 3 drop jumps: the same as the countermovement jump, but dropping from a step

Abs

- Crunch (also with variations) 1 series × 12 reps (also twisted, or with fitball)
- Leg raises; hollow man; V-up; V-sit
- On fitball: egg forward and lateral
- On fitball: Russian twist, also with weight

Core

- Plank (with all variations, based on the ability of the performer) frontal, dorsal and lateral: 12 seconds × 1 set × position (also on fitball)
- Plank knee cross; elbow plank twist; plank shoulder tap; bridge; Superman pull

Shoulders

- Prone exercises on fitball, in isotonic and/or isometric form: 1 set × 6 reps and/or 1 × 10 seconds
- Intra- and external rotation with elastic bands: 1 set × 6 reps x exercise
- Dumbbell anterior deltoid: front raises, 1 set × 6 reps
- Dumbbell lateral deltoid: lateral raises, 1 set × 6 reps
- Dumbbell rear deltoid: rear raises (torso leaned forward), 1 set × 6 reps
- Interscapular with elastic bands: isotonic and/or isometric, 1 set × 6 repetitions and/or 1 × 10 seconds

Continues

Continued

Lats and biceps

- 6 pullups with elastic bands, back stretches (5 seconds)
- 6 pushups with elastic bands, biceps stretches (5 seconds)
- 6 pulldowns with bands, lats stretches (5 seconds)
- 6 pushups with dumbbells, biceps stretches (5 seconds)

Pectorals and triceps

- 4-6 pushups (hands shoulder-width apart, elbows out), kneeling stretch, sitting on heels, bending torso forward, stretching arms forward, on floor (5 seconds)
- 4-6 pushups (hands wider than shoulders, elbows out), kneeling stretch, sitting on heels, lean forward by stretching arms forward on the floor (5 seconds)
- 4-6 pushups (hands with thumbs touching), triceps stretches (5 seconds)
- 4-6 pushups (hands shoulder-width apart, elbows tucked in at sides), triceps stretches (5 seconds)
- 4-6 jump pushups, kneeling stretching, sitting on heels, bending the torso forward by stretching the arms forward on the floor (5 seconds)
- 6 kickbacks with dumbbells or elastic bands, triceps stretches (5 seconds)

Specific warm-ups

Specific warm-ups must be based on the chosen sport. In our case, bodybuilding. **The approach to the chosen exercise for the session** must in any case be equally **gradual** and, in the case of complex exercises, it must also refer to the technical movement. **The external load must be increased, maintaining the most correct execution. Cooling down** at the end of a session is also very important, which I talked about in Chapter 32.

Conclusions

After reading this book, you will have likely realized that the road to muscle building is not so simple and that, especially regarding training, there are many possible ways, sometimes even seemingly opposite. There are actually many factors that induce muscle growth and one type of training can have a greater influence on one individual compared to another, without mentioning the influence of individual genetic characteristics. The large number of workouts and exercises that have been covered must not be a source of uncertainty and confusion, they must enrich your cultural baggage and allow you to make the best choice for you.

However, to recap the most crucial suggestions for increasing muscle mass, we find it appropriate to present you with this sort of handbook:

1. Focus mainly on multi-joint exercises, such as squats, deadlifts, bench presses, rows, and overhead presses, since, in addition to affecting larger muscle areas, they induce a greater secretion of GH and testosterone, and they stimulate the nervous system more.
2. You cannot develop large muscle mass with light weights: the use of heavy loads must be favored, provided that they do not contribute to the detriment of correct execution.
3. Recovery times of 90 to 120 seconds after heavy multi-joint exercises promote testosterone production, recovery times of 30 to 60 seconds promote GH production. Both are anabolic hormones involved in the muscle growth process.
4. In bodybuilding, the eccentric phase of the movement is extremely important, unlike weightlifting. Thus, it must last at least twice as long as the concentric one and is essential to promote the release of GH, IGF-1 and MGF (mechanical growth factor).
5. Use techniques like forced reps and negative reps to increase the intensity of your workout. Forced reps increase GH and testosterone production and stimulate protein synthesis for up to 72 hours after the training session.

6. If you increase the loads, decrease the recovery time between sets or introduce intensity techniques, your body reacts to the stress by overcompensating, so that you can handle the same stress again in the future easily, allowing you to increase the weights even further. This is why beginners in this discipline see great improvements as soon as they start their training programs.
7. At the beginning, we recommend following the first of the three principles mentioned in the previous point, i.e. trying to increase the load in each session compared to the previous one, without ever "spoiling" the execution of the movement. This is also the principle by which athletes will stabilize with weight gains and will have to resort to specific techniques to overcome the obstacle. It will become increasingly difficult to stress the muscle to a point it has never been stressed before.
8. In more advanced athletes it has been found that the use of a load around 80-85% of the maximum load, with which failure is reached, followed by some forced, negative and isometric repetitions, all interspersed with short rest periods and lightened by a few lighter lifts, is the most comprehensive method of working the muscle fiber and causing chronic sarcoplasmic inflammation, as well as muscle fiber tearing that stimulates IGF-1 and MGF.
9. You must be able to recognize when you are doing too much, when you are asking too much of your muscles and your body, risking overtraining and, therefore, losing muscle tone and fullness. When you train too long or too heavily, or without ever reducing the intensity of work, you can hit a plateau, i.e. a stop in muscle growth, and even activate systems of muscle destruction. In these cases, pulling back on intensity with a deload week will be beneficial.
10. Plan the achievement of your long-term goal and include sub-goals along the way which will be your checkpoints, in order to understand if you are on the right track or if you need to make some changes.

Suggested readings and websites

Chapters 1-15, 19, 20, 22, 24-30, 35

- Abdessemed D, Duche P et al. Effect of recovey duration on muscular power and blood lactate during the bench press exercise. *Int J Sports Med* 1999;20:368-373.
- Abraham WM. Factors in delayed muscle soreness. *Med Sci Sports* 1977 Spring;9(1):11-20.
- Ahtiainen JP, Pakarinen A et al. Acute hormonal responses to heavy resistance exercise in strength athletes versus nonathletes. *Can J Appl Physiol* 2004;29(5):527-543.
- Ahtiainen JP, Pakarinen A et al. Short vs. long rest period between the sets in hypertrophic resistance training: influence on muscle strenght, size, and hormonal adaptations in trained men. *J Strength Cond Res* 2005;19:572-582.
- Armeni M. *ACSM-ISSA. Research Manual.* 2001-2007s.
- Armstrong RB. Mechanisms of exercise-induced delayed onset muscular soreness: a brief review. *Med Sci Sports Exerc* 1984 Dec;16(6):529-538.
- Baechle TR, Earle RW. *Essentials of strength training and conditioning.* Human Kinetics, Champaign (IL), 2008.
- Bergeron MF. Lactic acid production and clearance during exercise. *National Strength and Conditioning Association Journal* 1991;13(5):47-50.
- Binzen CA et al. Postexercise oxygen consumption and substrate use after resistance exercise in women. *Med Sci Sports Exerc* 2001 Jun;33(6):932-938.
- Bodine SC, Stitt TN et al. Akt/mTOR pathway is a crucial regulator of skeletal muscle hypertropy and can prevent muscle atrophy in vivo. *Nat Cell Biol* 2001;3:1014-1019.
- Bolster DR, Kubica N et al. Immediate response of mammalian target of rapamycin (mTOR)-mediated signalling following acute resistance exercise in rat skeletal muscle. *J Physiol* 2003;553:213-220.
- Bompa TO. *Periodization: theory and methodology of training.* Human Kinetics, Champaign (IL), 1999.
- Bompa TO. *Theory and methodology of training: the key to athletic performance.* Kendall/Hunt Publishing Company, Dubuque (IA), 1983.
- Børsheim E, Bahr R. Effect of exercise intensity, duration and mode on post-exercise oxygen consumption. *Sports Med* 2003;33(14):1037-1060.
- Bottaro M et al. Effects of rest duration between sets of resistance training on acute hormonal responses in trained women. *J Sci Med Sport* 2009 Jan;12(1):73-78. Epub 2008 Feb 21.
- Brooks D. *The complete book of personal training.* Human Kinetics, Champaign (IL), 2004.
- Burd NA et al. Low-load high volume resistance exercise stimulates muscle protein synthesis more than high-load low volume resistance exercise in young men. *PLoS One* 2010;5(8):e12033.
- Burd NA et al. Resistance exercise volume affects myofibrillar protein synthesis and anabolic signalling molecule phosphorylation in young men. *J Physiol* 2010;588:3119-3130.
- Buresh R et al. The effect of resistive exercise rest interval on hormonal response, strength, and hypertrophy with training. *J Strength Cond Res* 2009 Jan;23(1):62-71.
- Chek P. *Program design: choosing reps, sets, loads, tempo, and rest periods.* C.H.E.K. Institute, 2002.
- Coburn JW, Malek MH. *NSCA's essentials of personal training.* Human Kinetics, Champaign (IL), 2011.
- De Salles BF et al. Rest interval between sets in strength training. *Sports Med* 2009;39(9):765-777.
- Farthing JP, Chilibeck PD. The effects of eccentric and concentric training at different veloc-

ities on muscle htpertrophy. *Eur J Appl Physiol* 2003;89:578-586.

- Fleck SJ, Kraemer WJ. *Designing resistance training programs.* Human Kinetics, Champaign (IL), 2004.
- Fleck SJ. Periodized strength training: a critical review. *J Str Cond Res* 1999;13:82-89.
- Frankel CC, Kravitz L. Periodization. Latest studies and practical applications. *IDEA Personal Trainer* 2000;11:15-17.
- Friedmann B, Kinscherf R et al. Muscular adaptations to computer-guided strength training with eccentric overload. *Acta Physiol Scand* 2004;182:77-88.
- Goto K et al. Effects of resistance exercise on lipolysis during subsequent submaximal exercise. *Med Sci Sports Exerc* 2007 Feb;39(2):308-315.
- Goto K et al. Muscular adaptations to combinations of high- and low-intensity resistance exercises. *J Strength Cond Res* 2004;18(4):730-737.
- Gotshalk LA et al. Hormonal responses of multiset versus single-set heavy-resistance exercise protocols. *Can J Appl Physiol* 1997 Jun;22(3):244-255.
- Gray H. *Gray's Anatomy: the anatomical basis of medicine and surgery.* Pearson Professional, London, 1995.
- Guglielmini C, Paolini AR, Conconi F. Variations of serum testosterone concentrations after physical exercises of different duration. *Int J Sports Med* 1984;5:246-249.
- Haennel RG et al. Effects of hydraulic circuit training following coronary artery bypass surgery. *Med Sci Sports Exerc* 1991 Feb;23(2):158-165.
- Häkkinen K et al. Selective muscle hypertrophy, changes in EMG and force, and serum hormones during strength training in older women. *J Appl Physiol* 2001 Aug;91(2):569-580.
- Hansen K et al. The effects of exercise on the storage and oxidation of dietary fat. *Sports Med* 2005;35(5):363-373.
- Harris RC et al. The time course of phosphorylcreatine resynthesis during recovery of the quadriceps muscle in man. *Pflugers Arch* 1976;367(2):137-142.
- Hather BM et al. Influence of eccentric actions on skeletal muscle adaptations to resistance training. *Acta Physiol Scand* 1991 Oct;143(2):177-185.
- Hawley JA, Hopkins WG. Aerobic glycolytic and aerobic lipolytic power systems. A new paradigm with implications for endurance and ultraendurance events. *Sports Med* 1995 Apr;19(4):240-250.
- Heydari M, Freund J et al. The effect of high-intensity intermittent exercise on body composition of overweight young males. *J Obes* 2012;2012:480467.
- Heyward VH. *Advanced fitness assessment and exercise prescription.* Human Kinetics, Champaign (IL), 2006.
- Higbie EJ, Cureton KJ et al. Effects of concentric and eccentric training on muscle strength, cross-sectional area, and neural activation. *J Appl Physiol* (1985) 1996;81:2173-2181.
- Hoffman J. Growth hormone. *National Strength and Conditioning Association Journal* 1990;12(5):78-81.
- Hoffman J. *NSCA's guide to program design.* Human Kinetics, Champaign (IL), 2011.
- Holman S. Train, eat, grow: the positions-of-flexion muscle-training manual, ed ital. Sandro Ciccarelli Editore, Figline Valdarno (FI), 2011.
- Hurley CF et al. The effect of caffeine ingestion on delayed onset muscle soreness. *J Strength Cond Res*, Post Acceptance, 3 sept. 2013 (archiviato dall'url originale il 19 aprile 2014).
- Jo E et al. Influence of recovery duration after a potentiating stimulus on muscolar power in recreationally trained individuals. *J Strength Cond Res* 2010;24(2):343-347.
- Jones D, Round J, de Haan A. *Muscle from molecules to movement: a textbook of muscle physiology for sport, exercise, physiotherapy and medicine.* Elsevier Health Sciences, London, 2004.
- Kaminsky LA, Bonzheim KA (ACSM). *ACSM's guidelines for exercise testing and prescription*, 7th ed. Lippincott Williams & Wilkins, Philadelphia, 2006.
- Karbaleifar S et al. The effects of caffeine on perceived pain of muscles. *Annals of Biological Research* 2011;2(6):16-21.
- Kawakami Y. The effects of strength training on muscle architecture in humans. *International Journal of Sport and Health Science* 2005.
- Kenney WL, Wilmore JH, Costill DL. *Physiology of sport and exercise.* Human Kinetics, Champaign (IL), 2011.
- Komi PV. *Strength and power in sport.* Wiley-Blackwell, Hoboken (NJ), 2001.
- Kosek DJ et al. Efficacy of 3 days/wk resistance training on myofiber hypertrophy and myogenic mechanisms in young vs. older adults. *J Appl Physiol* 2006 Aug;101(2):531-544.
- Kraemer WJ. Influence of the endocrine system on resistance training adaptations. *National Strength and Conditioning Association Journal* 1992;14(2):47-54.

- Kraemer WJ. Periodization in resistance training. *IDEA Personal Trainer* 1998;(9):27-34.
- Kraemer WJ et al. Hormonal and growth factor responses to heavy resistance exercise protocols. *J Appl Physiol* 1990 Oct;69(4):1442-1450.
- Kraemer WJ et al. Compatibility of high-intensity strength and endurance training on hormonal and skeletal muscle adaptations. *J Appl Physiol* (1985) 1995 Mar;78(3):976-989.
- Kraemer WJ et al. Physiologic responses to heavy-resistance exercise with very short rest periods. *Int J Sports Med* 1987;8(4):247-252.
- Kraemer WJ, Fleck SJ. *Optimizing strength training: designing non-linear periodization workouts*. Human Kinetics, Champaign (IL), 2007.
- Kraemer WJ, Ratamess NA. Hormonal responses and adaptations to resistance exercise and training. *Sports Med* 2005;35(4):339-361.
- Kravitz L. Resistance training: adaptations and health Implications. *Idea Today Health Publications* 1996;14:38-46.
- Krieger JW. Single versus multiple sets of resistance exercise: a meta-regression. *J Strength Cond Res* 2009 Sep;23(6):1890-1901.
- Krieger JW. Single vs. multiple sets of resistance exercise for muscle hypertrophy: a meta-analysis. *J Strength Cond Res* 2010 Apr;24(4):1150-1159.
- Lorenz DS et al. Periodization: current review and suggested implementation for athletic rehabilitation. *Sports Health* 2010 Nov.
- Luzi L. *Biologia cellulare nell'esercizio fisico*. Springer, Milano, 2009, p. 91.
- Manilal KP. *Science of strength training*. Pinnacle Technology, 2006.
- Maridakis V et al. Caffeine attenuates delayed-onset muscle pain and force loss following eccentric exercise. *J Pain* 2007 Mar;8(3):237-243. Epub 2006 Dec 11.
- Marx JO et al. Low-volume circuit versus high-volume periodized resistance training in women. *Med Sci Sports Exerc* 2001 Apr;33(4):635-643.
- Matveyev L. *Fundamentals of sports training*. Progress, Moscow, 1981.
- McArdle W, Katch FM, Katch V. *Exercise physiology: energy, nutrition, and human performance*. Lippincott Williams & Wilkins, Philadelphia, 2010, pp. 698-739.
- McCarty MF. Optimizing exercise for fat loss. *Med Hypotheses* 1995 May;44(5):325-330.
- Melov S et al. Resistance exercise reverses aging in human skeletal muscle. *PLoS One* 2007 May 23;2(5):e465.
- Mulligan SE et al. Influence of resistance exercise volume on serum growth hormone and cortisol concentrations in women. *J Strength Cond Res* 1996;10:256-262.
- Naclerio F et al. Effects of different resistance training volumes on strength and power in team sport athletes. *J Strength Cond Res* 2013 Jul;27(7):1832-1840.
- Ogasawara R, Sato K et al. The order of concurrent endurance and resistance exercise modifies mTOR signaling and protein synthesis in rat skeletal muscle. *Am J Physiol Endocrinol Metab* 2014.
- Ozolin NG. *Sovremennaja Systema Sportivnoj Trenirovky*. Fizkul'tura i Sport, Moskva, 1971.
- Paoli A, Moro T, Marcolin G et al. High-intensity Interval Resistance Training (HIRT) influences resting energy expenditure and respiratory ratio in non-dieting individuals. *J Transl Med* 2012 Nov 24;10:237.
- Paoli A, Neri M. *Principi di metodologia del fitness*. Elika, Cesena, 2010.
- Peterson M et al. Applications of the dose-response for muscular strength development: a review of meta-analytic efficacy and reliability for designing training prescription. *J Strength Cond Res* 2005 Nov;19(4):950-958.
- Peterson M et al. Maximizing strength development in athletes: a meta-analysis to determine the dose-response relationship. *J Strength Cond Res* 2004 May;18(2):377-382.
- Plowman SA, Smith DL. *Exercise physiology for health, fitness, and performance*. Lippincott Williams & Wilkins, Philadelphia, 2007.
- Poehlman ET, Melby C. Resistance training and energy balance. *Int J Sport Nutr* 1998 Jun;8(2):143-159.
- Raastad T et al. Hormonal responses to high- and moderate-intensity strength exercise. *Eur J Appl Physiol* 2000 May;82(1-2):121-128.
- Rahimi SSBR. Acute GH and IGF-I responses to short vs. long rest period between sets during forced repetitions resistance training system. *South African Journal for Research in Sport, Physical Education and Recreation* 2008;30(2).
- Ratamess NA et al. American college of sports medicine position stand. Progression models in resistance training for healthy adults. *Med Sci Sports Exerc* 2009;41:687-708.
- Rhea MR et al. A comparison of linear and daily undulating periodized programs with equated volume and intensity for strength. *J Strength Cond Res* 2002.

- Rhea MR et al. A meta-analysis to determine the dose response for strength development. *Med Sci Sports Exerc* 2003 Mar;35(3):456-464.
- Rhea MR, Alderman BL. A meta-analysis of periodized versus nonperiodized strength and power training programs. *Res Q Exerc Sport* 2004.
- Sarti MA, Monfort M et al. Muscle activity in upper and lower rectus abdominus during abdominal exercises. *Arch Phys Med Rehabil* 1996;77:1293-1297.
- Schoenfeld BJ. *Science and development of muscle hypertrophy*. Human Kinetics, Champaign (IL), 2016.
- Schumann M, Walker S et al. The order effect of combined endurance and strength loadings on force and hormone responses: effects of prolonged training. *Eur J Appl Physiol* 2014;114:867-880.
- Scotto di Palumbo A, Guerra E. Effect of combined resistance and endurance exercise training on regional fat loss. *Journal Sports Medicine Physical Fitness* 2017 June;57(6):794-801.
- Shepstone TN et al. Short-term high- vs. low-velocity isokinetic lengthening training results in greater hypertrophy of the elbow flexors in young men. *J Appl Physiol* (1985) 2005 May;98(5):1768-1776.
- Shing CM, Webb JJ et al. Circulating adiponectin concentration and body composition are altered in response to high-intensity interval training. *J Strength Cond Res* 2013;27(8):2213-2218.
- Smilios I et al. Hormonal responses after various resistance exercise protocols. *Med Sci Sports Exerc* 2003 Apr;35(4):644-654.
- Smith LL. Acute inflammation: the underlying mechanism in delayed onset muscle soreness? *Med Sci Sports Exerc* 1991 May;23(5):542-551.
- Spineti J et al. Comparison between different periodization models on muscular strength and thickness in a muscle group increasing sequence. *Rev Bras Med Esporte* 2013.
- Staron R et al. Muscle hypertrophy and fast fiber type conversions in heavy resistance-trained women. *Eur J Appl Physiol Occup Physiol* 1990;60(1):71-79.
- Stone MH et al. Health- and performance-related potential of resistance training. *Sports Med* 1991 Apr;11(4):210-231.
- Stoppani J. *Encyclopedia of muscle & strength*. Human Kinetics, Champaign (IL), 2006, pp. 12-14.
- Tesch P et al. Skeletal muscle glycogen loss evoked by resistance exercise. *Journal of Strength and Conditioning Research* May 1998;12(2).
- Thomas DQ, Kotecki JE. *Physical activity & health: an interactive approach*. Jones & Bartlett Learning, Burlington (MA), 2006.
- Todd IC et al. Cardiac rehabilitation following myocardial infarction. A practical approach. *Sports Med* 1992 Oct;14(4):243-259.
- Trapp EG, Chisholm DJ et al. The effects of high-intensity intermittent exercise training on fat loss and fasting insulin levels of young women. *Int J Obes* 2008;32:684-691.
- Villanueva MG et al. Influence of rest interval length on acute testosterone and cortisol responses to volume-load-equated total body hypertrophic and strength protocols. *J Strength Cond Res* 2012;26(10):2755-2764.
- Villanueva MG, Lane CJ, Schroedere ET. Short rest interval lengths between sets optimally enhance body composition and performance with 8 weeks of strength resistance training in older men. *Eur J Appl Physiol* 2015;115:295-308.
- Wakahara T, Fukutani A et al. Nonuniform muscle hypertrophy: its relation to muscle activation in training session. *Med Sci Sports Exerc* 2013 Nov;45(11):2158-2165.
- Wakahara T, Miyamoto N et al. Association between regional differences in muscle activation in one session of resistance exercise and in muscle hypertrophy after resistance training. *Eur J Appl Physiol* 2012;112:1569-1576.
- Weiss LW. The obtuse nature of muscular strength: the contribution of rest to its development and expression. *National Strength and Conditioning Association* November 1991;5(4).
- Willardson JM. The application of training to failure in periodized multiple-set resistance exercise programs. *Journal of Strength and Conditioning Research* May 2007;21(2):628-631.
- Willis LH, Slentz CA. Effects of aerobic and/or resistance training on body mass and fat mass in overweight or obese adults. *J Apll Physiol* (1985) 2012;113:1831-1837.
- Wolfe BL et al. Quantitative analysis of single- vs. multiple-set programs in resistance training. *J Strength Cond Res* 2004 Feb;18(1):35-47.
- Galimberti D. et al. *Nutrigenomica e Epigenetica: dalla biologia alla clinica*, 2017 Edra Ed.
- Garatachea N, Pareja-Galeano H, et al. Exercise attenuates the major hallmarks of aging. *Rejuvenation Res.* 2015 Feb;18(1):57-89. doi: 10.1089/rej.2014.1623. PMID: 25431878; PMCID: PMC4340807.
- Serra-Rexach JA, Bustamante-Ara N, Hierro

Villaran M, et al. Short-term, light- to moderate-intensity exercise training improves leg muscle strength in the oldest old: A randomized controlled trial. *J Am Geriatr Soc* 2011;59:594–602.
- Lustosa LP, Silva JP, Coelho FM, et al. Impact of resistance exercise program on functional capacity and muscular strength of knee extensor in pre-frail community-dwelling older women: A randomized crossover trial. *Rev Bras Fisioter* 2011;15:318–324.
- Sullivan DH, Roberson PK, Smith ES, Price JA, Bopp MM. Effects of muscle strength training and megestrol acetate on strength, muscle mass, and function in frail older people. *J Am Geriatr Soc* 2007;55:20–28.
- Haskell WL, Lee IM, et al. Physical activity and public health: Updated recommendation for adults from the American College of Sports Medicine and the American Heart Association. *Circulation* 2007;116:1081–1093.
- Villareal DT, Smith GI, et al. Regular multicomponent exercise increases physical fitness and muscle protein anabolism in frail, obese, older adults. *Obesity (Silver Spring)* 2011;19:312–318.

- https://journals.physiology.org/journal/jappl
- https://journals.lww.com/nsca-jscr/pages/default.aspx
- https://journals.lww.com/acsm-msse/pages/default.aspx
- https://news.harvard.edu/gazette/story/2014/12/using-weights-to-target-belly-fat/
- www.ergo-log.com – Moderate and intensive training equally good with weight-loss diet. Article, 16.05.2009.
- www.ergo-log.com – Cardio in two parts burns more energy. Article, 31.08.2009.
- www.ergo-log.com – Trained body burns more fat with gentle endurance exercise. Article, 09.01.2010.

Chapters 16-18, 21

- Cianti G. *Allenati e alimentati con i cicli naturali*. Elika, Cesena, 2005.
- Cianti G. *More! Di più, sempre di più*. MuscleHead, Firenze, 1997.
- Darden E. *Super high intensity bodybuilding*. G.P. Putnam's Sons, New York, 1986.
- Delavier F. *Guida agli esercizi di muscolazione*. Arcadia, Milano, 2008.
- Gold J, Kennedy R. *The World Gym*. Contemporary Books Inc., 1987.
- Hatfield FC. *Bodybuilding: a scientific approach*. McGraw-Hill, New York, 1984.
- Kennedy R, Weis DB. *Mass!* Contemporary Books Inc., 1986.
- Kennedy R, Weis DB. *Raw Muscle!* Contemporary Books Inc., 1989.
- Michalik S. *Atomic fitness*. Basic Health Publications Inc., Laguna Beach (CA), 2006.
- Parascandolo S. *Il bodybuilding scientifico in America*. Bodybuilding Concepts, New York, 1988.
- Pedemonte J. *Tecniche di bodybuilding*. Genova, 1994.
- Poliquin C. *The Poliquin principles*. Dayton Writers Group, Napa (CA), 1997.
- Weider J, Reynolds B. *Ultimate bodybuilding*. Contemporary Books Inc., 1988.
- Yates D, Wolff B. *Blood and guts*. Wolff Creative Group, 1993.

- https://www.t-nation.com – Training articles by Christian Thibaudeau.

Chapter 23

- Beaudry KM et al. Sex-based differences in hepatic and skeletal muscle triglyceride storage and metabolism. *Appl Physiol Nutr Metab* 2019 Aug;44(8):805-813. Epub 2019 Jan 31.
- Caplan AI. Mesenchymal stem cells. *J Orthop Res* 1991 Sep;9(5):641-650.
- Dumont NA et al. Satellite cells and skeletal muscle regeneration. *Compr Physiol* 2015 Jul 1;5(3):1027-1059.
- Galfano V et al. Ormoni e plasticità delle fibre del muscolo scheletrico. Ruolo nella patogenesi della sarcopenia. *L'Endocrinologo* 2018;19:243-246.
- Jorgenson KW et al. Identifying the structural adaptations that drive the mechanical load-induced growth of skeletal muscle: a scoping review. *Cells* 2020 Jul 9;9(7):1658.
- Piras A et al. Peripheral Heart Action (PHA) training as a valid substitute to high intensity interval training to improve resting cardiovascular changes and autonomic adaptation. *Eur J Appl Physiol* 2015 Apr;115(4):763-773.
- Staron RS et al. Fiber type composition of the vastus lateralis muscle of young men and women. *J Histochem Cytochem* 2000;48: 623-629.

Chapter 31

- Ahtiainen JP, Pakarinen A, Alen M et al. Muscle hypertrophy, hormonal adaptations and strength development during strength training in strength-trained and untrained men. *European Journal of Applied Physiology* 2003;89(6):555-563.

- Atherton PJ, Smith K. Muscle protein synthesis in response to nutrition and exercise. *Journal of Physiology* 2012;*590*(5):1049-1057.
- Baker D, Wilson G, Carlyon R. Periodization: the effect on strength of manipulating volume and intensity. *J Strength Cond Res* 1994;8(4):235-242.
- Blaauw B. Reggiani C. The role of satellite cells in muscle hypertrophy. *Journal of Muscle Research And Cell Motility* 2014;35(1):3-10.
- Bosco C. *La forza muscolare: aspetti fisiologici ed applicazioni pratiche*. Società Stampa Sportiva, Roma, 1997.
- Feriche B. et al. Resistance training using different hypoxic training strategies: a basis for hypertrophy and muscle power development. *Sports Medicine-Open* 2017;3(1):12.
- Fry AC, Kraemer WJ et al. Endocrine responses to overreaching before and after 1 year of weightlifting. *Canadian Journal of Applied Physiology* 1994;19(4):400-410.
- González-Badillo JJ et al. Maximal intended velocity training induces greater gains in bench press performance than deliberately slower half-velocity training. *European Journal of Sport Science* 2014;14(8):772-781.
- Graham J. Periodization research and an example application. *Strength and Conditioning Journal* 2002;24(6):62-70.
- Haff GG, Hobbs RT, Haff EE et al. Cluster training: a novel method for introducing training program variation. *Strength and Conditioning Journal* 2008;30(1):67-76.
- Häkkinen K, Keskinen KL. Muscle cross-sectional area and voluntary force production characteristics in elite strength-and endurance-trained athletes and sprinters. *European Journal of Applied Physiology and Occupational Physiology* 1989;59(3):215-220.
- Hodge AJ, Huxley HE, Spiro D. Electron microscope studies on ultrathin sections of muscle. *Journal of Experimental Medicine* 1954;*99*(2):201-206.
- Hornberger TA. Mechanotransduction and the regulation of mTORC1 signaling in skeletal muscle. *International Journal of Biochemistry & Cell Biology* 2011;43(9): 1267-1276.
- Jones K, Hunter G, Fleisig G et al. The effects of compensatory acceleration on upper-body strength and power in collegiate football players. *Journal of Strength and Conditioning Research* 1999;13(2):99-105.
- Juneau CE, Tafur L. Over time, load mediates muscular hypertrophy in resistance training. *Current Opinion in Physiology* 2019;11:147-148.
- Kadi F, Schjerling P et al. The effects of heavy resistance training and detraining on satellite cells in human skeletal muscles. *Journal of Physiology* 2004;558(3):1005-1012.
- Kraemer WJ, Fleck SJ, Evans WJ. Strength and power training: physiological mechanisms of adaptation. *Exercise and Sport Sciences Reviews* 1996;24:363-397.
- Kraemer WJ, Fleck SJ. *Optimizing strength training: designing nonlinear periodization workouts*. Human Kinetics, Champaign (IL), 2007.
- MacKenzie MG, Hamilton DL, Pepin M et al. Inhibition of myostatin signaling through Notch activation following acute resistance exercise. *PloS One* 2013;*8*(7):e68743.
- Mansor DA, Kadir ZA, Azidin RFR. A comparison of periodization models on muscular strength. In: *Proceedings of the International Colloquium on Sports Science, Exercise, Engineering and Technology 2014 (ICoSSEET 2014)*. Springer, Singapore, 2014, pp. 335-347.
- Mobley CB, Haun CT et al. Biomarkers associated with low, moderate, and high vastus lateralis muscle hypertrophy following 12 weeks of resistance training. *PLoS One* 2018;13(4):e0195203.
- Morales-Artacho AJ, Padial P, García-Ramos A et al. Influence of a cluster set configuration on the adaptations to short-term power training. *Journal of Strength and Conditioning Research* 2018;32(4):930-937.
- Petrella JK, Kim JS et al. Potent myofiber hypertrophy during resistance training in humans is associated with satellite cell-mediated myonuclear addition: a cluster analysis. *Journal of Applied Physiology* 2008.
- Rhea MR, Alderman BL. A meta-analysis of periodized versus nonperiodized strength and power training programs. *Research Quarterly for Exercise and Sport* 2004;75(4):413-422.
- Rhea MR, Ball SD, Phillips WT, Burkett LN. A comparison of linear and daily undulating periodized programs with equated volume and intensity for strength. *Journal of Strength and Conditioning Research* 2002;16(2):250-255.
- Schoenfeld BJ. The mechanisms of muscle hypertrophy and their application to resistance training. *Journal of Strength and Conditioning Research* 2010;24(10):2857-2872.
- Squillante A. *Allenamento della forza*. Giacomo Catalani Editore, Arezzo, 2020.

- Stone MH. et al. Periodization: effects of manipulating volume and intensity. *Strength and Conditioning Journal* 1999;21(2):56.
- Verkhoshansky Y, Verkhoshansky N. *Special strength training: manual for coaches*. Verkhoshansky Sstm., Roma, 2011, p. 274.
- Zatsiorsky VM, Kraemer WJ, Fry AC. *Science and practice of strength training*. Human Kinetics, Champaign (IL), 2020.

Chapter 32

- Cerretelli P. *Fisiologia dell'esercizio. Sport, ambiente, età, sesso*. Società Editrice Universo, Roma, 2001.
- Dal Monte A, Faina M. *Valutazione dell'atleta – Analisi funzionale e biomeccanica della capacità di prestazione*. UTET, Torino, 2003.
- Feldenkrais M. *Le basi del metodo per la consapevolezza dei processi psicomotori*. Casa Editrice Astrolabio, Roma, 1991.
- Kapandji IA. *Fisiologia articolare*. Marrapese Editore, Roma, 1983.
- Lacôte M, Chevalier AM, Miranda A, Bleton JP, Stevenin P. *Valutazione clinica della funzione muscolare*. Marrapese Editore, Roma, 1984.
- Massara G. *Attualità in chinesiterapia*. Marrapese Editore, Roma, 1991.
- Monari G. *Facilitazioni neuromuscolare propriocettive (P.N.F.). Schemi, tecniche e applicazione pratica*. IBS Sud, Roma, 1987.
- Pirola V. *Cinesiologia – Il movimento umano applicato alla rieducazione e alle attività sportive*. Edi.Ermes, Milano, 2002.
- Souchard PE. *Basi del metodo di rieducazione posturale globale*. Marrapese Editore, Roma, 1994.
- Souchard PE. *La respirazione*. Marrapese Editore, Roma, 1996.
- Thie JF. *Manuale di cinesiologia applicata con il "Touch for Health" metodo di integrazione energetica e posturale*. Red Edizioni, Como, 1985.
- Thompson CW. *Manuale di chinesiologia strutturale*. Medical Books, Palermo, 1986.
- Umili A. *Chinesiologia applicata per fitness e bodybuilding*. Società Stampa Sportiva, Roma, 1999.

Chapter 34

- Axler CT, McGill SM. Low back loads over a variety of abdominal exercises: searching for the safest abdominal challenge. *Med Sci Sports Exerc* 1997;29:804-810.
- Daggfeldt K, Thorstensson A. The role of the intra-abdominal pressure in spinal unloadning. *Journal of Biomechanics* 1997;30(11-12):1149-1155.
- Genovese E (a cura di). *Le sindromi da iperuso in atletica leggera*. Ravizza, 2002.
- Hansen T. Core stability training in low-back rehabilitation, 2004.
- Hodges PW, Gandevia SC, Richardson CA. Contractions of specific abdominal muscles in postural tasks are affected by respiratory maneuvers. *J Appl Physiol* 1997;83(3):753-760.
- Hodges PW, Kippers V, Richardson CA. Validation of a technique for accurate fine-wire electrode placement into posterior gluteus medius using real-time ultrasound guidance. *Electromyogr Clin Neurophysiol* 1997;37:39-47.
- Hodges PW, Richardson C, Jull G. Evaluation of the relationship between laboratory and clinical tests of transversus abdominis function. *Physiotherapy Research International* 1996;1:30-40.
- Hodges PW, Richardson CA. Contraction of the abdominal muscles associated with movement of the lower limb. *Physical Therapy* 1997;77(2):132-144.
- Hodges PW, Richardson CA. Feedforward contraction of transversus abdominis is not influenced by the direction of arm movement. *Exp Brain Res* 1997;114:362-370.
- Hodges PW, Richardson CA. Inefficient muscular stabilization of the lumbar spine associated with low back pain. A motor control evaluation of transversus abdominis. *Spine* 1996;21:2640-2650.
- Hodges PW, Richardson CA. Relationship between limb movement speed and associated contraction of the trunk muscles. *Ergonomics* 1997 Nov;40(11):1220-1230.
- Janda V, Va'Vrova M. Sensory motor stimulation. In: Liebenson C. *Rehabilitation of the spine: a practitioner's manual*. Williams and Wilkins, Baltimore, 1996, pp. 319-328.
- Konrad P et al. Neuromuscular evaluation of trunk-training exercises. *J Athl Train* 2001:36(2):109-118
- Kravitz L. Low-back stability training. Article review: McGill SM. Low back stability: from formal description to issues for performance and rehabilitation. *Exerc Sport Sci Rev* 2001;29(1):26-31.
- Kurt T. *Anatomia funzionale dell'uomo applicata all'educazione fisica ed allo sport*. Edi.Ermes, Milano, 1997.
- Lee D. *Terapia fisica del cingolo pelvico*. UTET, Torino, 2000.
- Lehman GJ, Hoda W, Oliver S. Trunk muscle activity during bridging exercises on and

off a swissball. *Chiropratic and Osteopathy* 2005;13:14.
- *Manuale di formazione*. Isokinetic, 2005.
- Marasco M. *Archi funzionali e biomeccanica vertebrale di John Martin Littlejohn. Le connessioni posturali cranio-rachidee*. Marrapese Editore, Roma, 2009.
- Marshall PW, Murphy BA. Core stability exercises on and off a swiss ball. *Archives of Physical Medicine and Rehabilitation* 2005;86:242-249.
- McGill SM, Cholewicki J. Mechanical stability of the in vivo lumbar spine: implication for injury and chronic low back pain. *Clinical Biomechanics* 1996;11(1):1-15.
- McGill SM. Stability: from biomechanical concept to chiropratic practice. *Journal of Canadian Chiropractic Association* 1999.
- Merritt L. Exercise compliance and the gym ball: a case study. *Journal of Canadian Chiropratic Association* 2001;45(4):221-224.
- O'Sullivan PB, Twomey L, Allison GT. Altered abdominal muscle recruitment in patients with chronic back pain following a specific exercise intervention. *JOSPT* 1998;27(2):114-124.
- O'Sullivan PB, Twomey L, Allison GT. Dynamic stabilisation of the lumbar spine. *Critical Reviews in Physical and Rehabilitation Medicine* 1997;9(3-4):315-330.
- Panjabi MM. The stabilizing system of the spine. Part I. Function dysfunction, adaptation and enhancement. *J Spinal Disorders* 1992.
- Panjabi MM. The stabilizing system of the spine. Part II. Neutral zone and instability hypotesis. *J Spinal Disorders* 1992.
- Pivetta S. *Tecnica della ginnastica medica. Cinesiterapia dei vizi posturali. Cifosi – Lordosi – Arti inferiori*. Edi.Ermes, Milano, 1996, pp. 117-130.
- Rasmussen-Barr E, Nilsson-Wikmar L, Arvidsson I. Stabilizing training compared with manual treatment in sub-acute and chronic low-back pain. *Journal of Manipulative and Physiological Therapeutics* 2003;8:233-241.
- Shirado O, Ito T, Kaneda K, Strax TE. Electromyographic analysis of four techniques for isometric trunk muscle exercises. *Arch Phys Med Rehabil* 1995 Mar;76(3):225-229.
- Spinal stabilization training: the transverse abdominus. *Journal of Bodywork and Movement Therapies* 1998;2(4):218-223.
- Stuge B et al. The efficacy of a treatment program focusing on specific stabilizing exercises for pelvic girdle pain after pregnancy. A randomized controlled trial. *Spine* 2004;29:351-359.
- Travell JG, Simons DG. *Il dolore muscolare: diagnosi e terapia*, vol. 1. Ghedini, Milano, 1996.
- Willett GM et al. Relative activity of abdominal muscles during commonly prescribed strengthening exercises. *J Strength Cond Res* 2001;15(4);480-485.
- Wisbey-Roth T. Grading and progressing a dysfunction specific core stability program. *Sportslink* 2000.
- Workman JC, Docherty D, Parfrey KC, Behm DG. Influence of pelvis position on the activation of abdominal and hip flexor muscles. *J Strength Cond Res* 2008 Sep;22(5):1563-1569.

Chapter 37

- Alexander DM et al. Using imagery to enhance performance in powerlifting: a review of theory, research, and practice. *Strength and Conditioning Journal* 2019 Aug.
- Bouguetoch A et al. Does partial activation of the neuromuscular system induce cross-education training effect? Case of a pilot study on motor imagery and neuromuscular electrical stimulation. *European Journal of Applied Physiology* 2021;121(8).
- Buck D et al. The effects of mental imagery with video-modeling on self-efficacy and maximal front squat ability. *Sports* 2016;4(2).
- Castaneda C. *The teachings of Don Juan: a yaqui way of knowledge*. University of California Press, Berkeley, 1968.
- Chaiwanichsiri D. et al. Effects of imagery-weight exercise. *J Med Assoc Thai* 2006 Aug;89.
- Dello Iacono A et al. Ain't just imagination! Effects of motor imagery training on strength and power performance of athletes during detraining. *Medicine & Science in Sports & Exercise* May 2021.
- Ghorbani M et al. The effect of three methods of kinesthetic imagery, active, and combined exercises on electromyographic pattern of hip hyperextension and the muscle strength of gluteus maximus and abdominal in women with lumbar hyperlordosis. *Physical Treatments* 2021;11(3):145-156.
- Hope E et al. A mindful lift-benefits of mindful meditation in strength and conditioning, part 1. *National Strength and Conditioning Association Journal* 2020 Nov.
- Jacobson E. *Progressive relaxation: a physiological and clinical investigation of muscular states and their significance in psychology and medical practice*. University of Chicago Press, Chicago, 1938.

- Kosslyn SM et al. New foundations of imagery. *Nature Reviews Neuroscience* 2001 Oct;2.
- Kubistant T. *Mind pump*. Leisure Press, Champaign (IL), 1988.
- Ladda AM et al. Using motor imagery practice for improving motor performance – A review. *Brain and Cognition* 2021 Feb;150.
- Lebon F et al. Benefits of motor imagery training on muscle strength. *Journal of Strength and Conditioning Research* June 2010;24(6).
- Leonard G. *The ultimate athlete*. North Atlantic Books, Berkeley, 2001.
- Lodge J et al. Children' s self-talk under conditions of mild anxiety. *J Anxiety Disord* Mar-Apr 1998;12(2):153-176.
- Marchant DC et al. Attentional focusing instructions influence force production and muscular activity during isokinetic elbow flexions. *Journal of Strength and Conditioning Research* 2009 Nov;23(8):2358-2366.
- Martin KA et al. Imagery use in sport: a literature review and applied model. *The Sport Psychologist* 1999;13.
- Neige C et al. Pain, no gain: acute pain interrupts motor imagery processes and affects mental training-induced plasticity. *Cerebral Cortex* July 2021.
- Newberg A, Waldman MR. *Words can change your brain*. Avery, New York, 2012.
- Nicassio P, Bootzin R. A comparison of progressive relaxation and autogenic training as treatments for insomnia. *Journal of Abnormal Psychology* 1974;83(3).
- Pakulanon S. The effective imagery use for athletes. *Journal of Sports Science and Health* Jan-Apr 2016;17(1).
- Papeo L et al. The default computation of negated meanings. *Journal Of Cognitive Neuroscience* 2016;28(12).
- Paravlic AH et al. Effects and dose-response relationships of motor imagery practice on strength development in healthy adult populations: a systematic review and meta-analysis. *Sports Medicine* 2018;48.
- Pascual LA et al. Modulation of muscle responses evoked by transcranial magnetic stimulation during the acquisition of new fine motor skills. *Journal of Neurophysiology* Oct 1995.
- Richter J et al. Maximizing strength training performance using mental imagery. *Strength and Conditioning Journal* Oct 2012;34.
- Schoenfeld BJ et al. Attentional focus for maximizing muscle development. *Strength and Conditioning Journal* Feb 2016.
- Schoenfeld BJ et al. Differential effects of attentional focus strategies during long-term resistance training. *European Journal of Sport* 2018.
- Schultz JH, Luthe W. *Autogenic training. A psychophysiologic approach in psychotherapy*. Grune & Stratton, New York, 1959.
- Silbernagel MS et al. Athletes' use of exercise imagery during weight training. *J Strength Cond Res* 2007 Nov;21(4):1077-1081.
- Singh A et al. Autogenic training and progressive muscle relaxation interventions: effects on mental skills of females. *European Journal of Physical Education and Sport Science* 2018;5(8).
- Slimani M et al. Effects of mental imagery on muscular strength in healthy and patient participants: a systematic review. *Journal of Sports Science & Medicine* 2016.

Chapter 38

- Bosco C et al. Adaptive responses of human skeletal muscle to simulated hypergravity condition. *Acta Physiol Scand* 1985;124:507-513.
- Brinkman AK et al. Management of type 1 diabetes. *Nurs Clin North Am* 2017 Dec;52(4):499-511.
- Daxenbichler G et al. Recent advances in steroid biochemistry and molecular biology. *Journal Steroid Biochemistry And Molecular Biology* 2009 Mar;114:195-199.
- Goldstein MS et al. Humoral nature of the hypoglycemic factor of muscular work. *Diabetes* 1961;10:232-234.
- Guo W et al. Testosterone plus low-intensity physical training in late life improves functional performance, skeletal muscle mitochondrial biogenesis, and mitochondrial quality control in male mice. *PLoS One* 2012;7(12).
- Haff GG et al. *Essentials of strength training and conditioning*, 4th ed. NSCA – National Strength and Conditioning Association 2015 Sept;4.
- Hoffmann C et al. Skeletal muscle as an endocrine organ: the role of myokines in exercise adaptations. *Perspect Med* 2017 Nov 1;7(11).
- Kraemer WJ et al. Hormonal and growth factor responses to heavy resistance exercise protocols. *J Appl Physiol* (1985) 1990 Oct; 69(4):1442-1450.
- Kraemer WJ et al. Muscle mass, strength training and testosterone. *J App Physiol* 1999 sep;87(3):982-992.
- Kraemer WJ et al. The endocrine system in sports and exercise. *The Encyclopaedia of Sports* 2008 Mar;11:110-112.

- Kumagai H et al. Increased physical activity has a greater effect than reduced energy intake on lifestyle modification-induced increases in testosterone. *J Clin Biochem Nutr* 2016 Jan;58(1):84-89.
- Morgentaler A et al. The history of testosterone and the evolution of its therapeutic potential. *Sex Med Rev* 2020 Apr;8(2):286-296.
- Nicholls AR et al. Growth hormone and insulin-like growth factor-1. *Front Horm Res* 2016;47:101-114.
- Ostrowski J et al. Stimulation of p85/RING3 kinase in multiple organs after systemic administration of mitogens into mice. *Oncogene* 1998;16:1223-1227.
- Pedersen BK et al. Muscle-organ crosstalk: the emerging roles of myokines. *Endocr Rev* 2020 Aug 1;41(4):594-609.
- Pedersen BK et al. Muscles, exercise and obesity: skeletal muscle as a secretory organ. *Nat Rev Endocrinol* 2012 Apr 3;8(8):457-465.
- Ronald JS. Effects of aerobic training, resistance training, or both on control of blood sugar in type 2 diabetes. *Ann Intern Med. Ann Intern Med* 2007 Sep 18;147(6):357-369.
- Schnyder S et al. Skeletal muscle as an endocrine organ: PGC-1alpha, myokines and exercise. *Bone* 2015 Nov;80:115-125.
- Sokoloff N et al. Exercise, training, and the hypothalamic-pituitary-gonadal axis in men and women. *Sports Endocrinology* 2016;47(27-43).
- Spattini M, Bevacqua E. *Guida alla medicina funzionale. La medicina del domani*. Edra, Milano, 2019.
- Stanton SJ et al. Testosterone and sport: current perspectives. *Horm Behav* 2012 Jan;61(1):147-155.
- Steensberg A et al. Interleukin-6 production in contracting human skeletal muscle is influenced by pre-exercise muscle glycogen content. *Journal of Physiology* 2001;537(2):633-639.
- Werlang Coelho C et al. Muscle power increases after resistance training in growth-hormone-deficient adults. *Med Sci Sports Exerc* 2002 Oct;34(10):1577-1581.

Chapter 39

- Alfonso J et al. Strength training versus stretching for improving range of motion: a systematic review and meta-analysis. *Healthcare (Basel)* 2021 Apr 7;9(4):427.
- Aristizabal JC et al. Effect of resistance training on resting metabolic rate and its estimation by a dual-energy X-ray absorptiometry metabolic map. *Eur J Clin Nutr* 2015 Jul;69(7):831-836.
- Arsenis NC, et al. Physical activity and telomere length: Impact of aging and potential mechanisms of action. *Oncotarget*. 2017 Jul 4;8(27):45008-45019.
- Beato M et al. Implementing strength training strategies for injury prevention in soccer: scientific rationale and methodological recommendations. *Int J Sports Physiol Perform* 2021 Jan 27;16(3):456-461.
- Beck BR et al. Exercise and Sports Science Australia (ESSA) position statement on exercise prescription for the prevention and management of osteoporosis. *J Sci Med Sport* 2017 May;20(5):438-445.
- Benedetti MG et al. The effectiveness of physical exercise on bone density in osteoporotic patients. *Biomed Res Int* 2018;2018:4840531.
- Bull FC et al. World Health Organization 2020 guidelines on physical activity and sedentary behaviour. *Br J Sports Med* 2020 Nov25;54(24):1451-1462.
- Calatayud J et al. Tolerability and muscle activity of core muscle exercises in chronic low-back pain. *Int J Environ Res Public Health* 2019 Oct;16(19):3509.
- Canuto Wanderley FA et al. Aerobic versus resistance training effects on health-related quality of life, body composition, and function of older adults. *J Appl Gerontol* 2015 Apr;34(3):NP143-165.
- Chakraborty D et al. Fibroblast growth factor receptor is a mechanistic link between visceral adiposity and cancer. *Oncogene* 2017 Nov 30;36(48):6668–6679.
- Choi JH et al. Comparison of trunk muscle activity between traditional plank exercise and plank exercise with isometric contraction of ankle muscles in subjects with chronic low back pain. *J Strength Cond Res* 2021 Sep 1;35(9):2407-2413.
- Chupel MU et al. Strength training decreases inflammation and increases cognition and physical fitness in older women with cognitive impairment. *Front Physiol* 2017 Jun 12;8:377.
- Ciccolo JT et al. Muscular strength is associated with self-esteem in college men but not women. *J Health Psychol* 2016 Dec;21(12):3072-3078.
- Colberg SR et al. Physical activity/exercise and diabetes: a position statement of the american diabetes association. *Diabetes Care* 2016 Nov;39(11):2065-2079.
- Collins H et al. The effect of resistance training interventions on "the self" in youth: a sys-

tematic review and meta-analysis. *Sports Med Open* 2019 Dec;5:29.

- Costa RR et al. Effect of strength training on lipid and inflammatory outcomes: systematic review with meta-analysis and meta-regression. *J Phys Act Health* 2019 Jun 1;16(6):477-491.
- D'Aurea Carolina VR et al. Effects of resistance exercise training and stretching on chronic insomnia. *Braz J Psychiatry* 2019 Jan-Feb;41(1):51-57.
- De Camargo Smolarek A et al. The effects of strength training on cognitive performance in elderly women. *Clin Interv Aging* 2016 Jun 1;11:749-754.
- De Mutsert R et al. Associations of abdominal subcutaneous and visceral fat with insulin resistance and secretion differ between men and women: the netherlands epidemiology of obesity study. *Metab Syndr Relat Disord* 2018 Feb;16(1):54-63.
- De Sousa EC et al. Resistance training alone reduces systolic and diastolic blood pressure in prehypertensive and hypertensive individuals: meta-analysis. *Hypertens Res* 2017 Nov;40(11):927-931.
- Edouard P et al. The athletics injury prevention programme can help to reduce the occurrence at short term of participation restriction injury complaints in athletics: a prospective cohort study. *Sports (Basel)* 2020 Jun 4;8(6):84.
- Elavsky S et al. Physical activity enhances long-term quality of life in older adults: efficacy, esteem, and affective influences. *Ann Behav Med* 2005 Oct;30(2):138-145.
- Fragala MS et al. Resistance training for older adults: position statement from the national strength and conditioning association. *Journal of Strength and Conditioning Research* 2019 Aug;33(8):2019-2052.
- Gareth Burt D et al. Effects of exercise-induced muscle damage on resting metabolic rate, sub-maximal running and post-exercise oxygen consumption. *Eur J Sport Sci* 2014;14(4):337-344.
- Gordon BR et al. Association of efficacy of resistance exercise training with depressive symptoms: meta-analysis and meta-regression analysis of randomized clinical trials. *JAMA Psychiatry* 2018 Jun 1;75(6):566-576.
- Gordon BR et al. Resistance exercise training for anxiety and worry symptoms among young adults: a randomized controlled trial. *Sci Rep* 2020;10:17548.
- Gordon BR et al. The effects of resistance exercise training on anxiety: a meta-analysis and meta-regression analysis of randomized controlled trials. *Sports Med* 2017 Dec;47(12):2521-2532.
- Gordon R, Bloxham S. A systematic review of the effects of exercise and physical activity on non-specific chronic low back pain. *Healthcare (Basel)* 2016 Jun;4(2):22.
- Hart PD, Buck DJ. The effect of resistance training on health-related quality of life in older adults: systematic review and meta-analysis. *Health Promot Perspect* 2019;9(1):1-12.
- Hong AR, Kim SW. Effects of resistance exercise on bone health. Endocrinol Metab (Seoul) 2018 Dec;33(4):435-444.
- Ihalainen JK et al. Strength training improves metabolic health markers in older individual regardless of training frequency. *Front Physiol* 2019 Feb 1;10:32.
- Jaggers JR et al. Aerobic and resistance training improves mood state among adults living with HIV. *Int J Sports Med* 2015 Feb;36(2):175-181.
- Jones RG 3rd, et al. A molecular signature defining exercise adaptation with ageing and in vivo partial reprogramming in skeletal muscle. *The journal of Physiology*. First published: 19 December 2022.
- Joseph RP et al. Physical activity and quality of life among university students: exploring self-efficacy, self-esteem, and affect as potential mediators. *Qual Life Res* 2014 Mar;23(2):659-667.
- Kekäläinen T et al. Effects of a 9-month resistance training intervention on quality of life, sense of coherence, and depressive symptoms in older adults: randomized controlled trial. *Qual Life Res* 2018;27(2):455-465.
- Lauersen JB et al. Strength training as superior, dose-dependent and safe prevention of acute and overuse sports injuries: a systematic review, qualitative analysis and meta-analysis. *Br J Sports Med* 2018 Dec;52(24):1557-1563.
- Lee JH et al. Resistance training for glycemic control, muscular strength, and lean body mass in old type 2 diabetic patients: a meta-analysis. *Diabetes Ther* 2017 Jun;8(3):459-473.
- Leite TB et al. Effects of different number of sets of resistance training on flexibility. *Int J Exerc Sci* 2017;10(3):354-364.
- Li Z et al. The effect of resistance training on cognitive function in the older adults: a systematic review of randomized clinical trials. *Aging Clin Exp Res* 2018 Nov;30(11):1259-1273.
- Liu Y et al. Resistance exercise intensity is correlated with attenuation of HbA1c and insulin in patients with type 2 diabetes: a systematic re-

view and meta-analysis. *Int J Environ Res Public Health* 2019 Jan;16(1):140.

- MacDonald HV et al. Dynamic resistance training as stand-alone antihypertensive lifestyle therapy: a meta-analysis. *J Am Heart Assoc* 2016 Sep 28;5(10):e003231.
- MacKenzie-Shalders K et al. The effect of exercise interventions on resting metabolic rate: a systematic review and meta-analysis. *J Sports Sci* 2020 Jul;38(14):1635-1649.
- Maestroni L et al. The benefits of strength training on musculoskeletal system health: practical applications for interdisciplinary care. *Sports Med* 2020 Aug;50(8):1431-1450.
- Mason C, Risques RA, et al. Independent and combined effects of dietary weight loss and exercise on leukocyte telomere length in postmenopausal women. *Obesity (Silver Spring)* 2013;21:E549–554.
- Mavros Y et al. Mediation of cognitive function improvements by strength gains after resistance training in older adults with mild cognitive impairment: outcomes of the study of mental and resistance training. *J Am Geriatr Soc* 2017 Mar;65(3):550-559.
- Mcleod JC et al. Resistance exercise training as a primary countermeasure to age-related chronic disease. *Front Physiol* 2019;10:645.
- McMurray RG et al. Examining variations of resting metabolic rate of adults: a public health perspective. *Med Sci Sports Exerc* 2014 Jul;46(7):1352-1358.
- McPherron AC et al. Increasing muscle mass to improve metabolism. *Adipocyte* 2013 Apr 1;2(2):92-98.
- Mekary RA et al. Weight training, aerobic physic (al activities, and long-term waist circumference change in men. *Obesity (Silver Spring)* 2015 Feb;23(2):461-467.
- Mosti MP et al. Maximal strength training improves bone mineral density and neuromuscular performance in young adult women. *J Strength Cond Res* 2014 Oct;28(10):2935-2945.
- Nam GE et al. Association between abdominal obesity and incident colorectal cancer: a nationwide cohort study in korea. *Cancers (Basel)* 2020 May 26;12(6):1368.
- Pallarés JG et al. Effects of range of motion on resistance training adaptations: a systematic review and meta-analysis. *Scand J Med Sci Sports* 2021 Oct;31(10):1866-1881.
- Park BS et al. Effects of elastic band resistance training on glucose control, body composition, and physical function in women with short- vs. long-duration type-2 diabetes. *J Strength Cond Res* 2016 Jun;30(6):1688-1699.
- Pereira ES et al. Significant acute response of brain-derived neurotrophic factor following a session of extreme conditioning program is correlated with volume of specific exercise training in trained men. *Front Physiol* 2018;9:823.
- Roberts CK et al. Untrained young men have dysfunctional HDL compared with strength-trained men irrespective of body weight status. *J Appl Physiol* (1985) 2013 Oct 1;115(7):1043-1049.
- Rowe P et al. *Physiology, bone remodeling.* StatPearls Publishing, Treasure Island (FL), 2021 Jan.
- Sadler S et al. Gluteus medius muscle function in people with and without low back pain: a systematic review. *BMC Musculoskelet Disord* 2019 Oct 22;20(1):463.
- SantaBarbara NJ et al. A systematic review of the effects of resistance training on body image. *J Strength Cond Res* 2017 Oct;31(10):2880-2888.
- Schoenfeld BJ, Grgic J. Effects of range of motion on muscle development during resistance training interventions: a systematic review. *SAGE Open Med* 2020;8:2050312120901559.
- Sherrington C et al. Exercise for preventing falls in older people living in the community. *Cochrane Database Syst Rev* 2019 Jan 31;1(1):CD012424.
- Shiroma EJ et al. Strength training and the risk of type 2 diabetes and cardiovascular disease. *Med Sci Sports Exerc* 2017 Jan;49(1):40-46.
- Sieczkowska SM et al. Effects of resistance training on the health-related quality of life of patients with rheumatic diseases: systematic review with meta-analysis and meta-regression. *Semin Arthritis Rheum* 2020 Apr;50(2):342-353.
- Silveira EA et al. Visceral obesity and its shared role in cancer and cardiovascular disease: a scoping review of the pathophysiology and pharmacological treatments. *Int J Mol Sci* 2020 Dec;21(23):9042.
- Sözen T et al. An overview and management of osteoporosis. *Eur J Rheumatol* 2017 Mar;4(1):46-56.
- Srikanthan P, Karlamangla AS. Muscle mass index as a predictor of longevity in older adults. *The American Journal of Medicine* 2014 June 1;127(6):547-553.
- Srikanthan P, Karlamangla AS. Relative muscle mass is inversely associated with insulin

resistance and prediabetes. Findings from the third national health and nutrition examination survey. *J Clin Endocrinol Metab* 2011 Sep;96(9):2898-2903.
- Strickland JC, Smith MA. The anxiolytic effects of resistance exercise. Front Psychol 2014;5:753.
- Suchomel TJ et al. The importance of muscular strength: training considerations. *Sports Med* 2018 Apr;48(4):765-785.
- Thomas MH, Burns SP. Increasing lean mass and strength: a comparison of high frequency strength training to lower frequency strength training. *Int J Exerc Sci* 2016;9(2):159-167.
- Vechetti IJ et al. Mechanical overload-induced muscle-derived extracellular vesicles promote adipose tissue lipolysis. *The FASEB Journal* 2021;35(6).
- Villareal DT et al. Aerobic or resistance exercise, or both, in dieting obese older adults. *N Engl J Med* 2017 May 18;376(20):1943-1955.
- Volpi E et al. Muscle tissue changes with aging. *Curr Opin Clin Nutr Metab Care* 2004 Jul;7(4):405-410.
- Walters BK et al. The effects of resistance training, overtraining, and early specialization on youth athlete injury and development. *J Sports Med Phys Fitness* 2018 Sep;58(9):1339-1348.
- Wilke J et al. Acute effects of resistance exercise on cognitive function in healthy adults: a systematic review with multilevel meta-analysis. *Sports Med* 2019 Jun;49(6):905-916.
- Xu C et al. Visceral adiposity index as a predictor of NAFLD: a prospective study with 4-year follow-up. *Liver Int* 2018 Dec;38(12):2294-2300.
- Yand J et al. Association between push-up exercise capacity and future cardiovascular events among active adult men. *JAMA Network Open* 2019;2(2):e188341.
- Yarizadeh H et al. The effect of aerobic and resistance training and combined exercise modalities on subcutaneous abdominal fat: a systematic review and meta-analysis of randomized clinical trials. *Adv Nutr* 2021 Feb 1;12(1):179-196.
- Yoon DH et al. Effects of resistance exercise training on cognitive function and physical performance in cognitive frailty: a randomized controlled trial. *J Nutr Health Aging* 2018;22(8):944-951.
- Zamani Sani SH et al. Physical activity and self-esteem: testing direct and indirect relationships associated with psychological and physical mechanisms. *Neuropsychiatr Dis Treat* 2016;12:2617-2625.

Acknowledgments

It's been a long time since my days of training in a garage with little more than improvised weights, but my passion for "iron" has accompanied me to this day.

While it is true that bodybuilding is an individual sport, I have believed in the importance of having a groupever since I opened the New Center Gym, so much so that I created a team so that which has churned out dozens of champions, who grew up and trained in the gym itself, and even hundreds more if you consider those who came from other gyms to be trained by me. When I opened my medical center and school, I always tried to build a group with the intention of helping others grow by passing on my knowledge and, in return, growing myself because teaching is unquestionably a two-way discipline.

Thus, for each of my books (we have now reached the tenth, not counting the English editions), I have always found it necessary and useful to involve the people I am surrounded with. The idea for this book periodically popped into my head, but The idea for this book Riccardo Gaspari, so it was only natural to involve esteemed professional friends, collaborators, and trainees, who are all instilled with a fervent passion for resistance training and for studying and being constantly up-to-date. The only *prerequisite is to practice what you preach.*

I believe, and hope, that this book is fundamentally different from all the others that can be found on the market for this sport, because here Riccardo, Federico, and I approach training through our direct experiences in the field, with what worked (and still works today) better for us and for the countless athletes (professional and amateur) we have trained with and have trained and whom we have personally followed over the years. Furthermore, the impact that this sport has on the entire body, including the brain and heart, has also been taken into consideration. Even the WHO, finally heartily recommends regular training with weights at all ages to better manage training, even in the presence of any type of disease (if it is not disabling).

Now, before the dutiful citations for the work done by all those who have contributed to the realization of this work, I would like to say a few words on behalf of my friend, collaborator, and exceptional professional, Davide Antoniella, who died prematurely before this book could see the light of day.

I met Davide many years ago and it was his thirst for knowledge that led him to contact me.

As, an athletic trainer, he also wanted to learn about sports medicine and the world of nutrition and supplements. From the beginning, a deep connection was born, as I recognized his great passion and his impressive preparation. Therefore, I added him to the teaching staff of my Functional Academy of Fitness Wellness and Antiaging (AFFWA) and subsequently a working collaboration was born with the opening of the Motor Evaluation Center, to complete my medical studies. But if Davide's technical qualities were, I would say, unique and exceptional, his human ones were even more so. He was always ready to help anyone and went out of his way for patients and friends. He was able to create an atmosphere of consideration and benevolence around him which, I believe, only a few can enjoy in equal measure. Davide, we will miss you very much, but your technical and human teaching will always be with us.

Massimo Spattini

Below is a brief presentation of the three co-authors of this volume.

Massimo Spattini Former Italian bodybuilding champion (born in Parma, in 1957), medical doctor, university professor, speaker at international congresses, journalist, popularizer, and best-seller writer. He has been President of AFFWA for years, organizing and teaching courses for Fitness and Bodybuilding instructors, Personal Trainers, and Athletic trainers. He opened the New Center Gym in Parma, of which he was also technical and health director; this gym was the "mecca" of bodybuilding in Italy in the 80s and 90s. From the early 80s, he he has travelled every year to Los Angeles, where he has friends, and collaborates with the leading exponents of international bodybuilding and anti-aging medicine. He works in Parma at the Massimo Spattini medical office. He specializes in Sports Medicine, Food Science and Dietetics, and is certified in Antiaging Medicine, Functional Medicine and Peptide Therapy in the USA.

Publications

- 2012: author of the book *La dietaCOM® e il dimagrimento localizzato*, Tecniche Nuove.
- 2013: author of the book *Antiaging e lo stile di vita integrato*, Tecniche Nuove.
- 2014: author of the book *La DietaCOM® in pratica*, Tecniche Nuove.
- 2014: author of the book *The COMdiet & spot reduction – ChronohOrMorpho Diet*, self-publishing.
- 2016: author of the book *Alimentazione e integrazione per lo sport e la performance fisica*, Edizioni LSWR.
- 2019: co-author of the book *Guida alla medicina funzionale. La medicina del domani*, Edizioni Edra.
- 2020: author of the book *Alimentazione e integrazione per lo sport e la performance fisica*, 2a edizione aggiornata e ampliata, Edizioni LSWR.
- 2020: author of the book *La Dieta Antivirus. Come potenziare il tuo sistema immunitario*, Edizioni LSWR.
- 2021: author of the book *Alimentazione e Integrazione per gli Ormoni e la Mente*, Edizioni LSWR.
- 2022: author of the book *Nutrition and supplementation for sport and physical performance*, Edizioni Edra.
- 2022: co-author of the book *Guida al Controllo Glicemico. Il trattamento non farmacologico dell'insulino-resistenza nella prevenzione del diabete*, Edizioni Edra.

Sports sector

- 1981: Emilian IFBB Heavyweight Champion.
- 1984: winner of the IFBB "Notte dei Campioni".
- 1986: Italian IFBB Heavyweight Champion.
- 1986: winner of the IFBB "Notte dei Campioni".
- 1988: winner of the selection for the IFBB World Championships.

Riccardo Gaspari Former Italian bodybuilding vice-champion (born in Cremona, in 1983), he is CEO founder of Personal Point Fitness&Nutrition, a personal training center and consulting firm where the author, working with a team of collaborators at an international level, follows any client from anywhere the world with a comprehensive approach.

Being a wellness consultant at various facilities throughout Italy, he is often requested as a fitness manager to organize the technical and managerial work of the most exclusive companies in the world of fitness and spas in Italy.

He organizes and participates as a speaker in conferences and themed seminars to spread the habit of well-being. He specializes in body recomposition and athletic preparations and also provides advice online. Hundreds of articles on the web bear his signature, ranging between practical and scientific arguments. Certified One to One Personal Trainer, he was an international fitness champion and has done product endorsement for market-leading companies, and also includes in his training course the rosette assigned by the Supplement Research Foundation; he still does intense research and study to always provide up-to-date data and cutting-edge services which, combined with passion and professionalism, represent his best calling card. Listed below are a few of the many competitions he has entered with WABBA:

- Podium GP Cercenasco 2010 HP/169 cm.
- Podium GP Cercenasco 2011 HP/169 cm.
- Triveneto champion HP/168 cm BB short 170 cm 2015.
- Hercules Olympia BB short 170 cm 2016 champion.
- Italian runner-up BB short 170 cm 2016.
- World podium BB short 170 cm 2016.
- Podium GP Planet BB short 170 cm 2016.

Currently, every day with enthusiasm, he makes his 20 years of experience in the world of fitness available to his customers, accompanying them on their path to success.

Author of the book *Beating cellulite with nutrition, supplements, and training* (LSWR Editions), he collaborates with some of the most prominent figures in the fitness and wellness sector and with market-leading companies in the production of fitness equipment and food supplements.

Federico Focherini Former Mr. Universe (born in Modena, in 1967) and One to One Personal Trainer with enormous experience in the field of competitions. Because of his cultural background in the field of training methodologies, his help is particularly requested by both Italian and foreign professionals. He has never stopped experimenting with the various existing training techniques and keeps training every day, with unchanged passion, offering his many clients only what can be functional to their success.

In his track record, he can boast about being NABBA Italian champion in 1989, NABBA European champion in 1995, NABBA world champion in 1995, and NABBA Absolute Mr. Universe in 1996. He was an IFBB professional bodybuilder in the 1997-2002 period, twice IFBB South African over 40 champion in 2008-2009, the 2018 NABBA Asian champion over 50, and bronze at the 2018 Australian National Championships.

From 1986 to 2018 he participated in 80 official competitions, of which 20 were in South Africa and 20 were between the European Championships, World Championships, Mr. Universe, and Mr. Australasia.

In his career, he has represented three different nations in international competitions: Italy, South Africa, and Kuwait.

The following are the key moments of his 32-year competing career:

- October 1996, Birmingham (UK): winning the Amateur Overall Mr. Universe (the first Italian to win it);

- October 1998, Germany and Finland: IFBB professional debut together with Ronnie Coleman (according to Federico, to date the greatest bodybuilder in history) and the top 10 bodybuilders in the world;
- December 2010: he was selected for the South African national bodybuilding team for the IFBB World Championships in Turkey, obtaining the official recognition of "Springbok" by the Government of the Republic of South Africa;
- October 2017: in Kuwait City, he was inducted into the Hall of Fame by the former NABBA World President Graeme Lancefield.

Certified Master Trainer in Italy and South Africa, he has worked as a bodybuilding and fitness coach in Italy, 1 year in Tucson (Arizona, USA), 9 years in Pretoria (South Africa), and 4 years in Salmiya (Kuwait). As we are writing these lines, he is back in Kuwait, invited directly by the Minister of Defense (the king's nephew), to train him personally, with the future option of training the local special forces.

His presence is often requested as a speaker in seminars with a strong practical connotation, where he illustrates in detail the correct execution of the exercises and various training techniques.

You can follow and contact him on social media on his Instagram channel: @federicofocherini.

Before contributing to this work, he wrote and published three other books: *El bonito crimen de los carabineros*, Eumeswil Edizioni, Broni (PV), 2006, in Italian; *The law of contempt*, CIESSE Edizioni, Montegrotto Terme (PD), 2014, in Italian; *Outrage of law*, CIESSE Edizioni, Montegrotto Terme (PD), 2015, in English.

At this point the time has finally come to introduce one by one, in strict alphabetical order, all those who have collaborated to the creation of this bodybuilding "encyclopedia".

Davide Antoniella has contributed, together with Ivan Martellato, to the drafting of Chapter 33 and previously collaborated in the drafting of the volumes *Antiaging and the integrated lifestyle, and Guide to Functional Medicine – The medicine of tomorrow*, for which he wrote a whole chapter.

As mentioned above, our dear friend and collaborator Davide passed away during the proofreading of the book, following an illness that left him with no future. We dedicate to his memory the affection of all those who knew and esteemed him as a highly trained professional. Below are his achievements.

He graduated in 1986 from the Higher Institute of Physical Education with a score of 110/110 cum laude: the D.O. Osteopathy, the multipurpose post-university specialization for teaching Support, the specialization of AIPAC professional Athletic Trainer and FIDAL youth and third-grade Volleyball Coach (Serie A), the specialization in physical exercise with patients suffering from chronic pathologies at the ASL 16 M.D.S.; the specialization at the International Society of Health Prevention – USA: Physical, functional evaluation and exercise prescription for physical fitness and recovery.

He attended the Open Academy of Medicine School of Medical Specialization and Continuing Medical Education: I-II-III-IV-V-VI annual Training Course on Neuroimmunomodulation, Metabolism, Clinic Nutrition, and Physical Rehabilitation.

He was Antiaging Advisor (AFFWA graduate) and had the Lifestyle Medicine & Functional Medicine Certification (AFFWA). He worked in the field of professional athletic training and rehabilitation at the Motor Evaluation Center of Parma. He collaborated with sports medicine and research centers for evaluation tests and application protocols, and for the functional evaluation and cardiological rehabilitation. He was co-author of several books and various articles in Italian scientific-popular journals. He was a lecturer at universities, federations, institutes, and promotional bodies.

Samir Bannout wrote the preface. Nicknamed the "Lion of Lebanon", he moved to the United States in 1978. In 1979 he won the IFBB World Amateur Championships, and in 1983 he won the IFBB Mr. Olympia title, the most important title for bodybuilding professionals. In 1984 he finished sixth at Mr. Olympia; convinced of having been penalized in the placement, in 1985 he moved to WABBA and won the World Championship for professionals in 1985 and 1986. In 1988 he competed again at Mr. Olympia but finished in eighth place. The following year he competed in the NABBA World Championships Professional, finishing in second place.

Subsequently, he returned to the IFBB and won his last competition as a professional: the 1990 Pittsburgh Pro Invitational. His last time on stage was in 2011, at the IFBB Pro World Masters Bodybuilding. He was the first bodybuilder from a Middle Eastern country to win Mr. Olympia. He was the only bodybuilder to defeat eight-time Mr. Olympia Lee Haney in a Mr. Olympia contest (Dr. Spattini, in 1988, when he was his training partner during his Mr. Olympia comeback, was also present in an interview ("The road to the Olympia") during which the interviewer pointed out that Lee Haney had stated that the only competitor he feared was Samir Bannout). He was the last Mr. Olympia to weigh less than 90 kg, the last of aesthetic bodybuilding.

Marco Tullio Cau contributed to the drafting of Chapter 37 and, previously, wrote some chapters of the volumes *Antiaging and the integrated lifestyle, Nutrition and supplementation for sport and physical performance, Guide to Functional Medicine – The medicine of tomorrow,* and *Nutrition and supplementation for hormones and the mind.* He obtained a degree in Clinical Psychology at the "Sapienza" University of Rome and subsequently a degree in Communication Sciences and Sociology at the same university. In addition, he attended numerous masters, including the master's degree in Clinical Nutrition at the Niccolò Cusano University, Rome, the two-year master's degree in Sport Psychology (Scuola Superiore di Psicologia dello Sport, Rome), the master's degree in Psychology of Food Behavior SPICAP also in Rome. He participated in the advanced training course in Antiaging and Antistress Methodology at the "Sapienza" University, in the "Lifestyle Expert over 60" specialization course at the University of Bari, in the two-year course as a sexual consultant (ISC-Rome) and has obtained various certifications, such as the AMFPC (Metabolic and Functional Approach in Clinical Practice) of AFFWA, the ECPS (EFS-ESSM Qualified Psycho-Sexologist, first world certification, Istanbul, Turkey) and others in the USA, where he also attended university courses at the Faculty of Psychology and Sociology of the University of California, Santa Barbara.

He is a lecturer at AFFWA, AMIA, Sanis, Issa-Italia, NABBA, for the Scuola dello Sport del Coni and for the training course "Wellness and lifestyles", held at the " La Sapienza" University. He has obtained the Lifestyle Medicine & Functional Medicine Certification (AFFWA). He was Italian junior bodybuilding champion (NABBA) in 1983 and, in accordance with the motto "practice what you preach", he still competes in discus throwing competitions, a discipline in which he competes for the Principality of Monaco, after having been multi-time champion and national Masters record holder.

Ciro di Cristino was the contributing author to Chapters 32 and 40.

Previously, he contributed to the drafting of chapters for the volumes *Antiaging and the integrated lifestyle* and *Guide to Functional Medicine – The medicine of tomorrow.* An ISEF graduate, he is Educator, Physical and Athletic Trainer. He was a rugby player in Noceto (PR) and later a coach and physical-athletic trainer of the youth sector, he was also the physical-athletic trainer for the FIR (Italian Rugby Federation) Youth National Teams. Over time he has refined his knowledge by participating in various in-depth courses: Connective tissue massage, Podalic massage, Touch for Health, Hemispheric integration, Wellbach (Pancafit), Use of the Fitball (in the kinesiological, sports, and fitness fields), Corrective Gymnastics, Ortho-Bionomy. In state schools, in addition to teaching, he has carried out projects for the recovery and enhancement of cognitive abilities through motor activity, health education through correct lifestyles, and psychomotricity, also collaborating with the Department of Sport of the Municipality of Parma. He was a lecturer at the "Sapienza" University of Rome in the training course "Wellness and Lifestyles"; he held a seminar at the University of Cassino: "The use of bodybuilding equipment in the athletic preparation of team sports"; and was a tutor in "Sports Medicine", Faculty of Medicine, Motor Sciences course at the University of Parma. He has also been a bodybuilding teacher at courses of various associations and competition judge at NABBA, AINBB, IFBB, WABBA, AIF, SIFe-SM, IFSB, FIH/P, Due Torri, Miss Fitness, Body Fitness. He has participated as a speaker at national and international conferences and congresses. He has collaborated with the magazines *New Vigor, Sportman e Fitness, Cultura Fisica, Sport e Salute, Gli Speciali dell'Accademia del Fitness, Olympian's News* and *L'Accademia del Fitness Wellness Antiaging*. He is co-author of the volumes: *Antiaging and integrated lifestyle* (Tecniche Nuove), for the chapter *Posture, Work environment, and functional capacities; Guide to Functional Medicine* (Edra Editions), for the chapter *Structural imbalances affecting the musculoskeletal system*. An expert in kinesiology and posturology, he has never stopped studying and practicing body-building.

Fernando R. Finardi was the contributing author to Chapter 39. He is Lifestyle Medicine and Functional Medicine Advisor, Personal Trainer, Food Educator with a master's degree in Antiaging Nutrition (AFFWA Academy). Over time he has practiced judo, athletics, cycling, jogging, and pilates, but bodybuilding is the sport that, after 39 years, he still carries on with passion and perseverance, supporting it with a balanced diet, anti-aging supplementation, and a correct lifestyle. As an insatiable reader of books, medical literature, and scientific articles relating to health and well-being, and as a firsthand practitioner of the acquired concepts, he wanted to help explain how bodybuilding, in the light of current scientific knowledge, is able to impact health in general and can contribute to successful age management. He collaborated in the revision of the texts of this volume and in maintaining relations with the co-authors and various collaborators, the publishing house, and the editorial studio. A great friend of Dr. Spattini, he has practically always joined him as first reader and trusted travel companion in his long and exciting publishing adventure.

Valeria Galfano was the contributing author to Chapter 23. She has a degree in Medicine and Surgery, specializing in Food Science, and she is an expert in metabolic pathologies, eating disorders, nutrition and sports supplementation.

She obtained her specialization at the "Sapienza" University of Rome and worked at the CASCO center (Centre of High Specialization for the Treatment of Obesity) at the Policlinico Umberto I. She has been interested in nutrition and sports supplements for many years, teaching at SIFA with the course "Training, nutrition and integration for women". She is a CSEN and OPES teacher for basic, advanced, and elite-level Personal Trainer courses. She has organized two university masters for SISDCA (Italian Society for the Study of Eating Disorders), dealing with topics related to bulimia nervosa and orthorexia nervosa. She holds the Lifestyle Medicine & Functional Medicine Certification (AF-FWA). She is co-author of the book *Guide to glycemic control* (EDRA Editions) and has written some chapters of the volumes *Nutrition and supplementation for hormones and the mind* (LSWR Editions), *Dietary prevention and therapy* (Il Pensiero Scientifico), *Nutrition and supplementation for sport and physical performance, 2nd edition* (LSWR Editions) and *Hidden and lesser-known eating disorders*. She is a co-author of scientific articles for the *L'Endocrinologo* journal and author of health news articles for the newspapers *Assocarenews* and *NurseTime*. In 2015 she became passionate about bodybuilding and since then she competes regularly in the bikini category. Winner of Miss Etruria BBF 2015 and of the BBF World Championship 2015, she currently competes in the IFBB federation, qualifying among the top positions and obtaining qualification for the Italian Championship for 3 consecutive years. In 2020 she obtained the OPES national diploma of advanced level Personal Trainer and the qualification of Competition Judge for bodybuilding.

Steven Giuffrida was the contributing author to Chapter 34. He has a competitive background in swimming and martial arts and has a passion for bodybuilding. He started his training course at the Italian Fitness Federation whuich awarded him the qualification of Top Trainer and Personal Trainer. Graduating in Motor and Sports Activity Sciences, he began to develop a passion for medical issues, earning various masters in the rehabilitation sector, up to a specialization in Medical Wellness.

He obtained the title of *massage therapist*, and specialized in therapeutic, sports, trigger point, postural massage, cranio-mandibular disorders and joint mobilization techniques. Being the technical director of numerous sports centres, he is also dedicated to the consultancy and athletic training of athletes who have achieved international titles. He began his training in Posturology by obtaining a master's degree in Functional Clinical Posturology under the patronage of the "Sapienza" University of Rome and the University of Palermo, until he held the role of speaker at various conferences, as well as lecturer in Posturology, specializing in shoulder, knee and ankle rehabilitation, and training methodologies applied to spinal column pathologies. He is a speaker at numerous conferences in the medical field: Angiology ("The skin ulcer in the center of the Mediterranean"), Diabetes ("Wellness and diabetes mellitus"), Orthopedics ("Videosurgery on the main orthopedic pathologies"), Posturology. He is a member of the medical-scientific committee of ADAS (Association for the Defense of the Environment and Health) and writes numerous articles on the subject of health and well-being. He currently dedicates his training and work activity to Medical Wellness, i.e. the training of subjects suffering from metabolic pathologies, alternating this activity with sports and rehabilitation massage therapy as well as postural gymnastics. Passionate about bodybuilding, he began his career as a WABBA athlete and then as a judge. His career culminates with the position of Chief Judge of WABBA International; moreover, he attends the most important national and international competitions. Today he continues his activity as a competitive athlete as a Master FIN swimmer.

Ivan Martellato contributed to the description of some of the exercises reported in Chapter 42 and is the co-author, together with Davide Antoniella, of Chapter 33. Previously he wrote a chapter for the book *Nutrition and supplementation for sport and physical performance*, 2nd edition. He is the author of the book *The secrets for muscle growth and antiaging* (self-publishing). He has a degree in Sports Science and Food Science, he is the scientific manager and co-founder of the genetic testing company VitaeDNA, bodybuilding and fitness instructor, and a nutritional biologist. In 2019 he obtained a master's degree in Functional Medicine at the IFM (Institute of Functional Medicine) and, in 2020, a master entitled "Peptides Therapy: Modules I and II" at A4M (American Academy of Anti-Aging Medicine), in California. He is the author of two scientific articles on muscle physiology: "Mechanical, molecular myofibrillar and proteomic modifications in muscle aging: a pilot study" (2018) and "Are muscle fibers of bodybuilders intrinsically weaker? A comparison with single fibers of aged-matched controls" (2020). His passion for dissemination has allowed him to be a speaker at various conferences, including Spazio Nutrizione, in Milan, and a lecturer in functional medicine masters organized by Vivereinforma S.r.l. and Italian School of Fitness and Nutrition (SIFA) S.r.l. Below is a glimpse at his achievements:

With the IFBB

- 3rd place Ludus Maximus Rome 2014;
- 2nd place in Northern Italy Verona 2015;
- 2nd place Ludus Maximus Rome 2015;
- 5th place in the Italian Championships Rome 2016;
- 3rd place Ben Weider Classic Pro Padova 2018.

With the WABBA

- 1st place in the Natural Cesena 2019 Italian Championships.

Andrea Militello contributed as co-author, together with Massimo Spattini, to the drafting of Chapter 38. He has a degree in Medicine and Surgery and specializes in Andrology with a second-level master's degree in Andrology and Seminology, Reconstructive Surgical Andrology, and Prosthetic Implantology.

He obtained the Lifestyle Medicine & Functional Medicine Certification (AFFWA) and is DietaCOM® Advisor. He is a lecturer at the Federiciana Università Popolare (Rome, Cosenza) in urological and translational sciences, and at the University of Ostrava (Rome branch) and the ASOMI College of Sciences in Malta. He is a member of the Technical-Scientific Committee of the Academy of Bio-Regenerative Medicine and Surgery Bo.Ri. He is a member of TopDoc GLOBAL The Strongest Expert Network in the World. He is an honorary member of the Argentine Society of Andrology.

Despite multiple clinical and teaching commitments, he has never stopped practicing bodybuilding.

Luca Silvestrini was the contributing author to Chapter 36. He graduated in Medicine and Surgery at the "Sapienza" University of Rome, specialized in Sports Medicine at the Catholic University of Rome "Agostino Gemelli" Polyclinic, and became a PhD candidate at the University of Rome Tor Vergata with a focus on exercise with overloads and benefits in ischemic heart disease in the diabetic and in the osteopenic patient. From the years at the Sant'Andrea Hospital to service at the local level for ASL RMB, to the direction of a research project on the relationship between the heart and resistance training, he has always focused his attention on the heart and the great vessels, in the cardiopathic patient and in the sportsman with pathology. It all started with an innate passion for bodybuilding and the need to understand the body's physiological response mechanisms after more than twenty years dedicated to these pillars of his life.

Below is a glimpse at his competitive achievements in bodybuilding.

- 1994: regional vice-champion, Central Italy, and 2nd place in the NABBA Italian Junior Championship.
- 1997: regional champion, Central Italy and Italian NABBA vice-champion, 4th place Colosseum IFBB.

- 1999: IPF-WABBA Italian champion, 3rd place in the IPF-WABBA European Championship.
- 2000: 3rd place in the NABBA World Championship, NABBA Mr. Universe finalist.
- 2007: IFBB Italian Championship finalist, 7th place at the Due Torri Gran Prix.
- 2008/2009: IFBB Italian Championship finalist, IFBB European Championship finalist, 3rd place at IFBB Notte dei Campioni.
- 2010: Italian IFBB vice-champion, participation in the IFBB World Championship (top 10).
- 2015: 4th place in the IFBB Italian Championship, 4th place in the IFBB Notte dei Campioni.
- 2018: 2nd place Ludus Maximus Master category, NABBA World Championship finalist, participation in the NABBA Mr. Universe.
- 2019: participation in the NABBA Mr. Universe, 4th place in the NABBA European Championship.

Antonio Squillante was the contributing author to Chapter 31 and, previously, authored a chapter of the book *Nutrition and Supplementation for Sport and Exercise Performance*, 2nd Edition. He is an athletic trainer, nutritionist, and researcher. He graduated in Motor Sciences and followed a specialization course in Food and Human Nutrition. After earning a master's degree in Athletic Training and Rehabilitation, he currently teaches in the United States at the University of Southern California in Los Angeles, where he is in the process of completing a Ph.D. in Sports Physiology.

He has over 10 years of experience in the world of athletic training as a Certified Strength and Conditioning Specialist (NSCA CSCS*D RSCC) and is registered in the register of sports nutritionists (CISSN SENr). He has worked for various college teams in the United States and Canada, and has coached in both track and field and professional weightlifting. He also teaches at Setanta College, Tipperary (Ireland), is a faculty member of the National Strength and Conditioning Association (NSCA), and is chairman of the Olympic Weightlifting Committee (NSCA Weightlifting SIG).

As an author, he has published studies in scientific journals of the sector (including the *Journal of Strength and Conditioning Research* and the *European Journal of Physical Education and Sport Science*) and has written several books dedicated to strength training in athletic preparation.

In powerlifting, he has competed and won in the United States participating in national and international competitions. In 2018, he finished third in the California State Championship, qualifying for the second year in a row to the national championships. More recently, he competed in endurance sports winning the duathlon and qualifying for the Track Cycling Masters World Championships in the Match Sprint category.

Further acknowledgments

We would like to thank to thank photographers Alex Ardenti, Angelo Bani, Terenzio Maggio, Danny D'Mello, Giorgio Mesghetz, Giorgio Sottile, and Art Zeller.